The Bioethics Reader
Editors' Choice

The Bioethics Reader
Editors' Choice

Edited by

Ruth Chadwick
Helga Kuhse
Willem Landman
Udo Schüklenk
Peter Singer

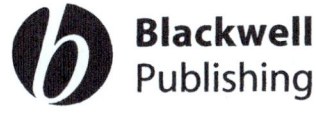
Blackwell
Publishing

Editorial organisation © 2007 Blackwell Publishing Ltd.

BLACKWELL PUBLISHING LTD.
350 Main Street, Malden, MA 02148-5020, USA
9600 Garsington Road, Oxford OX4 2DQ, UK
550 Swanston Street, Carlton, Victoria 3053, Australia

The right of Ruth Chadwick, Helga Kuhse, Willem Landman, Udo Schüklenk and Peter Singer to be identified as the Authors of the Editorial Material in this Work has been asserted in accordance with the UK Copyright, Designs, and Patents Act 1988.

First published in 2007 by Blackwell Publishing Ltd.

Library of Congress Cataloging-in-Publication Data

The bioethics reader : editors' choice / edited by Ruth Chadwick . . . [et al.].
   p. ; cm.
'Articles reprinted from Bioethics.'
Includes index.
ISBN 978-1-4051-7522-7 (alk. paper)
1. Bioethics. 2. Medical ethics. I. Chadwick, Ruth F. II. Bioethics.
[DNLM: 1. Bioethical Issue–Collected Works. WB 60 B615476 2007]

QH332.B5157 2007
174′.957–dc22

                2007018719

Set in 11 on 13 pt Times NRMT
by SNP Best-set Typesetter Ltd., Hong Kong

The publisher's policy is to use permanent paper from mills that operate a sustainable forestry policy, and which has been manufactured from pulp processed using acid-free and elementary chlorine-free practices. Furthermore, the publisher ensures that the text paper and cover board used have met acceptable environmental accreditation standards.

For further information
on Blackwell Publishing, visit our website:
www.blackwellpublishing.com

THE BIOETHICS READER
Editors' Choice

Contents

Contents

Contents

INTRODUCTION

20 Years of *Bioethics*

When *Bioethics* started more than two decades ago its founding editors described it as a publication aiming to be different from existing journals in the field. They promised that it would make a significant contribution to the discussion of crucial questions in health care and the biological sciences. *Bioethics* remains true to its founding editors' challenging objectives. They are worth re-stating. *Bioethics* is

> A truly international journal which does not assume that its readers are especially interested in developments in one particular country;
>
> An interdisciplinary journal, publishing articles which are of interest to, and readily understood by, readers from any discipline or from no discipline at all;
>
> A journal committed to publishing original articles which have passed through a careful process of screening by independent referees;
>
> A journal concerned with presenting practical contributions to the solution of real problems; and
>
> Above all, a journal which prizes rigorous argument and hence will constantly be on guard against the all-too-prevalent tendency for high-flow rhetoric and unsubstantiated assertion to dominate discussions of ethical issues in health care and the biological sciences.

Since its inception *Bioethics* has become one of the premier journals in a rapidly growing field. From its fledgling beginnings as a quarterly it has, together with its companion journal *Developing World Bioethics*, become one of currently three journals in the field that publishes on a monthly basis. Its initial print-run counting in the hundreds is a thing of the past. The journal's current subscriber base counts several thousand university libraries as well as many individuals. On-line accesses to individual articles are probably replacing the time-honoured, old-fashioned browsing through new journal issues in the library. We wonder how many readers have actually held a copy of the journals in their hands in recent years.

The journals experienced close to 100,000 downloads of individual articles last year. The internet (r)evolution has certainly not bypassed *Bioethics*.

As the past and current editors of the journal we thought it might be a good idea to compile a collection of some of the best articles we published. We chose them on the basis of various criteria, including our subjective 'liking' of a particular article, as well as on the basis of more objective criteria such as the imprint the article left in the field in terms of citations by others. We also aimed to provide a reasonable 'feel' for what happened in the field over the last decades by means of covering a whole range of issues, from conceptual questions to traditional topics, such as beginning and end-of-life issues to up-and-coming concerns such as public health. This introduction is meant to provide you with a brief overview of the contents of this volume.

Health care

While the development of bioethics as a distinct field of study is normally traced to the 1960s, *Bioethics* the journal began in 1986. Although bioethics is broader as a field than health care ethics, including work on developments in the life sciences, a major focus remains the professional–patient relationship, and this is represented in a major section of this volume. For instance, in their article Draper and Sorrell discuss patients' responsibilities. Over time the professional issues have arguably become more specialised, and we have illustrated this trend by including articles by Kuhse, on nursing ethics, and Radden, on psychiatric ethics.

Beginning and end of life

As with the field itself, the journal has had a major input to matters of life and death, including issues surrounding both the beginning and ending of life. Reproduction and abortion, on the one hand, and euthanasia and brain death, on the other, have continued to be well represented in submissions to the journal. We have selected here, for example, Gibson and van Bogaert providing very different ethical perspectives on abortion, Purdy on surrogate mothering, Savulescu on procreative beneficence, as well as McMahan on brain death. In another paper, reminding us again of the need to reflect on the global nature of the serious pressing ethical issues that we are facing, Henley discusses end-of-life care in children with AIDS in South Africa. Naturally the focus of the discussion – at the beginning of life, at least – has evolved with scientific developments, so that, for example, embryos and stem cells (the latter here discussed in the article by Holm) have arguably become more prominent as a focus of discussion than the moral status of foetuses. Where scientific developments are concerned, however, what has perhaps had most influence on the development of bioethics as a field has been the Human Genome Project. This has partly been a matter of available funding for projects in this area, and funding for bioethics has become a subject of discussion in its own right, but it has also had more far-reaching influence from a theoretical point of view.

The 'geneticization' of bioethics

The term 'geneticization' was coined to describe the ways in which explanations were increasingly being offered – first in the medical context and then in others – in genetic terms. The application of the concept in bioethics could be interpreted in a number of ways, including a tendency to focus on certain questions, but also the implications of genetics for ethics. The much-contested thesis of genetic exceptionalism holds that there is something about genetics which makes it special, for example that genetic information about one person has implications for their blood-relatives, and the fact that it is predictive and independent of time. This led to suggestions that ethical principles which were appropriate in health care as traditionally understood, where the focus was the individual patient, might not be appropriate for genetics. Specifically, long cherished notions such as the importance of individual informed consent have come under fresh scrutiny. Towards the end of the 1990s this trend was exacerbated by the turn towards biobanking. To the pre-existing concerns about relatedness in genetics were added features specific to population-wide genetic research and long-term storage of samples. These issues gave rise to a considerable amount of study of the implications for topics such as informed consent and privacy, illustrated in this volume by the article by Arnason on the Icelandic database project. Other papers in this section address the question of whether or not it would be acceptable to modify the human genome if we could (Agar), and the case of wrongful disability (Brock).

The public health turn

The move towards centre stage of the biobanking issue could be seen, however, not simply as part of the geneticization of bioethics, but as part of what might be called 'the public health turn'. It has sometimes been said that bioethics in its early days was too much concerned with the individual and not enough with public health, but the latter has in recent years attracted more attention from those working in the field, as shown by the inclusion here of the papers on the genesis of public health ethics (Bayer), vaccination (Dawson) and infectious disease (Selgelid). The latter category is arguably a special case because of high-profile concerns about the rise of new infectious diseases such as SARS, as well as the resurgence of old ones such as TB, in addition to the ongoing issues about long-standing diseases that remain prevalent in some parts of the world.

The global turn

It might be argued that bioethics has always been concerned with public health to a certain extent, in so far as it has had to confront issues of resource allocation in conditions of scarcity. The context of globalisation however has given a new emphasis to this in terms of increasing recognition of the problems of injustice in allocation of health care opportunities internationally. Our section on Just Health Care includes an article by Sterckx on patents and access to drugs in developing countries. Farmer and Gastineau's paper argues that bioethics must address what they call the growing 'outcome gap' between rich and poor patients. These are pieces from the sister journal of *Bioethics, Developing World Bioethics.* The very fact that this second journal was launched is testament to the growing recognition of the global context in which bioethical controversies are played out. The papers we have selected for the Research Ethics section are also very much to be seen in this light, concerned as they are with international human subjects research (London) and developing drugs for the developing world (Resnik). Schüklenk and Ashcroft review two of the predominant issues in international research ethics, namely the question of standards of clinical care in trials conducted in the developing world, as well as the politics involved in the production of international ethical guidelines.

The empirical turn

It has always been the case that academics from a number of disciplines have worked in bioethics, primarily philosophers, lawyers and theologians. From the earliest beginnings of the field it was recognised that no one discipline could deal with the full extent of the issues in bioethics, although there may be disputes about which discipline is primary and this has given rise to some controversy. In the last decade of the twentieth century, work in the social sciences in bioethics became more prominent and gave rise to what has been called an empirical turn. Work of this type included, at one level, surveys of attitudes to developments in the life sciences, including xenotransplantation and genetic modification. Programmes to facilitate public understanding of science also became popular, leading to what counts as 'public understanding' itself becoming a topic of study, eventually giving way to work on public *engagement* or *participation*, following criticism of the 'deficit model' implied by 'public understanding of science'. From the policy-making perspective of bioethics it is important to be responsive to public concerns about new developments and for policy to be informed by data about the extent to which people's decision-making about e.g. reproduction will be affected by advances in genetics. But 'public attitudes' do not of course determine what is right. Empirical research is also important, however, from a theoretical point of view in bioethics. The ways in which social context is relevant in ethics is an important issue: the prominence of certain principles, such as autonomy, may not be suitable for societies or social groups with a less individualistic culture. At an early stage *Bioethics* did include work with an empirical component; in later years the question of the respective contributions of different disciplines to bioethics has itself become an object of study by those working in the field, including authors in the journal, and we have here selected the article by Haimes, 'What can the Social Sciences Contribute to the Study of Ethics? Theoretical, Empirical and Substantive Considerations'.

Reflexivity

What all these trends and turns demonstrate is the need for bioethics as a field of study to be reflexive and constantly reconsider its own methods and theoretical approaches. In our first section of this volume, in addition to the Haimes article already mentioned, we have selected papers such as those by Rachels and Bostrom, which engage in that activity. Challenging problems remain, including the question of what method(s) are appropriately deployed within theoretical bioethics.

The future

There can be little doubt that the field is growing rapidly and, as success breed envy, it has its fair share of detractors. Some question whether bioethicists or other academics should be the preferred supplier of normative reasoning in the field. Others suggest that bioethicists have a habit of 'following the money' (funding or otherwise) and that they are beholden to corporate or other sponsors' interests. Whether or not this is true for the wide field that encompasses bioethics, or whether it may or may not be true only for certain areas of investigation is undoubtedly worthy of investigation.

No doubt areas of specialisation will develop a sharper profile within bioethics, most notably bioethical inquiries into questions of a global nature. Equally, the ever-changing landscape of ethical questions triggered by developments within genetics guarantees bioethics' constructive engagement with matters of public policy. This anthology provides you with a good overview of the most significant contributions published in *Bioethics* over the last two decades.

Acknowledgements

Udo Schüklenk is very grateful to Kyle Wilson who, at the time, worked at Witwatersrand University, in Johannesburg, South Africa, for superb research assistance during the early stages of this project.

Ruth Chadwick
Helga Kuhse
Willem Landman
Udo Schüklenk
Peter Singer

PART I: DOING BIOETHICS

Chapter 1

A Report from America

WHEN PHILOSOPHERS SHOOT FROM THE HIP

JAMES RACHELS

These days moral philosophers often find themselves in the heady position of being called upon by newspapers to comment on the latest public controversies. Being treated as quotable experts by the media may be old stuff for economists, and a few other academic types, but it is a new experience for philosophers, a visible result of the applied ethics movement that began twenty years ago. Sometimes the newspapers want columns of commentary. The op-ed page, pioneered by the *New York Times*, has now become a regular feature of most large metropolitan dailies. Op-ed columns aren't much like articles in *Bioethics*, but for the general public they are a good substitute. They allow enough space, and writing them allows one enough time, for serious reflection.

Sometimes, however, the newspapers want something different. The telephone rings, and a reporter rattles off a few 'facts' about something somebody is supposed to have done. Ethical issues are involved – something alarming is said to have taken place – and so the 'ethicist' is asked for a comment to be included in the next day's story, which may be the first report the public will have seen about the events in question.

Usually when this happens the reporters aren't interested in detailed analysis or lengthy qualifications. A short, pithy quote is what's wanted. Nor are the reporters eager to hear reassurances that the alarming events really aren't alarming. That doesn't make good copy. What makes good copy is the idea that the events being reported are morally troubling, or worse. And frequently philosophers are willing to provide just such comments. The story then appears, with a pronounced moral slant: 'Such-and-such has happened, and the ethicists say it's bad.' More often than not, this combination of reporters' interests and philosophers' snap judgments has a conservative effect. The new developments are viewed as troubling against the background, not of careful analysis, but of accepted wisdom.

In March 1990 a story appeared in American newspapers about a Los Angeles couple who had decided to have another child in the hope that the baby's bone marrow cells could be used to save the life of their teenaged daughter. Abe and Mary Ayala, who are in their forties, had not intended to have an additional child; in fact, Abe Ayala had had a vasectomy. But their 17-year-old daughter, Anissa, was dying of leukemia, and a bone marrow transplant was her only hope. After two years of searching in vain for a suitable donor, they decided to have another child because there was a one-in-four chance that the new family member would be a suitable donor. So Abe Ayala had his vasectomy reversed and Mary Ayala became pregnant. The baby, a girl named Marissa, was born on April 6 and she is indeed a compatible donor. The transplant procedure, which will be accomplished sometime in the fall, will involve little risk for the baby, and Anissa's chances of surviving will rise from zero to between 70 and 80 percent.

The Ayalas were understandably elated to learn that Anissa's life might be saved. However, the newspaper stories prominently featured quotations from medical ethicists who labelled their decision 'troublesome' and even ('outrageous': 'The ideal reason for having a child,' said a well-known figure in the field, 'is associated with that child's own welfare – to bring a child into being and to nurture it. One of the fundamental precepts of ethics is that each person is an end in himself or herself, and is never to be used solely as a means to another person's end without the agreement of the person being used.' The Ayalas' baby 'is not seen as an end in itself, but as a means to another end. The fact that the other end is laudable doesn't change that.' Another expert was quoted as saying that the Ayalas' decision means 'we're willing to treat people like objects' – and, he added, 'I don't think we ought to do that.'[1]

The Ayalas are real people, not characters in a made-up classroom example, and they didn't care much for the ethicists' comments. Mrs. Ayala said that the ethicists ought to be worrying more about the shortage of marrow donors, and less about their decision. Anissa herself was asked what she thought about all this, and she said that she was 'sort of troubled' by the criticism, but added that 'We're going to love our baby.'

If Anissa were trained in philosophy, she might find the criticisms less troubling. She might observe that people have always had

---

[1] *The New York Times*, 17 February, 1990, 1.

babies for reasons other than the 'ideal' one. Real life rarely measures up to philosophers' expectations. People have children so that the children can share in the family's work, to please the grandparents, or just because it's expected of them. They sometimes have second children because they don't want the first to be an 'only child'. None of this is strange or unusual; it's just the way life is. What is important is, as Anissa insists, that once born the children are loved and nurtured within good families. Anissa might also point out that her mother, in fact, had wanted another baby anyway – it was only her father's wish to have no more children. And finally, she might express some appropriate scepticism about the idea that an individual 'is never to be used solely as a means to another person's end without the agreement of the person being used.' Does this mean that, if Anissa already had a baby sister, the baby could not be used as a donor because the baby was not old enough to give permission? Should Anissa herself be left to die, for the sake of respecting this principle? Perhaps the ethicist quoted in the *New York Times* thinks so; he was quoted as saying 'It's outrageous that people would go to this length.'

Curiously, there is an argument, proceeding from principles endorsed by the most conservative pro-life advocates, that supports the Ayalas' decision. This argument invokes the idea that we are conferring a benefit on someone by bringing them into existence. The new baby, not Anissa, seems the really big winner here: after all, if her parents had not decided to have her, the baby would have not got to exist. Those who oppose abortion sometimes ask: Aren't you glad your mother didn't have an abortion? The answer, of course, is that most of us are happy that our mothers didn't do that; otherwise we wouldn't be here now. The people who ask this question think that something follows about the morality of abortion, although it isn't clear what; but they usually fail to notice that we could just as well ask: Aren't you glad that your parents didn't practice birth control? (Orthodox Catholics, at least, are consistent on this point.) We should be equally happy that contraceptives were not used by our parents, and for the same reason: otherwise, we wouldn't be here now. Similarly, Anissa's little sister might someday be asked: Aren't you glad that your parents decided to have you? Aren't you fortunate that Anissa needed those stem cells? Perhaps this means that conservatives who take a pro-life view ought to be happy with the Ayalas' decision, rather than being critical of it.

It might be doubted, however, that this is a sound argument. The idea that we are conferring a benefit on someone by bringing them into existence is easily disputed. I would rather rest my defense of the Ayalas' decision on a different sort of reasoning. First we may consider two separate questions:

1. Suppose a couple, before having any children at all, is trying to decide whether to have one child or two. They slightly prefer having only one. But then they are told that if they have only one child it will die when it is a teenager. However, if they have two, both will probably live full lives. Would it be wrong for the couple to decide, for this reason, to have two children?

2. Suppose a couple already has two children, one a teenager dying of leukemia, and the other an infant who is the only available bone marrow donor. The infant cannot give its permission, of course, but then again it would not be harmed at all by the procedure. Would it be wrong, under these circumstances, to use some of the infant's stem-cells to save the teenager's life?

It seems to me that it would be easy enough to argue that the answer to both these questions is no. Then the inference to the permissibility of the Ayalas' decision would be obvious.

But this is a peripheral point. My subject here is in the performance of philosophers – 'ethicists' – as commentators on public events. Sometimes they do what we might think philosophers ought to do: challenge the prevailing orthodoxy, calling into question the assumptions that people unthinkingly make. But just as often they function as orthodoxy's most sophisticated defenders, assuming that the existing social consensus must be right, and articulating its theoretical 'justification'. And when all else fails, there is another familiar argument that can be relied upon: the slippery slope. Any departure from business-as-usual can be pronounced 'troubling' because of what it might lead to. The Ayalas' decision was also criticised on this ground. It was said that it might lead to 'fetus farming,' or to abortions so that the aborted fetus can be used for life-saving purposes.

Of course we don't know exactly what will happen to the Ayala family, or to social values, in consequence of decisions such as theirs. But two comments seem relevant. First, there is nothing new about their sort of decision. In the publicity surrounding the Ayala

Chapter 2

RETHINKING MEDICAL ETHICS: A VIEW FROM BELOW

PAUL FARMER AND NICOLE GASTINEAU CAMPOS

I. INTRODUCTION

Bioethics and medical ethics are necessarily a contentious enterprise. These fields have the potential to embrace not only empiric research, but also philosophical commentary, informed opinion, and essay as well. The best scholarship in these related fields often addresses 'unresolved issues' of moral conflict. Some issues are unresolved because they stem from novel developments, such as xenotransplantation or the latest in stem-cell research; other issues are unresolved because too little attention has been paid to them in recent decades, in part because the discipline of medical ethics has arisen in certain social contexts and not in others. We argue here that lack of access to the fruits of modern medicine and the science that informs it is an important and neglected topic within bioethics and medical ethics. This is especially clear to those working in what are now termed 'resource-poor settings' – to those working, in plain language, among populations living in dire poverty.

AIDS research has been a case in point. In a recent commentary on the ethics of HIV vaccine trials, physician Joia Mukherjee voiced in print what many who do not read or write are saying about the ethics of AIDS research within settings in which AIDS is now the leading infectious cause of adult death:

> When asked, 'Have you no morals?' Alfred Doolittle, in George Bernard Shaw's *Pygmalion*, answered, 'Can't afford them, governor. Neither could you if you was as poor as me.' The modern concept of human rights underpins a moral society and holds government responsible for fulfilling those rights. From informed consent to the right to privacy, civil and political rights have dominated the human rights focus of the HIV-1 epidemic. Yet, the economic and social rights of people with HIV-1 infection, in particular the rights to health care and to share in scientific

advances, are glaringly disparate between rich and poor countries. This disparity has become the focus of debate in transnational HIV-1 vaccine research.[1]

Mukherjee's commentary will resonate with some and rankle others. But many of those who would find her views compelling are those who will never read a medical journal because they do not read; others read but do not have access to journals. These are the people whose views we seek to echo in offering a view of medical ethics 'from below.'

First, what is meant by 'a view from below'? What is not intended by this expression? Elsewhere, we have elaborated a critique of the scholarship of suffering from the perspective of those living in great poverty.[2] Here we will note in passing that dissymmetries of power are present in all medical exchanges: between well and sick, expert and non-expert, white and black – the list goes on. But these dissymmetries are often masked in the language of academic medicine and public health. In a 1992 book, Howard Brody notes that 'the word *power* is essentially absent from the vocabulary that scholars of medical ethics have constructed for their discipline and that has been accepted by almost everyone who does work in the field or tries to apply medical-ethic insights to the clinical context.'[3] This honest assessment serves as a stepping stone for our essay, which moves far beyond the boundaries of the world's most affluent nations, the birthplace of professional societies of medical ethicists and bioethicists. Since the topic of medical rationing, which implies scarcity, is a staple of the medical ethics literature,[4] we add at the outset that we refer in this essay to the world's poor, especially the poor of the poorest countries. When the question 'Who shall live?' was posed, these people were not yet in the consciousness of those building a new field.

Subaltern populations within rich and middle-income countries have long been caught up in the key dramas of medical ethics: witness the Tuskegee Syphilis Study, which followed 600 African

---

[1] J.S. Mukherjee. HIV-1 Care in Resource-Poor Settings: A View from Haiti. *Lancet* 2003; 362: 994–995, at 994.

[2] P. Farmer. On Suffering and Structural Violence: A View from Below. *Dædalus* 1995; 125: 261–283.

[3] H. Brody. 1992. *The Healer's Power*. New Haven & London. Yale University Press: 12.

[4] V. Fuchs. 1975. *Who Shall Live? Health, Economics, and Social Choice*. New York. Basic Books.

American men in Alabama from 1932 to 1972, and continues to have its echoes even today.[5] Similar experiences have been documented in Europe, South Africa, and Brazil.[6] But, to this day, the poorest people in the poorest countries are likely to appear only in the margins of the bioethics literature if they appear at all. We have seen their critiques of research ethics dismissed as confused and ill-informed commentary or as 'conspiracy theories.' But much is to be gleaned from such critiques, as more in-depth and sympathetic explorations of them suggest.[7] This paper is meant as a constructive critique of bioethics and medical ethics, not only from the point of view of those living in great poverty but from the perspectives advanced by the 'socialising disciplines.' These include anthropology, history, political economy and the sociology of knowledge; few would regard philosophy, for years the parent discipline of ethics, as a socialising discipline. It is our hope, here, to help 'resocialise' medical ethics as part of a broader intellectual and social project that is necessary as dominant cultures, academic and otherwise, increasingly favour psychological or individualist readings of social problems ranging from addiction to AIDS to 'non-compliance' with medical regimens.[8] We will draw on our experience in Haiti and the United States in order to offer an overview of what is lacking not only in ethics but also in conventional human rights discourses, which have also influenced medical ethics and bioethics.

As a physician-anthropologist and a specialist in health policy, our views may be regarded as suspect by some within the field of medical ethics. For this reason, we start our review by relying on certain voices from within the discipline of medical ethics. After pointing to deficiencies underlined from within the discipline, we

---

[5] Roughly 400 of these men had syphilis, and most lived in poverty. Despite the 1947 discovery of a cure for the disease – to this day, syphilis is treated with penicillin – subjects were never offered that very inexpensive drug, even though they had joined the study assuming that they would be treated. Nor were they informed of the study's real purpose. (S.M. Reverby, ed. 2000. *Tuskegee Truths: Rethinking the Tuskegee Syphilis Study*. Chapel Hill. University of North Carolina Press. A.M. Brandt. 1987. *No Magic Bullet: A Social History of Venereal Disease in the United States Since 1880*. New York. Oxford University Press.)

[6] See, for example, commentary on Norplant trials in Brazil. A.R. Dos Reis. Norplant in Brazil: Implantation Strategy in the Guise of Scientific Research. *Issues in Reproductive & Genetic Engineering: Journal of International Feminist Analysis* 1990; 3: 111–118.

[7] P. Farmer. 1992. *AIDS and Accusation: Haiti and the Geography of Blame*. Berkeley & Los Angeles. University of California Press.

[8] G. Lipovetsky. 1993. *L'Ere du vide: Essais sur l'individualisme contemporain*. Paris. Gallimard.

turn to problems occurring right now in the course of efforts to respond to AIDS and tuberculosis, among other modern plagues.

II. WHAT'S WRONG WITH MEDICAL ETHICS?

In the social field in which bioethics and medical ethics have emerged – affluent industrialised countries, by and large, and within the past few decades – practitioners of these disciplines are seen, by themselves and by others, as liberal reformers. Three major and overlapping groups may be discerned. Within clinical settings, ethicists are the guardians of morally sound practice and a safeguard against abuses. By the close of the last century, most major teaching hospitals had ethics committees; many boasted in-house ethicists active in addressing the quandary ethics of individual patients. As often as not, ethics consults in such hospitals take into consideration discord between patients' families and medical staff or withdrawal of care for those deemed unlikely to be saved by 'heroic interventions.' The salutary impact of these developments is not disputed.

A second major stream of medical ethics is constituted by the everyday practice of ethics within modern biomedical research. The research arena has been home to an explosive growth of institutional review boards (IRBs); human subjects committees abound. Disclaimers regarding potential personal gain are required in the publishing of data and it is not possible to publish even photographs or the comments of patients without 'ethical clearance.' In the university with which we are affiliated, students cannot undertake research involving human subjects without going through an ethics course and filling out an application. Again, many regard these as positive developments. But some would note that it is not easy to link the proliferation of such committees and regulations with a rise in ethical treatment of the destitute sick, especially if we take a global perspective.

It is possible to read, for example, front-page exposés of research projects conducted by first-world universities in Africa and learn that, although research subjects have signed informed-consent forms, they have no clear notion about what the research explores or about how they figure in the endeavour.[9] Other research projects,

---

[9] H. French. AIDS Research in Africa: Juggling Risks and Hope. *New York Times* 9 October, 1997: A1, A14.

duly blessed by multiple review boards in both the research university and the host country, are so manifestly unethical in the eyes of some leaders of modern medicine that they can be termed reminiscent of Tuskegee in the world's leading medical journals. Consider studies involving what many argue are unethical placebo controls in AZT trials attempting to develop a cheaper drug regimen to prevent mother-to-child transmission of HIV.[10] Despite the fact that the US Public Health Service began recommending the use of zidovudine to prevent MTCT in 1994, a review by Lurie and Wolfe in 1997 counted 15 studies taking place in developing countries in which some or all of participants were not receiving antiretroviral therapy to prevent MTCT.[11] Editor of the *New England Journal of Medicine* Marcia Angell explicitly compared such studies to Tuskegee, and chastised the NIH and CDC for contributing funds to several projects:

> The fact remains that many studies are done in the Third World that simply could not be done in the countries sponsoring the

[10] Also consider the more recent example of a randomised-control trial conducted between November 1994 and October 1998, which examined the relationship between serum viral load, concurrent sexually transmitted diseases, and other known and putative HIV risk factors. The research team screened 15 127 individuals in a rural district of Uganda, of whom 415 were identified as HIV-positive with an initially HIV-negative partner. The researchers then tracked these serodiscordant couples for thirty months, following the viral load of the infected partner and the rate of seroconversion among the previously uninfected partners. The study concludes that 'viral load is the chief predictor of the risk of heterosexual transmission of HIV-1.' (T.C. Quinn, M.J. Wawer, N. Sewankambo, D. Serwadda, C. Li, F. Wabwire-Mangen, M.O. Meehan, T. Lutalo & R.H. Gray. Viral Load and Heterosexual Transmission of Human Immunodeficiency Virus Type I. *New England Journal of Medicine* 2000; 342: 921–929.) In an accompanying editorial, *New England Journal of Medicine* editor Marcia Angell voiced her hesitation about publishing the study and was quite pointed in her criticism: 'It is important to be clear about what this study meant for the participants. It meant that for up to 30 months, several hundred people with HIV infection were observed but not treated.' Furthermore, 'the very condition that justified doing the study in Uganda in the first place – the lack of availability of antiretroviral treatment – will greatly limit the relevance of the results there.' (M. Angell. Investigators' Responsibilities for Human Subjects in Developing Countries. *New England Journal of Medicine* 2000; 342: 967–969.) Explicit comparisons to Tuskegee were made in the popular press; in the electronic magazine *Slate*, one writer asked: 'The . . . volunteers in the sample were not offered treatment nor were their healthy sex partners informed that the research subjects were HIV positive. Excuse please, but why isn't this like the [*New England Journal of Medicine*] supporting the Tuskegee experiments?' (S. Shuger. Supreme Court Cover-Up. *Slate* 30 March, 2000. Available at: http://slate.msn.com/?id=1004976.)

[11] P. Lurie & S.M. Wolfe. Unethical Trials of Interventions to Reduce Perinatal Transmission of the Human Immunodeficiency Virus in Developing Countries. *New England Journal of Medicine* 1997; 337: 853–856.

work. Clinical trials have become a big business, with many of the same imperatives. To survive, it is necessary to get the work done as quickly as possible, with a minimum of obstacles. When these considerations prevail, it seems as if we have not come very far from Tuskegee after all.[12]

The majority of such international biomedical research has inequality as its foundation, and ethical codes developed in affluent countries are quickly ditched as soon as affluent universities undertake research in poor countries. Then come a series of efforts to develop alternative (read, less stringent) codes 'appropriate' to settings of destitution.

A third strand of work is less closely tied to clinical care or research endeavours: teaching and scholarship on bioethics and medical ethics. Again, the explosive growth of these fields is easy to gauge simply by looking at journals, publications, and the number of faculty appointments within schools of medicine, nursing, and public health. Many of these scholars have formal training in both medicine and philosophy.

What is the primary purpose of these three overlapping strands of medical ethics and bioethics? An anthropologist might ask, what are the social fields in which they emerge? Whose interests are they intended to protect? What ends do they serve?

Such questions, which admit to multiple answers in multiple arenas, are not always welcome. None of the answers are facile ones, since even the quandary ethics of clinical practice are disputed terrain. But even more disputed are research ethics when projects span vertiginous social inequalities. The ethical dilemmas stemming from such research are almost invariably about the haves and the have-nots, and this is as true today as it was during the long decades in which the Tuskegee experiment was being conducted. But much professional commentary on medical ethics appears divorced from straightforward discussion of racism and the yawning gulf between researchers and subjects. Larry Churchill notes this at times absurd divorce between ethical dilemmas that arise in everyday life and the professional commentary they spawn:

> Bioethical disputes – as measured by the debates in journals and conferences in the United States – often seem to be remote from

[12] M. Angell. The Ethics of Clinical Research in the Third World. *New England Journal of Medicine* 1997; 337: 847–849.

the values of ordinary people and largely irrelevant to the decisions they encounter in health care. In this sense, philosophical theorizing might be considered harmless entertainment, which if taken too seriously would look ridiculous, as several Monty Python skits have successfully demonstrated.[13]

Churchill's critique of philosophical theorising is even more poignant when the 'ordinary people' in question do not have access to modern health care. What 'decisions' are taken by the world's poorest, who are also, by any honest accounting, the globe's sickest? One of the ways to answer this question would be to spend time interviewing the destitute sick about what they regard as their ranking problems; it is also possible, we have discovered, to interview them about the ethics of research.

We draw on our experience with infectious diseases in some of the poorest communities in the world to interrogate the central imperatives of bioethics and medical ethics. AIDS, tuberculosis, and malaria are the three leading infectious killers of adults in the world today. Because each disease is treatable with already available therapies, the lack of access to medical care is widely perceived in heavily disease-burdened areas as constituting an ethical and moral dilemma. In settings in which research on these diseases is conducted but there is little in the way of therapy, there is much talk of first world diagnostics and third world therapeutics.[14] To quote a woman who had returned to central Haiti, dying of AIDS, after years in the city, 'We're good enough to study but not good enough to care for.' This woman, who later received therapy for her disease and stopped dying, was nonetheless passionate about the topic well after her own lack of care was addressed and she began to respond to antiretroviral therapy. In another interview, conducted in her home, she expounded at some length:[15]

---

[13] L. Churchill. Are We Professionals? A Critical Look at the Social Role of Bioethicists. *Dædalus* 1999; 128: 253–274, at 255.

[14] Emanuel et al. have suggested guidelines for 'what makes clinical research ethical.' Among their criteria is 'fair subject selection' – subjects should not be vulnerable individuals and must have the potential to experience the benefits of any ethical research project. (E.J. Emanuel, D. Wendler & C. Grady. What Makes Clinical Research Ethical? *Journal of the American Medical Association* 2000; 283: 2701–2711.)

[15] Several patients being treated for HIV at the Clinique Bon Sauveur in rural Haiti are quoted throughout this article. These interviews are not part of a formal ethnographic study, but rather an effort to convey patient stories in their own words.

I was diagnosed [with HIV infection] because of a research project that [a US research university] was doing. That was ten years ago. This was in [a slum in Port-au-Prince]. I went back a lot to have my blood drawn but I never got any treatment. And I knew from the radio that other people received treatment. These were people who could pay $200 a month. They were people who could go and make a deposit at a bank and then they'd get their medicines for a month . . . I came home [to central Haiti] to die, but even now that I'm better I'm still angry about it. Ten years of them sucking my blood and nothing! I was a skeleton sitting on the bench waiting for them to call my name. It's when I got to be a skeleton that the nurse told me that I didn't have to come any more. It's as if poor people were animals. But we won't serve as their guinea pigs [*Men nou p'ap sevi kom kobay yo*].[16]

Although the expression 'first-world diagnostics and third-world therapeutics' may not be the term commonly used in Haiti, the idea behind the expression has wide currency among patients and non-patients there. This is because, with many infectious diseases, the research enterprise is fundamentally a transnational one. It is also a fundamentally inegalitarian exercise in the sense that medicine and science are expanding rapidly, but in a social context of growing global inequality, which ensures that the fruits of medicine and science are not available to many who need them most.[17]

Medicine, public health, and research are all caught up in a web of unequal relations. The link between research on AIDS and access to therapy for HIV has been the most scrutinised, perhaps, of this troubling aspect of modern medicine. But other startling examples abound. Organ transplantation is a disturbing case in point. This is not because the clamour for access to organs by those living with, say, renal failure and poverty has reached the ears of most who write about the ethics of the rapidly expanding practice of organ transplantation. It is rather because, globally, the poor are more likely to serve as donors, rather than recipients, of organs.

Organ transplantation is altogether unknown in countries as poor as Haiti, but is common in wealthier but inegalitarian countries and regions throughout the developing world. And almost everywhere we look, trafficking in organs occurs in predictable ways

---

[16] The research project mentioned has, by report, since been terminated.
[17] On the growth of global inequality since 1980, see: J.K. Galbraith. A Perfect Crime: Global Inequality. *Dædalus* 2002; 131: 11–25.

– predictable, that is, to those who look at social inequalities across borders. To quote one anthropologist who works on this topic, 'the flow of organs follows the modern routes of capital: from South to North, from Third to First World, from poor to rich, from black and brown to white, and from female to male.'[18]

The seamy underbelly of organ donation in the poor world has been noted by other anthropologists and by adventurous ethicists as well; an 'organs watch' website has even been established.[19] Although egregious violations of rights are a major problem – the literature is already rife with stories of organs, from kidneys to corneas, quite literally stolen – a far greater problem is the legal and 'ethically approved' transfer of organs across social gradients. In other words, the ethical codes currently in place have not prevented abuses grounded, however subtly, in growing inequalities. When someone living in destitution 'opts' to sell a kidney and signs all informed-consent forms in front of multiple witnesses, is the term 'informed consent' really meaningful? Rather, what does such informed consent really mean? That the donor is a priori informed about his or her chances of survival without the money disbursed upon donation?

So it is with much AIDS research. If individuals living in slums in African cities, unable to read and write, are to participate in clinical trials, what sort of process must they go through in order to provide informed consent? Or is there a darker possibility: that research across such deep gradients of inequality means that the research enterprise is itself fundamentally coercive unless special measures are taken?

These questions, which are not meant as rhetorical, get at one of the oldest and most fraught debates within social theory: the reticulated relationship between structure and agency. A 'view from below' would ask how poverty, racism, and gender inequality come to constrain agency, the ability to make choices. If one believes in the ability of research to lessen misery and suffering – as we do – what 'special measures' might one envision as we seek to conduct research in settings of great poverty? How might we ensure that the measures are not in and of themselves coercive, as many incentives are deemed to be?

---

[18] N. Scheper-Hughes. The Global Traffic in Human Organs. *Current Anthropology* 2000; 41: 191–224, at 193.
[19] Organs Watch. University of California, Berkeley. Available at: http://sunsite.berkeley.edu/biotech/organswatch/

To answer these and related questions, we note again that it is necessary to resocialise the problems at hand – the quest for vaccines, say, or novel therapeutics or organ transplantation – in order to have a broader view of the inequalities in which such endeavours are grounded, whether researchers see them or not. Efforts to resocialise problems allow all concerned to have a more meaningful understanding of what it is the research subjects (or organ donors) hope to gain from participating in what are, often enough, their only encounters with modern biomedicine. And even a preliminary attempt to consider these topics in their broader social contexts allows us to come to a preliminary conclusion: the more desperate the poverty of subaltern populations (research subjects or organ donors who live in poverty, sick prisoners), the greater the constraint on their agency. In other words, the steeper the gradient of social inequality across which such transactions occur, the greater the risk of abuse without the 'special measures' we discuss below.

One of the ways of rethinking medical ethics is to place the 'outcome gap' front and centre as an ethical issue. The term 'outcome gap' admits to many meanings, but here we follow the example of paediatrician Paul Wise, who some years ago interrogated conventional wisdom regarding low birth weights in urban United States, where race and class are strongly associated with rates of premature delivery, with weight at birth, and with rates of infant mortality. These oft-noted disparities of outcome had led, in the last quarter of the previous century, to a movement to divert money from neonatal intensive care units to social conditions for African-American women. But Wise noted that such a diversion would not get to the heart of the matter:

> Too often, those who elevate the role of social determinants indict clinical technologies as failed strategies. But devaluing clinical intervention diverts attention from the essential goal that it be provided equitably to all those in need. Belittling the role of clinical care tends to unburden policy of the requirement to provide equitable access to such care.[20]

Arguments about resource allocation – another staple, as noted, of commentary within medical ethics – are not really 'socialised' since they do not include an honest accounting of how an affluent society,

[20] P. Wise. Confronting Racial Disparities in Infant Mortality: Reconciling Science and Politics. *American Journal of Preventive Medicine* 1993; 9: 7–16, at 9.

or even a city, chooses to spend available resources. Resocialising the problem of low birth rate would require frank discussion of racism, subsidies for the rich and shrinking resources for the poor, military expenditures, and, again, the growing gap between the rich and the poor. It would also require careful consideration of equitable access to clinical care. These topics, like the term 'power', are rarely encountered in professional journals devoted to medical ethics.

And so it is with each of the problems mentioned in this essay: AIDS, chronic renal failure, prison-seated epidemics of tuberculosis, and racial disparities in infant mortality. Each problem has generated debates within medical ethics, and new technologies to address them may generate debates within bioethics. But it is possible to discern in scholarly discourse what might be termed a 'Luddite approach' to the problem: we should halt AIDS research in resource-poor settings, we should stop performing kidney transplants, we should focus exclusively on prison reform rather than treating epidemic tuberculosis within prisons, and we should stop building NICUs. These unwelcome conclusions are reflected not only within scholarship in medical ethics but also its pious echoes in clinical medicine, medical education, and public health.

We are opposed to these Luddite traps. Each of the dilemmas discussed here calls for new and better technologies, whether they are for managing renal failure or for developing a vaccine for AIDS. To argue, as we do, that the primary ethical issue of modern medicine and public health is the outcome gap, itself rooted in transnational and growing social inequalities, is not to argue for merely shuffling around research and service priorities with decisions based on primitive notions of cost-effectiveness, the latest fashion in policy making. The problem is much deeper. Indeed, we have argued elsewhere that the growing outcome gap constitutes the chief human rights challenge of the 21st century.[21] This assertion will seem odd to many who term themselves experts in the field of human rights, accustomed, as they are, to exhorting governments to respect civil and political rights. But the importance of social and economic rights is paramount in settings of poverty, which are also settings of excess morbidity and mortality.

---

[21] P. Farmer. 2003. *Pathologies of Power: Health, Human Rights, and the New War on the Poor*. Berkeley. University of California Press.

But what does it mean, for both bioethics and human rights, when a person living in poverty is able to vote, is protected from torture or from imprisonment without due process, but dies of untreated AIDS? What does it mean when a person with renal failure experiences no abuse of his or her civil and political rights, but dies without ever having been offered access to dialysis, to say nothing of transplant? What does it mean when an African-American neonate does not have ready access to the care only afforded in a NICU?

The world's poor do not live on another planet; nor do they live in countries in which such technologies are unavailable. Surveys have shown that in the world's poorest countries, the affluent have ready access to both antiretroviral agents and therapy for renal insufficiency; NICUs are close at hand for infants born to affluent families. At the same time, the world's poor, even those living in wealthy nations, do not have reliable access to good medical care or to the fruits of medical science. And if this is regarded as an ethical problem, then it is one that is growing rapidly and worsened by the development of new and more effective therapies. It is new because some of the diseases and all of the technologies are new: impossible to imagine the key philosophers of yesteryear pondering these technologies because they did not yet exist. Whenever more effective technologies are introduced there will be, in the absence of an equity plan, a growing outcome gap – the unmentioned elephant in the room of medical ethics.

III. LINKING BIOETHICS TO SOCIAL ANALYSIS: RETHINKING THE CASE OF TUBERCULOSIS IN PRISONS

We have underlined two steps that would make medical ethics more compelling in settings of great poverty: using the socialising disciplines to contextualise fully ethical dilemmas in settings of poverty and, a related gambit, the systematic participation of the destitute sick. A third step is to link research across steep gradients with the interventions that are demanded by the poor or otherwise marginalised. Examples of the fruits of linking better analysis and better interventions have been offered elsewhere. In the cases cited above, understanding the ethics of AIDS research in Africa or Haiti would rely heavily on interviewing people living with both poverty and this disease. But what is true for AIDS is true for most other maladies afflicting the poor disproportionately.

Elsewhere, we have offered the example of prisoners in Russia who are sick with drug-resistant tuberculosis in order to underline the shortcomings of current approaches to these problems.[22] To summarise a complex biosocial process for the purposes of the current exercise, it is important to know that a doubling of incarceration rates occurred after the collapse of the Soviet Union. The infamous gulag came to be more than three times as full in 'democratic' Russia, with Siberian incarceration rates exceeding, at one point, 1000 per 100 000 population (only the United States rivals this ratio). Overcrowding, poor ventilation, interruption of medical supplies and salaries for overworked prison staff, and malnutrition led to explosive epidemics of tuberculosis within Russia's prisons. But this was not the sort of tuberculosis seen in Haiti or sub-Saharan Africa. In some senses, the Russian epidemics were more reminiscent of the prison-seated outbreaks documented in New York beginning in the late 1980s: although HIV was not a factor in the Russian epidemics, they were, as in New York, prison-based and involved strains of highly drug-resistant *Mycobacterium tuberculosis*, the organism that causes the disease.[23]

Into this dramatic and novel situation came, for the first time, non-Russian aid agencies and non-governmental organisations. To date, there have been few thorough studies of this stunning development, but such analyses are important to our understanding of what is occurring within prison walls today.[24] By the mid 1990s, such organisations were prominent players in post-Soviet states, all of which had seen catastrophic deterioration in their social safety nets and medical systems. The nongovernmental organisations were mostly European and North American, and in the post-perestroika

[22] P. Farmer & N. Gastineau. Rethinking Health and Human Rights: Time for a Paradigm Shift. *Journal of Law, Medicine & Ethics* 2002; 30: 655–666.

[23] For a review see: P.E. Farmer, A.S. Kononets, S.E. Borisov, A. Goldfarb, T. Healing & M. McKee. 1999. Recrudescent Tuberculosis in the Russian Federation. In *The Global Impact of Drug-Resistant Tuberculosis*. Program in Infectious Disease and Social Change, ed. Boston. Program in Infectious Disease and Social Change: 39–83. See also: V. Stern & R. Jones. 1999. *Sentenced to Die? The Problem of TB in Prisons in East and Central Europe and Central Asia*. London. International Centre for Prison Studies, King's College.

[24] For one such study, see: G. Bukhman. 2001. *Reform and Resistance in Post-Soviet Tuberculosis Control*. Doctoral Dissertation, University of Arizona. Ann Arbor. University Microfilms.

disarray they had something their Russian (and Azeri and Georgian and Kazakh, etc.) partners did not then have: money and clout. The ability of these aid organisations to shape responses to epidemic tuberculosis in Siberia was significant, and they insisted on what they termed the most 'cost-effective' approach, the one endorsed by international tuberculosis experts, including the World Health Organization: directly observed therapy with 'first-line' anti-tuberculous drugs. But some of the Russian prison physicians objected, as did members of Russia's large and crumbling tuberculosis-treatment infrastructure: the prisoner-patients had drug-resistant tuberculosis and would not be cured by standard first-line regimens; some Russian specialists made other objections. These voices were drowned in an undercurrent of censorious opinion from the international experts and the non-governmental agencies, which, flush with resources and backed by international expert opinion, insisted on giving all prisoners the same doses of the same first-line drugs.

In Siberia and in other pilot sites, treatment outcomes were nothing short of catastrophic: less than half of all patients were deemed cured (expected cure rates for supervised therapy of drug-susceptible tuberculosis exceed 95%).[25] Worse, prisoner-patients who were not cured by therapy with first-line drugs emerged from this treatment, if they survived, with 'amplified' resistance. That is, their prognosis had worsened dramatically even if they were to be afforded care with the right drugs.[26] But the non-Russian groups, whether international tuberculosis experts or aid groups, did not concede that they had made an error. Instead, they pressed on, delivering precisely the same medications even to prisoner-patients with documented multi-drug-resistant tuberculosis.

More delegations visited Siberia in 1998. Members of at least one delegation pointed out that drug resistance was not the *likely* cause of treatment failure, it was the cause *already documented*. Somewhat discreetly, it would seem, the lead non-governmental organisation had sent sputum samples for drug-susceptibility testing to at least two reference laboratories in Western Europe. Both laboratories

[25] M.E. Kimerling, H. Kluge, N. Vezhnina, T. Iacovazzi, T. Demeulenaere, F. Portaels & F. Matthys. Inadequacy of the Current WHO Re-Treatment Regimen in a Central Siberian Prison: Treatment Failure and MDRTB. *International Journal of Tuberculosis and Lung Disease* 1999; 3: 451–453.

[26] P. Farmer. Managerial Successes, Clinical Failures. *International Journal of Tuberculosis and Lung Disease* 1999; 3: 365–367.

confirmed that patients within Siberian prisons were sick from highly resistant strains of *M. tuberculosis* – strains resistant to precisely those drugs being administered, under direct supervision, by the non-governmental organisations who had been chastising Russian experts for their lack of knowledge of modern tuberculosis control.

Well before 2000, tuberculosis had become the leading cause of death in Russian prisons. In Siberian facilities, surviving prisoners had become less and less treatable, and those with multi-drug-resistant tuberculosis were cohorted behind barbed wire and declared altogether 'untreatable.' But this was not the case: multi-drug-resistant tuberculosis is treatable with other, more expensive drugs; data from a slum in Peru and rural Haiti have made it clear that such efforts can succeed in settings far poorer than Siberia.[27] The real debate was not about the efficacy of therapy but about its costs.

By 2001, the lead non-governmental organisation appeared to yield to growing pressure from prisoners, their guards, and expert opinion: it would work with its Russian partners to treat patients with multi-drug-resistant tuberculosis with the drugs to which their strains had been shown to be susceptible. It took the organisation well over a year to procure the drugs, but early in 2002 it announced the programme was to commence treatment right away. The need was great: in a single oblast in Western Siberia, an estimated 2000 prisoner-patients were warehoused with active multi-drug-resistant tuberculosis. But although the drugs began to arrive in Siberia, no treatment occurred in the ensuing year. In September 2003, the lead organisation issued a press release: they were pulling out of Siberia. As of today, not a single prisoner has been treated, by non-governmental organisations based in Siberia for a decade, for multi-drug-resistant tuberculosis, although thousands, perhaps more, have died of this disease. The press release blames Russian officials, particularly those in the Ministry of Health, for their intransigence,

[27] P. Farmer, J. Bayona, S. Shin, L. Alvarez, M. Becerra, E. Nardell, C. Nuñez, E. Sanchez, R. Timperi & J.Y. Kim. Preliminary Results of Community-Based MDRTB Treatment in Lima, Peru. *International Journal of Tuberculosis and Lung Disease* 1998; 2 (Suppl. 2): S371. C. Mitnick, J. Bayona, E. Palacios, S. Shin, J. Furin, F. Alcantara, E. Sanchez, M. Sarria, M. Becerra, M.C. Fawzi, S. Kapiga, D. Neuberg, J.H. Maguire, J.Y. Kim & P. Farmer. Community-Based Therapy for Multidrug-Resistant Tuberculosis in Lima, Peru. *New England Journal of* Medicine 2003; 348: 119–128.

but it is likely that careful study of what occurred will come to a somewhat different conclusion.[28]

The story is a sad one, but it will become sadder: circulating strains of multi-drug-resistant *M. tuberculosis* will mean that prisoner detainees are exposed to epidemic strains of highly drug-resistant tuberculosis and then do not receive care when they need it. But that will not change the fact that the initial approach of the non-governmental organisations was incorrect: multi-drug-resistant tuberculosis cannot be cured with regimens based on the very drugs to which infecting strains are resistant, but these patients' prognosis can be worsened by such practices, even if proper therapy later becomes available. Since international authorities had endorsed these practices they should have been the first to acknowledge the error and to make pledges to help correct it. But no mea culpa has been issued from any interested party.

All interested parties, including those willing to underline the ethical lapses involved, must be part of a broader movement not merely to point to such lapses, masked or acknowledged, but also to address them. In the case of multi-drug-resistant tuberculosis in Russian prisons, that means staying and seeing these patients through treatment that is effective, not 'cost-effective.' The fact that prisoners with drug-resistant tuberculosis were given drugs that were wholly ineffective is a reminder that concepts such as 'cost-effectiveness' are in fact ideological constructs. The example is one of many and serves, too, as a reminder of the most pressing questions for modern medical ethics.

IV. ALTERNATIVE AND COMPLEMENTARY FRAMEWORKS: PRAXIS MAKES PERFECT?

The examples offered above have received scant attention in the medical ethics literature and much of that attention has been inaccurate. To blame a lack of HIV care on beleaguered and cash-poor African governments is similar to blaming tuberculosis outbreaks in Siberia on prolonged pre-trial detention or the malfeasance of local prison officials. Such observations are superficial and also

---

[28] MSF Ends Tuberculosis Treatment in Kemerovo Region, Russia. 30 September, 2003. Available at: http://www.msf.org/countries/page.cfm?articleid=D657393B-C8E6-4CD7-9835259FD4F8AFEF

convenient, since they deflect attention from the truly powerful forces and actors that, respectively, shape epidemics and declare which interventions are cost-effective and which are not. These actors are more likely to be found in New York, Washington, Geneva or London than they are to be found in Siberia, Port-au-Prince, or Pretoria. It is also superficial to spend time underlining the shortcomings of any one particular field, and we add that our goal here is not to denigrate what constitutes a robust enough intellectual enterprise, but rather to point to ways in which the medical and bioethics communities might illuminate complex and transnational ethical problems. Such analysis would prove useful across steep gradients of social inequality, the context and driving force of the world's great epidemics.[29] One cautionary lesson of Tuskegee is that it may take decades for ethics to catch up with observations that come quite naturally to those marginalised by poverty, racism, and other forces that are not often the subject of polite conversation within medical ethics.

One reason for this selective silence is that ethics in general has until recently relied heavily on philosophy, its parent discipline, and very little on the social sciences relevant to medicine. Bioethics is fundamentally socially constructed. To resocialise medical ethics – as part of a broader project, which includes critique of dominant modes of thinking in a broad variety of fields – would mean a turn towards disciplines such as anthropology, history, and political economy. But even within philosophy, John Rawls has laid out a framework that might be applied fruitfully to problems such as those now gathering force within Siberian prisons and African slums. Rawls is, of course, famous for his difference principle, which requires preferential treatment for the most disadvantaged, regardless of the social costs this principle can entail.[30] Critics have rightly

---

[29] P. Farmer. 1999. *Infections and Inequalities*. Berkeley. University of California Press.

[30] J. Rawls. 1999. *A Theory of Justice*. Revised edition. Cambridge, MA. Harvard University Press: § 26, pp. 130–139; § 13, pp. 65–73. Rawls's more precise definition of the difference, or maximin principle, is that society must choose the scheme of institutions that most advantages the least advantaged persons in society. In practice, this emphasis on the absolute position of the most disadvantaged in society may force society to forgo schemes that produce lesser aggregate wealth or utility. Other scholars have cited the tensions between distributive 'injustice' and over-consumption by the wealthy, which may lead to such harms as environmental degradation and exploitation of the poor. See: A. Jameton & J. Pierce. Environment and Health: Sustainable Health Care and Emerging Ethical Responsibilities. *Canadian Medical Association Journal* 2001; 164: 365–369.

noted the principle's underemphasis on health,[31] but one can read Rawls as making a broader point about how we should view social practices. For if we take Rawls seriously, we have to ask ourselves if we truly care about the most disadvantaged when we give prisoners ineffective therapy that is declared 'cost-effective.'[32]

Sociologists of knowledge will one day point to the competing paradigms that have led important ethical dilemmas to remain invisible or little noted, but in the short term much more could be said simply by restoring to these problems more of the social and historical complexities inherent in each of them. A certain humility is warranted, as philosopher Caputo wryly suggests:

> Far be it from me to make ethics tremble. I tremble even at the prospect that I will be found guilty of spreading the word that the pants of the great man are split. For that I have already prepared a defense aimed at exonerating me of all responsibility ... The result is that it will be very hard to identify the guilty party, to find anyone who is singularly responsible, if we are all rounded up by the police and charged with inciting a riot against ethics.[33]

The sociology of knowledge is another field full of promise in the broader project to resocialise medical ethics.[34] Our understanding of science, for example, is given a significant boost when the

---

[31] D. Brock. Broadening the Bioethics Agenda. *Kennedy Institute of Ethics Journal* 2000; 10: 21–38. Philosopher Norman Daniels has also contributed significantly to bioethical literature by applying Rawlsian principles to justify the right to health (see, for example: N. Daniels. 2002. Justice, Health, and Health Care. In *Medicine and Social Justice*. R. Rhodes, M. Battin & A. Silvers, eds. Oxford. Oxford University Press: 6–23). Both Brock and Daniels discuss resource prioritisation for the worst off.

[32] This attitude toward prisoners is also hard to square with an equally important, though largely forgotten, aspect of Rawls's theory of justice – the inviolability of each person. As Rawls himself elegantly states, '[e]ach person possesses an inviolability founded on justice that even the welfare of society as a whole cannot override.' Rawls, *op. cit.* note 26, § 1, p. 3.

[33] J.D. Caputo. 1993. *Against Ethics: Contributions to a Poetics of Obligation with Constant Reference to Deconstruction*. Bloomington. Indiana University Press.

[34] Berger and Luckmann note that 'The sociology of knowledge must concern itself with whatever passes for "knowledge" in a society, regardless of the ultimate validity or invalidity (by whatever criteria) of such "knowledge". And in so far as all human "knowledge" is developed, transmitted and maintained in social situations, the sociology of knowledge must seek to understand the processes by which this is done in such a way that a taken-for-granted "reality" congeals for the man in the street. In other words, we contend that the sociology of knowledge is concerned with the analysis of the social construction of reality.' (P. Berger & T. Luckmann. 1966. *The Social Construction of Reality: A Treatise on the Sociology of Knowledge*. Garden City, NY. Anchor Books.)

non-rational procedures that lead to paradigm shifts come into clear relief. 'Given a paradigm, interpretation of data is central to the enterprise that explores it', writes Thomas Kuhn. 'Paradigms are not corrigible by normal science at all.'[35] Most would argue that medical ethics and philosophy are not the sorts of science that Kuhn had in mind; many practitioners of anthropology and, to a lesser extent, sociology, are willing to admit that the term 'social science' may be a bit grand. And although economists are unwilling, often, to point to the ideological frameworks that undergird their work, they are at least willing to call theirs 'the dismal science.'

In addition to the invaluable insights of sound epidemiology, which suggests the mechanisms by which social inequalities serve as the leading risk for both falling ill with infectious disease and then being denied access to adequate care, there is a special role for ethnography and for detailed case studies. If ethicists were to interview patients and sick *non*-patients – for many of the destitute sick never become patients and are never offered the chance to confront ethical dilemmas – as often as they interrogate philosophical treatises, the resocialisation of medical ethics would be well underway. Here we quote another Haitian woman, whose commentary easily spans the gulf from access to AIDS therapies to the right to employment. She made these comments in 2001 after gaining more than 20 pounds on antiretroviral medications:

> We're always sick here. If we're not dying of AIDS, we're dying of hunger, or both. Now that I am better, it's not as if my problems have disappeared. It's that I can wake up and fight them again. For two years I lay in bed, my children watching me die, bringing me sips of water . . . [Their father] is gone – my sister has seven children of her own. All I could think about was what will happen to my children when I die? My sister had already purchased my coffin but then [the clinic] gave me these [antiretroviral] medicines. Someone comes to see me everyday, to make sure I take them. The first thing that hit me was hunger. The medicines started killing the virus and then I became hungry. But we had no food in the house – how would that be possible, if [the father of her children] were gone and I was dying? Charity food does not allow you to regain your strength and to feed your

---

[35] T. Kuhn. 1970. *The Structure of Scientific Revolutions*. Second edition. Chicago. University of Chicago Press: 122.

children at the same time. That's why we always reach the same conclusions in our [support-group meetings]. If you want to prevent AIDS among poor women, give them jobs . . . I'm happy I'm better, and I'd rather be alive than dead. But all I do every day, still, is worry about how I'm going to feed my children. I don't want to become a thief.

In our own writing on these topics we have sought to echo and amplify such commentaries, writing about the need to re-mediate inequalities of access to health care as a fundamental human right. Are such calls – for the right to health care and to jobs – merely grandstanding when echoed by academics, broadsides dressed in scholarly guise? We would answer by insisting that both bioethics and medical ethics have a long way to go on this score before scholars in these fields can object that the views of the destitute sick receive too much emphasis in the literature.

Listening to the afflicted is not merely moral praxis, although it is that. It affords us rich insights into the sorts of problems that we have outlined in this essay. Because the poor quite literally *embody* many of the ethical dilemmas stemming from injustices within medicine and public health, they add insights that cannot be obtained through reference to philosophy. For ethical reflection is part of everyday life, and when the stakes are high – in a squatter settlement in Haiti, say, or a prison in Western Siberia – soliciting these views are central to the quest for understanding. With the exception of sociopaths, as Churchill notes, '[the capacity to think critically about moral values and direct our actions in terms of such values] is common to all of us.'[36] The same is not true of particle physics or evidence-based medicine, which do not figure prominently in everyday discourse and reasoning. But herein lies the great promise of a resocialised ethics: seeking the views of the destitute sick will breathe new life into medical ethics.

The call to rely more heavily on the views of the afflicted is not a call to turn our backs on philosophy but rather a call to turn our attention to those who suffer most. It is also a call to turn towards the disciplines that can illuminate the social production, and maintenance, of that suffering. Just as history and political economy can show us how science and medicine have grown but not in tandem with ethical approaches to global health equity, so too can history

[36] Churchill, *op. cit.* note 13, p. 259.

and political economy in turn illuminate ethnography and other 'experience-near' disciplines.

Each of the problems mentioned above is an obvious example. The distribution of HIV infection is as surely sculpted by social inequalities as is access to both HIV care and to what might be called prevention equity. To engage in ethical debate about vaccine trials or ethically sound clinical research in 'resource-poor settings', as many have done in recent years, it is necessary to understand the social inequalities that sculpt both the AIDS epidemic and social responses to it. Indeed, it is these very inequalities of risk and access that make it attractive to conduct research on diseases endemic among the world's poor. As for organ transplants, there can be no honest understanding of international movement of organs without acknowledging the steep social gradients across which they move. Such observations, even when undergirded by robust research, cause those involved in the enterprise to bristle, but that makes these observations no less true.

There are other paradigms and bodies of knowledge that can help to resocialise bioethics. Within the human rights movement is a small but growing effort to underline the importance of social and economic rights, which are the rights commonly demanded by the poorest populations. These include the right to health care, schooling, housing, and clean water. Some have attempted to listen to the poorest and restore these rights to their proper place in the hierarchy of rights, and also to underscore the impossibility of understanding current debates in global medical ethics without understanding the extreme disparities that underpin the 'ethical' dilemmas of the destitute sick.[37]

Medical ethics also stands to gain from insights from liberation theology, as noted by Marcos Fabri dos Anjos. Although ethics and philosophy have long been entangled in religious reflection, there is thus far very little synergy between medical ethics and the one branch of theology that concerns itself chiefly with the problem of poverty in the modern world. The conclusions of dos Anjos are worth citing here:

First, to what level of quality can medical ethics aspire, if it ignores callous discrimination in medical practice against large

[37] P. Farmer. Pathologies of Power: Rethinking Health and Human Rights. *American Journal of Public Health* 1999; 89: 1486–1496.

populations of the innocent poor? Second, how effective can such theories be in addressing the critical issues of medical and clinical ethics if they are unable to contribute to the closing of the gap of socio-medical disparity?[38]

Regardless of which or how many of the socialising disciplines are used, modern medical ethics would stand to benefit from another dramatic change. We argue here that those who study ethical dilemmas will be called increasingly to have a hand in re-mediating them. These calls will come from 'below', from the afflicted themselves. The concept of 'pragmatic solidarity' is instructive as medicine, science, and public health stumble and fall in the very regions most in need of them. AIDS in Africa and tuberculosis in prisons are cases in point. Pragmatic solidarity is a cumbersome term, perhaps, and one that makes many academics uncomfortable. Anthropologists, for example, have long argued that their task is to observe rather than intervene, but this claim is undermined by the arguments that anthropology's supposed neutrality was in fact perceived by others, including those studied, as a small but at times integral part of the colonial project.[39]

The social sciences, if that is what we are to term them, cannot claim neutrality. There is no social variant of Heisenberg's principle, and it is possible to argue that no field of inquiry can span such dizzying social inequalities and not influence the very topic it proposes to study. Researchers from the modern university are invariably actors in a social field and medical ethicists who work across steep gradients of inequality are, all objections to the contrary notwithstanding, powerful actors when compared to those they study.

Listening to the poorest will lead us back, inevitably, to the outcome gap. The 'special measures' mentioned above will vary from place to place and from problem to problem, but medical ethicists should expect to become part of teams seeking to lessen the outcome gap by remediating access to effective medical care. And once that step is taken, we will have the option of trying to ignore what we are being told by the afflicted, or to take seriously the challenge of linking the struggle for social and economic rights

---

[38] M. dos Anjos. Medical Ethics in the Developing World: A Liberation Theology Perspective. *Journal of Medicine and Philosophy* 1996; 21: 629–637.

[39] T. Asad, ed. 1975. *Anthropology and the Colonial Encounter*. London. Ithaca Press & Humanities.

– the right to food, housing, clean water, education, and jobs – to scholarly inquiry that breaches the frighteningly deep gap between the haves and the have-nots.

V. CONCLUSIONS OR NEW DIRECTIONS?

Like any established fields of scholarly inquiry, bioethics and medical ethics are broad and large enough to contain their own internal critics. And like many practitioners of an academic discipline, ethicists are not always eager to embrace critiques from beyond the field. But this essay is meant merely to complement ongoing research and reflection within bioethics and medical ethics.

Writing of AIDS, historian Allan Brandt astutely notes that, 'In the years ahead we will, no doubt, learn a great deal more about AIDS and how to control it. We will also learn a great deal about the nature of our society from the manner in which we address the disease. AIDS will be a standard by which we may measure not only our medical and scientific skill but also our capacity for justice and compassion.'[40] When Brandt writes of 'our society', he refers to the global village through which HIV has raced. Access to AIDS care has yet to follow. Surely this constitutes a daunting ethical problem.

Research in medical ethics has thus far been conducted largely in affluent and industrialised nations. Yet these 'resource-rich' settings are tied, and intimately so, to the poorest parts of the world. Haiti, the Western Hemisphere's most HIV-burdened nation, is the classic case in point: born of late 15th-century European expansion, Haiti was, by the 18th century, the world's most profitable slave colony. It is now commonly termed the poorest country in the Western Hemisphere. But the creation of this poverty over time is seen within Haiti as a result of the historical processes that created one of the most brutal slave colonies on record. The key events in Haitian history, from the slave revolt that led to the founding of Latin America's oldest republic to the 20th-century US military occupation of Haiti and subsequent generous support of military dictators, are as familiar to Haitians as they are forgotten by French and US citizens. So too was Tuskegee all but forgotten by modern medicine and yet remembered by African Americans. Indeed, historians and

---

[40] A. Brandt. 1988. AIDS: From Social History to Social Policy. In *AIDS: The Burdens of History*. E. Fee & D.M. Fox, eds. Berkeley. University of California Press: 147–171, at 168.

medical ethicists are to be thanked for having kept this issue alive until a formal presidential apology was obtained in 1997, 50 years after penicillin was found to be effective therapy for syphilis, and 25 years after the cessation of the experiment. Research in South Africa, similarly, is necessarily fraught, in part because the scars of apartheid are forgotten by newly arrived AIDS researchers but not by those who endured apartheid and now see their communities attacked by yet another foe. The Haitians have a saying, '*bay kou bilye, pote mak chonje*': he who delivers the blow forgets; he who bears the scar remembers.

Injustices of one sort or another are very often central to the modern ethical problems in medicine, public health, and science. Rawls was correct to underline the centrality of justice in considerations of ethical problems, and the process of resocialising medical ethics and bioethics is in part a process of restoring the historically deep and geographically broad analysis that comes naturally to the world's destitute sick, who bear the scars of history.

Another way of putting this is best saved for the end of this essay: medical ethics must grapple more persistently with the growing problem posed by the yawning gap between rich and poor. The central topics of bioethics and medical ethics need to be linked to questions of social justice and to consideration of how inequalities of all sorts are linked to the inequalities studied by sociologists, anthropologists, and epidemiologists. In almost all countries in which medical ethics and bioethics have taken root – which is to say in most countries, at this writing – access to care, even access to informed participation in clinical trials, is determined as much by social standing as by disease process. This basic epidemiological and social fact emboldens us to close with a warning: if social inequalities persist and grow, we will no longer be welcome to conduct research or even to comment on it. To cite Joia Mukherjee again, 'If the medical community is to use data generated in high-burden and vulnerable populations to develop an HIV-1 vaccine, we must ensure that the global community will help governments fulfill the right to health and share the fruits of research with the world's poorest communities.'[41]

---

[41] Mukherjee, *op. cit.* note 1, p. 995.

Chapter 3

WHAT CAN THE SOCIAL SCIENCES CONTRIBUTE TO THE STUDY OF ETHICS? THEORETICAL, EMPIRICAL AND SUBSTANTIVE CONSIDERATIONS

ERICA HAIMES

INTRODUCTION[1]

Since the late twentieth century the Euro-American mass media have given a great deal of coverage to debates over topics such as abortion, euthanasia, fertility treatment, surrogacy, organ donation, genetic screening and access to medical treatment. Topics outside the medical field such as genetically modified crops, investment policies, child labour and environmental issues have also been thoroughly aired. Since the debates have been primarily concerned with the ethics of such practices it could be argued that their prominence represents an increase in awareness of ethical issues. However, the voice of sociology and the other social sciences is rarely heard in these debates. Is this because (i) the social sciences have little to say on these issues, or is it because (ii) though it has much to say, the voice of the social sciences has had little impact, and is this, in turn, because (iii) the social sciences are not usually associated with the study of ethics and ethical issues?

On the first point, some writers claim that the social sciences have not had a major interest in ethics, or in medical ethics and bioethics in particular.[2] However, although there may not (yet) be a 'sociology of ethics', for example, there is a substantial body of theoretical

[1] The ideas presented in this article are an extensive development of those that I first presented at the British Sociological Association Annual Conference in 1999 as an invited member of a Wellcome Trust panel. A version of the panel's discussion can be found in Pat Spallone et al. 2000. Putting sociology on the bioethics map. In *For Sociology*. J. Eldridge et al., eds. Durham. Sociology Press: 191–206.
[2] For example, T. Osborne. Sociology, liberalism and the historicity of conduct. *Economy and Society* 1994; 23: 484–501; and R. Zussman. The contributions of Sociology to medical ethics. *Hastings Center Report* 2000; January–February: 7–11.

and empirical work in the field of ethics from sociology and the social sciences in general. It is part of the purpose of this paper to identify that body of work and to suggest ways in which it might contribute to the study of ethics. It has to be acknowledged that, so far, this work has had only limited impact beyond its own disciplinary walls. This is surprising given the increasing use of the acronym, ELSA (a reminder to scientists and policymakers to consider the ethical, legal and social aspects of developments in medicine and science) that would appear openly to invite social scientists to join law and philosophy in contributing to these debates. Several countries, including the United States and Sweden, have nationally funded programmes to encourage research in the ELSA fields. However it appears that the voices of ethicists and lawyers have dominated those of the social scientists, possibly because of their more precise focus: what after all is included in the rather vague term, 'social aspects'? Social scientists are not frequently cited by these other disciplines and they are not often called upon to participate in public debates or to contribute to the policymaking arenas. Thus another purpose of this article is to try to make the voice of the social sciences heard more clearly, though not by drowning out those other voices. The aim is not sociological imperialism but rather a dialogue with other disciplines.[3] Thus, even though I am writing primarily as a sociologist I shall be using sociology and 'social sciences' as broadly interchangeable terms. The boundaries between them are blurred in much of the relevant work so it is more useful to emphasize their shared interests in the conceptual, cultural, political and practical aspects of the social world, and the contributions that these can make to the study of ethics, than to get caught up in their differences.

On the third point, it probably is true to say that the social sciences are not associated in the lay, scientific or political mind with ethics and ethical debates. Indeed most ethicists probably do not associate social science with ethics other than in the somewhat arbitrary distinction between normative and descriptive ethics. Nelson questions this presumption of a linear relationship between ethicists and social scientists, in which the latter provide the data upon which the former make judgements: 'Moral theories, informed by facts, judge practices'. He argues instead for an

---

[3] D. Silverman. 1985. *Qualitative Methodology and Sociology.* Gower. Aldershot: 194–195.

interactive model between the two.[4] Another purpose of this paper is to develop Nelson's argument further and to demonstrate that, by virtue of their theoretical as well as their empirical interests, the social sciences have more to contribute than just 'the facts'. The social sciences see legal and ethical issues as primarily social issues and, because of this encompassing perspective, can contribute not only to the understanding of ethical issues but also to the understanding of the social processes through which those issues become constituted as ethical concerns.

In brief, therefore, the overall aim of this article is to contribute to the hitherto limited discussion[5] on the contributions of the social sciences to the study of ethics. I shall frame the discussion through a consideration of three broad questions:

(i)   What theoretical work can the social sciences contribute to the understanding of ethics?

(ii)   What empirical work can the social sciences contribute to the understanding of ethics?

(iii)   How does this theoretical and empirical work enhance the understanding of how ethics, as a field of analysis and of debate, is socially constituted and situated?

It may well be that some colleagues reading this article see no objection to Nelson's description of the relationship between ethicists and social scientists since they see (bio)ethics as a branch of moral philosophy which aims to evaluate ethical arguments in order thereby to eliminate poor quality reasoning. They therefore might have little interest in the above questions, seeing them primarily as matters of social practice, which might be of interest to social scientists but which are of little relevance to ethicists.[6] However I should like to suggest several reasons why these three questions are of direct relevance to bioethicists, beyond the point of making a case for the inclusion of social science in ethical debates.

---

[4] J.L. Nelson. Moral teachings from unexpected quarters. Lessons for bioethics from the social sciences and managed care. *Hastings Center Report* 2000; January–February: 12–17, esp. p. 12, p. 16.

[5] Although see also R. DeVries and J. Subedi, eds. 1998. *Bioethics and Society*. New Jersey. Prentice-Hall; B. Hoffmaster. Can ethnography save the life of medical ethics? *Social Science and Medicine* 1992; 35: 1421–1431; Spallone et al., *op. cit.* note 1.

[6] I am grateful to one of the anonymous reviewers of this article for encouraging me to make these points explicitly.

First, ethics is no longer a purely abstract discipline since there is a growing interest within bioethics in conducting empirical investigations and, within philosophy more broadly, with applied work. This alone suggests that there is potential for a fruitful collaboration between ethicists and social scientists. Therefore a clearer understanding of each other's perspective on the same issues of substantive interest would be of mutual benefit. At the very least these three questions, and their answers, provide an indication of how social scientists approach ethics and ethical issues. Second, whilst there is still a legitimate case to be made for seeing ethics as an abstract formal discipline, distanced from matters of actual social practice, it is not possible to posit the same view of ethicists themselves. As individual and collective practitioners of their discipline, however varied in their approaches and interests, they are members of professional and other social groupings and are thus subject to the influences of, and in turn influence, broader social changes and developments. At the very least I would argue that there is some interest for bioethicists in seeing themselves in a social context, even if there is a resistance to seeing their subject in such a way. All three questions above, but particularly (i) and (iii), suggest ways in which the practitioners of ethics might be understood in terms of broader social patterns and organisations. Third, I suggest that there is more to be gained than mere interest from understanding this social identity of ethicists, since one of the consequences of the growing lay and media interest in ethics and ethical issues is the increased scrutiny, and even criticism, social and political, of ethicists themselves.[7] This is part of what it means to see ethicists in a social context. From a social science point of view, to understand more about ethics is to understand more about ethicists, and vice versa, as the answers to the questions above will indicate. A clearer understanding of how this social identity affects their influence on the conduct of ethical matters is, I would suggest, a matter of practical as well as theoretical interest for ethicists.

I shall take each question in turn though the first will be treated at greater length since it has received the least attention in previous writings. The division between theoretical and empirical work is somewhat artificial (can one conduct good quality empirical research without being informed by a particular theory of knowledge; equally can one understand theoretical claims without an

---

[7] See Pat Spallone et al., *op. cit.* note 1.

understanding of how the everyday empirical world operates?) but, given the tendency hitherto to see the social sciences as having only a limited, empirical, contribution to make it is important to consider these two inter-linked strands separately for the moment. This both ensures clarity and expands the understanding of the social science contribution.

WHAT THEORETICAL WORK CAN THE SOCIAL SCIENCES CONTRIBUTE TO THE UNDERSTANDING OF ETHICS?

Social theory covers a wide array of approaches to the analysis of the social world. These can be broadly delineated as: theories of the subject and the relationship between the individual and society; theories of social structure, organization and institutions, including explanations for change in these and for their changing relationship with the individual; critical theory, which examines the relationships between social life, politics and the ordering of society through processes of rationalisation and bureaucracy; the sociology of difference, defined in a number of ways such as multiculturalism, ethnicity, gender and, finally, theories of modernity and postmodernity.[8] Within this body of work, a number of theorists (primarily though not exclusively sociologists) have taken an explicit interest in ethics, either as the subject of their investigations or as part of their explanatory repertoire in the analysis of broader social phenomena.

(i) Weber's writings contain two[9] possible lines that might shape a sociology of ethics. First, he demonstrated that a concern with how one ought to be and how one ought to act can influence a broader cultural trend towards the emergence of certain types of society and away from other possible lines of development. He coined the term 'economic ethics' in describing the effects of religion on economic affairs.[10] Second, he was interested in the practice

---

[8] A. Elliot. 1999. Introduction. *Contemporary Social Theory.* A. Elliott, ed. Oxford. Blackwell: 1–31.

[9] First, in *The Protestant Ethic and the Spirit of Capitalism* (1958. New York. Free Press.) and second in 'Science as a vocation'. In *From Max Weber.* 1946. H. Gerth and C.W. Mills, eds. New York. Oxford University Press.

[10] T. Osborne. 1998. Constructionism, authority and the ethical life. In *The Politics of Constructionism.* I. Velody and R. Williams, eds. London. Sage: 221–234.

of scholarly life itself. These two strands (the first a broadly defined notion of ethics as a field of sociological study, and the second, a narrower view of ethics that informs a reflection on how one's values affect how one acts as a sociologist) have varying degrees of prominence in later work.[11]

(ii) Theorists such as Hobhouse and Ginsberg saw ethics as central to their work in the analysis of systems of government. Helmes-Hayes claims that they saw sociology's 'real or first purpose' as being 'to formulate a general, historically informed theory of social and moral development'.[12] Ginsberg in particular was interested in the 'sociologically related issues of ethics' and saw 'no grounds for assuming that [a moral judgement] is not susceptible of investigation by rational methods' even though this went against the prevailing practice of separating ethics from social science.[13]

(iii) Foucault's interest in 'practices of the self' spanned a concern with individualism, liberalism and modernity: 'the heart of this problem being how to construct oneself ethically without recourse to overriding moral norms'.[14] He identified a continuity from Ancient Greece to contemporary Europe and argued that in both societies there is a reluctance to relate ethics to religious beliefs and to accept that legal systems have a part to play in personal, private lives. In contemporary life, ethics becomes an aesthetics of the self, a process in which one crafts oneself into being a 'moral agent'. This approach is expanded in Osborne's own work on 'ethical stylizations'. 'This means I want to connect ethics to the issue of person-formation. Ethical styles are to ethics what styles of reasoning are to scientific truth; that is, before one can be ethical or unethical, one needs a style of ethical judgement, or rather a particular stylization of the person that is equipped to make ethical judgements'. For example, he claims that Victorian ideals of altruism had less to do with one's conduct towards others and more to do with the need to sustain an acceptable sense of self by avoiding

[11] For example, R. Dingwall. Ethics and ethnography. *Sociological Review* 1980; 28: 871–891; and Silverman, *op. cit.* note 3.

[12] R.C. Helmes-Hayes. From universal history to historical sociology: a critical comment. *British Journal of Sociology* 1992; 43: 333–344, esp. p. 340.

[13] M. Ginsberg. 1942. Reason and Unreason in Society. London. Longman's Green and Co: 127–128, as quoted in Helmes-Hayes.

[14] Osborne, *op. cit.* note 2, p. 487; see also P. Rabinow, ed. 1997. *Michel Foucault: Ethics, Subjectivity and Truth.* London. Allen Lane: esp. pp. 255–256.

sloth and misery, altruistic acts being one way whereby this was achieved. Turning to contemporary society he suggests that we do not now live in an immoral world, as some argue, but rather that we live in a world of many ethical stylizations but with few rules about 'ethical content'.[15]

(iv) Giddens seeks to understand the relationship between the self and society without privileging either concept. His structurationist work on life politics links substantive concerns (the environment, biological reproduction, globalisation, and self-identity) with a view of trends distinctive to societies at a stage of late modernity: '. . . life politics concerns political issues which flow from processes of self-actualisation in post-traditional contexts, where globalising influences intrude deeply into the reflexive project of the self, and conversely where processes of self-realisation influence global strategies . . . Life politics is a politics of life decisions'. These decisions are a feature of everyday life for individuals who no longer have the certainties and rules of traditional society to guide their actions and to tell them who they are and what their place is within society. Thus, 'how should we live?' is the question at the centre of life politics. 'Life political issues . . . call for a remoralising of social life and they demand a renewed sensitivity to questions that the institutions of modernity systematically dissolve'.[16]

(v) A concern with ethics has been taken up in more recent debates in cultural theory. Lash acknowledges that 'ethical debates have become so central in recent years to social and cultural theory that they can no longer be ignored' which implies that though they have been present they have not yet received adequate attention. One failing of early social scientific work on ethics was, according to Lash, the tendency to see ethics as part of the superstructure, 'to be explained through a set of social causes and in terms of social interests. The cultural turn itself brought, thankfully, a departure from such positivist notions of causation and problematized the utilitarian assumptions of the notions of interests'. He characterises these debates as being between liberal theorists such as Rawls and Habermas, and communitarian writers such as Charles Taylor and Alisdair MacIntyre.[17]

---

[15] Osborne, *op. cit.* note 10, pp. 221, 231.

[16] A. Giddens. 1991. *Modernity and Self-Identity.* Cambridge. Polity Press: esp. pp. 214–224.

[17] 5. Lash. Introduction to the ethics and difference debate. *Theory, Culture and Society* 1996; 13: 75–78.

(vi) This debate has now been expanded by the postmodern ethics of writers such as Bauman whose work is particularly useful for advancing the sort of discussion advocated in this article. He notes how important the notions of universality and foundation have been to philosophers and legislators in modernity as they have sought to eliminate ambiguity and conflict and to achieve order and uniformity, in morality and ethics as in everything else. He observes, '. . . the moral thought and practice of modernity was animated by the belief in the possibility of a non-ambivalent, non-aporetic ethical code . . . It is the disbelief in such a possibility that is postmodern . . . The foolproof – universal and unshakeably founded – ethical code will never be found'.[18] Whilst some have seen this as a precursor of social collapse,[19] Bauman is more optimistic, seeing possibilities for individuals and communities to formulate new ideas of responsibility and ethics: 'a radically novel understanding of moral phenomena has been opened'.[20]

(vii) Feminist ethics, based on a confluence of feminism, the social sciences and philosophy, has been developed by a number of writers. As Bennett observes, 'Feminist theory provides an alternative theoretical framework for bioethical decision-making by providing an analysis that is based on interpersonal relations and connections rather than individualised rights. Feminists have argued the need for greater acknowledgement and valuing of the role of caring and nurturing relationships . . .' Such work challenges what it argues are male-centred theories of ethics, specifically the communitarian writers who assume shared understandings of the social world and of social order. Such challenges have implications for how central ethical concepts such as autonomy might be understood. For example, Bennett argues that we should talk of 'embodied autonomy', which depends on understanding 'individuals whose lived realities are mediated through the embodied intersections of race, class, gender, sexuality, disability and fertility. Autonomy is not found in an extra-corporeal individual carrying a bag full of rights as a safeguard against the world. Instead, autonomy is articulated by an embodied self, through relationships with others.'[21]

---

[18] Z. Bauman. 1993. *Postmodern Ethics.* Oxford. Blackwell: 2–27.
[19] Elliott, *op. cit.* note 8, p. 27.
[20] Bauman, *op. cit.* note 17.
[21] B. Bennett. Posthumous reproduction and the meanings of autonomy. *Melbourne University Law Review* 1999; 23: 286–307, esp. pp. 300–301.

As these different strands of work suggest, not only has there been a great deal of social science interest in the concept of ethics, there has also been sufficient space and liveliness within that work for debates and opposition to arise. Just on the one topic of social change, social theory has produced two tales about the transition to modernity and the effects of the growth of science, the market and bureaucracy upon notions of morals and ethics. First, the tale that 'modernity was ushered in by forces inimical to ethics, to community, to values' so that there was a fragmentation of moral and ethical life, and, second, the tale that there was 'an erosion of all values by the uniform, levelling and monolithic forces of bureaucratic culture and rationalization'.[22] In the transition from modernity to either late modernity or even postmodernity, the focus has changed again. As Lash puts it, 'Now no longer were questions of rights and justice necessarily pivotal in ethics. No longer was ethics necessarily a question of moral agency. Now the moral self was a singular ethical subjectivity finding itself in face of the unbounded demands of "the other" '.[23]

It would be inappropriate to try to make unified claims about the cumulative contributions of such a diverse body of work. However what is clear is that ethics is a part of what needs to be explained when analysing the key areas of social science interest. From these diverse theories we gain an understanding of ethics as shaping, and being shaped by, major social forces; of ethics being historically and culturally located; of ethics working in association with key social institutions, such as religion, government and the family; of ethics defining particular social groups, such as genders, professions, communities or sexualities; of ethical values being both reflective and constitutive of the self. That is, of ethics as being embedded within those aspects of the social world that tend to be taken as given, or as unproblematic, features of the world, by the normative statements of ethicists in general.

There is a danger that, with such diversity of interests, contexts and uses, the very notion of ethics disappears in a myriad of diverse meanings. However whilst it could be argued that that is true of the field of ethics more generally (how precisely do most writers employ this term?) it is a charge that warrants more serious response. There

---

[22] Osborne, *op. cit.* note 2, pp. 493–493.
[23] Lash, *op. cit.* note 16, p. 76.

are at least two possible responses. The first is to say that the key contribution of the social science work considered so far lies in its very diversity, since we can see if our understanding and usage of that term is extended, clarified or even challenged by the uses presented here. In that respect, this work can be said to have made a contribution to rigorous thought.

The second response to the charge of the disappearing concept of ethics is provided in the next section, where examples of empirical research on ethical issues are presented. Much of the work reviewed hitherto, with the exception of feminist sociology, tends to lack an empirical engagement with the practices of ethics or, more precisely, with the practices of what becomes designated as 'ethics', and this makes it easier for the concept to become even more elusive. Several commentators from within the discipline have noted the tendency for the social sciences to become somewhat abstract when dealing with such issues. Ginsberg called for small-scale studies to provide empirical content in order to achieve the goal of understanding social life as a whole; Osborne calls for a 'plurality of sober-minded forms of analysis and critique' of ethical issues; Lash, in a somewhat different style, declares, 'We want to bring ethics out into the streets'.[24]

WHAT CAN EMPIRICAL SOCIAL SCIENCE CONTRIBUTE TO THE UNDERSTANDING OF ETHICS?

As already mentioned, empirical social science could be seen as providing descriptive 'facts' to go alongside normative statements. And there is an acknowledged need for this, since, as Zussman claims, many ethicists' propositions are based on empirical claims that are usually unsupported by evidence.[25] However besides resisting being seen as the 'handmaiden' of ethics, as it was once seen as the handmaiden of medicine, sociology in particular would question this simplistic division. As Nelson points out, empirical inquiry is not just an exercise in 'scooping up the facts'.[26] Social scientists would argue that those 'facts' are inherently tied to theories of

[24] Osborne, *op. cit.* note 2, p. 494; Lash, ibid.

[25] Zussman, *op. cit.* note 2, p. 8.

[26] Nelson, *op. cit.* note 4, p. 13.

knowing the world and to a repertoire of techniques and skills for accessing that world (or indeed for constructing that world through an ongoing set of social processes[27]).

Therefore in this section it is useful to consider the contributions of empirical work from the social sciences in a number of different ways. First, examples of the empirical work that has been done; second, the potential within that existing work to give rise to a number of further questions and third, in terms of the epistemological and methodological techniques for gaining empirical access to the social world. The purpose in bringing this material together is not to try to impose a false unity on existing work but to establish that such work exists and to identify a web of connections between that work, to assist in the identification of new questions about the relationship between the social sciences and ethics.

Examples of empirical work

Given the breadth of theoretical work it is perhaps not surprising that there is also a wide range of empirical work within the social sciences that has the potential to enhance our understanding of ethical issues. Just a few examples shall be covered to illustrate this claim. Much of this work did not set out to be an explicit investigation of ethical issues per se, but it nonetheless touches upon and reveals how ethics are 'done' (identified, thought about, acted upon) in everyday life, across a range of substantive examples.

Given the prominence of assisted conception and embryology in ethical debates over the last twenty years this is a familiar and useful place to begin to lodge certain claims about the potential of social science work in this field; one can then move from that point to consider 'medical ethics', 'bioethics' and 'ethics' more generally. Others might want to argue for a different starting point, although it is worth noting Toulmin's claim that 'medicine saved the life of ethics'[28] as an additional reason for focusing on medical contexts.

Commenting on reproduction and on the technological malleability of the body more generally, Giddens remarks, 'The more we reflexively "make ourselves" as persons, the more the very category

[27] I. Velody & R. Williams. 1998. Introduction. In *The Politics of Constructionism*. Velody and Williams, eds. London. Sage: 1–12.
[28] S. Toulmin. How medicine saved the life of ethics. *Perspectives in Biology and Medicine* 1982; 25: 736–750.

of what "a person" or "human being" is comes to the fore'.[29] These and related issues lie at the heart of concerns over the new reproductive technologies and assisted conception. It is usually at this point in a public or policymaking discussion that philosophers are invited in, to explain the different forms that answers to such questions might take. Whilst there is a place for abstract principlism, there is also a place for the social sciences to throw further light both on the questions themselves and on the contexts in which they arise. Examples of empirical investigations of what issues come to the fore in the field of assisted conception, and how they are reasoned through and handled by everyday actors, can be seen in the work of several social scientists.

Franklin conducted an ethnographic study of couples' experiences of the in vitro fertilisation (IVF) treatment process. On the question of what counts as a person Franklin found that some women blurred the boundaries between chemical pregnancies, embryos and actual babies. As one woman said at the point of embryo replacement, 'well, they are my babies 'cos they are my embryos'.[30] This blurring provided support for couples and gave them the stamina to sustain the arduous treatment. Thus we have here a highly contextualised definition of what is a person: one that is given meaning and consequentially acted upon. This study reveals other aspects of JVF treatment that raise ethical questions. Franklin's couples found that the rigours of WF treatment dominated their lives but were hard to resist as the promise of resolution (of their infertility or of their difficulties in coming to terms with their infertility) beckoned. However as they proceeded with treatment it became apparent that for most couples there would be no resolution in either sense. The paradox was that the ethical arguments advanced in support of IVF ('helping desperate couples') as a response to ethical concerns about the process (experimentation on human embryos), are shown, by empirical investigation, to be open to challenge, as the evidence from Franklin's study suggests that 1VF creates a desperation to succeed that had not been there in the first place. Also TVF is shown to create other ethical difficulties, such as women being sold or pursuing IVF treatment when there are reducing levels of likely success. However the data also show

---

[29] Giddens, *op. cit.* note 15, p. 217.
[30] S. Franklin. 1997. *Embodied Progress.* London. Routledge: 182.

that despite acknowledging these costs most of the women interviewed strongly endorsed the treatment. As Franklin concludes, '. . . women's experiences of WF . . . are far from simple. They are composed of feelings and perceptions that are equivocal and ambivalent, positive and negative, empowering and disempowering. These paradoxical dimensions of the experience of the IVF procedure are fundamental to many of the ways of making sense of it . . .'[31]

Price's work also shows additional ethical dilemmas created by IVF that are rarely discussed: that of treatment succeeding 'too well', resulting in multiple births. In her study of parents coping with triplets, quads or quins,[32] Price found a vast range of practical and emotional problems associated with multiple births. The practical problems included: not being able to pick up all babies at any one time; coping with different sleeping patterns amongst the children; isolation because of the difficulties of taking three or more small babies out at any one time; financial difficulties; the sheer amount of work and the lack of formal or informal assistance on a regular basis from family, friends or social services. Emotional problems arose between the parents who had little time or energy to deal with each other's needs and from the difficulties of treating any of the children as individuals given the demands they made as a group. Therefore, the risks of a multiple birth require serious consideration between doctor and patient before IVF is provided. However, this entails other ethical considerations, such as should doctors prioritise the avoidance of a triplet birth by only replacing two embryos (rather than the three allowed in UK legislation). Thus, the impact of this research has been that exposure of the practical difficulties of coping with higher order births has added ethical considerations to the physiological considerations of whether it is more effective to transfer three or only two embryos. This in turn raises other ethical dilemmas for practitioners, such as the question of balancing, on the one hand, their patients' desires for a baby (and their own needs to produce satisfactory IVF success rates) with the now known problems of a multiple birth. A question that Price's study did not attempt to answer but which she raises as part of the discussion is the possibility of using selective reduction

---

[31] Ibid., p. 194.
[32] F. Price. 1992. Having triplets, quads or quins: who bears the responsibility? In *Changing Human Reproduction*. M. Stacey, ed. London. Sage: 92–118.

as a solution to a multiple pregnancy. The paradox here is that the very success of IVF creates further ethical dilemmas over abortion. Therefore what is learned from Price's study is that ethical questions about assisted conception are rarely confined to single treatment contexts but are likely to impinge on, and be affected by, the broader social context of the interplay between families, medicine, the state and reproductive issues.

Both Price's and Franklin's work point to questions about what counts as informed consent. Should information include the consequences of going through the treatment process itself? Should information include detailed consideration about whether a multiple birth is actually something parents have seriously considered and know that they can cope with? The social science research described here suggests that the answer to both questions is 'yes'. Clearly both sets of data can be challenged but only by other empirical findings.

A different type of study is reported by Haimes. This is an empirical examination of the normative statements (taken from documents and interviews) that comprise the two sides of the debate over whether children conceived through donated gametes should be told information about their genetic parents. The aim of the analysis is to 'prise open those unstated assumptions upon which the debate rests, to see what process of reasoning, and what repertoire of concerns, are available to those participating in such discussions'. This is another example of the success of assisted conception creating further ethical difficulties, since the process of helping people to have children creates the situation where those children have their genetic origins rendered unknowable. These difficulties are usually hidden from most bioethicists' gaze since they lie within the communities and families rather than within the more visible context of the clinic. The analysis shows that the apparently virulently opposed sides of the debate share a large amount of common ground, including: a view of families as needing to be discrete, self-contained units; uncertainty about the place of genetics and biology in making the family, and uncertainty about prioritising the needs of one member of the family over another. These in turn show that the debate depends upon notions of 'ordinary' and 'extraordinary' families, which are themselves statements of ethical values and are thus open to challenge from other value positions, for example claims about the legitimacy of diverse family forms. This study demonstrates that 'the handling of genetic origins is not a simple matter, but can be shown, through a sociological analysis, to have consequences for and connections to, other aspects of the wider society'.[33]

A final example of empirical work comes from Edwards who provides valuable insight into how ordinary people, with no direct involvement with assisted conception, think about these ethical and social issues. In her ethnographic study of 'Alltown',[34] she discovered that residents identified three related sets of dangers with these practices: psychological (in terms of worrying about the effects on the children conceived), biological (in terms of the risks of incest which was used as a 'conceptual brake . . . a boundary, a limit which ought not to be traversed') and relational (the impact of reproductive technologies on wider social relationships). Edwards found that her informants located the ethical complexities raised by assisted conception within other complex family relationships that they had either experienced themselves or had heard about, such as remarriage, step-relatives or co-habitations. If those pre-existing frameworks raised no concerns then their parallels within assisted conception were also accepted; if there were concerns in the pre-existing scenarios, such as fears about incest, then the parallel case in assisted conception caused concern. One aspect that worried respondents was the possibility that a child might not be able to make full kinship claims (for example, for unquestioned support throughout life) on his/her relatives because of being conceived through donated gametes. This worry was explained through the examples provided by half-relatives or step-relatives who might feel not fully attached to a family. However there was also the experience in existing families of marginal individuals (such as long-lost fathers or other relatives) wanting to stake unjustified kinship claims on children. This example was used to explain the dangers of a donor wanting to make a claim on a child that s/he had helped to conceive (or indeed the dangers of the child making claims on the donor). These dangers were thought to increase if the donor was already related, for example a sister donating an egg. However, other experiences such as the closeness of sisters, and the need to keep things in the family were also used to justify that practice.

---

[33] E. Haimes. 1992. Gamete donation and the social management of genetic origins. In *Changing Human Reproduction*. M. Stacey, ed. London. Sage: 119–147.

[34] J. Edwards. 1998. Donor insemination and 'public opinion'. In *Donor Insemination: International Social Science Perspectives*. K. Daniels and E. Haimes, eds. Cambridge. Cambridge University Press: 151–172.

Elsewhere, in reference to the same study, Edwards concludes, 'People interpret what they see as the implications of NRT not through what they know of the techniques and philosophies of reproductive medicine, but through what they know about the practice and predictabilities of kinship'.[35]

This study shows that new technical possibilities do not always create new ethical dilemmas but when they do, everyday actors are seen to have other cultural reference points through which they resolve such difficulties. In this case, that which is usually presented as an issue of medical ethics, is seen by everyday actors as an issue of family ethics. That is, the 'same' ethical issues are located in different contexts by different sets of actors and are accordingly seen to have different implications and meanings. It is these differences that are open to empirical investigation.

Questions raised by empirical investigations

The studies cited here have a contribution to make beyond their own individual empirical findings. They have the potential to stimulate further questions about the ethical context of reproductive technologies since they provide an empirical basis to Giddens' observation that reproduction 'is now a field where plurality of choice prevails'.[36] This theme is further analysed by the social anthropologist, Marilyn Strathern: 'Choice is a significant value to which Euro-Americans give weight in setting up families . . . developments in new reproductive technology have made newly explicit the possibility of choosing whom and what one desires to call family. In opening up ways of thinking, they offer a cultural enablement of a kind.'[37] This claim can be pursued through further empirical research. For example, taking the aforementioned studies as a guide, one might ask to what extent do different groups (patients, clinicians, policymakers, ordinary people) share a view of the importance of choice in specific reproductive circumstances? In the

[35] J. Edwards. 1993. Explicit connections: ethnographic enquiry in north-west England. In *Technologies of Procreation*. J. Edwards, S. Franklin, E. Hirsch, F. Price and M. Strathern, eds. Manchester. Manchester University Press: 42–66, esp. pp. 63–64.

[36] Giddens, *op. cit.* note 15, p. 219.

[37] M. Strathern. 1996. Enabling identity? Biology, choice and the new reproductive technologies. In *Questions of Cultural Identity*. S. Hall and P. du Gay, eds. London. Sage: 37–52, esp. p. 47.

case of preimplantation genetic diagnosis, for example, in what sense does a woman 'choose' to have her embryos screened: is this perceived to be a choice by the woman or does she see it as an obligation, in order to avoid what are said to be the personal and social costs of a disabled child? Also does choice in such situations include the option of the woman actively choosing to have a child with disabilities, and rejecting those embryos that have been shown not to have disabilities? Equally how are certain views of choice curtailed by other 'ethical' considerations, such as the welfare of the child?[38] And how much are such choices constrained by the exercise of professional power and authority?[39] As we have seen, these questions, when subjected to empirical investigation, expand our repertoire of what counts as an 'ethical' question by alerting us to the possibility of multiple perspectives on ethics.

Therefore, such empirical studies both complement the broader theoretical sweeps outlined in the previous section (by revealing yet further 'ways of thinking' and by showing what 'cultural enablement' might look like in specific contexts) and stimulate further theoretical and empirical lines of investigation. Such an empirical grounding also sheds further light on how the 'politics' of life politics might be enabling in some contexts but also constraining in others.

The findings of these empirical studies and the additional questions and lines of investigation that they give rise to suggest that if we are to understand more clearly how individuals 'act ethically' we have to engage in the detailed, contextualised dilemmas. As Bauman argues, 'Human reality is messy and ambiguous – and so moral decisions, unlike abstract ethical principles, are ambivalent. It is in this sort of world that we must live; and yet, as if defying the worried philosophers who cannot conceive of an "unprincipled" morality, a morality without foundations, we demonstrate day by day that we can live or learn to live, or man age to live in such a world, though few of us would be ready to spell out, if asked, what the principles that guide us are, and fewer still would have heard

[38] R. Burbidge & E. Haimes. 1996. Infertility treatment and the welfare of the child. Paper presented to the British Sociological Association Medical Sociology Group Annual Conference.

[39] See for example, E. Freidson. 1975. *Profession of Medicine*. New York. Dodd, Mead and Co.; T. Osborne, *op. cit.* note 2; R.B. Pippin. Medical practice and social authority. *Journal of Medicine and Philosophy* 1996; 21: 417–437.

about the "foundations" which we allegedly cannot do without, to be good and kind to each other.'[40]

The contributions of social science methodology

A third feature of the contributions of empirical social science is the epistemological frameworks and the methodological skills and techniques that provide the means for accessing and engaging with messy human reality. As the above studies demonstrate, methodological strategies such as ethnographic research and participant observation, and research methods, such as in-depth interviewing, are particularly powerful in revealing the details of how people think and act ethically in everyday life.[41] Other techniques have also been fruitfully deployed to reveal empirical data on ethical considerations. Also in the field of reproductive technologies these have included the documentary analysis of Hansard debates,[42] survey research to elicit clinician's strategies for implementing the welfare of the child clause in the UK's Human Fertilisation and Embryology Act, 1990[43] and historical methods to analyse the debates over the provision of fertility services on the NHS.[44] These techniques provide access to (i) the locations and institutions (for example, clinics, hospitals, courts, government committees, ethics committees) in which ethical dilemmas arise, (ii) the actors (for example, professionals, lay people, policy makers, family members) involved in the activities and discussions around these dilemmas, (iii) the diverse range of definitions and meanings that underpin both the dilemmas themselves and the answers proffered (and that underpin the diversity of responses from different actors in different locations and institutions, at different periods in history), and finally, (iv) the broader socio-cultural frameworks (of family, health, community, economy, religion, law, politics and so on) which both shape the

[40] Bauman, *op. cit.* note 17, p. 32.
[41] Hoffmaster, *op. cit.* note 5; S. Holm. 1997. *Ethical Problems in Clinical Practice.* Manchester. Manchester University Press.
[42] E. Haimes. 1990. *Family Connections.* (Doctoral thesis, University of Newcastle); S. Franklin. Making representations. In *Technologies of Procreation, op. cit.* note 34; M. Mulkay. Rhetorics of hope and fear in the great embryo debate. *Social Studies of Science* 1993; 23: 721–742.
[43] Burbidge & Haimes, *op. cit.* note 37.
[44] N. Pfeffer. From private patients to privatisation. In *Changing Human Reproduction, op. cit.* note 31, pp. 48–74.

repertoire of possible responses and which are shaped by the actual responses given in actual cases.

It is of course not the case that other disciplines lack either an interest, or skills, in conducting such empirical work: Zussman points to the work done by doctors, nurses and health administrators.[45] Similarly, Holm is one of several bioethicists now conducting empirical research, taking as his subject the ethical reasoning of health care professionals.[46] However, besides providing many of the methodological tools used by others, the social scientist has the broad range of theoretical and epistemological resources and interests that assist him/her to make further sense of those situated practices, by asking questions that go beyond those that are immediately apparent in the situation itself, to connect these dilemmas to broader debates about social and cultural development, as outlined in the section on social theory. Such broader perspectives enhance the growing empirical research of bioethicists and others, in a number of ways. First, by providing opportunities for fruitful collaboration between the disciplines, and, second, by providing further insights into the nature and provenance of particular situations and into the wider social and cultural vicissitudes that will have an impact on those settings and on the groups and individuals that populate the settings. It is these attempts to connect the empirical data with theoretical explanations that make the social science enterprise distinctive and which take it beyond the handmaiden, 'scooping up' role. It is this disciplinary imperative, to connect the particular to the general, that also leads the social sciences beyond the specific ethical questions of particular practices, to ask further questions about the very designation of certain issues as being 'ethical issues'. The next section examines this.

HOW CAN SOCIAL SCIENCE RESEARCH ENHANCE THE UNDERSTANDING OF HOW ETHICS AS A FIELD OF STUDY IS SOCIALLY CONSTITUTED AND SITUATED?

As the above empirical examples show, assisted conception practices have been culturally, professionally and politically packaged

---

[45] Zussman, *op. cit.* note 2, p. 11.
[46] Holm, *op. cit.* note 40, chs. 3 and 4.

as 'ethical issues' but it is important to ask whether alternative packaging is possible. For example, one study suggests the 'yuk' reaction that greets practices such as the use of ovarian tissue from foetuses or cadavers for egg donation is as much stimulated by a sense of 'social impropriety' (that is, a sense that anyone having to identify this as part of their biography would be seen as drawing undue attention to the more unseemly aspects of procreation) as by any particular ethical stance.[47] Thus, detailed empirical analyses such as these provide insight into how ethical issues are so packaged. However, there is much less work, empirical or theoretical, on this aspect so this section is much more speculative than the previous two sections. The focus is on trying to identify the likely directions that such work might take in the future.

Still within the field of medical ethics, answers to this question might be found through an exploration of the social processes of labelling, whereby certain matters are designated 'ethical', and others 'economic' or 'political'. For example, what is 'being done' when decisions about embryo experimentation are routinely categorised as ethical questions and when issues such as the funding of fertility treatment on the National Health Service are routinely labelled economic or political questions? Where do such labels come from? What are the consequences of such labels? What alternative arguments and actions are constrained by the application of such labels? What would happen if alternative labels were applied?

Other lines of inquiry are likely to be equally fruitful. For example, there is a need to ask what is the relationship between the history of medical ethics and state policies, such that some fields have become highly legislated, for example, abortion, and others, such as euthanasia, are not. The history of medical ethics is important since as Osborne points out, its current focus on patient care is a relatively recent development; its first and long-term concern has been with the etiquette of inter-professional rivalry.[48] Mackenzie, drawing on the work of Hacking, demonstrates how to do an historically informed social constructionist analysis of morality 'by "taking a look" at the local, empirical facts that surround their emergence as problems'[49] An exploration of the history of medicine

---

[47] B. Haimes & R. Williams. Social constructionism and the new technologies of reproduction. In *The Politics of Constructionism, op. cit.* note 10, pp. 132–146.
[48] T. Osborne. Power and persons. *Sociology of Health and Illness* 1994; 16: 514–535.
[49] C. Mackenzie. Social constructionist political theory. In *The Politics of Constructionism, op. cit.* note 10, pp. 200–220; esp. p. 201.

and ethics would also be useful to document the ways in which certain cases have provided a forum for particular formulations of ethical positions, such as the Tony Bland case in the UK. An awareness of the history of medical ethics would also be useful in documenting the transition of certain practices from being 'ethical concerns' to 'mundane practices', and back again, as has happened to some extent with donor insemination.[50] Turning to contemporary medicine, the increasingly influential role of 'the four principles' (autonomy, beneficence, non-maleficence and justice) in guiding clinical decisions may shed light on the notion of 'ethics as mantra': some suggest that rather than assisting clinicians in clarifying their possible courses of action these principles simply tend to reproduce 'normative frameworks' instead.[51] It has already been shown how 'autonomy' can be challenged.

Other questions require systematic theoretical and empirical examination, for example, what, if anything, is distinctive about the different ethical domains? Are medical ethics different from ethics of the environment, or issues around ethical investment, or legal ethics, and so on? Some would argue that there are profound differences.[52] For Schenck it is the 'radical responsibility' and the 'radical threat' of medicine that gives rise to intense ethical debates, mainly because of the bodily concerns of medicine. 'Going into discussions of medical ethics attending only to ethical theories, without attention to the phenomenon of embodiment, would be like going into a discussion of the rules governing ball games without paying attention to the differences between football, basketball and baseball, focusing only on abstract discussions of the nature of "rules" and "games" as such. Too often ethicists of medicine seem lost in just this way; and that is because they tend to ignore that which distinguishes medical ethics from business ethics or legal ethics which is of course the centrality of the body for the practice of medicine and the texture of embodiment of human life itself'.[53]

Such claims are of course open to empirical investigation; for example, returning to Osborne's claims about ethical stylizations, is

---

[50] K. Daniels & B. Haimes. 1998. *Donor Insemination*. Cambridge. Cambridge University Press.

[51] R. Chadwick & M. Levitt. 1996. Comment. In *Cultural and social objections to biotechnology*. Biocult Project Team Report. University of Central Lancashire: 160–173.

[52] Freidson, *op. cit.* note 38, p. 342.

[53] D. Schenck. The texture of embodiment: foundation for medical ethics. *Human Studies* 1986; 9: 43–54, esp. p. 50.

there evidence of different professionals in different fields (for example, law, medicine, academia) displaying distinctive stylizations? These claims lead on to other questions: what impact does singling out ethical domains in this way have on the practices within those domains; how are the boundaries between different ethical domains established, challenged, penetrated, or changed? What happens when different ethical domains clash (for example, the legal and the medical[54])? Equally, what happens when it is assumed that two domains are so different that ethical concerns about practices in one field are not reflected to the same extent as in another domain?[55] Whilst some work is being conducted on these sorts of questions, much of it needs to be more clearly theoretically framed if it is to contribute to broader understandings of social life.

In other words, the task here is to conduct a social science analysis of the social processes, meanings and institutions that frame and produce 'ethics' and ethical problems. Some of these questions might be addressed through a 'genealogy of ethics': how has it become possible to talk of ethical concerns; how have matters become so designated; how do they become attached to particular fields of activity (and not to others); what institutions have formed to deal with ethical issues; what ideologies, knowledges, webs of power have arisen around these institutions; how has the notion of 'ethical expertise' arisen; what is the history of its attachment to particular disciplines? Nelson suggests that the social sciences might mount an implicit challenge to bioethicists in asking why they attend to the questions they do and 'even whose interests they think it appropriate to serve'.[56]

Work has already begun on other lines of analysis that will help to situate ethics in a socio-historical context, including: the possibility of cross-cultural ethics,[57] the notion of ethics in developing countries[58] and the multiplicity of ethical positions, including the framing of ethics for particular religions and so on. Each of these in turn raises further questions about the framing of ethical debates

---

[54] M. Stacey. 1992. *Regulating British Medicine*. London. Wiley.
[55] See for example, L. Gofton and B. Haimes. Necessary Evils? *Sociological Research Online 1999*; 1. http://www.socresonline.org.uk.
[56] Nelson, *op. cit.* note 4, p. 14.
[57] See for example G.R. Gillet. Medical ethics in a multicultural context. *Journal of Medical Ethics* 1995; 238: 531–537.
[58] See for example B. du Jardin. Health and human rights. *Social Science and Medicine* 1994; 39: 1261–1274.

in certain conceptual terms (such as lying, truth, trust, autonomy, personhood) and the tendency to ignore or exclude other terms (such as power, politics, authority). Again Nelson is pointed in his commentary: 'The social sciences might make a contribution to bioethics by helping the field's practitioners understand better what's behind its deeply installed respect for individual autonomy and whether it has assumed more the character of an ideology than a moral philosophy.'[59]

Such a conceptual analysis would allow for the possibility of alternative models emerging.[60] The historical perspective might cause alertness to a consideration of whether the twenty-first century is particularly challenging in terms of ethical dilemmas or whether each period sees itself as confronting new and more difficult dilemmas than previous eras. Such work would lend an empirical base to Bauman's wish that '. . . the sources of moral power which in modern ethical philosophy and political practice were hidden from sight, may be made visible, while the reasons for their past invisibility can be better understood'. It is also likely that such studies would reveal evidence for Bauman's claim about the relativism of ethical codes and of recommended moral practices.[61] Clearly, at this point it is only possible to identify some of the questions that might provide analytical purchase: others will arise as the discussions and explorations progress.

CONCLUSION

Silverman suggests that 'The social, political and cultural contexts of health communication and ethics is a crucial area which raises central questions about the relevance to society of sociological research'.[62] This article has at least outlined the relevance of the social sciences to the study of ethics. A review follows, showing how the four broad purposes proposed in the introduction have been fulfilled, with a brief indication where this leads, in terms of the relationship between social science and ethics.

---

[59] Nelson, *op. cit.* note 4, p. 15.
[60] V. Shame. Justice and care: the implications of the Kohlberg-Gilligan debate for medical ethics. *Theoretical Medicine* 1992; 13: 295–318.
[61] Bauman, *op. cit.* note 17, pp. 3, 14.
[62] D. Silverman. Review: social science perspectives on medical ethics. *British Journal of Sociology* 1992; 43: 506.

The first purpose was to identify the various strands in the social science work on ethics. These fall broadly into theoretical and empirical contributions from a wide range of social scientists. The second purpose was to identify how this body of work contributes to the study of ethics. The theoretical work expands the questions one can ask about the study of ethics by relating it to the dominant themes in the social sciences. The empirical work contributes at several levels. It provides the data on particular substantive issues; that is, the 'facts' about what people say or do on particular topics. This in turn provides data on how individuals and groups think and act ethically; that is the 'how' and the 'why' of what people say and do, that fall outside the frameworks of formal philosophy. In addition, the empirical work demonstrates and refines the techniques for gaining access to the 'what', 'how' and 'why' of ethical behaviour. Together, the theoretical and empirical work provide knowledge on the social processes that lie behind the designation of certain areas of social life as being 'to do with' ethics, and the exclusion of other areas as not being of concern for the study of ethics.

The third purpose was to try to make the voice of the social sciences heard more clearly. However, it is perhaps a weakness of the work that has been done hitherto that its proponents have not made full use of each other's contributions, which might be part of the reason why the voice has not been heard. It is hoped that this identification and delineation of existing work will assist the voice of social science to be heard more clearly, both in communication with each other and in communication with ethicists and other disciplines. Equally the identification of a number of so far unanswered questions should help this dialogue since it both preempts any sociological imperialism and presents a task in common for a number of disciplines to work on together.[63] In that sense there is a dialogue that arises out of the intellectual space created by questions, which in turn generate further questions and collaborative work.[64]

The cumulative impact of this existing and potential work helps to fulfil the fourth purpose of this article, which is to establish that

[63] I am grateful to one of the anonymous reviewers of this article for pointing out that it will probably be as necessary for the social sciences to engage (more fully than they currently do) with the legal arena as much as with ethics, if their voice is to be heard, given the intertwining of law and ethics in countries such as the United States and Uganda.

[64] Silverman, *op. cit.* note 3, pp. 194–195.

social science has more to contribute than just the 'facts'. Zussman expresses reservation about sociology being the junior partner to medical ethics yet he does not really make a strong enough case for seeing it as other than this because he fails to embed the empirical work of social scientists within their theoretical roots and hence their analytical framework. It is the theoretical framework that provides the future direction for the relationship between the social sciences and ethics: one that puts ethics centre stage as the subject of social science enquiiy. This is a quite different focus and approach to work than that of examining a series of substantive topics (euthanasia, abortion, informed consent etc.) to provide empirical data for ethicists to use to refine their normative analysis. The advantage of putting ethics and ethicists centre stage, as the subjects of sociological research, is that they can then be located in a broader socio-historical context, which enables new questions to be asked. (Such as, why are these issues defined as ethical concerns by these people in these times and these places?) That is, more precise questions that are at the same time more general in so far as they are indicators of broader concerns and trends of particular societies at particular times. It is the recognition of this potential that supports the claim that it is indeed possible to have a 'sociology of ethics'.

One feature this particular article does not lack is questions. It is hoped it too will stimulate a dialogue since it contains the beginnings of an exploration in the sociology of knowledge, in a field where social science perspectives can contribute to the central focus of concerns rather than merely stand on the sidelines.

Acknowledgements

I should like to thank the two anonymous reviewers for *Bioethics*, plus Ruth Chadwick, Paul Johnson, Main Levitt, Peter Phillimore, Pat Spallone, Michael Whong-Barr and Tom Wilkie for their encouragement with this paper.

Chapter 4

IN DEFENSE OF POSTHUMAN DIGNITY

NICK BOSTROM

TRANSHUMANISTS VS. BIOCONSERVATIVES

Transhumanism is a loosely defined movement that has developed gradually over the past two decades, and can be viewed as an outgrowth of secular humanism and the Enlightenment. It holds that current human nature is improvable through the use of applied science and other rational methods, which may make it possible to increase human health-span, extend our intellectual and physical capacities, and give us increased control over our own mental states and moods.[1] Technologies of concern include not only current ones, like genetic engineering and information technology, but also anticipated future developments such as fully immersive virtual reality, machine-phase nanotechnology, and artificial intelligence.

Transhumanists promote the view that human enhancement technologies should be made widely available, and that individuals should have broad discretion over which of these technologies to apply to themselves (morphological freedom), and that parents should normally get to decide which reproductive technologies to use when having children (reproductive freedom).[2] Transhumanists believe that, while there are hazards that need to be identified and avoided, human enhancement technologies will offer enormous potential for deeply valuable and humanly beneficial uses. Ultimately, it is possible that such enhancements may make us, or our descendants, 'posthuman', beings who may have indefinite health-spans, much greater intellectual faculties than any current human being – and perhaps entirely new sensibilities or modalities – as well as the ability to control their own emotions. The wisest approach *vis-à-vis* these prospects, argue transhumanists, is to embrace

[1] N. Bostrom. 2003. The Transhumanist FAQ, v. 2.1. *World Transhumanist Association.* Webpage: www.transhumanism.org/resources/FAQv21.pdf
[2] N. Bostrom. Human Genetic Enhancements: A Transhumanist Perspective. *Journal of Value Inquiry*, Vol. 37, No. 4, pp. 493–506.

technological progress, while strongly defending human rights and individual choice, and taking action specifically against concrete threats, such as military or terrorist abuse of bioweapons, and against unwanted environmental or social side-effects.

In opposition to this transhumanist view stands a bioconservative camp that argues against the use of technology to modify human nature. Prominent bioconservative writers include Leon Kass, Francis Fukuyama, George Annas, Wesley Smith, Jeremy Rifkin, and Bill McKibben. One of the central concerns of the bioconservatives is that human enhancement technologies might be 'dehumanizing'. The worry, which has been variously expressed, is that these technologies might undermine our human dignity or inadvertently erode something that is deeply valuable about being human but that is difficult to put into words or to factor into a cost-benefit analysis. In some cases (for example, Leon Kass) the unease seems to derive from religious or crypto-religious sentiments, whereas for others (for example, Francis Fukuyama) it stems from secular grounds. The best approach, these bioconservatives argue, is to implement global bans on swathes of promising human enhancement technologies to forestall a slide down a slippery slope towards an ultimately debased, posthuman state.

While any brief description necessarily skirts significant nuances that differentiate between the writers within the two camps, I believe the above characterization nevertheless highlights a principal fault line in one of the great debates of our times: how we should look at the future of humankind and whether we should attempt to use technology to make ourselves 'more than human'. This paper will distinguish two common fears about the posthuman and argue that they are partly unfounded and that, to the extent that they correspond to real risks, there are better responses than trying to implement broad bans on technology. I will make some remarks on the concept of dignity, which bioconservatives believe to be imperiled by coming human enhancement technologies, and suggest that we need to recognize that not only humans in their current form, but posthumans too could have dignity.

TWO FEARS ABOUT THE POSTHUMAN

The prospect of posthumanity is feared for at least two reasons. One is that the state of being posthuman might in itself be degrading, so that by becoming posthuman we might be harming ourselves. Another is that posthumans might pose a threat to 'ordinary' humans. (I shall set aside a third possible reason, that the development of posthumans might offend some supernatural being.)

The most prominent bioethicist to focus on the first fear is Leon Kass:

> Most of the given bestowals of nature have their given species-specified natures: they are each and all of a given *sort*. Cockroaches and humans are equally bestowed but differently natured. To turn a man into a cockroach – as we don't need Kafka to show us – would be dehumanizing. To try to turn a man into more than a man might be so as well. We need more than generalized appreciation for nature's gifts. We need a particular regard and respect for the special gift that is our own given nature[3]

Transhumanists counter that nature's gifts are sometimes poisoned and should not always be accepted. Cancer, malaria, dementia, aging, starvation, unnecessary suffering, and cognitive shortcomings are all among the presents that we would wisely refuse. Our own species-specified natures are a rich source of much of the thoroughly unrespectable and unacceptable – susceptibility for disease, murder, rape, genocide, cheating, torture, racism. The horrors of nature in general, and of our own nature in particular, are so well documented[4] that it is astonishing that somebody as distinguished as Leon Kass should still in this day and age be tempted to rely on the natural as a guide as to what is desirable or normatively right. We should be grateful that our ancestors were not swept away by the Kassian sentiment, or we would still be picking lice off each other's backs. Rather than deferring to the natural order, transhumanists maintain that we can legitimately reform ourselves and our natures in accordance with humane values and personal aspirations.

If one rejects nature as a general criterion of the good, as most thoughtful people nowadays do, one can of course still acknowledge that particular ways of modifying human nature would be

---

[3] L. Kass. Ageless Bodies, Happy Souls: Biotechnology and the Pursuit of Perfection. *The New Atlantis* 2003; 1.

[4] See e.g. J. Glover. 2001. *Humanity: A Moral History of the Twentieth Century*. New Haven. Yale University Press.

debasing. Not all change is progress. Not even all well-intentioned technological intervention in human nature would be on balance beneficial. Kass goes far beyond these truisms, however, when he declares that utter dehumanization lies in store for us as the inevitable result of our obtaining technical mastery over our own nature:

> The final technical conquest of his own nature would almost certainly leave mankind utterly enfeebled. This form of mastery would be identical with utter dehumanization. Read Huxley's *Brave New World*, read C. S. Lewis's *Abolition of Man*, read Nietzsche's account of the last man, and then read the newspapers. Homogenization, mediocrity, pacification, drug-induced contentment, debasement of taste, souls without loves and longings – these are the inevitable results of making the essence of human nature the last project of technical mastery. In his moment of triumph, Promethean man will become a contented cow.[5]

The fictional inhabitants of *Brave New World*, to pick the best known of Kass's examples, are admittedly short on dignity (in at least one sense of the word). But the claim that this is the *inevitable* consequence of our obtaining technological mastery over human nature is exceedingly pessimistic – and unsupported – if understood as a futuristic prediction, and false if construed as a claim about metaphysical necessity.

There are many things wrong with the fictional society that Huxley described. It is static, totalitarian, caste-bound; its culture is a wasteland. The brave new worlders themselves are a dehumanized and undignified lot. Yet posthumans they are not. Their capacities are not super-human but in many respects substantially inferior to our own. Their life expectancy and physique are quite normal, but their intellectual, emotional, moral, and spiritual faculties are stunted. The majority of the brave new worlders have various degrees of engineered mental retardation. And everyone, save the ten world controllers (along with a miscellany of primitives and social outcasts who are confined to fenced preservations or isolated islands), are barred or discouraged from developing individuality, independent thinking, and initiative, and are conditioned not to desire these traits in the first place. *Brave New World* is not a tale of human enhancement gone amok, but is rather a tragedy of

---

[5] L. Kass. 2002. *Life, Liberty, and Defense of Dignity: The Challenge for Bioethics.* San Francisco. Encounter Books: p. 48.

technology and social engineering being deliberately used to cripple moral and intellectual capacities – the exact antithesis of the transhumanist proposal.

Transhumanists argue that the best way to avoid a *Brave New World* is by vigorously defending morphological and reproductive freedoms against any would-be world controllers. History has shown the dangers in letting governments curtail these freedoms. The last century's government-sponsored coercive eugenics programs, once favored by both the left and the right, have been thoroughly discredited. Because people are likely to differ profoundly in their attitudes towards human enhancement technologies, it is crucial that no single solution be imposed on everyone from above, but that individuals get to consult their own consciences as to what is right for themselves and their families. Information, public debate, and education are the appropriate means by which to encourage others to make wise choices, not a global ban on a broad range of potentially beneficial medical and other enhancement options.

The second fear is that there might be an eruption of violence between unaugmented humans and posthumans. George Annas, Lori Andrews, and Rosario Isasi have argued that we should view human cloning and all inheritable genetic modifications as 'crimes against humanity' in order to reduce the probability that a posthuman species will arise, on grounds that such a species would pose an existential threat to the old human species:

> The new species, or 'posthuman,' will likely view the old 'normal' humans as inferior, even savages, and fit for slavery or slaughter. The normals, on the other hand, may see the post-humans as a threat and if they can, may engage in a preemptive strike by killing the posthumans before they themselves are killed or enslaved by them. It is ultimately this predictable potential for genocide that makes species-altering experiments potential weapons of mass destruction, and makes the unaccountable genetic engineer a potential bioterrorist.[6]

There is no denying that bioterrorism and unaccountable genetic engineers developing increasingly potent weapons of mass

---

[6] G. Annas, L. Andrews & R. Isasi. Protecting the Endangered Human: Toward an International Treaty Prohibiting Cloning and Inheritable Alterations. *American Journal of Law and Medicine* 2002; 28, 2&3: p. 162.

destruction pose a serious threat to our civilization. But using the rhetoric of bioterrorism and weapons of mass destruction to cast aspersions on therapeutic uses of biotechnology to improve health, longevity, and other human capacities is unhelpful. The issues are quite distinct. Reasonable people can be in favor of strict regulation of bioweapons, while promoting beneficial medical uses of genetics and other human enhancement technologies, including inheritable and 'species-altering' modifications.

Human society is always at risk of some group deciding to view another group of humans as being fit for slavery or slaughter. To counteract such tendencies, modern societies have created laws and institutions, and endowed them with powers of enforcement, that act to prevent groups of citizens from enslaving or slaughtering one another. The efficacy of these institutions does not depend on all citizens having equal capacities. Modern, peaceful societies can have large numbers of people with diminished physical or mental capacities along with many other people who may be exceptionally physically strong or healthy or intellectually talented in various ways. Adding people with technologically enhanced capacities to this already broad distribution of ability would not need to rip society apart or trigger genocide or enslavement.

The assumption that inheritable genetic modifications or other human enhancement technologies would lead to two distinct and separate species should also be questioned. It seems much more likely that there would be a continuum of differently modified or enhanced individuals, which would overlap with the continuum of as-yet unenhanced humans. The scenario in which 'the enhanced' form a pact and then attack 'the naturals' makes for exciting science fiction, but is not necessarily the most plausible outcome. Even today, the segment containing the tallest ninety percent of the population could, in principle, get together and kill or enslave the shorter decile. That this does not happen suggests that a well-organized society can hold together even if it contains many possible coalitions of people sharing some attribute such that, if they ganged up, they would be capable of exterminating the rest.

To note that the extreme case of a war between humans and posthumans is not the most likely scenario is not to say that there are no legitimate social concerns about the steps that may take us closer to posthumanity. Inequity, discrimination, and stigmatization – against, or on behalf of, modified people – could become serious issues. Transhumanists would argue that these (potential) social problems call for social remedies. One example of how contemporary technology can change important aspects of someone's identity is sex reassignment. The experiences of transsexuals show that Western culture still has work to do in becoming more accepting of diversity. This is a task that we can begin to tackle today by fostering a climate of tolerance and acceptance towards those who are different from ourselves. Painting alarmist pictures of the threat from future technologically modified people, or hurling preemptive condemnations of their necessarily debased nature, is not the best way to go about it.

What about the hypothetical case in which someone intends to create, or turn themselves into, a being of such radically enhanced capacities that a single one or a small group of such individuals would be capable of taking over the planet? This is clearly not a situation that is likely to arise in the imminent future, but one can imagine that, perhaps in a few decades, the prospective creation of superintelligent machines could raise this kind of concern. The would-be creator of a new life form with such surpassing capabilities would have an obligation to ensure that the proposed being is free from psychopathic tendencies and, more generally, that it has humane inclinations. For example, a future artificial intelligence programmer should be required to make a strong case that launching a purportedly human-friendly superintelligence would be safer than the alternative. Again, however, this (currently) science fiction scenario must be clearly distinguished from our present situation and our more immediate concern with taking effective steps towards incrementally improving human capacities and health-span.

IS HUMAN DIGNITY INCOMPATIBLE WITH POSTHUMAN DIGNITY?

Human dignity is sometimes invoked as a polemical substitute for clear ideas. This is not to say that there are no important moral issues relating to dignity, but it does mean that there is a need to define what one has in mind when one uses the term. Here, we shall consider two different senses of dignity:

1. Dignity as moral status, in particular the inalienable right to be treated with a basic level of respect.
2. Dignity as the quality of being worthy or honorable; worthiness, worth, nobleness, excellence.[7]

On both these definitions, dignity is something that a posthuman could possess. Francis Fukuyama, however, seems to deny this and warns that giving up on the idea that dignity is unique to human beings – defined as those possessing a mysterious essential human quality he calls 'Factor X'[8] – would invite disaster:

> Denial of the concept of human dignity – that is, of the idea that there is something unique about the human race that entitles every member of the species to a higher moral status than the rest of the natural world – leads us down a very perilous path. We may be compelled ultimately to take this path, but we should do so only with our eyes open. Nietzsche is a much better guide to what lies down that road than the legions of bioethicists and casual academic Darwinians that today are prone to give us moral advice on this subject.[9]

What appears to worry Fukuyama is that introducing new kinds of enhanced person into the world might cause some individuals (perhaps infants, or the mentally handicapped, or unenhanced humans in general) to lose some of the moral status that they currently possess, and that a fundamental precondition of liberal democracy, the principle of equal dignity for all, would be destroyed.

The underlying intuition seems to be that instead of the famed 'expanding moral circle', what we have is more like an oval, whose shape we can change but whose area must remain constant. Thankfully, this purported conservation law of moral recognition lacks empirical support. The set of individuals accorded full moral status by Western societies has actually increased, to include men without property or noble decent, women, and non-white peoples. It would seem feasible to extend this set further to include future

[7] J.A. Simpson & E. Weiner, eds. 1989. *The Oxford English Dictionary*, 2nd ed. Oxford. Oxford University Press.
[8] F. Fukuyama. 2002. *Our Posthuman Future: Consequences of the Biotechnology Revolution*. New York. Farrar, Strauss and Giroux: p. 149.
[9] Fukuyama, *op. cit.* note 8, p. 160.

posthumans, or, for that matter, some of the higher primates or human-animal chimaeras, should such be created – and to do so without causing any compensating shrinkage in another direction. (The moral status of problematic borderline cases, such as foetuses or late-stage Alzheimer patients, or the brain-dead, should perhaps be decided separately from the issue of technologically modified humans or novel artificial life forms.) Our own role in this process need not be that of passive bystanders. We can work to create more inclusive social structures that accord appropriate moral recognition and legal rights to all who need them, be they male or female, black or white, flesh or silicon.

Dignity in the second sense, as referring to a special excellence or moral worthiness, is something that current human beings possess to widely differing degrees. Some excel far more than others do. Some are morally admirable; others are base and vicious. There is no reason for supposing that posthuman beings could not also have dignity in this second sense. They may even be able to attain higher levels of moral and other excellence than any of us humans. The fictional brave new worlders, who were subhuman rather than posthuman, would have scored low on this kind of dignity, and partly for that reason they would be awful role models for us to emulate. But surely we can create more uplifting and appealing visions of what we may aspire to become. There may be some who would transform themselves into degraded posthumans – but then some people today do not live very worthy human lives. This is regrettable, but the fact that some people make bad choices is not generally a sufficient ground for rescinding people's right to choose. And legitimate countermeasures are available: education, encouragement, persuasion, social and cultural reform. These, not a blanket prohibition of all post-human ways of being, are the measures to which those bothered by the prospect of debased posthumans should resort. A liberal democracy should normally permit incursions into morphological and reproductive freedoms only in cases where somebody is abusing these freedoms to harm another person.

The principle that parents should have broad discretion to decide on genetic enhancements for their children has been attacked on the grounds that this form of reproductive freedom would constitute a kind of parental tyranny that would undermine the child's dignity and capacity for autonomous choice; for instance, by Hans Jonas:

Technological mastered nature now again includes man who (up
to now) had, in technology, set himself against it as its master . . .
But whose power is this – and over whom or over what?
Obviously the power of those living today over those coming
after them, who will be the defenseless other side of prior choices
made by the planners of today. The other side of the power of
today is the future bondage of the living to the dead.[10]

Jonas is relying on the assumption that our descendants, who will
presumably be far more technologically advanced than we are,
would nevertheless be defenseless against our machinations to
expand their capacities. This is almost certainly incorrect. If, for
some inscrutable reason, they decided that they would prefer to be
less intelligent, less healthy, and lead shorter lives, they would not
lack the means to achieve these objectives and frustrate our designs.

In any case, if the alternative to parental choice in determining
the basic capacities of new people is entrusting the child's welfare
to nature, that is blind chance, then the decision should be easy.
Had Mother Nature been a real parent, she would have been in jail
for child abuse and murder. And transhumanists can accept, of
course, that just as society may in exceptional circumstances override parental autonomy, such as in cases of neglect or abuse, so too
may society impose regulations to protect the child-to-be from genuinely harmful genetic interventions – but not because they represent choice rather than chance.

Jürgen Habermas, in a recent work, echoes Jonas' concern and
worries that even the mere *knowledge* of having been intentionally
made by another could have ruinous consequences:

> We cannot rule out that knowledge of one's own hereditary fea-
> tures as programmed may prove to restrict the choice of an
> individual's life, and to undermine the essentially symmetrical
> relations between free and equal human beings.[11]

A transhumanist could reply that it would be a mistake for an
individual to believe that she has no choice over her own life just
because some (or all) of her genes were selected by her parents. She
would, in fact, have as much choice as if her genetic constitution

---

[10] H. Jonas. 1985. *Technik, Medizin und Ethik: Zur Praxis des Prinzips Verantwortung*.
Frankfurt am Main. Suhrkamp.
[11] J. Habermas. 2003. *The Future of Human Nature*. Oxford. Blackwell: p. 23.

had been selected by chance. It could even be that she would enjoy significantly *more* choice and autonomy in her life, if the modifications were such as to expand her basic capability set. Being healthy, smarter, having a wide range of talents, or possessing greater powers of self-control are blessings that tend to open more life paths than they block.

Even if there were a possibility that some genetically-modified individuals might fail to grasp these points and thus might feel oppressed by their knowledge of their origin, that would be a risk to be weighed against the risks incurred by having an unmodified genome, risks that can be extremely grave. If safe and effective alternatives were available, it would be irresponsible to risk starting someone off in life with the misfortune of congenitally diminished basic capacities or an elevated susceptibility to disease.

WHY WE NEED POSTHUMAN DIGNITY

Similarly ominous forecasts were made in the seventies about the severe psychological damage that children conceived through *in vitro* fertilization would suffer upon learning that they originated from a test tube – a prediction that turned out to be entirely false. It is hard to avoid the impression that some bias or philosophical prejudice is responsible for the readiness with which many bioconservatives seize on even the flimsiest of empirical justifications for banning human enhancement technologies of certain types but not others. Suppose it turned out that playing Mozart to pregnant mothers improved the child's subsequent musical talent. Nobody would argue for a ban on Mozart-in-the-womb on grounds that we cannot rule out that some psychological woe might befall the child once she discovers that her facility with the violin had been prenatally 'programmed' by her parents. Yet when, for example, it comes to genetic enhancements, eminent bioconservative writers often put forward arguments that are not so very different from this parody as weighty, if not conclusive, objections. To transhumanists, this looks like doublethink. How can it be that to bioconservatives almost any anticipated downside, predicted perhaps on the basis of the shakiest pop-psychological theory, so readily achieves that status of deep philosophical insight and knockdown objection against the trans-humanist project?

Perhaps a part of the answer can be found in the different attitudes that transhumanists and bioconservatives have towards posthuman dignity. Bioconservatives tend to deny posthuman dignity and view posthumanity as a threat to human dignity. They are therefore tempted to look for ways to denigrate interventions that are thought to be pointing in the direction of more radical future modifications that may eventually lead to the emergence of those detestable posthumans. But unless this fundamental opposition to the posthuman is openly declared as a premise of their argument, this then forces them to use a double standard of assessment whenever particular cases are considered in isolation: for example, one standard for germ-line genetic interventions and another for improvements in maternal nutrition (an intervention presumably not seen as heralding a posthuman era).

Transhumanists, by contrast, see human and posthuman dignity as compatible and complementary. They insist that dignity, in its modern sense, consists in what we are and what we have the potential to become, not in our pedigree or our causal origin. What we are is not a function solely of our DNA but also of our technological and social context. Human nature in this broader sense is dynamic, partially human-made, and improvable. Our current extended phenotypes (and the lives that we lead) are markedly different from those of our hunter-gatherer ancestors. We read and write, we wear clothes, we live in cities, we earn money and buy food from the supermarket, we call people on the telephone, watch television, read newspapers, drive cars, file taxes, vote in national elections, women give birth in hospitals, life-expectancy is three times longer than in the Pleistocene, we know that the Earth is round and that stars are large gas clouds lit from inside by nuclear fusion, and that the universe is approximately 13.7 billion years old and enormously big. In the eyes of a hunter-gatherer, we might already appear 'posthuman'. Yet these radical extensions of human capabilities – some of them biological, others external – have not divested us of moral status or dehumanized us in the sense of making us generally unworthy and base. Similarly, should we or our descendants one day succeed in becoming what relative to current standards we may refer to as posthuman, this need not entail a loss dignity either.

From the transhumanist standpoint, there is no need to behave as if there were a deep moral difference between technological and other means of enhancing human lives. By defending post-human dignity we promote a more inclusive and humane ethics, one that will embrace future technologically modified people as well as humans of the contemporary kind. We also remove a distortive double standard from the field of our moral vision, allowing us to perceive more clearly the opportunities that exist for further human progress.[12]

[12] For their comments I am grateful to Heather Bradshaw, John Brooke, Aubrey de Grey, Robin Hanson, Matthew Liao, Julian Savulescu, Eliezer Yudkowsky, Nick Zangwill, and to the audiences at the Ian Ramsey Center seminar of June 6th in Oxford 2003, the Transvision 2003 conference at Yale, and the 2003 European Science Foundation Workshop on Science and Human Values, where earlier versions of this paper were presented, and to two anonymous referees.

PART II: HEALTH CARE PROFESSIONAL–PATIENT RELATIONSHIP

Chapter 5

PATIENTS' RESPONSIBILITIES IN MEDICAL ETHICS

HEATHER DRAPER AND TOM SORELL

INTRODUCTION

Medical ethics is one-sided. It dwells on the ethical obligations of doctors to the exclusion of those of patients. This one-sidedness may have something to do with the use in standard medical ethics of the concept of autonomy. We begin by calling attention to some of the limitations of that use of the concept. We then turn to the responsibilities that we think patients have to doctors: those that arise from general ethical obligations, and those that arise from the doctor-patient relationship. Finally, we consider how doctors ought to respond when patients fail in their duties to them.

THE ONE-SIDEDNESS OF MEDICAL ETHICS

Medical ethics tends to focus on only one side of the doctor-patient relationship. One reason for this is that standard writing in medical ethics is directed at a professional audience. Although it is hard for anyone to claim that patients can do no wrong, the wrong they do seems to be out of place in writing or teaching directed to doctors. In this respect, medical ethics resembles business ethics, which often overlooks the immorality and unreasonableness that customers can be guilty of.[1] Even though doctors are likely to remain the main audience for medical ethics, it does not follow that medical ethics

---

[1] There are special reasons why in business ethics the transgressions of customers may not only be overlooked but denied. The belief that the customer is always right dies hard in both professional ethics and the wider consumer culture from which most of us sometimes benefit. For a discussion of the onesidedness of this belief, see T. Sorell. The Customer is not Always Right. *Journal of Business Ethics* 1994; 13: 913–918. For applications of this line of thought to consumerism in thinking about patients in the National Health Service in the UK, see T. Sorell. Morality, Consumerism and the Internal Market in Health Care. *Journal of Medical Ethics* 1997; 23: 71–76.

is solely the ethics of the doctor's role or even the ethics of the more inclusive role of the health care professional. It extends to patients as well.

An analogy may make this clearer. In the UK, the rule-book for users of public roads is called the Highway Code. In practice, the Highway Code is only studied by learner car drivers, and most of the code is addressed to people in charge of motor vehicles. Drivers have to pass a test of their knowledge of the Highway Code before being given a licence. Pedestrians are never required to learn the code unless they are also drivers, and in the UK many pedestrians who own no cars are probably entirely ignorant of its provisions for those who travel the roads on foot. But the fact that pedestrians are ignorant of the rules and have no incentive to learn them, does not mean that rules addressed to pedestrians do not exist or that they cannot be broken, still less that they are out of place in a rule-book for road users. Pedestrians stand to the rules of the road in the UK as patients stand to the rules of the health care system. Doctors are like drivers. They have to pass examinations for professional qualifications that require knowledge of, or even evidence of, ethical conduct. Patients are like pedestrians. They do not have to pass a test to qualify as patients, but how they behave affects others involved in the health care system, sometimes adversely. Just as the Highway Code does not consist simply of provisions relevant to those of its audience who need to pass tests, so medical ethics may have an audience beyond doctors or health care professionals. Just as the compilers of the rules of the road have good reasons for including rules for pedestrians, so writers of medical ethics have reason to recognise obligations on patients. Text books like the best-selling *Principles of Biomedical Ethics* by Tom Beauchamp and James Childress – which we shall take in this paper to embody 'mainstream medical ethics' – should either be re-named or else find principles of biomedical ethics that can be applied to takers and givers of health care alike.

The one-sidedness of mainstream medical ethics in respect of the doctor-patient relationship is more than a matter of being directed at an overly narrow audience. There is also an unevenness in the distribution of the moral burdens. Mainstream medical ethics puts a big and largely unconditional responsibility on doctors to treat patients 'no questions asked'. This obligation can take either of two forms. In wartime, doctors are obliged to treat everyone equally – friend or foe. The peacetime counterpart of this is that paedophiles, rapists and murders are supposed to be treated without reference to their crimes or moral character. Again, doctors treat patients without making judgements about the cause of their illness. Unless it affects their treatment, doctors are not expected to ask how patients came to be ill or damaged. What is learned during the history taking should not be permitted to colour the doctor's view of the patient, who must be treated impartially. Nor can doctors turn away patients who are in acute need of treatment but who cannot pay. In this respect, medical ethics is quite unlike business ethics. It is reasonable for a plumber, even in an emergency, to ensure that he can be paid before starting a job, and it is reasonable for a shop to ask how the goods came to be faulty before offering a replacement.

In comparison to what it asks of doctors, mainstream medical ethics makes very few demands of patients, and these usually begin and end with consent. Traditionally, medical ethics has asserted that, as autonomous agents, competent patients must be allowed to decide for themselves the course of their medical treatment, and even whether to be treated at all. It is for the doctor to communicate effectively all the relevant information, assess the patient's competence, persuade without coercing, and abide by whatever decision the patient makes. Little or nothing is said about what kinds of decisions patients *ought* to make. Nor is much said about their responsibilities for making good rather than bad decisions. Indeed, with the exception of recent literature on responsible uses of resources (a topic to which we will return), mainstream medical ethics implies that a competent patient's decision is good simply by virtue of having been made by the patient. At times it seems as though patients never make, or cannot make, bad decisions. Bad decisions may be explained away – sometimes by the courts – as the doctor's failure to gain proper consent[2] or failing this, the doctor's failure to override the wishes of the patient and act in her best interests instead![3]

Yet if autonomy in medical ethics is to mean the same as in general ethics – and surely it is supposed to – autonomy must go hand in hand with taking responsibility for what is chosen. In

---

[2] For example, Sidway v Bethlem RHG [1985] 1 All ER 643.
[3] For an example see Unnecessary hysterectomy? *The Journal of the Medical Defence Union* 1999; 15: 20–22.

particular, if things go badly, a decision made by a patient cannot suddenly turn into a piece of negligence on the doctor's part. But in medical ethics the duty of care often trumps the need for autonomous patients to take the bad consequences of the bad choices they knowingly make. Even though one of the justifications for obtaining patient consent is that it is the patient who has to live with the consequences of her decision, doctors routinely rescue patients from the consequences of their decisions – such as decisions to drink and smoke too much – and in the process rescue patients from taking the consequences that their pretensions to autonomy are supposed to expose them to. In the same way, doctors are obliged to be blind to how the patient came to suffer those consequences, even if the current fix she is in results from autonomously choosing not to follow medical advice.

Is there any moral basis for this approach to patients? There is the undoubted vulnerability of patients to negligent or incompetent or insensitive treatment by doctors, and their relative powerlessness and ignorance when it comes to certain decisions about their treatment. These things call for the protection of patients against those treating them, or perhaps for measures – legal and educational – that make patients more equal in decision-making processes affecting them. But the key thing – the thing that seems to make intelligible the kinds of moral duties that doctors have to inform patients and to act only when necessary and on the best information – is the vulnerability of patients. There is sometimes a blind spot in moral thinking with regard to the vulnerable and weak. The blind spot manifests itself in a certain pattern of suspicion that seems natural when something goes wrong and the weak or vulnerable suffer as a result. The presumption is that when the weak or vulnerable suffer in a transaction in which the strong are also involved, the weak are innocent, and the strong are probably responsible or should be foremost in offering to compensate the weak or vulnerable for what has happened. But there are many counter-examples to this way of thinking. The vulnerability of patients does not mean that they cannot be negligent and contribute significantly to bad health outcomes, even though it is much easier for a negligent or incompetent doctor to do much more harm. Relative vulnerability does not confer inability to do wrong.

The analogy introduced earlier may help in this connection. Among road users, pedestrians are much more vulnerable, other things being equal, than car drivers, lorry drivers and even cyclists. Cyclists are a danger to pedestrians, but are vulnerable to drivers of heavier vehicles. These facts are reflected in the legal qualifying conditions for being a driver, and in certain rules of the road. You need a driver's license to operate a car, and a special licence to drive heavy lorries. Cars have to stop at pedestrian crossings, and they have to give cyclists a wide berth. These rules are justified by the relative vulnerability of pedestrians and cyclists. But it is not as if pedestrians and cyclists – the most vulnerable road users of all – are exempted from following the rules of the road, or as if they can't break them. It is just as possible for a drunk on foot to cross the road recklessly as for a drunk driver to turn into a road recklessly. Vulnerability, then, does not confer automatic innocence of wrongdoing on the vulnerable.

The vulnerability of patients does not confer innocence on them either. Nor does the autonomy of vulnerable people insulate them from responsibility for the consequences of decisions made jointly with doctors. This is indirectly acknowledged even by the conception of autonomy in mainstream medical ethics. The mainstream conception calls for the full consultation of patients by doctors in clinical decisions, and for the participation in clinical decision-making of patient advocates, and disinterested third parties – people who can make patients' views better heard and respected and who can prevent their being paternalistically overridden. The ideal that these arrangements apparently attempt to capture is that of a genuine *partnership* between clinician and patient in a course of treatment. The other side of the coin of treatment decisions reached in partnership, however, is joint responsibility for the outcomes, including cases where things go badly wholly as a result of these decisions, and the patient turns out to be harmed or disappointed. But, as we have already suggested, in actual cases where things go badly, the solidarity in decision-making is likely to break down: the fact that it is the patient and not the doctor who feels the bad effects, and the doctor and not the patient who emerges intact, seems to undo the partnership. A presumption of negligence can grow up that apparently frees the patient to sue, even when she is responsible for making the decisions that led to things going badly.

Perhaps the breakdown in solidarity is justified, because the patient and doctor can rarely *really* be equals in the decision-making process in the first place – it may be too much of an ideal.

But can it always be *so* much of an ideal that the patient never carries any responsibility? Autonomy without responsibility is not autonomy, even where the autonomy is a vulnerable patient's autonomy. There may be an obligation on patients in certain cases to live with certain decisions that leave them badly off.

PATIENTS AND GENERAL ETHICS: RESPECT FOR PERSONS AND DUTIES OF CITIZENS

Respect for persons

Some of the duties which patients have to their doctors (and other health care workers) come from a general obligation upon everyone to respect other people. Several examples of bad patient behaviour serve to illustrate:

- Whilst waiting for treatment in accident and emergency a patient complains constantly and abusively to the nurses and reception staff about having to wait his turn. When he sees the doctor he begins to swear again and finally punches the doctor.
- In order to get an earlier hospital appointment, a patient exaggerates her symptoms of abdominal pain to her GP.
- Following an emergency consultation with her GP on a Sunday, a patient promises to get her repeat prescription in good time in future. She doesn't and has to be seen as an extra at the end of a busy day.
- A patient decides not to keep a hospital out-patient appointment because a friend calls by unexpectedly.

In all these cases, the wrongdoing is the same and is of a kind dealt with in general ethics: the patient fails to show the respect for persons that is due to *anyone*, not just health care professionals. Anyone who swears at others or hits them without provocation is doing something wrong, regardless of the role of the person sworn at or attacked. And the basis of the wrong is disrespect. It is the same for anyone who breaks a promise, wastes another's time, or tells partial truths to get their own way. Of course there may be something particularly bad about abusive behaviour directed at people who are trying to give help, as in the first example, but even there part of the wrong is the wrong of disrespect.

Competent patients have a responsibility to look after their own health

Patients not only have obligations to health care professionals that flow from an obligation to respect others. They have obligations to themselves to promote their own health. Or so we shall argue. These obligations in their turn ground obligations to seek medical advice and listen to it. Patients have further obligations to take publicly-provided medical advice if they are citizens of welfare states. We shall come to this later on.

We begin, however, with obligations of patients to themselves. Medical ethicists who otherwise agree about the importance of autonomy are sceptical about responsibilities to one's self, especially when this responsibility is understood as preserving and promoting one's own health. But this responsibility can readily be justified within a Kantian ethical framework. Within this framework moral mistreatment is often connected with a failure fully to recognise humanity or personhood. And for Kant this was as much a possibility in the treatment of oneself as the treatment of others. To take an example from outside medical ethics, the Kantian framework readily explains the intuition that servility is wrong, and wrong in a way related to the wrong of enslavement. Enslaving another is the strongest denial possible of their autonomy, of their capacity to make choices for themselves. Servility is wrong, because it denies or undercuts the same thing as enslavement – a person's autonomy. The fact that the person doing the undercutting is oneself does not make it all right.[4] Now since Kant regarded autonomy as a possibility even in a being who is physically incapacitated, there is no direct argument in Kant's own terms from the need to preserve autonomy to the need to preserve one's health and avoid incapacitation. Nevertheless, there is a perfectly clear sense in which people who connive in the loss of their physical capacity or who damage their health are reducing the means they have to accomplish their ends, and this counts for Kant as a piece of practical irrationality that morality must recognise. Kant himself ascribed autonomy to a noumenal agent not identifiable with the human being. For Kantians other than Kant, who may want to think of autonomy as a property primarily of naturally realised agents, like embodied

[4] For an extended discussion of servility from a Kantian perspective, see T. Hill. 1991. *Autonomy and Self-Respect.* Cambridge. Cambridge University Press.

human beings, a deliberate reduction in physical capacity might be regarded as a direct assault on autonomy itself. Kant, for his part, recognises moral duties to oneself as a natural (or animal) being:

> There are impulses of nature having to do with man's animality. Through them nature aims at a) his self-preservation, b) the preservation of the species, and c) the preservation of his capacity to enjoy life, though still on the animal level only. The vices that are here opposed to man's duty to himself are *murdering himself*, the unnatural use of his *sexual inclination*, and such *excessive consumption of food and drink* as weakens his capacity for making purposive use of his powers.[5]

Kant goes on to define a sense of 'mutilation' according to which any wilful reduction of one's physical powers counts as the wrong of self-mutilation.[6] In this sense it might count as mutilation to continue in a life-style that one knows (after being given medical advice) will severely damage one's health. Although this is 'mutilation' in an unusual sense, there seems no strain in saying that reducing one's powers gratuitously is a way of harming oneself for no good reason, and that harming oneself for no good reason is wrong.

We are not claiming that there can be no conflict between avoiding damage to one's health and discharging other duties. Asserting that autonomous individuals have duties not to incapacitate themselves or reduce their capacities gratuitously is compatible with accepting that sometimes individuals have to make hard choices that require them to make personal sacrifices for the good of others. A mother, for instance, may neglect her own health because she lacks the resources both to promote her own health and that of her children. In a case such as this, the harm to self might be taken as justified. Asserting that individuals have duties to themselves may also be compatible with refusing treatment or ignoring medical advice in cases where there is little evidence of success of treatment or where there is a genuine clash of values – such as occurs when attempting to balance quantity and quality of life in terminal illnesses. But these cases are likely to be exceptional. In many more

---

[5] I. Kant. 1991. (1797) *Metaphysics of Morals*. M. Gregor, trans. Cambridge. Cambridge University Press. Akademie edition, vol. 6: 420.
[6] Ibid. p. 421. Kant appears to mean a permanent reduction of one's powers.

cases, patients harm their own health when the welfare of others is not at stake and where doing so is unreasonable.[7]

In utilitarianism, it is the collective welfare that morally justifies action or inaction, and health is an important component of welfare. Public health counts for more than individual health where there is a conflict between the two, but often it will promote the public health to do what one can to stay healthy oneself. And this can mean following good medical advice. Utilitarianism would also justify certain exceptions to this rule, similar to those outlined for Kantian ethics. Utilitarianism may permit us to sacrifice our own health if by so doing, greater health for others is achieved. Likewise, utilitarianism may permit us to refuse a procedure where there is little evidence that it will succeed, or where there was some genuine disagreement between doctor and patient about whether the good of health translates best into longevity or quality of life. But typically both utilitarianism and Kantianism will argue morally for not damaging one's health and for undoing habits or ways of life that *are* damaging.

Patients as citizens

In welfare states, discussion about the use of limited resources extends naturally to a consideration of whether citizens have some sort of moral obligation, other things being equal, to limit their demands on these resources. If the answer is 'Yes', then there may be a civic obligation to follow preventive health measures recommended by one's doctor. If one is advised to stop smoking or overeating, and one disregards that advice, so that one's condition deteriorates to the point that expensive treatment is required to keep one alive, one may be doing something doubly wrong – breaking obligations to oneself and breaking civic obligations not to use public resources unnecessarily.

Patients may attempt to justify their negligence by saying that the taxes they pay on cigarettes or their contributions to national insurance mean that they have paid for the treatment they need as the result of ignoring medical advice. This argument is often used in an unsophisticated way, for it overlooks all the tax-financed benefits

---

[7] The law in the UK conspires to support the mainstream medical ethics position by claiming that patients have the right to refuse treatment for irrational reasons, as well as no reason at all (Sidway v Bethlem RUG [1985] 1 All ER 643).

that go beyond health care that people enjoy. But even if all patients who ignored medical advice were net contributors to the welfare state, the argument would still be flawed. The justification for the welfare state is not only that of egoism (I pay my taxes so that I will benefit if the need arises). It is also justified by the belief that a decent society ought to use what resources it can to support the weakest and the poorest. It runs counter to this latter justification for people to assess their obligations solely in terms of whether they pay in more than *they* get out. The relevant question is whether the neediest get all they might.

How important is the fact that those who ignore medical advice and make themselves ill voluntarily put themselves in need of a scarce good? In many welfare states penalties operate for those citizens who become voluntarily homeless or voluntarily unemployed. Sometimes they become ineligible for housing or unemployment benefits. Yet, if doctors were required to operate the same kind of penalty system when allocating health care – namely to withhold medical care from those who became ill through their own choices – this would be deemed unethical from a medical ethics perspective.[8] There are good reasons why the distribution of medical resources cannot be treated in every respect like the distribution of housing and unemployment insurance. For one thing it would be difficult to prove in all cases that neglect was the source of ill-health. The more we understand about genetics, the more we know that environmental factors are only partly to blame for ill-health, and it would be wrong to penalise an individual for her genes since her genetic make-up is beyond her control. It is also difficult to prove that an individual *knowingly* endangered her health. This might be offered as a partial defence for smokers, for instance, who might argue that at the time they started smoking the harmful effects were unknown, or that they were non-autonomous minors who succumbed to peer pressure. Moreover, the penalty that may be paid by those who have contributed to their own ill-health could be out of proportion to the wrongdoing – a delay in medical treatment may not just cause short-term inconvenience or straightened circumstances. None of this, however, justifies people in contributing knowingly to a deterioration in their health and expecting everyone else to pay the bill.

[8] For a discussion of the general issues in the spirit of tolerance for patients whose lifestyles are 'unhealthy', see I. de Beaufort. 1999. Individual Responsibility for Health. In R. Bennett and C. Erin, eds. *HIV and AIDS: Testing, Screening and Confidentiality.* Oxford. Oxford University Press: 107–124.

In short, there are duties not to use health services casually. And the duties become more unbreakable the closer the services abused get to being acute medical services. Someone who indulges their hypochondria by frequent visits to the GP, or who summons an ambulance after getting a sunburn; someone who knowingly presents himself at an emergency room with nothing more than severe indigestion; or who calls out a doctor because he needs a repeat prescription that could be filled in office hours next day; all of these patients do something morally wrong, wrong primarily because they take away time and resources better spent on more urgent cases. The obligations that these patients fail to respect or make good are their obligations as citizens to the health care system and other patients.[9]

The counselling relationship

Doctor-patient relationships in general practice are certainly changing. Patients register with the whole practice, rather than with a particular doctor, and which doctor they see may depend crucially on availability in an appointment system. Nonetheless, perhaps the greatest continuity of care is still provided in general practice. For even if the entire history of the patient is not personally known to a general practitioner (GP), the GP notes generally offer by the far the most complete patient history. Suppose that this history is one of gradually declining health, reasonably thought by the GP to be due to over-eating, smoking, drinking to excess, or something else to do with lifestyle. Suppose that the patient is becoming obese and is in danger of developing diabetes, for example. He is advised to diet, but ignores the advice. Or suppose that a patient is sent for tests to establish whether or not he is suffering from bowel cancer, and is too embarrassed to go. Let us assume that there is no doubt in either the patient's or the health care practitioner's mind that the course of action recommended makes sense. There is simply a failure on the patient's part to follow through. Is this another case of patient wrong-doing? Yes, because not only does he knowingly aggravate his own condition, doing himself harm, but he

---

[9] Sorell, 1997, *op. cit.* note 1, notes that these obligations do not exist only within a public health care system open to everyone, though clearly such a health care system is of a kind it is easiest to misuse or overuse. The obligations also exist where the health care system is small and private and open only to the few. The fact that the system is small and exclusive may make its overuse less likely; it does not make the obligation not to overuse it otiose or unintelligible.

unreasonably refuses to play by the rules of situations in which people seek and are given medical advice. These rules can be taken to assume that both patient and doctor have a serious stake in some sort of health gain for the patient, and that so long as the means of achieving the gain seem reasonable to both parties, the patient will fall in with them. This is another duty that the patient has that flows from general ethics. This duty is not just another version of the duty to self – though it could be – it is also a duty owed to the doctor. This duty may have something in common with a duty it is arguable people have in counselling relationships in general, at least where there is no doubt that the counsellor puts the best interests of the advice-seeker foremost. If the advice-seeker asks for advice, then he should be prepared to listen seriously to it. That is why it is wrong, and not just imprudent, for someone who asks for advice to dismiss it angrily when he does not like what he hears – because he has asked for advice and not e.g. flattery. The advisee should take what he hears seriously if there is no reason to think it is not offered in good faith. And if he genuinely agrees with the advice, and is not just saying he does, he should – morally should – follow through with it, other things being equal.

Perhaps only the listening is strictly owed to the counsellor in the counselling situation, while the following through is owed to oneself. But in the medical situation it may be different. The same GP who gives the advice that is apparently accepted and not acted upon may have to pick up the pieces when, as a result, the condition of the patient worsens later. And picking up the pieces may consist in trying to get a patient to take advice a second or third or fourth time. The worse the condition becomes, the more the duty of care limits the room for manoeuvre of the doctor. He becomes a sort of captive helper. And so the duty of the patient may be a duty not to conspire in bringing this captivity about. In this sense, the duty that one has as an advisee in a doctor-patient relationship begins in general ethics, and, as a result of the ethical constraints upon doctors, ends up in medical ethics.

PATIENTS' DUTIES TO DOCTORS AS CAPTIVE HELPERS

The captivity of doctors works on two levels: on the one hand, individual doctors are only exceptionally allowed to break off a relationship with a patient; on the other hand, even if a particular doctor-patient relationship proves impossible or is brought to an end, the profession as a whole will continue to provide care for the patient.

Ought doctors be captive helpers?

One question about the captivity is whether it is fair; another is whether it protects an interest so vital that the one-sidedness is acceptable. One reason why it may be fair for doctors to guarantee to pick up the pieces for patients is that the patients are the vulnerable party in a relationship that can only ideally ever be an equal one. But to suggest that doctors have to persevere with patients simply because they are, as a group, vulnerable, seems to suggest either a very paternalistic view – patients are never to be given true autonomy that would hold them accountable for their actions – or else it suggests that the vulnerability of patients is sufficient to ensure that they are never truly autonomous, and are not therefore moral agents with responsibilities for their health. We have already argued that the relative vulnerability of patients is not a good reason to assume that they cannot also have responsibilities to doctors, or to others jointly with doctors. Further, to suggest that no patient is actually autonomous is incompatible with the emphasis that mainstream medical ethics has placed on autonomy. Clearly, some patients are not autonomous – but we take it that these patients are already catered for in mainstream medical ethics, which requires doctors to act in the best interests of patients who are brain-damaged, mentally ill, unconscious, infants etc. We also acknowledge that some patients face very restricted life choices or have a genetic pre-disposition for disease. But, these exceptions aside, patients who are generally able to consent or refuse consent to medical treatment or to follow medical advice are presumed by mainstream medical ethics to be autonomous.[10] If genuinely

---

[10] At this point we are assuming that mainstream medical ethics is correct to equate competence and autonomy. We would argue that this should not always be the case – and Gillick competent children might be a case in point. The Gillick case in the UK established that children under the age of 16 can give consent, provided that they are sufficiently mature and intelligent to understand the medical intervention in question and its implications. However, according to other UK case law, children under 16 do not have the right to refuse medical intervention and their parents can over-rule any refusal of consent, by consenting on their behalf.

autonomous, they must be expected to take responsibility for the decisions that they make – including responsibility for any resulting ill health, and responsibility for the long-term breakdown of their relationship with their doctor and its eventual cessation. This argument suggests that captive doctors should be freed.

Another objection to our claim about the unfairness of doctors' captivity is that doctors enter the profession *knowing* that there will be difficult patients, including patients who repeatedly ignore important medical advice. It is a problem that goes with the territory; so it cannot be counted a kind of unfairness. Although this objection is natural enough, it is question-begging. The fact that a kind of behaviour is to be expected is not justification for the behaviour. Until men were criticised for leaving all domestic labour and childcare to their wives, women thinking of getting married could predict that their husbands would leave such things to them. But this does not justify those unenlightened husbands in refusing to share the burdens, and it does not remove the impression that women intending to get married had a certain unfair division of labour to look forward to.

We now turn to the best interests of patients. There are perhaps two ways of justifying doctors' captivity on the basis of the interests of patients: it might be justified on the grounds that we are better off when this obligation is generally observed, even if it is unfair in some individual cases. Or it might be justified as a protection for patients against unwarranted discrimination. Let us begin with the possibility that captivity leaves patients better off. Though it has a different basis, the captivity of doctors might be likened to the captivity of friends and relations of dependent adults. Adults are generally expected to fend for themselves and run their lives – mishaps and all – unaided. Sometimes, however, they get into trouble and turn for support and various kinds of assistance to their nearest and dearest. The nearest and dearest are under some sort of obligation to pick up the pieces if the mishaps are serious, even if the person who suffers them gets into trouble persistently. They are under an obligation because friendship involves loyalty, and therefore a willingness to help even when it is difficult or inconvenient to do so, and because belonging to a family is often supposed to be a necessary last line of defence against a sometimes hostile world of strangers. This defence is more urgently needed the younger one is, but it does not disappear when one grows up, and very late adulthood may reintroduce it in a powerful form. So the devotion of friends and relations can be morally necessary, even if the people who depend on it do not always deserve it. The doctor/patient relationship may be like this kind of relationship. It is generally better for doctors to be – like the friends and relatives – captive helpers because it is an important aspect of doctoring that patients in need are not abandoned, even when some of these patients are undeserving in the sense that they perpetually put themselves in need of care.

The captivity of doctors may also be justified in another way, for there is a danger that unjustified discrimination may occur if doctors are required to become unblinded to the behaviour of patients. Unblinding doctors would mean that they would have to judge whether patients should be left untreated as a consequence of the autonomous decisions they have made. This raises several concerns. Doctors are only human and humans are fallible in many different ways. Some are racist, ageist or sexist etc. Such doctors might all too readily act on questionable judgements about patients' behaviour if they were free to break off their relationship with patients too easily. Likewise, some doctors might be bad judges of how responsible or irresponsible a patient had been. All of these are reasons why it is better, on balance, to tolerate the captivity of doctors.

What duties for patients flow from benefiting from a captive relationship?

The analogy between doctors' captivity and the captivity of friends and relations extends to the limits on this captivity. For there *are* limits. The devotion of friends and relations can be strained to breaking point, and the people who make use of it are under some obligation to try and limit their calls on it and return to the adult norm of looking after themselves as far as possible. The captivity of the nearest and dearest is not then an unconditional and permanent captivity. Neither should the captivity of doctors be: as adults who can be expected to regain or acquire their independence and keep to a minimum the burdens they avoidably create, autonomous patients are under an obligation to do what they can to limit the captivity of doctors. The upshot of this is that in medical ethics, patients should have an obligation to follow reasonable medical advice – especially the kind of medical advice we referred to earlier, namely that with which the patient actually agrees before something like weakness of will sets in. Doctors, like the friends and relations, have an obligation to persevere in the hope that patients will eventually be able to achieve or return to the norm of taking proper care of their own health. But patients also have an obligation to enable doctors whose sound advice is ignored to withdraw from this obligation. The main duty of patients who need care from doctors they keep captive is to do their part in reducing their need for medical care and in co-operating with doctors so that doctors are *willing* rather than captive helpers in the doctor-patient relationship.

WHAT CAN DOCTORS DO WHEN PATIENTS DO NOT ACT RESPONSIBLY?

If patients also have duties in medical ethics, then presumably doctors should have some recourse when patients fail in these duties, just as patients do when doctors fail. The difficulty here is that, in releasing themselves from the role of captive helper, doctors abandon patients to their fate, and there will inevitably be hard cases.

Consider a patient on dialysis who ignores sound advice to limit his fluid intake. This is necessary because patients on dialysis tend to retain fluid that is then removed as part of the dialysis process. Only so much fluid can be safely removed in a single dialysis session – removing too much can lead to heart failure. Patients who do not comply may, therefore, have to be given additional dialysis sessions in order to prevent this. But dialysis is often in short supply, and providing additional sessions for one patient inevitably means that other patients will receive no dialysis at all.

Let us suppose that the patient has no good reason for his failure to comply with the advice to limit his fluid intake; he just keeps giving into the temptation to drink. What action could the doctors reasonably take against this patient? One possibility is that they could issue an ultimatum: since he is persistently not complying with the recommendations for fluid intake, they will no longer be providing him with additional sessions. They would have to explain that the consequences of continuing to abuse fluids without the additional sessions would be discomfort and eventually heart failure. Such an ultimatum would force the patient to accept the consequences of his autonomous behaviour. In effect, the patient would be required to act as the responsible adult he is. Arguably this action shows greater respect for his autonomy then does providing the additional sessions. But what if, after several months of adult behaviour, the resolve of our patient begins to weaken, his fluid retention gradually worsens and he is eventually admitted to accident and emergency with heart failure for which immediate dialysis is the obvious solution? Under these circumstances would it be ethical for the doctors to continue to refuse to give additional dialysis? In this case, we have to conclude that it would not. In an acute, life-threatening situation, the safety net of captivity would return because it would be wrong not to save a life, even one endangered through stupidity or weakness of will.

This answer suggests that doctors ultimately remain captive. If this is so, are there any measures that doctors can take to free themselves from captivity? Perhaps not. But in this case doctors might continue to refuse more than routine dialysis once the crisis has past. This may in time lead to another acute admission (though it is to be hoped that the patient may be shaken into compliance by his brush with death), when yet again emergency dialysis will be provided. However, it would not be wrong of the doctors to stick to this cycle even if it damages the patient's health in the long run. As a result of his behaviour, the patient's longevity and quality of life will inevitably be affected and from this there is no one to rescue him but himself.

Finally, let us look at another, less unusual, example – that of the patient who is persistently and unjustifiably very rude or violent toward his GP. Clearly, the GP may remove this patient from her list: medical ethics does not require an individual doctor to be captive in the face of physical or verbal abuse. But suppose the patient repeats this behaviour with several other GPs. Here it is not the captivity of the individual doctor that is being tested, but the captivity of the profession as a whole. What can be done in this case to free the profession from captivity? One solution might be that the patient be denied access to *any* kind of one-to-one relationship with any doctor. Instead he would only be given emergency treatment in an accident and emergency unit, with a policeman or security guard present. Certainly the profession can be unblinded to the behaviour of this individual so that nothing more than the basic minimum was given and he would be excluded from minor or preventative care/advice. In some sense the profession remains captive – the patient is never abandoned – but he is being denied any meaningful doctor/patient relationships as a result of his very unreasonable behaviour.

CONCLUSION

Autonomous patients do have duties – most of which are left out of mainstream medical ethics. Some of these duties flow from the obligations all persons have to each other; others are the responsibilities citizens have in a welfare state. More specifically, patients have duties corresponding to those that render doctors captive helpers. Patients have to – morally have to – do their best to ensure that they minimise this captivity and enable doctors to be willing helpers. Although doctors remain captive in the face of acute or life-threatening illness, it is not unethical for doctors to free themselves from this captivity in cases that fall short of life or death.

Chapter 6

CLINICAL ETHICS AND NURSING: 'YES' TO CARING, BUT 'NO' TO A FEMALE ETHICS OF CARE

HELGA KUHSE

I. INTRODUCTION: ETHICS, PRINCIPLES, WOMEN AND NURSES

Is ethics gendered? Do women and men approach ethics differently? The answer of many thinkers has been 'yes'.

Rousseau thought that abstract truths and general principles are 'beyond a woman's grasp . . .; woman observes, man reasons'.[1] Schopenhauer bluntly proclaimed: '. . . the fundamental fault of the female character is that it has *no sense of justice'*. This 'weakness in their reasoning faculty', Schopenhauer continued, 'also explains why women show more sympathy for the unfortunate than men'.[2] Finally, to give just one more example, Freud believed that 'for women the level of what is ethically normal is different from what it is in men'. Women, he wrote, 'show less sense of justice than men'.[3]

On these views, then, men and women not only approach ethics differently, but insofar as women were thought to lack a head for abstract principles, and a sense of justice, their ethical approach was also regarded as somewhat defective and inferior to that of men. At the same time, and rather paradoxically, women's traits and moral dispositions were often seen as somewhat purer, and more worthy, than those of men. For Rousseau, for example, women who had

---

[1] Jean-Jacques Rousseau: *Emile*, trans. Barbara Foxley, London: Dent, 1966, pp. 349, 350.

[2] Arthur Schopenhauer: 'On Women' in Mary Mahowald (ed): *Philosophy of Woman – An Anthology of Classic and Current Concepts*, Indianapolis: Indiana, 1983, p. 231 (emphasis in original).

[3] Sigmund Freud: 'Some Psychical Consequences of the Anatomical Distinction Between the Sexes', in *The Standard Edition of the Complete Psychological Works of Sigmund Freud*, trans. and ed. James Strachey, London: The Hogarth Press, 1961, Vol. XIX, pp. 257–58. (I owe this reference to Carol Gilligan: *In a Different Voice*, Cambridge, Mass.: Harvard University Press, 1982, p. 7.)

developed the distinctively feminine traits of gentleness, tenderness, compassion, self-sacrifice and mental passivity, were only a 'little lower than the angels';[4] and the poet Lord Tennyson called women the 'interpreters between gods and men'.[5]

Nursing has always been a predominantly female profession and there was, and probably still is, a widespread belief that nursing, like few other professions, allows women to develop and express their specific feminine virtues. As one writer put it as recently as 1980:

> [N]urses were . . . angels! Angels of mercy! They were with him constantly, these women figures. They were gentle and good. They fixed his pillows. They came when he called for help. They said: "This will make you feel better" and ("There, isn't that better?" They touched him with their hands, flesh to flesh. His succor. His life savers. His lifelines.[6]

Mary Wollstonecraft, a contemporary of Rousseau's, saw a firm link between the feminine virtues of gentleness and docility, and the subjection of women. She charged that Rousseau and some other 'specious reasoners', consistently recommended 'gentleness, docility and a spaniel-like affection . . . as the cardinal virtues of the sex', but ultimately regarded women as 'gentle, domestic brutes', incapable of the kind of reason that distinguishes human beings from the beast. 'The nature of reason', she said, 'must be the same in all'.[7]

Many modern feminists still accept Wollstonecraft's basic point that there is but one ethics for women and men. There is, however, also another school of thought which holds that traditional male thinkers, while wrong on much else, were right on at least one point: that women and men do approach ethics differently. This school of thought rejects the idea that women are *incapable* of abstract, principled thinking; rather, and much more fundamentally, it claims that principled ethical thinking is not the only valid (or best) approach to ethics. There is, according to this view, an alternative 'female' approach to ethics which is based not on abstract 'male' ethical principles or wide generalisations, but on 'care', that is, on receptivity and responsiveness to the needs of others.

---

[4] Jean-Jacques Rousseau: *Emile, op. cit.*, p. 359.
[5] Alfred Lord Tennyson: 'The Princess'. (The poem can be found in various anthologies.)
[6] Martha Lear: *Heartsounds*, New York: Simon and Schuster, 1980, pp. 38–39.
[7] Mary Wollstonecraft: *A Vindication of the Rights of Women*, New York: Norton, 1967, pp. 50, 68, 69.

Nurses have taken a keen interest in these female approaches to ethics. Drawing on the views expounded by Carol Gilligan[8] and Nel Noddings,[9] nurses claim that a female 'ethics of care' better captures their moral experiences than a traditional male 'ethics of justice'.[10] The latter approach, a prominent proponent of a nursing ethics of care proclaims, regards principles as more important than people; nurse-caring, on the other hand, is patient-centered: 'it ties us to the people we serve and not to the rules through which we serve them'.[11]

The claim that women and men approach ethics differently is not the focus of my paper, although I will briefly return to it at the end of my discussion. I will be addressing the second issue, that is, the claim that nurses should adopt a female ethics of care because this is preferable to the justice approach. Since different writers have distinct ideas about what constitutes a (nursing) ethics of care, all I can do in this paper is introduce and then briefly discuss one common central theme: that a female ethics of care has no use for, and does not need, universal principles or rules.

As my discussion will show, I very much doubt that such an ethics will serve either patients or nurses well. Rather, nurses who decide to conduct their professional lives in accordance with an ethics of care are likely to find themselves in a position where they, like generations of nurses and women before them, may be praised for their caring feminine traits and dispositions, but will be unable to assert their moral claims, or to speak on behalf of those for whom they care.

Let me begin my critique by taking a closer look at the notion of 'care'.

---

[8] Carol Gilligan: *In a Different Voice*, Cambridge: Harvard University Press, 1982.

[9] Nel Noddings: *Caring – A Feminine Approach to Ethics and Moral Education*, Berkeley: University of California Press, 1984.

[10] See, for example, the articles in the collection by Jean Watson and Marilyn A. Ray (eds.): *The Ethics of Care and the Ethics of Cure: Synthesis in Chronicity*, New York: National League for Nursing, 1988; Mary Carolyn Cooper: 'Gilligan's Different Voice: A Perspective for Nursing', *Journal of Professional Nursing*, Vol. 5, No. 1, 1989, pp. 10–16; Sara T. Fry: 'Toward a theory of nursing ethics', *Advances in Nursing Science*, Vol. 11, No. 4, pp. 9–22; Randy Spreen Parker: 'Nurses' stories: The search for a relational ethics of care', *Advances in Nursing Science*, Sept. 1990, pp. 32–40; Dena S. Davis: 'Nursing: An Ethics of Caring', *Hum. Med.*, 1985, Vol. 2, No. 1, pp. 19–25.

[11] Jean Watson: 'An Introduction: An Ethics of Caring/Curing/Nursing' *qua* Nursing: in Jean Watson and Marilyn A. Ray (eds.): *The Ethics of Care . . .* , *op cit.*, p. 2. Jean Watson is here citing Nel Noddings: *Caring . . .* , *op. cit.*, no page number given.

II. CARING AS A MORAL DISPOSITION[12]

'Care' is a rich and highly ambiguous notion. Caring for another person – the notion that will occupy us in the present context – has connotations of concern, compassion, worry, anxiety, and of burden; there are also connotations of inclination, fondness and affection; connotations of carefulness, that is, of attention to detail, of responding sensitively to the situation of the other; and there are connotations of looking after, or providing for, the other.[13]

For the purposes of understanding and evaluating an ethics that has care as its central concept, it would be important to know which understanding of 'care' its exponents have in mind. Unfortunately the nursing literature is not of any great help. Nurses use the term 'care' in many different and potentially contradictory ways.[14] As Howard Curzer notes, proposals include 'presence', 'empathy plus expression of feeling', 'truth-telling and touch', 'showing concern', and 'enabling or assisting'.[15] Underlying these different understandings is some general agreement that 'care' must involve more than mere caring behaviour; there must also be some empathy, attachment or connectedness, in the sense of 'caring about' the patient.

What precisely 'caring for/caring about' amounts to is, however, none too clear. Definitions and explanations are imprecise, obscure and sometimes even mystical. One prominent writer in the field, Sally Gadow, for example, defines 'care'

> as an end in itself. While it may serve as a means of reaching a further state, it is always and above all a state that itself can be fully inhabited. While it may serve as a vessel for reaching a remote shore, it is at the same time and above all a vessel in which one can live even when – especially when – there is no destination in sight or in mind.[16]

---

[12] This section contains some passages drawn from Helga Kuhse: 'Against the Stream: Why Nurses Should Say 'No' to a female Ethics of Care', forthcoming in *Revue Internationale de Philosophique*.

[13] On the richness of the notion of 'caring', see Nel Noddings: *Caring . . .*, *op. cit.*, pp. 9–16.

[14] For a thorough critique of Sara Fry's concept of care (in 'The role of caring in a theory of nursing', *Hypatia*. Vol. 4, No. 2, 1989, pp. 88–103) see Howard J. Curzer: 'Fry's Concept of Care in Nursing Ethics, *Hypatia*, Vol. 8, No. 3, 1993, pp. 174–183.

[15] Howard J. Curzer: 'Fry's Concept of Care . . .', ibid., p. 175.

[16] Sally Gadow: 'Covenant Without Cure: Letting Go and Holding On in Chronic Illness', in (eds.) Jean Watson and Marilyn A. Ray (eds.): *The Ethics of Care and the Ethics of Cure . . .*, *op. cit.*, pp. 5–6.

Similarly Jean Watson. Watson holds that true 'transpersonal caring' entails that

> the nurse is able to form a union with the other on a level that transcends the physical . . . [where] there is a freeing of both persons from their separation and isolation . . .[17]

Other writers speak of nurse-caring as 'a feeling of dedication to the extent that it motivates and energizes action to influence life constructively and positively by increasing intimacy and mutual self-actualization';[18] an 'interactive process', which is achieved by 'a conscious and intuitive opening of self to another, by purposeful trusting and sharing energy, experiences, ideas, techniques and knowledge';[19] or as 'the creative, intuitive or cognitive helping process for individuals and groups based upon philosophic, phenomenologic, and objective and subjective experiential feelings and acts of assisting others'.[20]

Writers in the field generally recognize that the notion of 'care' is as yet inadequately understood, and that there is as yet no satisfactory ethics of care that can serve as a foundation for nursing.

Despite these inconsistencies and obscurities, and my doubts about the feasibility of building an ethical theory on the concept of care alone, there is value in focusing on care as an important, but often neglected, component of ethics.

A sympathetic reading of the nursing literature will reveal a number of common threads. As also in Nel Noddings' approach,[21] there is emphasis on relationship, on attachment, openness, and on attentiveness and responsiveness to the needs of the cared-for. 'Caring' is thus not so much a matter of actions, task, or processes, as a mode of being, a virtue, or a stance or attitude towards the object of one's attention. In other words, in attempting to articulate an ethics of care, writers are not so much trying to answer the traditional ethical question of right action: 'What should I do?'; but

[17] Jean Watson: *Nursing – Human Science and Human Care: A Theory of Nursing*, Norwalk, Conn.: Appleton-Century Crofts, 1985, p. 66.
[18] E.O. Bevis: 'Caring: A Life Force', in (ed.) M. Leininger: *Caring: An Essential Human Need*, Thorofare, NJ: Slack, 1981, p. 50.
[19] B. Blattner: *Holistic Nursing*, Englewood Cliffs, NJ: Prentice Hall, 1981, p. 70.
[20] M. Leininger: 'Caring: A Central Focus of Nursing and Health Care Services', *Nursing and Health Care*, October 1980, p. 143, as cited by Hilde L. Nelson: 'Against Caring', *The Journal of Clinical Ethics*, Vol. 3, No. 1, Spring 1992, p. 9.
[21] Nel Noddings: *Caring . . .* , *op. cit.*

rather the question: 'How should I, the carer, meet the cared-for'. I shall refer to this understanding of care as 'dispositional care'.

Dispositional care presupposes not only commitment and motivation, but also openness and receptivity to the needs of the other – a state that Nel Noddings calls 'engrossment'. Engrossment entails a putting aside of the self so that the carer can perceive, and then sensitively respond to, the particular and unique experiences and needs of the other.

The ideas of dispositional care and of engrossment are far from unproblematical. Various criticisms have been raised against current articulations of them – that they are, for example, based on an impractical ideal, that they employ a notion of care that, while suited to characterise personal relationships of great intimacy and depth, is ill-suited for the nurse-patient encounter, or that they are potentially exploitative of women.[22] While these criticisms cannot easily be dismissed, I take it as given that there is *some* sense in which our attitudes or dispositions matter and that a caring disposition or stance, loosely understood as sensitive openness and responsiveness to the needs of particular others, will contribute to better patient care. It emphasises the importance of receptivity and responsiveness, as well as the uniqueness of particular persons and situations. Health-care professionals who are 'dispositional carers' are more likely to be receptive to the needs of patients, where these patients are recognised as *particular others*, that is, as individuals, with special needs, beliefs, desires and wants – rather than, say, as 'the cancer' in Ward 4. This entails that dispositional care is not only an appropriate part of nursing ethics, but of medical ethics as well.

When dispositional care is lacking, patients' needs may not be met. This view gets some support from a recently published observational study reporting on the interaction of nurses and doctors with dying patients. The non-participant observer reported one case, where nurses failed to notice that a dying patient was thirsty, that the patient could not reach the drink that was placed before

---

[22] See, for example, Stan van Hooft: 'Caring and professional commitment', *The Australian Journal of Advanced Nursing*, Vol. 4, No. 4, 1987, pp. 29–38; Helga Kuhse: 'Caring is not enough: reflections on a nursing ethics of care', *The Australian Journal of Advanced Nursing*, Vol. 11, No. 1, 1993, pp. 32–42. Catharine A. MacKinnon: *Feminism Unmodified: Discourses on Life and Law*, Cambridge: Harvard University Press, 1987. Janice G. Raymond: 'Reproductive Gifts and Gift Giving: The Altruistic Woman', *Hastings Center Report*, November/December 1990, pp. 7–11.

her, and that she could not sit up unaided and would fall back when no support was provided. While many factors other than the lack of dispositional care could also explain why this patient's needs were not met, the case description suggests that the nurses, rather than simply being callous, were not receptive and sensitive enough to recognize that this particular patient needed additional help.[23]

As Lawrence Blum has observed, moral philosophy's traditional preoccupation with action-guiding rules and principles, and focus on such notions as universalizability and impartiality, have masked the importance of what he calls 'moral perception and particularity' – that is, the important role that is played by our ability to recognise the morally salient features of a situation. For all the moral principles in the world (and our willingness to employ them) will not help if we lack the kind of 'moral perception' necessary to tell us when to employ them.[24]

To sum up, then, it seems that Blum and proponents of a nursing ethics of care are right when they say that such traits as perceptivity, sensitivity and responsiveness are morally significant. Blum is also right, it seems to me, when he says that philosophy's traditional preoccupation with sometimes blunt rules and principles, and with universalizability and impartiality, has resulted in less than adequate attention being paid to this aspect of ethics. Proponents of a care approach do, however, often want to go much further than that. They are saying that care alone should be playing a role – that there is no place, or only a very limited place, in an ethics of care for abstract universal principles or rules.

III. THE REJECTION OF PRINCIPLES

Caring is a good thing and everyone, not just nurses, should be more caring. If dispositional care can thus quite properly be regarded as a significant part of ethics, it is, however, not the whole of ethics. Ethics is also, and some would say, primarily, about the justification of actions. This aspect of ethics becomes particularly important in contexts, such as nursing and medicine, where there is frequent moral disagreement about the rightness or wrongness of actions:

---

[23] Mina Mills, Huw T.O. Davies, William A. Macrae: 'Care of dying patients in hospital', *British Medical Journal*, Vol. 309, Sept. 3, 1994, pp. 583–586.
[24] Lawrence Blum: 'Moral Perception and Particularity', *Ethics*, Vol. 101, July 1991, pp. 701–725.

whether a dying patient should, for example, be kept alive, or allowed to die; told the truth, or be protected from it for her own good.

Proponents of female ethics of care do, however, display a distaste for reasoned argument and justification. In her book *Caring*, Nel Noddings explicitly rejects abstract principles and the requirement of universalizabililty as an appropriate part of ethics. Ethics, she suggests, is not a matter of impartial and abstract principles and rules, but of relationships – of care for family, friends, and the 'proximate stranger'.[25] But, as Hilde Nelson notes, care is 'blind and indiscriminate'.[26] It cannot by itself tell us what to do.

The following 'personal narrative' by a nurse, Randy Spreen Parker, will illustrate what can happen when the rejection of principles is taken to its logical conclusion.[27] The narrator describes herself as a 'seasoned critical care nurse', who had abandoned '[t]he language of rights, duties and obligations' (which she experienced as 'alien' and 'detached from the experience' of nursing) to 'learn the lines of a different script – a script that was written in a universal, relational language' – the language of care.

Parker had cared in what appears to have been an admirable fashion for an aphasic patient, Mike, who had difficulties in speaking and understanding.

Mike was a diabetic. Due to poor blood circulation, it was necessary to perform a hip-disarticulation – a radical amputation of the leg at the hip. He was left with a deteriorating 'gaping cavernous wound that extended from his rib cage to his pelvis'. The wound needed dressing changes every three hours. This was excruciatingly painful, since Mike, who also had a lung problem, could not be given adequate pain medication.

When it became clear to both patient and nurse that 'further medical interventions served no meaningful purpose', Parker spoke to the attending physician and head nurse and told them that she 'did not feel' that Mike (who had difficulty speaking coherently) wanted to continue life-sustaining treatment.

Parker asked to remain Mike's primary nurse and to care for him, but, she explained, she could not participate in any further dressing changes or resuscitation measures.

---

[25] Nel Noddings: *Caring . . .* , *op. cit.*

[26] Hilde L. Nelson: 'Against Caring', *The Journal of Clinical Ethics*, Vol. 3, No. 1, 1992, p. 9.

[27] A similar description of this case also appears in Helga Kuhse: 'Against the Stream . . .', *op. cit.*

I tried to explain my rationale but found myself fumbling for the right words. How could I translate my own moral experience into traditional moral language? The scripts were different. After several meetings with the attending physician and other nurse managers, I was removed from intensive care and placed on a medical-surgical unit.

Over the next week, Mike was resuscitated several times, before he died 'in pain, frightened and alone'.[28]

Parker's realization that her 'moral experience' of caring and 'traditional moral language' have radically different scripts is of course quite correct. Moral experience is private, traditional moral language is not. One person's raw moral experience holds no persuasive powers for others, and should also be regarded critically by the person herself. After all, at times our feelings and experiences may seriously mislead us. They need testing against some standard that lies outside the experience itself.

When it comes to the justification of particular actions, we need to give reasoned arguments for our views. In the clinical context, such arguments will typically rely on certain universal principles, such as respect for autonomy or a health care professional's *prima facie* duty to act in the patient's best interests. To eschew all moral principles is to withdraw from moral discourse and to retreat into an essentially dumb world of one's own.

Of course, the assumption is that caring, in its sensitive attention to the particularities of the situation can give the right answer. But this is not so. Sensitivity and particularity alone can not guide action. We always must decide which particularities of a situation, which elements of the personal histories of those involved, are of moral significance and which are not.

To decide what she should do, the agent must first 'abstract' some particularities of the situation – those that she regards as morally significant – as her action guide. These abstractions – for example that Mike was suffering and wanted to die, that there was no hope, and so on – are the kind of stuff that principles are made of. Once stated in principled form (for example: 'Patients who are hopelessly ill, who are suffering and want to die, should be allowed to die') these abstractions can be tested, and accepted or rejected, as the case may be. Without principles of some sort – and it is of course

[28] Randy Spreen Parker: 'Nurses' Stories . . .', *op. cit.*, pp. 31–34.

an open question what these principles should be – there can be
no ethical discourse, no justification – only particularities and
unguided feelings; neither will have any persuasive powers for
others, nor should they have persuasive power for us.

Caring advocates' distaste for principles follows, of course, from
the requirement that the carer should be fully attentive to the
circumstances of each individual person, and the nuances of her
particular and unique situation. The assumption is that abstraction
presupposes sameness, where there is, in fact, uniqueness.

Nel Noddings provides an extensive critique of abstract principles by distinguishing the 'approach of the father' from that 'of
the mother':

> The first moves immediately to abstraction where . . . thinking
> can take place clearly and logically in isolation from the compli-
> cating factors of particular persons, places, and circumstances;
> the second moves to concretization where . . . feelings can be
> modified by the introduction of facts, the feelings of others, and
> personal histories.[29]

Noddings is correct when she suggests that additional facts,
feelings, and personal histories will, and should, often make a difference to our moral evaluation of a situation. Nonetheless, the
dichotomy she draws between an 'ethics of care' and an 'ethics of
principle' in terms of the distinction between 'concretization' and
'abstraction' is a false one.

In the passage just quoted, the contrast between 'abstraction' and
'concretization' seems to rest, at least in part, on the distinction
between 'thinking in isolation from complicating factors' and
'thinking modified by the introduction of facts . . .'. But could
ethical thinking *ever* proceed in isolation from concrete facts and
particular circumstances? Even Kant, rigidly holding that one must
never lie, even to a would-be-murderer, needs to refer to the facts:
do you really know whether the man's intended victim is in the
house? How sure do you have to be that he is there, for the statement
'I don't know where he is' to count as a lie?[30]

---

[29] Nel Noddings: *Caring . . .* , *op. cit.*, pp. 36–37.
[30] See I. Kant: 'On a supposed right to tell lies from benevolent motives' in *Kant's Critique of Practical Reason and Other Works on the Theory of Ethics*, trans. Thomas Kingsmill Abbott, London: Longman's, Green & Co., 1909, pp. 361–365.

By the same token, even those who take Noddings' 'mother's approach' will have to abstract some details from the infinitely many that describe a given situation. Noddings' reference to 'feelings' and 'personal histories' is already an abstraction of particular aspects of the situation: apparently a person's height, or hair colour can (always? usually?) be left out. But even then, it is simply not possible to take all the feelings, or each aspect of every personal history into account. This means that the question is not *whether* context is relevant, but rather *which* elements of that context ought to be 'abstracted' from the overall context as significant for ethical decision-making.[31]

What the morally relevant factors are is perhaps the most central and vexing question in traditional ethics. Those who approach ethics from the perspective of the justice tradition will focus on aspects relevant to the application of certain principles or rules; those who approach ethics from a consequentialist perspective will focus on certain goals – for example, how much pleasure or pain a given action will produce, or how well it satisfies the preferences of all those affected by the action; and those who approach ethics from the care perspective will focus on aspects related to the maintenance of relationships, that is, on care for family, friends, and the 'proximate stranger'.

This brings us to the next question: Is an ethics that focuses on our responsibilities to those with whom we stand in direct relationships adequate?

Nel Noddings regards concern for those distant from us – for example, those starving in Africa, those who are not our patients, or those who do not belong to our species – as a form of 'romantic rationalism'.[32] But this response will not do. It entails that a whole range of important ethical issues that go beyond personal human relationships and the lived experience of human care, such as the distribution and redistribution of wealth or the distribution of scarce health care resources, could not be challenged from within the care perspective.[33]

---

[31] This point is also made by George Sher: 'Other Voices, Other Rooms', in (eds.) Eva Federe Kittay and Diana Meyers: *Women and Moral Theory*, United States of America: Rowman and Littlefields Publishers, 1987, p. 180.
[32] Nel Noddings: *Caring . . .* , *op. cit.*, p. 3.
[33] See also Claudia Card: 'Caring and Evil', *Hypatia*, Vol. 5, No. 1, Spring 1990, pp. 101–108.

If women and nurses excessively devalue reasoned argument, if they dismiss ethical principles and norms and hold that notions of impartiality and universalizability have no place in a female ethics of care, then they will be left without the theoretical tools necessary to condemn some actions or practices, and to defend others. Bereft of a universal ethical language, women will be unable to participate in ethical discourse. They will not be able to speak on behalf of the patients for whom they care, nor will they be able to defend their own legitimate claims[34] – and the motto of the first Canadian school of nursing: 'I see and I am silent' would have continuing relevance for nurses.[35]

IV. CONCLUSION

I began my paper by asking whether women and men approach ethics differently. I myself am dubious about the claim that ethics is gendered and that women are inherently more caring than men. Rather, I am more persuaded by the general idea that social practices and roles give rise to particular moral experiences and visions of 'the good'. Women have traditionally tended the home, nurtured children, supported husbands, and nursed the sick. Men, on the other hand, have traditionally played more public roles. Their activities did not primarily involve care for 'concrete others' but rather dealings with strangers or 'abstract others'.[36]

Broad ethical principles and rules, notions of rights and justice have an appropriate role to play in the public sphere. Insofar as the public sphere is the realm of strangers, we cannot know the personal histories and particular circumstances of all those affected by our decisions, nor can we care for them in a personal way. But we can, and must, ensure that their rights and claims are protected, and that they are treated fairly.

Care, on the other hand, has a more central role to play in the private sphere, where people can respond to each other as 'concrete'

[34] See also L.M. Purdy: 'Feminist Healing Ethics' in *Hypatia*, Vol. 4, No. 2, Summer 1989, pp. 9–12.
[35] John O. Goden: 'Editorials – No Longer Silent', *Humane Medicine*, Vol. 4, No. 1, May 1988, p. 1.
[36] Jean Grimshaw: 'The Idea of a Female Ethic' in Peter Singer: *Companion to Ethics*, Oxford: Blackwell, 1991, pp. 496–499.

others, and where the maintenance of relationships requires sensitivity and responsiveness to the particularities of the situation and the needs and desires of those concerned.

Now, if it is the case that traditional ethical theories are based on the experiences of men in the public sphere, then we should not be too surprised to find that the insights of women, derived from their experience in the private sphere have often been ignored.[37] Nursing straddles the public and the private. It is a public enterprise, but 'care' is quite properly recognised as the – largely – appropriate mode for the one-to-one encounter between nurses and patients. Patients as a whole would not be well-served if they were regarded as 'abstract' individuals, as merely the bearers of certain rights or claims. Such an approach would leave many of their needs unmet. While 'care' is thus necessary for good patient care, it is not – as I have suggested above – an adequate foundational concept for a nursing ethics of care. Ethics, and women and nurses, need justice as well.

I started by quoting a number of traditional thinkers. Let me close with a quote from one other philosopher. 'Clearly', Aristotle maintained,

> . . . moral virtue belongs to all . . . but the temperance of a man and of a woman, or the courage and justice of a man and of a woman are not . . . , the same . . . "Silence is a woman's glory", but this is not equally the glory of man.[38]

One way to prove him wrong, is to reject a female (nursing) ethics of care.

---

[37] See also Jean Grimshaw: 'The Idea of a Female Ethic', *op. cit.*
[38] Aristotle: *Politics*, Book I, Chapter 13.

Chapter 7

PSYCHIATRIC ETHICS

JENNIFER RADDEN

INTRODUCTION

Psychiatric practice and psychiatric care seem to give rise to their own distinctive ethical dilemmas and issues, their own distinctive codes of conduct, and their own uses of moral theory and theorizing. Psychiatry is a medical sub-specialty, and as such is governed by the principles of biomedical ethics, but it is also a unique social and medical practice; arguably, its uniqueness means that those more general bioethical principles, while necessary, are not sufficient for a characterization of psychiatric ethics.

As the literature illustrates, psychiatric ethics spans several somewhat different domains: the guidelines governing ethical research in psychiatry,[1] the professional ethics required in the practice of psychiatry, and a broader set of moral and ethical problems and dilemmas distinctive to, or at least magnified by, the mental health care setting. Only the last two of these domains will be dealt with here. These two partially overlap. The ethical psychiatrist will be required to understand the way moral values such as autonomy, beneficence and confidentiality guide professional conduct. But professional ethics for psychiatric practice does not generally deal with the complex philosophical theorizing and debates – about paternalism (or, as it is sometimes known, parentalism), freedom, personal responsibility, agency, rationality, individual and community, self and other – which are raised by the application of these values to the mental health care setting.

Even narrowed to professional ethics, the scope of psychiatric ethics is shaped by the different purposes of psychiatric practice. In forensic settings where legal liability, professional censure and other legal and quasi-legal matters arise professional rules of conduct are

---

[1] See L.W. Roberts and B. Roberts. Psychiatric Research Ethics: An Overview of Evolving Guidelines and Current Ethical Dilemmas in the Study of Mental Illness. *Biological Psychiatry* 1999; 46: 1025–1038.

the single concern – those actions required, permitted and forbidden in professional practice. In the educational context attention can be paid not only to rules of conduct but to the ideals and values of the practice and the moral theoretical issues raised by mental disorder and mental health care. Dyer's separation between entry (and educational) and exit contexts suggests itself here.[2] Professional censure and evaluation and breaches of specific rules occur in the 'exit' setting; the practitioner's moral character and the broader moral framework receive attention in the entry setting. Issues of legal liability for treaters comprise only part of the scope of psychiatric ethics discussed in this review. Despite a recent tendency to reduce the notion of ethics and ethical inquiry in this way, ethical practice in psychiatry is practice consistent with ethical ideals, and not merely with prudential principles for avoiding lawsuit.[3]

The review which follows is organized into two parts: Part 1 contains a selection of problems in psychiatric ethics that remain of continuing concern. These problems are part of the nature and/or cultural history of mental disorder and mental health care. Although perhaps not recognized as such, it is safe to say they have existed as long as mental disorder and mental health care themselves. Part 2 reviews a group of issues and problems introduced by recent advances, trends, and policies in, or affecting, mental health care.

FOUR PERENNIAL PROBLEMS

The model of patient as autonomous agent

This model, derived from other medical sub-specialties and other professional relationships, appears to be problematic with the typical psychiatric patient. If only temporarily and partially, psychiatric patients are often deprived of capabilities required for an exercise of autonomy (as they are of their best defenses against exploitation): their judgement in matters concerning their long-term self interest; their reasoning ability, their self-control, and their capacity to communicate their concerns and needs to others. Unlike

---

[2] A. Dyer. 1999. Psychiatry as a Profession. In *Psychiatric Ethics*, Third Edition. S. Bloch, P. Chodoff, S.A. Green, eds. Oxford University Press.
[3] P. Malley & E. Reilly. 1999. *Legal and Ethical Dimensions for Mental Health Professionals.* Philadelphia. George Buchanan Co.

the patient seeking medical attention for almost every other condition (the exceptions are the dementias and organic brain diseases which similarly affect reasoning, decision making and judgement), the psychiatric patient often has diminished autonomy.

The philosophical and moral challenge, then, is to determine whether or to what extent, the autonomy model is applicable to psychiatric patients. This inquiry is a delicate one. Stigmatizing attitudes towards mental disorder have undeniably exaggerated the extent to which the mentally ill are imperfectly rational and autonomous agents, and modern day efforts to extend the presumption of autonomy (by replacing the designator 'patient' with that of 'client,' for example) have gone some way towards undoing the ill effects of such prejudicial attitudes. Nonetheless, it must be possible to acknowledge and avoid the wrongs associated with the cruel and discriminatory attitudes of the past without resorting to a misapplication of the autonomy model. Unwarrantedly attributing capabilities to the psychiatric patient when such capabilities are at least temporarily compromised involves its own inhumanity and injustice.

The model by which the patient is understood as an autonomous agent is integral to the principle of informed consent. To the extent that psychiatric patients elude the model, they will be deficient as autonomous agents capable of giving or withholding informed consent as to treatment or participation as research subjects.[4] The 'consumer' or negotiated contract principle by which the patient becomes a 'client' able to contract psychiatric services is similarly reliant on the model of patient as autonomous agent.[5]

This issue is far reaching. It underlies the 'protean'[6] problems with which psychiatric ethics still grapples, such as treatment refusal, involuntary hospitalization for care and protection, responsibility in the criminal setting, and the set of issues surrounding the criterion of competence (competence to stand trial, competence to

---

[4] L.W. Weiss. Informed Consent and the Capacity for Voluntarism. *American Journal of Psychiatry* 2002; 159: 705–712.
[5] R.M. Veatch. 1991. *The Patient-Physician Relation: The Patient as Partner, Part 2.* Bloomington Ind. Indiana University Press; L. Emmanuel, and E. Emmanuel. Four Models of the Physician-Patient Relationship. *Journal of the American Medical Association* 1992; 267: 2221–2226.
[6] R. Peele & P. Chodoff. 1999. The Ethics of Involuntary Treatment and Deinstitutionalization. In Bloch, Chodoff and Greene, *op. cit.* note 3.

refuse and consent to treatment, competence to undertake legal contracts, for example). Such problems are discussed in two recent, valuable anthologies[7] and the criterion of competence receives thoughtful analysis in the present volume (see Silver).

Careful recent work explores the alleged duty to provide care for those who, while not a threat to others, are a threat to themselves or otherwise in need of mental health care, even when this care is unwelcome.[8] Paternalist or 'parentalist' approaches to psychiatric patients includes those of Kultgen, Tjltveit, and Dunn.[9] One particular debate within the tangle of issues here presents itself as a kind of paradox or dilemma: sometimes, it may be morally necessary to violate the psychiatric patient's expressed wishes and thus her 'autonomy,' in order to restore or enhance her autonomy. As Dunn puts it:

> [P]aternalism need not be interpreted in a heavy-handed, authoritarian manner (even though it does involve substituting someone else's authority over that of an irrational person's). It can also be interpreted as caring enough for another to make difficult, probably unpopular decisions in the short-term in the hope that in the long-term genuine autonomy will be promoted.[10]

The opponents of such 'compassionate' or 'weak' paternalism invoke the traditional dangers voiced by Millian liberals such as that of ascertaining another's best interests: they stress the high standard of justification called for in other settings when an individual's freedom and bodily integrity are comparably interfered with; they point to the vulnerability of the psychiatric patient to exploitation and of psychiatric practice to misuse.[11] Advocating a contextualized and particularist approach, Hardcastle and Stewart

---

[7] R. Edwards, ed. 1997. *Ethics of Psychiatry: Insanity, Rational Autonomy, and Mental Health Care.* New York. Prometheus Books; Bloch, Chodoff and Greene, 1999, *op. cit.* note 3.

[8] D. Van De Veer. 1986. *Paternalistic Intervention.* Princeton NJ. Princeton University Press; J. Kultgen. 1995. *Autonomy & Intervention: Parentalism in the Caring Life.* Oxford. Oxford University Press.

[9] Ibid; A.C. Tjeltveit. 1999. *Ethics and Values in Psychotherapy.* London. Routledge; C. Dunn. 1998. *Ethical Issues in Mental Illness.* Brookfield USA. Aldershot: Avebury/Ashgate Publishing Limited.

[10] Ibid., pp. 20–21.

[11] T. Szasz. 1963. *Law, Liberty and Psychiatry.* New York. Collier Books; B. Gert & C.M. Culver. The Justification of Paternalism. *Ethics* 1989; 2: 199–210; P. Chodoff. 1999. Misuse and Abuse of Psychiatry: An Overview. In Bloch, Chodoff and Greene, *op. cit.* note 3.

raise some of these issues in their discussion of irrational suicide.[12] The unresolved applicability of the autonomous agent model will also influence the extent to which psychiatry is seen as requiring its own unique ethics, rather than subsumable under the principles and rubric of biomedical ethics.[13] If and to the extent that the autonomy model applies to psychiatric patients, practice concerning those patients will be expected to conform to those broader principles of biomedical ethics. (Obviously other factors such as the conviction that psychiatric disorder is the product of neurobiological states may also contribute to this judgment.)

Status and effects of diagnostic categories

The nature of psychiatric disorder, its epistemological status, and the social effects of diagnosis, have for long been the focus of psychiatric ethics and they remain so today.[14] The belief that diagnostic categories reflect arbitrary social constructions, rather than a taxonomy of biologically based deficits and/or dysfunctions of the brain, continues to challenge and subvert the tenets of biological psychiatry. This view finds support in a past history of misuses of diagnosis, most glaring the former Soviet Union's practice of pathologizing political dissidence.[15] Nearer to home, it points to the use of psychiatric diagnosis to affirm such exclusionary social norms as misogyny and homophobia in the diagnostic categories of masochistic personality disorder, and homosexuality, respectively.

Concerns about the epistemological status of psychiatric concepts occur at every level of generality. Notoriously, the category of

---

[12] Hardcastle and Stewart. Supporting Irrational Suicide. *Bioethics* 2002; 16: 425–438.

[13] Dyer, *op. cit.* note 3; American Psychiatric Association, Ethics Committee. 1995. Opinions of the ethics committee on the principles of medical ethics with annotations especially applicable to psychiatry. Washington DC. American Psychiatric Association; J. Radden. Notes Towards a Professional Ethics for Psychiatry. *Australian and New Zealand Journal of Psychiatry* 2002; 36: 2.

[14] T. Szasz. 1974. *The Myth of Mental Illness.* Revised Edition. New York. Harper Collins; P. Caplan. How *Do* They Decide Who is Normal? The Bizarre, But True, Tale of the DSM Process. *Canadian Psychology/Psychologie Canadienne* 1995; 32: 162–170; F.W.M. Fulford. 1989. *Moral Theory and Medical Practice.* Cambridge. Cambridge University Press; J. Sadler. Epistemic Value Commitments in the Debate over Categorical vs Dimensional Personality Diagnosis. *Philosophy, Psychiatry & Psychology* 1996; 3: 203–222; W. Reich. 1999. Psychiatric Diagnosis as an Ethical Problem. In Bloch, Chodoff and Greene, *op. cit.* note 3.

[15] Chodoff, *op. cit.* note 12.

mental disorder itself wants conceptually satisfactory definition.[16] From the broadest category of mental disorder itself, to the syndromal categories found in nosological systems such as the DSMs and the ICDs (hysteria, manic-depression, schizophrenia and so on), to the definitions of symptoms and symptom types (delusional thinking, hallucination, thought disorder, thought insertion), conceptual puzzles and confusion are to be found, and the disagreement they have engendered, has affected psychiatric patients.[17] Due to the controversial nature of almost every aspect of the conceptual basis of psychiatry, psychiatric ethics has been deemed the ugly duckling within biomedical ethics.[18] The dubious epistemological status of diagnostic concepts and categories affects not only the subjects of such labeling but the labelers, who remain ambivalent and unresolved over the meaning and purpose of these linguistic tools.[19] Because major disorders of psychiatry have as yet no known biological markers and want for a complete biological explanation, those skeptical of the scientific status – or of the social meaning and effects of – psychiatric diagnosis recognize its power, and remain troubled by its potential for abuse.

A professional ethics over and above biomedical ethics

Turning to the professional ethics guiding psychiatric treatment, we find another iteration of the disputed analogy between biological illness and psychiatric illness. Aspects of the psychiatric patient, the treatment offered that patient, and the therapeutic relationship each serve to distinguish psychiatric treatment from other medical treatment, despite the obvious and important

---

[16] T. Szasz. Second Commentary on Aristotle's Function Argument. *Philosophy, Psychiatry & Psychology* 2000; 7: 3–16; J. Wakefield. Disorder as Harmful Disfunction: A Conceptual Critique of DSM-IIIR's Definition of Mental Disorder. *Psychological Review* 1992; 99: 232–247; J. Wakefield. Aristotle as a Sociobiologist. *Philosophy, Psychiatry & Psychology* 2000; 7: 17–44; G. Megone. Mental Illness, Human Function, and Values. *Philosophy, Psychiatry & Psychology* 2000; 7: 45–76; T. Thornton. Mental Illness & Reductionism. *Philosophy, Psychiatry & Psychology* 2000; 7: 77–94; D. Dickenson & K.W.M. Fulford. 2000. *In Two Minds: A Casebook of Psychiatric Ethics*. Oxford. Oxford University Press.
[17] O. Wahl. 1999. *Telling is Risky Business: Mental Health Consumers Confront Stigma*. Rutgers, NJ. Rutgers University Press.
[18] K.W.M. Fulford & T. Hope. 1994. Psychiatric Ethics: A Bioethical Ugly Duckling? In *Principles of Health Care Ethics*. R. Gillon, ed. London. John Wiley & Sons.
[19] T. Luhrmann. 2000. *Of 2 Minds: The Growing Disorder in American Psychiatry*. New York. Knopf.

similarities and analogies between these different practices. In dispute are the extent of the difference and the extent to which that difference requires a distinctive ethics for psychiatry over and above the principles of biomedical ethics applicable to all medical treatment contexts.[20] In a far-sighted and influential document, *Principles of Medical Ethics: With Annotations Especially Applicable to Psychiatry*, the American Psychiatric Association has attempted to capture features distinguishing psychiatric practice and to explore their implications.[21]

Several features of the practice of psychiatry appear to generate distinctive ethical concerns. First, the degree of confidentiality required is more critical, both because of the subject matter raised in therapy, and because of continuing societal stigma branding and labeling the psychiatric patient. Second, the use of the relationship or alliance as a therapeutic tool places special demands on the behavior permitted by the treater. The more precise rules of conduct regulating therapist behavior are customarily expressed in the language of boundaries and boundary 'violations'.[22] Such rules of conduct and a means of identifying and codifying them appear to be an essential element of ethical psychiatric practice. Third, the patient's vulnerability is increased because the goals of therapy are so broad, far-reaching and potentially significant. This places a greater responsibility on the treater to act ethically and in the interests of the patient.[23] Fourth, a related vulnerability is associated with the patient, so frequently deprived of those traits most useful in combating exploitation. This vulnerability imposes a special burden on the treater. With greater opportunity to exploit and dominate, the treater must adhere to stricter standards of awareness and good conduct.[24]

---

[20] T. Beauchamp & J. Childress. 1994. *Principles of Biomedical Ethics.* Fourth Edition. New York. Oxford University Press.

[21] American Psychiatric Association, Ethics Committee. 1995. Opinions of the ethics committee on the principles of medical ethics with annotations especially applicable to psychiatry. Washington DC. American Psychiatric Association.

[22] G. Gabbard. 1999. Boundary Violations. In Bloch, Chodoff and Greene, *op. cit.* note 3; J. Radden. Boundary Violation Ethics: Some Conceptual Clarifications. *The Journal of the American Academy of Psychiatry and the Law* 2001; 29: 3.

[23] A.C. Tjeltveit. 1999. *Ethics and Values in Psychotherapy.* London. Routledge C. Dunn, *op. cit.* note 10; Radden, 2002, *op. cit.* note 14; F.W.M. Fulford, *op. cit.* note 15.

[24] Dunn, *op. cit.* note 10; G. Gabbard. 1999. Boundary Violations. In Bloch, Chodoff and Greene, *op. cit.* note 3.

A recent discussion of psychiatric euthanasia vividly illustrates the distinctiveness imposed by the psychiatric setting, demonstrating the way the traditional tools of bioethics which work well enough for issues about euthanasia in the rest of medicine fail to engage with the same issues as they arise in psychiatry.[25]

Gender and psychiatry

Gender is inescapably tied to psychiatric practice through epidemiology, associations, theories of psychosexual development, and as part of a systemic patriarchal culture.

Psychiatric diagnosis, practice and research have from their beginnings been influenced by widespread associations and attitudes that saw women as particularly prone to mental disorder. Even today women seem to make up a great, and perhaps (the data is ambiguous) disproportionate number of those seeking help from psychiatry and subject to psychiatric diagnosis; moreover recent studies reveal gender links – in incidence, age of onset, course, and response to therapy, in several mental disorders.[26]

The central categories within which mental disorder was understood in our Western traditions were all strongly associated with one sex or the other, or 'gendered,' for hundreds of years – rationality and the reasoning capabilities, the passions, the mind, beliefs, moods, emotions, the will, the self and self-control. Like madness itself, the feminine was associated with irrationality, lack of control, unbridled passion, immaturity, and so on, linking the feminine with madness by powerful strands of cultural influence.[27]

The categories of race, class and ethnicity, are also implicated in psychiatry. But this long cultural association in which madness and its seat in the mental faculties were all gendered categories arguably renders the question of gender especially unavoidable for psychiatric practice.

---

[25] S. Burgess, K. Hawton. Suicide, Euthanasia, and the Psychiatrist. *Philosophy, Psychiatry & Psychology.* 1998; 5: 113–126.

[26] E. Frank, ed. 2000. *Gender and its Effects on Psychopathology.* Washington DC. American Psychopathological Association.

[27] V. Skultans. 1979. *English Madness: Ideas on Insanity, 1580–1890.* London. Routledge & Kegan Paul; E. Showalter. *The Female Malady: Women, Madness and English Culture 1830–1980.* London. Virago; J. Usher. 1991. *Women's Madness: Misogyny or Mental Illness?* Amherst. University of Massachusetts Press; B. Wenegrat. 1995. *Illness and Power: Women's Mental Disorders and the Battle Between the Sexes.* NY. NYU Press.

Psychological theorizing has often propounded stereotypical assumptions about sex roles and supported differently valued criteria of mental health for men and women; less desirable traits such as dependency and passivity were attributed to women, while the more desirable traits of assertiveness and independence were judged normal for men.[28] As was noted earlier, gender bias has been identified in diagnostic categories such as Premenstrual Dysphoric Disorder, and Histrionic Personality Disorder.[29] Psychological theories also treated women's dissatisfaction with traditional roles as indicative of psychopathology.[30]

Finally, the pattern by which male therapists help female patients replicates within the therapeutic relationship the power arrangement in which women usually find themselves in the patriarchal structure of the broader society.[31] Because of this broader context, receiving care from a male practitioner is for a woman a different experience from that experienced by a male patient with the same therapist.[32]

The pervasive presence of gender within psychiatric theory and practice suggests a range of additional ethical strictures incumbent on the psychiatric professional, including sensitivity to gendered psychiatric diagnoses, and gendered theoretical models.

PART 2: ISSUES AND PROBLEMS RAISED BY RECENT ADVANCES, TRENDS, AND POLICIES IN OR AFFECTING MENTAL HEALTH CARE

The stimulus for bioethics as we know it today was largely technological and other advances in medicine. Such advances brought with them new challenges over beginning, ending and quality of life issues that were recognized to be inescapably and deeply

---

[28] I.K. Broverman, D.M. Broverman & F.E. Clarkson, et al. Sex-role Stereotypes and Clinical Judgements of Mental Health. *Journal of Consulting and Clinical Psychology* 1970; 34: 1–7.

[29] Caplan, *op. cit.* note 15; D. Russell. 1995. *Women, Madness and Medicine.* Cambridge MA. Polity Press.

[30] Ibid; J. Busfield. 1996. *Men, Women and Madness: Understanding Gender and Mental Disorder.* New York. New York University Press.

[31] T. Karasu. 1991. Ethical Aspects of Psychotherapy. In *Psychiatric Ethics.* S. Bloch and P. Chodoff, eds. Oxford. Oxford University Press.

[32] L. Brown. 1994. *Subversive Dialogues.* New York. Basic Books.

philosophical. Psychiatry also has been transformed by advances, trends and policies in the last few decades, and these changes have in the same way introduced new ethical problems, issues and dilemmas. In this brief review, I will focus on a selection of these changes and outline the response to them found in the literature on psychiatric ethics.

Psychoactive drugs

Psychopharmacology has given rise to innumerable ethical and value questions raised not only in the scholarly literature but also through mainstream journalism, talk shows, television, and patient literature – Prozac nation has arrived, and not gone unnoticed.

A primary ethical concern is that these drugs are over-prescribed – in schools, nursing homes and other institutions to solve management problems; among the well to enhance already enhanced life experience;[33] among the unwell who would be better treated with talk therapy. This is a polarizing issue. The proponents of these wonder drugs label as pharmacological Calvinists those who allege such overuse.[34] They are in turn accused of failing to measure the far-reaching effects of the rapid 'soma-tization' of our society.[35] They are also accused of being the witting or unwitting agents of the drug companies growing rich on the sale of such remedies.[36] (This economic argument is multifaceted, and includes recent concern that these drug companies profits far exceed an appropriate and just 'fair price' or even earnings from the lower price of such drugs in other countries.)

Psychopharmacology has also raised new forensic questions: should the defendant be subject (against his will or voluntarily) to psychoactive drugs to ensure competence to stand trial?[37] Does the knowledge of these medications' effects on behavior alter the time

---

[33] P. Kramer. 1993. *Listening to Prozac.* New York. Viking.
[34] D. DeGrazia. Prozac, Enhancement, and Self-Creation. *Hastings Center Report* 2000; 30: 34–40; C. Elliott. Pursued by Happiness and Beaten Senseless: Prozac and the American Dream. *Hastings Center Report* 2000; 30: 7–12.
[35] Ibid.
[36] D. Healy. 1997. *The Anti-Depressant Era.* Cambridge MA. Harvard University Press; R. Whitaker. 2002. *Mad in America: Bad Science, Bad Medicine, and the Enduring Mistreatment of the Mentally Ill.* Cambridge, MA. Perseus Publishing.
[37] P. Brown, C. Pantelis. 1999. Ethical Aspects of Drug Treatment. In Bloch, Chodoff and Greene, *op. cit.* note 3.

honored view that when a crime is committed because of mental disorder the person is not rightly held criminally responsible?[38] If medicating mentally disordered patients otherwise deemed too dangerous to be set free can ensure public safety, does the state have a duty to release those patients conditional upon their use of medications?[39]

Each of these moral questions is contested, controversial, and polemical in part because of more basic uncertainties about these new medications: data as to their actual effectiveness is contested, as are their long and even short term side-effects. Yet a genuine moral dilemma arises here: proof of effectiveness requires double blinded studies and other protocols [such as clearing the subject's system before introducing experimental drugs (the so-called 'wash-out')] incompatible with established ethical constraints on experimenting with human subjects whose competence to consent to such protocols is likely compromised. (This dilemma aside, there is suspicion that research directions may be determined less by a spirit of purely scientific inquiry than by the interests of drug manufacturers, and this has been a cause for concern.[40])

Treatment for prodromal conditions

A recent trend in the identification and treatment of mental disorder focuses on 'prodromal' states.[41] Studies offer early indication that by identifying and aggressively treating those whose behavior, 'signs' and/or genetic profile seem to indicate greater risk for developing schizophrenia before the disorder exhibits diagnosable symptoms can lessen the impact of the disorder in cases where it emerges.[42]

Serious ethical issues are raised by this trend. It imposes strong anti-psychotic medications on many 'false positive' adolescents who would not prove to have developed schizophrenia; a stigmatizing label is introduced early; and it involves medicating a group whose

---

[38] E.W. Mitchell. Madness and Meta-responsibility: the culpable causation of mental disorder and the insanity defense. *Journal of Forensic Psychiatry* 1999; 10: 597–622.

[39] Peele and Chodoff, *op. cit.* note 7.

[40] Healy, *op. cit.* note 37, Brown and Pantelis, *op. cit.* note 38.

[41] T.H. McGlashan. Early Detection and Intervention in Schizophrenia. *Schizophrenia Bulletin* 1996; 22: 197–199.

[42] A.R. Yung & P.D. McGorry. Is pre-psychotic intervention realistic in schizophrenia and related disorders? *Australian and New Zealand Journal of Psychiatry* 1997; 31: 806–807.

immaturity puts their informed consent status in doubt, to name a few of these.[43]

The controversy raised by the possibility of treating prodromal conditions is intense and the stakes high. Against the concerns raised by the regimen's opponents, its defenders speak of the possibility of preventing chronicity,[44] a goal that, because of the devastating nature of schizophrenia, is hard to dismiss.

Genetics and psychiatry

Recent work on psychiatric genetics must proceed mindful of the ugly history of the eugenics movement wherein the presence of alleged genetic defects justified policies violating fundamental rights of the mentally ill, including basic reproductive freedoms.[45] Even when these dangers are foresworn, however, the genetic risks of psychiatric illness and the nature and present state of psychiatric genetics are the subject of common misunderstandings that foster assumptions about the alleged 'taint' of psychiatric illness. Thus, it is sometimes naively implied that genetic testing could be appealed to in practical and public policy dilemmas. Tests for most mental illnesses are many years off, however. Today genetic screening relies on diagnosed or undiagnosed mental illness in the family medical record, not on evidence of propensities to suffer mental illnesses based on genetic testing. Even if genetic tests were available, the information they would provide seems likely to remain limited. This is because in the more common kinds of severe mental disorder such as schizophrenia and bipolar and unipolar affective conditions, there is not a simple one-to-one correspondence between genotype and phenotype. Rather than monogenic (involving only one gene) these disorders are polygenic (involving many genes of small effect) or oligogenic (involving a small group of genes). Because they do not have straightforward Mendelian patterns of inheritance, the accuracy of predictive testing will never approach anything close to 100%. (The upper limit of predictive accuracy is found in monozygotic twin concordance rates, now believed to be about 50% for

---

[43] M.L.A. Heinimaa. Conceptual Problems of Early Intervention in Schizophrenia. *Hong Kong Journal of Psychiatry* 1999; 9: 20–24.

[44] McGlashan, *op. cit.* note 42.

[45] A. Farmer & P. McGuffln. 1999. Ethics and Psychiatric Genetics. In Bloch, Chodoff and Greene, *op. cit.* note 3.

schizophrenia and 70% for manic-depression.)[46] A corollary of a disorder having this polygenic or oligogenic basis detracts further from the future usefulness of such testing: these conditions are likely to show genetic variants or alleles of high frequency in the general population. For example, a putative risk factor for schizophrenia is an allelic variant at the gene encoding for the 5-HT_{2A} serotonin receptor. But this variant is found in 60–70% of the population. Thus, compared with those without this variant, those with it apparently have a very modest increased risk: their greater likelihood of developing schizophrenia is only 1.5 times.[47]

A better understanding of the genetic aspects of mental disorder will have other important benefits, nonetheless. Although no cure is yet available for any of the major mental disorders and the effectiveness of current treatments is difficult to assess, research into the genetics of psychiatry is expected to help in the development of targeted treatments and is believed by many to be warranted for that reason alone.

Managed care

As Morreim predicted more than a decade ago[48] the economic overhaul of medicine undergone in the US (among other nations), with its imperatives of increasing profits and containing costs, has affected mental health care in a distinctive way and posed special ethical challenges for psychiatry.[49] A range of interconnected ethical tensions have been spawned by these changes in practice and policy, each of which affects not only patient rights and treater responsibilities but also the quality and effectiveness of mental health care; I will note only three kinds. First, and perhaps most important, managed care places new strains on confidentiality, privacy and trust. While apparently integral to effective therapy, the patient's

---

[46] D. Sullivan. 2000. Genetic Determinism, Free Will and Criminal Responsibility: Anticipating Genetic Excuses. (Unpublished manuscript)

[47] Ibid; J. Horgan. 1999. *The Undiscovered Mind: How the Human Brain Defies Replication, Medication and Explanation.* New York. The Free Press.

[48] E.H. Morreim. The New Economics of Medicine: Special Changes to Psychiatry. *Journal of Medicine and Philosophy* 1990; 15: 98.

[49] R. Meyer, C. McLaughlin. 1998. *Between Mind, Brain, and Managed Care: The Now and Future World of Academic Psychiatry.* Washington DC. American Psychiatric Press; M. Schlesinger, M. Wynia, and D. Cummins. Some Distinctive Features of the Impact of Managed Care on Psychiatry. *Harvard Review of Psychiatry* 2000; 8: 216–230; S. Green. 1999. The Ethics of Managed Mental Health Care. In Bloch, Chodoff and Greene, *op. cit.* note 3.

need to trust the treater with extremely sensitive information is put in jeopardy by increasingly bureaucratized systems of care and payment. Erosion of such trust in turn affects the therapeutic relationship, as do other aspects of the new regimens. Second, managed care requires a very different model of the compact established between treater and patient. It calls, for instance, for what has been dubbed 'fiscal informed consent': the effects of managed care on the course of treatment, the likely breaches of confidentiality, the possibility that treatment may be terminated before it is complete because of a denial of benefits, and so on, appear to be matters to be acknowledged and agreed upon at the beginning of therapy. Finally, managed care generates many new conflicts of role and ethical obligation for the treater.[50] In addition to acting as advocate for the patient and as exclusively committed to that patient's health and well being, a traditional medical role usually believed incompatible with any other, the treater now must act as health care rationer and gate keeper.[51] These and other conflicts of role and responsibility generate recurrent ethical dilemmas, and leave many working within psychiatry today frustrated, confused and resentful, a state itself affecting care.[52]

CONCLUSION

Managed care, psychiatric genetics, treatment of prodromal signs, and psychopharmacology represent only a fraction of the sources of ethical problems and dilemmas raised by early twenty-first century psychiatry. Others are the question of mental health care rationing and the injustices associated with uneven access to mental health care;[53] the issues of 'parity' between third party coverage of (other) medical and psychiatric conditions, respectively, now the subject of US legislation at the federal and state levels and the topic of an essay in the *Bioethics* special issue on Psychiatric Ethics;[54] the

---

[50] J.A. Lazarus, S.S. Shafstein, eds. 1998. *New Roles for Psychiatrists in Organized Systems of Care.* Washington, DC. APA Press.
[51] P. Appelbaum. Legal Liability and Managed Care. *American Psychologist* 1993; 48: 251–257.
[52] Luhrmann, *op. cit.* note 20.
[53] Ibid.; J. Sabin & N. Daniels. 1999. Ethical Issues in Mental Health Resource Allocation. In Bloch, Chodoff and Greene, *op. cit.* note 3.
[54] See Woolfolk and Doris. *Bioethics* 2002; 16: 469–485.

cluster of special considerations surrounding children's mental health, highlighted in a recent report from the Surgeon General's office;[55] the so-called global burden of mental disease understood as morbidity, mortality and disability and viewed as a public health crisis;[56] mental health policy dilemmas around deinstitutionalization and community psychiatry;[57] and mental disorder in relation to disability concepts and law.[58] Moreover, we can anticipate that new or newly critical ethical dimensions will emerge with each change in the understanding and treatment of mental disorder. Genetic tests for disorders would place extra pressure on issues of privacy and knowledge, for example, and invite new kinds of discrimination. Each scientific and social advance seems likely to bring its own ethical issues.

Similarly, science may eventually allow us to identify and explain states of mental disorder with reference to specific biological markers and underlying causes, thus eliminating much of the negativity, mystery and fear presently surrounding them. Yet some of the systemic prejudice and stigma attaching to such states seem likely to remain as long as our cultural values are unchanged, values which include autonomy, rationality, self-control, personal identity and psychological integrity. With roots deep in the Greek origins of Western culture, these values are entrenched, long lived and antithetical to the ravages wrought by mental disorder. Nothing less than the elimination of these states through prevention and cure, it would seem, could entirely end the negativity attaching to them.

---

[55] Department of Health and Human Services. 1999. *Report of the Surgeon General's Conference on Children's Mental Health: A National Action Agenda.* http://www.surgeongeneral.gov/cmh/childreport.htm#panl
[56] C. Murray & A. Lopez. 1996. *The Global Burden of Disease.* Cambridge MA. Harvard University Press.
[57] Peele and Chodoff, *op. cit.* note 7.
[58] R.J. Bonnie, J. Monahan, eds. 1997. *Mental Disorder, Work Disability, and the Law.* Chicago. University of Chicago Press.

Chapter 8

FEMALE GENITAL MUTILATION AND COSMETIC SURGERY: REGULATING NON-THERAPEUTIC BODY MODIFICATION[1]

SALLY SHELDON[2] AND STEPHEN WILKINSON[3]

INTRODUCTION

In this paper, our aim is to take seriously the reported anger of members of some communities at the prohibition of female genital mutilation in the face of the popular acceptance and toleration of other, Western practices involving harm to the individual.[4] This concern is expressed forcefully by Lois Bibbings, who notes a lack of consistency in the legal treatment of what might appear to be similar procedures. She argues that:

> . . . any legal regulation of body-altering practices should be consistent. In addition if restrictions are to be imposed, they should be constructed according to valid health concerns and should treat the practices according to the risks involved, rather than merely enforcing dominant notions of the acceptable body.[5]

[1] We are grateful to Doris Buss, Eve Garrard, Nick Dearden, David McNaughton, and Michael Thomson.
[2] Department of Law, University of Keele, UK.
[3] Department of Philosophy, University of Keele, UK.

[4] Speaking of Western 'horror and outrage' towards female genital mutilation, James notes that 'of course a non-Western woman might react similarly to the excesses of cosmetic surgeon (in, for example, California)', see Stephen James, 'Reconciling international human rights and cultural relativism: the case of female circumcision', *Bioethics* 8 (1994) pp. 1–26. See also Rhoda Howard cited in Lois Bibbings, 'Touch: socio-cultural attitudes and legal responses to body alteration', in *Law and the Senses*, ed. Lionel Bentley and Leo Flynn, London: Pluto, 1996, pp. 176–198; Alison Slack, 'Female circumcision: a critical appraisal', *Human Rights Quarterly* 10 (1988) pp. 437–486, at p. 463; Isabelle Gunning, 'Arrogant perception, world travelling and multicultural feminism: the case of female genital surgeries', *Columbia Journal of Human Rights Law Review* 23 (1991), pp. 189–248, at p. 213; Sandra Lane and Robert Rubinstine, 'Judging the other: responding to traditional female genital surgeries', *The Hastings Center Report*, 26 (1996), pp. 31–41.
[5] Bibbings, 'Touch', p. 188.

Careful attention must be paid to such arguments in multi-cultural democracies which pride themselves on laws which are fair and free of racial prejudice. In such a context, extra care and sensitivity is needed when governments legislate to outlaw the traditional practices of particular ethnic groups.

Our strategy in this paper will be to analyse whether the kinds of principles and arguments used to justify a general ban on female genital mutilation ought (if accepted in the case of female genital mutilation) to lead us to ban certain other widely accepted practices. Specifically, we shall deal with one example which seems particularly pertinent and topical: cosmetic surgery. This focus is suggested by the fact that those who have made the charge that prohibiting female genital mutilation may lay Western governments open to charges of 'cultural imperialism' often cite permissive attitudes towards cosmetic surgery as evidence of hypocrisy or inconsistency. Other practices which might equally have provided relevant points of comparison (such as male circumcision, boxing and tattooing) are not considered here due to confines of space.

We will discuss only female genital mutilation as performed on consenting adult women. This focus may seem strange given that most such procedures are performed on girls below the age of eighteen. However, this is not always the case[6] and, for our purposes, the focus on adult women is important because Western liberal democracies have traditionally espoused the aim of protecting the freedom of action of the competent adult provided that she does no harm to others. For this reason, the fact that some countries have banned female genital mutilation even when requested by an *adult* woman is particularly striking. A further reason for this focus is that other countries have *not* taken this stance and have chosen to differentiate between adult women and girls who are below the age of majority. This point of divergence in itself merits further scrutiny. The issue of what children may consent to, or of what responsible adults may consent to on their behalf, must therefore remain the subject of another paper.

Before proceeding to the main body of our argument, we will provide a clearer idea of what exactly we mean by the terms 'female

---

[6] According to a Minority Rights Group report, the age at which female genital mutilation is performed varies from a few days old to shortly before the birth of the first child. Minority Rights Group, *Report 47: Female Circumcision, Excision and Infibulation*, 2nd edn, London: Minority Rights Group, 1985.

genital mutilation' and 'cosmetic surgery' and briefly outline their legal status.

FEMALE GENITAL MUTILATION AND COSMETIC SURGERY: DEFINITIONS AND LEGAL STATUS

Female genital mutilation

Female genital mutilation is a generic term used to encompass a number of practices involving surgical removal of parts of the female genital organs.[7] These practices are very old and form an important part of the customs and traditions of some communities. According to a UN report, female genital mutilation is practised in at least 25 countries in Africa and in a number of other countries.[8] The degree of surgery involved ranges from 'Sunna' circumcision (understood here as the removal of the prepuce and the tip of the clitoris), excision or clitoridectomy (which involves the removal of the clitoris and often the labia minora) to infibulation or pharaonic circumcision (which involves excision plus the removal of labia majora and the sealing of the two sides through stitching or natural fusion of scar tissue; what is left is a very smooth surface, and a small opening – sometimes no bigger than the head of a match – to permit urination and the passing of menstrual blood).[9]

The health implications of female genital mutilation have been well documented.[10] Immediate consequences may include haemorrhage, septicaemia, infection and acute pain. Later effects may

---

[7] These practices are also known as female circumcision or female genital modification. This terminology has itself been a point of fierce contestation and dispute. We have retained the more common term of female genital mutilation in this paper to emphasise the received distinction between it and the acceptable practice of cosmetic surgery (which term in itself implies the respectability of a clinical procedure performed under medical control).

[8] United Nations, *Human Rights Fact Sheet 23: Harmful Traditional Practices Affecting the Health of Women and Children*, Geneva: United Nations, 1995.

[9] In some societies, 'ritual' circumcision is practised, involving nothing more than the pricking of the clitoris to draw a drop of blood, see United Nations, ibid. This would seem to involve no serious physical harm to the girl and is probably not covered by the legislation in the countries discussed. Although this might be construed as falling within general provisions which prohibit acts which 'otherwise mutilate' the female genitalia (for example s.1(1) (a) of the *Female Circumcision Act*), this seems to us to be unlikely.

[10] See United Nations, ibid; Minority Rights Group, *Female Circumcision*, and Efua Dorkenoo, *Cutting the Rose: Female Genital Mutilation, the Practice and its Prevention*, London: Minority Rights Group, 1995, esp. pp. 13–27.

include keloid formation, infertility as a result of infection, dysmenorrhea, obstructed labour and fistula formation leading to incontinence in later life. There is a broad (though not complete) consensus that even comparatively mild forms of female genital mutilation normally result in decreased sexual pleasure for the woman or, at worst, any form of intercourse being extremely painful. It also seems probable that serious psychological harm may result from the procedure, although little research has been done on this question. The most serious health consequences result from infibulation, although cataclysmic haemorrhage can also occur during circumcision with the removal of the clitoris.[11] The health risks and complications associated with female genital mutilation will vary according to the skill of the operator, the gravity of the mutilation, the (lack of) hygiene of the conditions in which the procedure is performed and the extent to which the girl or woman struggles. It is impossible to estimate with any degree of accuracy the number of deaths world-wide which result from female genital mutilation since the operation is often performed secretly and a very small proportion of the cases of immediate complication reach hospital. Nevertheless, a Minority Rights Group Report asserts that hospital staff in all the areas concerned are very familiar with last minute and often hopeless attempts to save bleeding, terrified little girls.[12]

Female genital mutilation has provoked strong reactions from both Western commentators and writers in the countries from whence it originates. The practices have been attacked as brutalising and sexist – being designed to control women's sexuality and to ensure female virginity before marriage.[13] Such authors have condemned female genital mutilation as an 'unspeakable atrocity'[14] which is both harmful to the health of women[15] and a violation of their human rights.[16] Similar sentiments influenced the British Parliament in its decision to ban female genital mutilation. In the Parliamentary discussions of the *Prohibition of Female Circumcision Bilk*, female genital mutilation was described as 'barbaric' and

---

[11] United Nations, *Human Rights Fact Sheet, No. 23.*

[12] Minority Rights Group, *Female Circumcision*, p. 5.

[13] For an account of the reasons why female genital mutilation is performed see Dorkenoo, *Cutting the Rose*, esp. pp. 34–41.

[14] Mary Daly, *Gyn/Ecology: the Metaethics of Radical Feminism*, Boston: Beacon Press, 1978.

[15] United Nations, *Human Rights Fact Sheet 23.*

[16] Alison Slack, 'Female circumcision'.

"atrocious",[17] a "terrible violation"[18] which is "against all humanity, kindness, respect and love".[19] Although it was recognised that these practices would probably be deemed unlawful under existing common law,[20] it was felt that this should be put beyond doubt by the introduction of specific legislation.[21]

Cosmetic surgery

'Cosmetic surgery' comprises an even broader range of practices. A recent report in an English newspaper listed the following cosmetic surgical interventions which had been performed on just one patient: eye widening, liposuction on the jaw line, abdomen, knees and thighs, a facelift, chemical peels, silicone breast implants, nose operations, a temple lift, lower eye revision, permanent upper lip enlargement, more liposuction on hips, thighs and knees, plus other 'minor' procedures.[22] The negative health impact of cosmetic surgery remains the subject of some debate, with silicone implants exciting particular attention.

The working definition of cosmetic surgery which we will adopt is as follows: a surgical intervention is cosmetic if and only if its primary aim is to change the appearance of the patient. What this definition attempts to capture is the 'common sense' idea that what is distinctive about purely cosmetic surgery is that it is supposed to change *only the way the patient looks*. Other forms of surgery, on the other hand, normally aim to affect *the patient's physical health*. Of course, many interventions (e.g. treatment for burns) have cosmetic and non-cosmetic parts or aspects. Hence, the distinction between cosmetic and other interventions may not be terribly clear in practice. Furthermore, it can be argued that the distinction between affecting someone's looks and affecting her health is not just practically, but also conceptually shaky, since (arguably) looking a certain way (e.g. being 'disfigured' or scarred) can sometimes

---

[17] Baroness Masham of Ilton, H.L. Deb. Vol. 441, Col 685 (21 April 1983).

[18] Baroness Ewart-Biggs, H.L. Deb. Vol. 441, Col. 690 (21 April 1983).

[19] Lord Kennet, H.L. Deb. Vol. 441, Col. 675 (21 April 1983).

[20] Lord Hailsham, H.L. Deb. Vol. 441 Col. 676 (21 April 1983), Lord Trefgarne, H.L. Deb. Vol. 441, Col. 679 (21 April 1983). For discussion of this point see R.D. Mackay, 'Is female circumcision unlawful?', *Criminal Law Review* (1983) pp. 717–722.

[21] Marion Roe, H.C. Deb. Vol. 77, Col. 583 (19 April 1985). See also, Lord Trefgarne, H.L. Deb. Vol. 441, Col. 679 (21 April 1983).

[22] Esther Oxford, 'The woman who fights plastic surgeons', *Independent on Sunday*, 8 April 1994.

itself be a negative health state – one which could (at least in principle) be *cured* by cosmetic surgery. Also, cosmetic surgery is sometimes used as a means of improving someone's *mental* health, in which case it again seems to be deliberately health-affecting.

The law regulating female genital mutilation and cosmetic surgery

Over the past two years, New Zealand, Australia,[23] the United States of America[24] and Canada[25] have all introduced legislation to ban female genital mutilation within their jurisdictions. These reforms all follow in the footsteps of legislation introduced in the United Kingdom in 1985 and are very similar to it in form. Here we will take the 1985 Act as a paradigm example of the kind of statute which has been introduced.

In the United Kingdom, under s.1(1) of the *Prohibition of Female Circumcision Act* it is illegal:

a)   to excise, infibulate or otherwise mutilate the whole or any part of the labia majora or labia minora or clitoris of another person; or

b)   to aid, abet, counsel or procure the performance by another person of any of those acts on that other person's own body.

S.1(2) provides that an operation which would be covered by the above wording should not be deemed unlawful where it is performed by a doctor on the grounds that it is necessary for the

[23] Female genital mutilation was criminalised in New South Wales in 1994, in South Australia in 1995, and in Victoria in 1966. Consent is expressly ruled out as a defence.

[24] Having noted that 'such mutilation infringes upon the guarantees or rights secured by Federal and State law, both statutory and constitutional', the US Congress outlawed the performance of female genital mutilation on girls under 18 years of age, introducing a maximum penalty of up to five years imprisonment for those who perform it. This measure was introduced as part of the controversial *Illegal Immigration Reform and Immigrant Responsibility Act*, 1996. See *Reproductive Freedom News*, V, 17, 25 October 1996.

[25] In Canada, a new section 268 to the Criminal Code, provides that 'wounds or maims' includes to excise, infibulate or mutilate, in whole or in part, the labia majora, labia minora or clitoris of a person except where:

a)   a surgical procedure is performed, by a person duly qualified by provincial law to practice medicine, for the benefit of the physical health of a person or for the purpose of that person having normal reproductive functions or normal sexual appearance or function; or

b)   the person is at least eighteen years of age and there is no resulting bodily harm.

The law specifically provides that the consent of a young person shall have no effect, except where the procedure is covered by the above sections.

physical or mental health of the person on whom it is performed; or where it is performed by either a doctor or a midwife on a woman who is in labour or has just given birth for purposes connected with the labour or birth. Attempting to plug an obvious potential loophole in the legislation, s.2(2) provides that in determining whether such an operation is necessary for the woman's health, no account shall be taken of 'the effect on that person of any belief . . . that the operation is required as a matter of custom or ritual'.[26]

It is noteworthy that the UK legislation makes no distinction between adults and minors. This is different from the US Federal legislation which only applies to under-18s,[27] and the Canadian law which refuses to criminalise procedures where 'the person is at least eighteen years old and where there is no resulting harm'.

As far as cosmetic surgery is concerned, the picture is very different. In the countries discussed above, cosmetic surgery has traditionally remained a matter of little concern to the criminal law (at least where procedures are performed by a registered medical practitioner).[28] In some places, this may be beginning to change. Following a number of complaints from women who have had breast implants in the 1980s and early 1990s, the US Food and Drug Administration has banned the use of silicone implants for women who want them strictly for cosmetic reasons.[29] Other cosmetic surgical interventions remain widely available. In the United Kingdom, although *technically* it would seem that a strong legal argument might be produced to the effect that many cases of cosmetic surgery are unlawful,[30] in practice its legality is broadly accepted and it seems highly unlikely in the face of a well-established toleration of such practices as breast enhancements, plastic surgery and

---

[26] That this legislation has not succeeded in eradicating female genital mutilation in the United Kingdom is widely accepted. See, for example, J.A. Black and G.D. Debelle, 'Female genital mutilation in Britain', *British Medical Journal*, 310, 17 June 1995, pp. 1590–1592.

[27] This does not prevent individual states from introducing laws which prohibit female genital mutilation for adult women.

[28] In the UK there is no legal requirement for the medical practitioner to acquire any specific training in cosmetic surgery. A report in *The Independent on Sunday* estimated that one in four surgeons practising cosmetic surgery had no specialist training in plastic surgery (1 April 1994).

[29] Mark Tran, 'Breast implant firm files for bankruptcy', *The Guardian,* 16 May 1995.

[30] Gerald Dworkin's seminal paper on the law relating to organ transplantation argues that there are four conditions which an operation must fulfil if it is not to be deemed unlawful. One of these is that it must be therapeutic, i.e. it must be expressly for the patient's benefit. See Gerald Dworkin, 'The law relating to organ transplantation in England', *Modern Law Review* 33 (1970), p. 353.

liposuction, that the lawfulness of these procedures could be successfully challenged.

CAN THE DIFFERENTIAL TREATMENT OF FEMALE GENITAL MUTILATION AND COSMETIC SURGERY BE JUSTIFIED?

Having set out what we mean by both 'female genital mutilation'
and 'cosmetic surgery', we can now proceed to our central question:
can the differential legal treatment outlined above be justified? Is it
right to be broadly tolerant of the latter and extremely restrictive
towards the former? In the rest of this paper, then, we examine
whether there are any convincing *arguments* which could be produced in support of this difference in treatment. Although we recognise that the vast majority of female genital mutilations are
performed on girls who are below the age of eighteen, for the
reasons given above, from now on we focus solely on adult women.

Our starting assumption is that for both cosmetic surgery and
female genital mutilation, given the value commonly attached to
the liberty of the adult individual, the onus is on those who wish to
put limits on this to provide justifications for so doing. This is not
to doubt that there are some occasions when it is permissible for
the state to intervene to impose such restrictions. Rather, it is to
assert that when an intervention seeks to impose significant limitations on individual freedom, such an intervention must always be
carefully considered, rationally justified and fairly applied. Accordingly, in the rest of the paper, we examine the main arguments for
the prohibition of female genital mutilation, assessing in each case
both **(a)** whether the argument succeeds in justifying the ban on
female genital mutilation with regard to adult women and, if so, **(b)**
whether a parallel argument would also support a ban on cosmetic
surgery. We shall focus on the following four claims which are
commonly made in support of prohibition:

(i)   that no woman could validly consent to female genital
        mutilation;
(ii)   that female genital mutilation is an oppressive and sexist
        practice;
(iii)   that female genital mutilation should be banned because it
        involves the intentional infliction of injury;

(iv)   that female genital mutilation should be banned because it causes offence.

1. Consent

Can the decision to be circumcised even when all the facts and risks are known, be considered truly voluntary when the only alternative is to be ostracized for such aberration?[31]

Opponents of female genital mutilation have argued that only someone who was coerced, manipulated, or highly irrational would agree to undergo female genital mutilation and that, therefore, valid informed consent to it is, in practice, impossible. Similarly, others have pointed to the problems of education and access to the information necessary to make a valid decision and social pressure which may vitiate the woman's consent.[32] The kind of pressure envisaged may take two forms. It may either be *direct* pressure from friends and family who seek to persuade or force women to undergo female genital mutilation or, alternatively, it may be *indirect* pressure to conform to deep-rooted, internalised social expectations.

If the pressure envisaged in this kind of argument is of the first (direct) kind, however, surely this would justify appropriate safeguards to ensure that consent was valid, rather than a complete ban on all female genital mutilation procedures. A good example of such an alternative legal regime would be the UK regulations governing organ transplantation which impose specific safeguards to ensure that consent is valid and uncoerced where a living donor is genetically unrelated to the donee.[33] On the other hand, if the concern is with general social pressures to conform, is it sustainable simply to *assume* that *no* woman could *ever* rationally consent to female genital mutilation? Whilst the debates around female genital mutilation have typically focussed on the most serious forms of female genital mutilation, it is important to remember that some forms – such as 'Sunna' – are comparatively mild. And there is no doubt that the decision whether or not to have female genital mutilation may have important social consequences (such as seriously affecting one's marriage possibilities).

[31]   Slack, 'Female circumcision', p. 472.
[32]   Slack, ibid, p. 471.
[33]   *The Human Organ Transplants (Unrelated Persons) Regulations* (1989), SI No 2480. These conditions are set out in regulation 3.

In any case, if the claim that consent to these procedures can never be valid holds true, then it may also hold true for many forms of cosmetic surgery where the decision to have such surgery results from overt or covert social pressure to conform to certain physical ideals. In fact, just such a picture of cosmetic surgery has been painted by some feminist writers who have cast women who elect to be surgically altered as 'cultural dopes'.[34] Kathy Davis summarises this stream of feminist writing in the following way:

> [Cosmetic surgery] tends to be regarded as an extreme form of medical misogyny, producing and reproducing the pernicious and pervasive cultural themes of deficient femininity. Consequently, it is difficult to imagine that any woman of sound mind and/or correct principles would willingly submit to a practice like cosmetic surgery. . . .[35]

Davis herself goes on to argue that such a view of those women fails to understand their reasons for going ahead with cosmetic surgery which are much more to do with 'being ordinary', with 'taking one's life into one's hands' and with determining how much suffering is fair.[36] If this is true, however, might a similar argument not also be made for why some women might voluntarily choose to submit to female genital mutilation? In societies where this is an important rite of passage, a sign of belonging or a perceived rendering of the female genitals more aesthetic, might the decision to undergo female genital mutilation not be a rational, considered choice? Is it possible simply to *assume* that it can never be so?

Ultimately, the question of whether valid consent to female genital mutilation is possible depends on how demanding one's standards for valid consent are. If we adopt a less demanding standard, then it is likely that (given appropriate safeguards) valid consent to female genital mutilation will be a possibility. But if we adopt a more demanding standard, such that even very general social pressures to conform are taken to rule out the possibility of valid consent to female genital mutilation, then it is likely that many cases of cosmetic surgery will also turn out not to be genuinely consensual. Hence, the attempt to differentiate female genital mutilation

---

[34] Kathy Davis, 'Remaking the she-devil: a critical look at feminist approaches to beauty', *Hypatia* 6 (1991), pp. 21–43.
[35] Davis, ibid, p. 22.
[36] Davis, ibid.

from cosmetic surgery in terms of arguments about consent does not succeed.

2. An oppressive practice?

> Women are victims of outdated customs, attitudes and male prejudice. This results in negative attitudes of women about themselves. There are many forms of sexual oppression, but this particular one [female genital mutilation] is based on the manipulation of women's sexuality in order to assure male domination and exploitation.[37]

The second argument that we consider says that female genital mutilation should be prohibited as it is part of a set of oppressive practices and attitudes towards women. This is most strongly encapsulated in the feminist critique that female genital mutilation is part of the 'global subordination of women'.[38] Thus it has been noted that female genital mutilation is designed to ensure virginity before marriage and sexual fidelity after it largely by decreasing female sexual pleasure and, in the case of infibulation, by rendering penetrative intercourse impossible.[39] Further, as was seen above, female genital mutilation has serious health consequences for those women who undergo it. According to the proponents of this argument, the role of law should be to discourage and prevent such practices and attitudes for '[i]f women are to be considered as equal and responsible members of society, no aspect of their physical, psychological, or sexual integrity can be compromised'.[40]

However, simply to say that female genital mutilation is oppressive to women seems not to provide a clear way of differentiating female genital mutilation from other things which are widely tolerated. Feminist writers have argued that a variety of widely accepted practices – such as marriage, current arrangements regarding child care, employment practices, prostitution and pornography – are oppressive towards women. Indeed, to return to our example of cosmetic surgery, this has been criticised as a part of female sexual oppression, casting women as

---

[37] Raqiya Haji Abdalla Dualeh, cited in Dorkenoo, *Cutting the Rose*, p. 29.
[38] Toubia, 'Female genital mutilation', p. 232.
[39] See Minority Rights Group, *Female Circumcision*, and Slack, 'Female Circumcision'.
[40] Toubia, 'Female genital mutilation', p. 235.

... the victims of oppressive masculinist ideologies of feminine beauty that demanded slender but voluptuous shapes, faces unmarked by the passage of time, and, above all, an irrevocably white and upper-class appearance.[41]

Once again, without anything more it seems inconsistent to legislate against female genital mutilation but not cosmetic surgery. A supporter of the current legislative *status quo* might argue that female genital mutilation is more serious than cosmetic surgery, but this is untenable if one opposes the least serious forms of the former against the most painful and risky forms of the latter. So again, there seems to be no relevant difference between all those practices prohibited together under the label of female genital mutilation and all those broadly tolerated as cosmetic surgery.

3. The injury argument

'The point to grasp, for the needs of the legislator, is that all these procedures are mutilations, and that the operation assaults, and attempts to cancel, the womanhood of a person.'[42]

The next argument that we consider is that female genital mutilation is importantly different from cosmetic surgery in that whereas most forms of female genital mutilation either necessarily involve permanent injury or are very likely to do so, this is not true of most forms of cosmetic surgery. Before we can scrutinise this argument, however, we need to provide a definition of injury which will distinguish it from mere modification. One such account, which we shall accept for the purposes of this argument, is provided by Clouser, Culver and Gert who define 'malady' (a category which includes illness, disease and injury) as follows:

Individuals have a malady if and only if they have a condition, other than their rational beliefs and desires, such that they are incurring, or are at a significantly increased risk of incurring, a harm or evil (death, pain, disability, loss of freedom, or loss of pleasure) in the absence of a distinct sustaining cause.[43]

---

[41] Davis, 'Remaking the she-devil', p. 25. See also Naomi Wolf, *The Beauty Myth: How Images of Beauty are Used against Women*, London: Vintage, 1991.

[42] Lord Kennet, H.L. Deb. Vol. 441 Col. 673 (21 April 1983).

[43] K. Danny Clouser, Charles Culver, and Bernard Gert, 'Malady', in *What is Disease?* ed. James Humber and Robert Almeder, Totowa, New Jersey: Humana Press, 1997 pp. 173–218, at p. 190.

Female genital mutilation and injury

On this account, whether a particular type of female genital mutilation involves permanent injury depends chiefly on whether the woman suffers one or more of the 'evils' listed above.[44] Infibulation arguably involves increased risk of *all* of the evils which Clouser, Culver and Gert list. For the less serious procedures, loss of pleasure and loss of freedom and/or opportunity are those which are most likely to be involved and, for the purposes of this argument, we focus just on these two evils. With this in mind, it is useful to divide female genital mutilation into three broad categories:

(a) Operations which *either* prevent the woman from having sexual intercourse *or* make it difficult and/or painful for her to have sexual intercourse (and/or other sexual activities).
(b) Operations which make sexual intercourse less pleasurable than they would otherwise have been.
(c) Neither (a) nor (b); the capacity to have sexual intercourse and to derive pleasure from sexual activity is unimpaired.

Both category (a) operations and category (b) operations involve injury. Category (a) operations involve loss of freedom/opportunity and category (b) operations involve loss of pleasure.[45] Most types of female genital mutilation involve the removal of the clitoris, which most accept would result in the loss of physical pleasure.[46] As such, operations which include its removal necessarily fall into category (b) and are, therefore, the cause of permanent injury. Many types of female genital mutilation make it physically impossible (or at least *extremely* difficult and/or painful) for the woman to have sexual intercourse. The most serious of these is

[44] When considering the ban on female genital mutilation, we assume that if it (or some forms of it) were permitted, then it could be carried out only by qualified doctors in sterile conditions. Arguments regarding harm due to insanitary conditions provide justification for the regulation of those conditions and not complete prohibition.
[45] Many operations will fall into both (a) and (b), in which case they are injurious in two different respects.
[46] Views vary about the *exact* role of the clitoris, especially when it comes to the question of its role in orgasm. Some, like Koedt, claim that it is essential for orgasm; others warn against over-estimating its role in sexual pleasure. See Anne Koedt, 'The myth of the vaginal orgasm', in *Living with Contradictions: Controversies in Feminist Social Ethics*, ed. Alison Jaggar, Oxford: Westview Press, 1994, pp. 481–486.

infibulation, which is an injury which falls into category (a) and category (b).

The only type of female genital mutilation which may not involve necessary/permanent injury is Sunna (understood here as the removal of the prepuce or hood of the clitoris). For Sunna, there is not necessarily any *direct physical effect* on the woman's ability to have sexual intercourse, although this does not of course preclude the possibility of there being negative *indirect* effects on the woman's sexuality (through psychological harm). However, we can say that, leaving psychological damage aside, Sunna does not fall into category (a). Whether Sunna falls into category (b) is a disputed issue.[47] As such, all that we can say with any confidence about the question of whether Sunna is an injury is the following. *If* it results in loss of pleasure, then it falls into the same category as full-scale clitoris removal (although the *degree* of injury involved would almost certainly be less for Sunna). If, on the other hand, it results in no loss of pleasure then it is not an injury.

There is, then, a strong argument for the view that most forms of female genital mutilation do indeed involve injury. However, since the aim of the argument was to show that there are important differences between female genital mutilation and other practices which are permitted we need now to turn our attention back to cosmetic surgery.

Female genital mutilation, cosmetic surgery and the doctrine of double effect

Although purely cosmetic surgical interventions do sometimes *cause* permanent physical injury, their defenders may claim (with some empirical support) that these injuries are merely foreseen (i.e. unintended) side-effects. Here they might rely on the doctrine of double effect to justify the procedure. According to the doctrine of double effect, acts which produce a bad effect as well as a good one are permissible, provided that the following conditions are met:

---

[47] Some have claimed that Sunna can actually *increase* sexual pleasure, see Morayo Atoki, 'Should female circumcision continue to be banned?', *Feminist Legal Studies* 2 (1995), pp. 223–235, at p. 230.

(i)   the intended act is not *wrong or bad in itself*;
(ii)   the foreseen good consequences of the act are sufficiently good to outweigh the foreseen bad consequences;
(iii) the foreseen bad consequences are *not means* of achieving what the agent intends.

Applying this to the example of breast implants might work as follows. Assuming both that the main aim of the operation is to change the woman's appearance so as to make her more attractive and that there are long-term health risks associated with such implants, the surgeon can use the doctrine of double effect to justify performing the operation:

(a)   Is it intrinsically *wrong to insert breast implants?* Leaving aside some of the more extreme views based on the 'unnaturalness' of such interventions, almost certainly not.
(b)   Are the foreseen bad consequences of the act sufficiently bad to outweigh the foreseen good consequences? This will depend on the degree of risk and the benefits to be derived. But it certainly seems conceivable that there will be many such cases where the answer is no.
(c)   Is the (risk of) injury involved a means of achieving what is aimed at? Leaving aside temporary risks involved in the surgery itself, almost certainly not. Why? Because the aimed-for consequences (greater attractiveness) and the long-term risk are both effects of a common cause (inserting the implants). Therefore, the former does not cause the latter and is, hence, not a means of achieving the latter.

Can defenders of female genital mutilation employ a similar strategy? They might argue that we can distinguish clearly between those effects that are aimed at and those that are merely foreseen. The aims involved will normally be socio-cultural (e.g. improved chances of marriage) or perhaps just aesthetic. Any injury is a mere *side*-effect foreseen but unintended.

However, there are serious problems with attempting to use the doctrine of double effect to justify female genital mutilation in this way. More specifically, most cases of female genital mutilation are likely to fall foul of condition (iii): injuring the woman is normally a *means* of achieving what is intended. For example, in the case of clitoridectomy, it seems clear that the removal of the clitoris is the *means of achieving* the intended increased social acceptability. And since (as previously established) this removal constitutes an injury, injuring the woman is a means. Hence, the doctrine of double effect will not work to justify female genital mutilation in such a case.[48]

We seem, then, to have discovered at least the first steps in an argument which will (if ultimately successful) justify differential legal treatment of cosmetic surgery and female genital mutilation. More specifically, there appear to be two (related) differences between cosmetic surgery and female genital mutilation. First, cosmetic surgery does not normally aim to inflict an injury, whereas female genital mutilation can and often does. Second, while both cosmetic surgery and female genital mutilation may *cause* injury, cosmetic surgery can (in such cases) normally be justified by using the doctrine of double effect; this is not true of female genital mutilation. However, although these first moves in the injury argument look promising, it ultimately fails for reasons that we shall now discuss.

---

[48] There is a further objection to the injury argument which is worth mentioning briefly here. Defenders of female genital mutilation might argue as follows. The relevant action (for the purposes of applying the doctrine of double effect) is removing the clitoris. This has some good effects (such as social benefits) and some bad effects (for example, loss of pleasure). The good effects are aimed at and the bad effects are not. Further, the bad effects are *side-effects* and *not means* of achieving the good effects, since both are effects of a common cause (removing the clitoris). Hence (provided that the good effects are sufficiently good) the doctrine of double effect is as applicable to female genital mutilation as it is to cosmetic surgery.

There seem to be two problems with this line of argument. The first is that, in at least some cases, loss of pleasure and/or opportunity (to have sexual intercourse) may in fact be *means* of achieving the social goods in question (and not, therefore, mere side-effects) because they are the very features of female genital mutilation which make it attractive. For example, infibulated women might be thought of as more desirable precisely *because* they have been unable to have vaginal intercourse. The second is that there seems to be the following difference between female genital mutilation and cosmetic surgery. To remove a woman's clitoris (in the kind of cases under consideration) is identical with (and not merely a cause of) her being injured, since it is (arguably) impossible for her to undergo the procedure without suffering one or more of the relevant evils (most obviously loss of pleasure). This, however, is not true of most forms of cosmetic surgery, since it is quite possible (in principle) to have one's appearance modified without being permanently injured. And even when people complain about the alleged dangers of cosmetic surgery, this is almost always in terms of its side-effects (the argument being that the risk of serious side-effects is significant enough to outweigh any cosmetic benefits accrued).

Of course, for this point to go through, one would have to think quite carefully about what sorts of practices might properly be called cosmetic surgery. For example, things like a 'cosmetically motivated' amputation of a limb would fall into the same category as female genital mutilation, since they are necessarily injurious. However, it seems that most real examples of cosmetic surgery are ones which are not necessarily injurious and where there is, at worst, a risk of injurious side-effects.

We would like to thank one of our anonymous referees for suggesting this line of argument.

A 'holistic' conception of injury?

One further objection to the injury argument is that, in deciding whether female genital mutilation necessarily involves injury, it takes into account an *unduly narrow* range of considerations. As was seen above, according to the injury argument, most forms of female genital mutilation involve injury, because they modify the woman's body in a way which causes her to have less pleasure and opportunity than she otherwise would have. However, defenders of female genital mutilation may argue as follows. They might concede that other things being equal, procedures like clitoridectomy and infibulation result in a reduction in pleasure and opportunity. Nonetheless, they might argue, other things are most certainly *not* equal. More specifically, undergoing female genital mutilation may, due to social attitudes and customs, provide the woman with a range of *additional* opportunities and pleasures which she would not otherwise have had (e.g. those related to marriage prospects). And if we take these social advantages into account, then there will turn out to be some (perhaps many) cases in which female genital mutilation generates a net gain in pleasure and opportunity. If we accept that there are some cases where these additional social benefits outweigh the direct physical harms *and* we accept that a modification is an injury only if it leads to an *overall net decrease* in pleasure and opportunity, then the claim that female genital mutilation involves injury will turn out to be false. For although it is true that it always involves, as it were, *prima facie* injury, whether it *really* involves injury, all things considered, will depend in each case on the extent to which the woman gains other social benefits.

However, this attempt to include social attitudes as considerations which partially determine whether an intervention is an injury is itself problematic, for there is a danger that the concept of injury will be collapsed into the more general concept of harm. To illustrate this, consider the following case:

> A and B are soldiers in a highly dangerous combat situation. Their chances of being seriously injured or killed in battle are extremely high. B asks A to shoot her. That way, B gets to be taken to a hospital in a safe area and her chances of serious injury or death will be dramatically reduced. Does A injure B?

Although in this case A clearly does something which benefits B, surely this is a paradigm case of injury? Shooting someone in the leg is injuring them, no matter what extrinsic social benefits they derive from that injury. What cases like this show is that, when considering the relationship between injury and general welfare, we have a basic choice to make. Either we can be *holists* about injury, adopting a *wide* conception of it which says that someone is injured only if they are harmed overall. Or we can adopt a *narrow* conception of injury, according to which injury may on occasion be good for an individual, all things considered. The wide conception includes in it social factors so that someone who is *prima facie* injured may turn out not to be when we weigh in social advantages of the 'injury'. On the narrow conception, though, cases like this would be described as ones where, although the individual really is injured, they have nevertheless benefitted overall. In short, the narrow conception allows there to be cases where being injured is good for you, whereas the wide conception does not. Those who suggest the injury argument as a way of distinguishing between cosmetic surgery and female genital mutilation need to choose between these two conceptions and whichever option they choose they face problems.

If they adopt a wide conception of injury, then their central premise – that female genital mutilation necessarily involves injury – will turn out to be false, since there are possible (and probably actual) cases in which the 'social' benefits of female genital mutilation outweigh the 'health' disbenefits. And in such cases, according to the wide conception, the individual is not injured. If, on the other hand, they adopt the narrow conception, then it does seem to us that their central premise is true. However, they then face a new problem. Namely, is it really plausible to suppose that intentionally injuring someone (in the narrow sense) is wrong and should be banned, even in those cases where it is in the injured person's interests to be injured?

There are two problems with this supposition. First, what normally motivates the view that injury is wrong is a thought about harm. Injuring normally amounts to harming (overall) and so goes against supposed duties of non-maleficence. However, if a desire to prohibit harming is what drives the prohibition on injury, it is hard to see why this should cover *all* injuries and, in particular, why it should be extended to cover injuries which are (overall) good for the injured person. It is unclear why we need to invoke the concept of injury at all if what we are trying to avoid is harm. Why not just prohibit harm?

The second problem is that committing ourselves to the view that injury (even when not harmful) should be prohibited will lead to extremely counter-intuitive results in other areas. One case in point is vasectomy. Like some forms of female genital mutilation, vasectomy seems to amount to the deliberate infliction of a permanent injury (narrowly conceived) in that it leads to a loss of opportunity (the opportunity to reproduce) and to a failure to function of part of the reproductive system.[49] However, providing vasectomies is normally thought to be justified because it provides a range of *social* opportunities and goods which are thought to outweigh significantly any *prima facie* harm inflicted. What cases like this show is that if we combine (i) the narrow conception of injury with (ii) the view that injurious practices should be banned, then we will be committed to an unpalatably restrictive view of many widely accepted practices.[50]

The injury argument: final conclusion

The injury argument ultimately fails. Either its proponents must adopt a wide conception of injury in which case their central claim about the difference between female genital mutilation and cosmetic surgery (that the former almost always involves an injury) is probably false. Or they must adopt the narrow conception, in which case they would have to hold that deliberately injuring should be prohibited, even if it is in the interests of the injured person. This latter assertion seems unsustainable given that (a) it is unmotivated (in particular, unsupported by thoughts about non-maleficence) and (b) it would lead to absurdly restrictive policies in other areas.

---

[49] The possibility of reversal, of course, makes vasectomy less serious. However, its effects are still permanent in the weaker sense: i.e. without further restorative intervention, the effects will persist.

[50] An interesting parallel is provided by the British Medical Association's guidance for doctors on male circumcision, which suggests that even if the practice does involve a minor injury (in the narrow sense) it may, in any case, be justified in terms of its social benefits: 'The practice of [male] circumcision has previously been considered to be morally neutral, that is, no harm was caused to the child . . . The neutrality of the procedure, however, is now being increasingly challenged although it is argued that it is in the best interest of the child to be circumcised, to be accepted into a religion or community. Arguably the procedure can confer social benefits in some such circumstances.' British Medical Association, *Circumcision of Male Infants: Guidance for Doctors*, (BMA: September 1996), p. 2.
Available at http://www.cirp.org/CIRP/library/statements/bma/ (26th June 1997).

4. Arguments from offence

> Migrant settlement is a process of give and take. If Australia finds a certain folk custom repulsive, a migrant has the duty to give this custom away. This is the price to pay for our common good.[51]

> The degree of abhorrence of these procedures felt by all can leave no room for uncertainty.[52]

The next type of argument we consider is based on the idea that female genital mutilation is somehow offensive in a way that cosmetic surgery is not. Therefore, if we accept that one proper function of the law is to protect the public from harms caused or constituted by offence, there seems to be a compelling argument for banning female genital mutilation, but not cosmetic surgery, since only the former harms the public (by disturbing and/or offending them).

The main problem with what one might call arguments from *actual* offence is that they can generate highly counter-intuitive conclusions. For if the *mere* fact that most people are offended by the existence of a practice is supposed to justify a ban on that practice, then given (for example) a widespread taboo regarding geriatric sexual intercourse, such an argument could be used to justify banning sex between (say) people in their seventies. Indeed, arguments from actual offence could be used to justify bans on *absolutely anything* (provided of course that enough people were offended) and we take this to be a decisive objection to arguments of this type.

There may, however, be a more acceptable kind of argument, one which says that we are justified in banning a practice if enough people are offended by it and if their offence is *reasonable* or *rational*. These arguments (which we shall term *arguments from reasonable offence*) are not vulnerable to the criticism just levelled at arguments from actual offence. For since (we presume) it would be unreasonable to be seriously offended by the existence of geriatric sex, arguments from reasonable offence would not justify banning

---

[51] Australian Legislative Council (21 February 1994) cited in David Fraser, 'The first cut is (not) the deepest: deconstructing "female genital mutilation" and the criminalization of the other', *Dalhousie Law Journal* 2 (1995), pp. 310–379, at p. 351.

[52] Marion Roe, H.C. Deb. Vol. 77, Col. 583 (19 April 1985). See also, Lord Trefgarne, H.L. Deb. Vol. 441, Col. 679 (21 April 1983).

it. Arguments from reasonable offence are, therefore, worth taking seriously.

The issue of whether or not there is such an argument for banning female genital mutilation hinges on two questions. First, are enough people seriously offended by its existence? And second, if there are enough such people, is their offence reasonable or rational? Let us grant that the answer to the first of these questions is yes. Then, the question of whether there is an offence-based argument which would justify banning female genital mutilation (while permitting cosmetic surgery) comes down to the question of whether it is reasonable for society to be offended by the existence of female genital mutilation.[53]

Once the argumentative state of play is viewed in this light, though, the argument from offence, which was at the outset supposed to be an *independent* argument for banning female genital mutilation seems to have lost all of its force and interest. For in order to know whether the argument from offence is sound, we also need to know (in advance, as it were) whether or not it is reasonable to be offended by the existence of female genital mutilation. There is, of course, an important distinction between being offended by *seeing* a particular practice and being offended by its *mere existence* and, here, by virtue of the nature of the procedure under discussion, we assume that it is only the latter which is relevant.[54] Since we are concerned here not with the kind of offence that one might have if one actually witnessed female genital mutilation but with the kind of offence someone might feel just by knowing that this practice existed in her country, we are presumably dealing with what might be termed *moral* offence – the feeling that such practices are deeply wrong and should not therefore be tolerated even in private.

What would make moral offence of this kind reasonable? Well, since providing a general account of reasonableness would be an enormous task, outside the scope of our present project, let us instead suggest just three ways (there are doubtless others) in which such offence might be *un*reasonable.

---

[53] We assume here that there is *not* an offence-based argument available for a ban on cosmetic surgery, simply because not enough people are seriously offended by it.

[54] In any case, even if one accepts arguments from reasonable offence, it is only reasonable offence of the second, 'even in private' kind which legitimates a *complete ban* on a practice. Offence of the first kind would only serve to justify restrictions on the circumstances under which the practice takes place (e.g. not in public).

1. It involves inconsistency, or arises from attitudes which are themselves inconsistent.
2. It is based on a false belief.
3. It is based on an ignorance of relevant facts and arguments.

Now precisely what all the *other* arguments in this paper are about are these things. Is someone who adopts very different moral stances towards cosmetic surgery and female genital mutilation being inconsistent? Is the desire to ban female genital mutilation based on a false belief (be that a non-moral, empirical mistake, or a moral one)? And are there arguments and facts which, if articulated, would provide compelling reasons for *not* treating cosmetic surgery and female genital mutilation as importantly different? So the problem with the argument from (reasonable) offence is this. *Either* it must just *assume* that all of these questions are to be answered in the negative, in which case it is hopelessly question-begging. *Or* it must involve tackling head-on all of the other arguments in this paper and, in so doing, lose all of its *independent* argumentative force.

We conclude, then, that even if we accept arguments from reasonable offence, they cannot add anything to this particular debate, since in order to know whether or not the offence in question was reasonable, we would need in any case to address all of the other arguments concerning the issue. If those arguments successfully showed why female genital mutilation (but not cosmetic surgery) should be banned, then the argument from offence may be sound. But it could only be known to be sound if we, in effect, no longer needed it – i.e. if some *other* argument had already been produced which showed why female genital mutilation was wrong and, therefore, why being morally offended by female genital mutilation was reasonable. And in this paper we have failed to find such an argument.

CONCLUSIONS: TOWARDS A CONSISTENT LEGAL FRAMEWORK?

In this paper we have attempted, and failed, to find any rationally sustainable means of legitimating the current legal *status quo* in a number of Western countries which prohibit all forms of female genital mutilation whilst being extremely tolerant of cosmetic surgery. This does not lead to any inevitable conclusion regarding policy recommendations other than to suggest that more careful thought be given to precisely why female genital mutilation is illegal for adult women, and if these reasons would not also provide justification for outlawing certain forms of cosmetic surgery.

In the absence of statutory intervention, both female genital mutilation and cosmetic surgery would have been regulated by the law of assault and battery. In the UK, doctrine provides that one can only agree to an operation which *prima facie* constitutes an injury when it is performed by a doctor with the patient's consent and is in the patient's best interests.[55] Thus the legality of any cosmetic surgical intervention or female genital mutilation would rely on a delicate legal balancing act, involving weighing the benefits to be derived from surgery against any risks and/or negative side-effects.[56] On this test, it seems probable that most forms of female genital mutilation (bar ritual circumcision and possibly 'Sunna' practised on adult women) would be deemed unlawful. And much cosmetic surgery would no doubt be seen as lawful, being justified by reason of the patient's mental health.[57] It seems highly unlikely, however, that this would be true for all cosmetic surgery procedures such as repeated face lifts and tummy tucks for individuals who are in no way beyond the range of the normal but merely want to improve their appearance for aesthetic reasons.

What a reversion to the common law position might achieve would be a challenging of the perception that female genital mutilation and cosmetic surgery are *fundamentally* different and the situating of both on a continuum of body modification practices.[58] Whether this would change the differential legal treatment they would receive in practice, however, remains debatable in the light of

---

[55] Dworkin, 'The law relating to organ transplantation in England'.

[56] It is probable from the case law regulating the removal of organs from live donors, that the courts would adopt here what we described above as a 'holistic' conception of injury. See *Strunk* v. *Strunk* (1969) 445 SW 2d 145 (Ky CA) and *Re Y* [1996] 2 FLR 791 allowing the removal of an organ from a live donor who is incapable of giving valid legal consent because of age or mental incapacity. In both of these cases, the benefit to the donor is described in psychological/emotional terms.

[57] For example, this might cover both the case for plastic surgery for a patient who was horribly disfigured as a result of an accident and felt unable to leave the house and face other people as a result, and a breast enhancement operation for a woman who suffered a severe lack of self-confidence due to a gross disparity between the size of her breasts.

[58] See Bibbings, 'Touch'.

the following statement, made *obiter dicta* in a recent decision of the House of Lords:

> Even when violence is intentionally afflicted and results in serious bodily harm the accused is entitled to be acquitted if the injury was a foreseen incident of a lawful activity in which the person injured was participating. Surgery involves intentional violence resulting in serious bodily harm but surgery is a lawful activity. Other activities carried on with consent by or on behalf of the injured person have been accepted as lawful not withstanding that they involve actual bodily harm or may cause serious bodily harm. Ritual [male] circumcision, tattooing, ear-piercing and violent sports including boxing are lawful activities.[59]

This seems to suggest that the courts' treatment of body modification practices may be no more consistent or rationally justifiable than that of the legislature.

---

[59] Per Lord Templeman, *R* v. *Brown* [1993] 2 All ER 75.

PART III: JUST HEALTH CARE

Chapter 9

PATENTS AND ACCESS TO DRUGS IN DEVELOPING COUNTRIES: AN ETHICAL ANALYSIS

SIGRID STERCKX

I. INTRODUCTION

The debate on the advisability of (certain aspects of) the patent system has a very long and turbulent history. The introduction of the WTO-TRIPs Agreement (1994) – which implies the quasi-worldwide implementation of high standards for the legal protection and enforcement of intellectual property rights, including patents – has by no means quieted down this debate, but rather, has intensified it. At the WTO, as well as in various other forums, a remarkable debate is going on about the potential impact of patents on access to health care. In August 2000, the UN Commission on the Promotion and Protection of Human Rights adopted a resolution declaring that there are apparent conflicts between the TRIPs regime, on the one hand, and human rights (including the right to health) on the other. Other commentators consider the property right of patent holders as a human right and argue for a further strengthening of those rights. Yet others, who do not frame the problem in terms of rights, defend patents with economic arguments or by invoking fairness. The main question of concern in this paper is to what extent these different arguments can justify the practice of patenting drugs, particularly in developing countries.

II. SOME FACTS ABOUT PATENTS IN THE TRIPS ERA

Patents form an example of intellectual property rights, next to, *inter alia*, copyrights and trade marks. A patent is a certificate delivered by or on behalf of the government, attesting that the object of the patent meets a number of requirements. The substantial requirements for patentability are novelty, inventiveness, utility and sufficient disclosure of the invention in the patent application.

The rights of patent holders are limited in two ways. Firstly, by time: in most countries a patent is valid for twenty years (counted from the date of application). Secondly, by space: its validity is limited to the jurisdiction of the Patent Office that granted the patent.

In the early 1980s, various industrial lobbies in the US reported enormous losses, which they attributed to infringements of their intellectual property rights (IPRs).[1] These infringements were said to be due to the 'inadequate' legal protection of IPRs in developing countries. Many developing countries note, however, that: (1) the evolution of IPR protection in industrialised countries has always been determined by what these countries regard as their national interest; and (2) in view of their economic development objectives, developing countries need lower protection standards.

In the traditional forum for intellectual property negotiations, the *World Intellectual Property Organisation* (WIPO), the developing countries were considered too influential (in number) by some industrialised countries. Therefore, the US, later followed by others, pushed for the introduction of the intellectual property topic on the agenda of the General Agreement on Tariffs and Trade (GATT).[2] After seven years of hard talks in the so-called *Uruguay Round* of GATT negotiations came about the TRIPs agreement (*Agreement on Trade-Related Aspects of Intellectual Property Rights*).[3] The TRIPs agreement significantly strengthens patent protection standards, and of course reduces the sovereign power of decision of national governments.

In the industrialised countries, TRIPs came into effect on January 1, 1996. In developing countries going through a transitional phase from a planned economy to a market economy, the Agreement entered into force on January 1, 2000. The so-called 'least-developed countries' were given respite until January 1, 2006.

---

[1] See e.g.: US International Trade Commission. 1988. *Foreign Protection of Intellectual Property Rights and the Effects on the US Industry and Trade*. Publication No. 2065.
[2] See e.g.: C.A.P. Braga. The Economics of Intellectual Property Rights and the GATT: A View from the South. *Vanderbilt Journal of Transnational Law* 1989; 22: 243–264.
[3] GATT Secretariat, ed. 1994. Annex 1C: Agreement on Trade-Related Aspects of Intellectual Property Rights. In *The Results of the Uruguay Round of Multilateral Trade Negotiations. The Legal Texts*. Geneva. WTO: 365–403. Also available at: docsonline.wto.org/DDFDocuments/t/UR/FA/27-trips.doc

During the WTO's ministerial conference held in Doha in November 2001, the decision was made to extend this transitional period with respect to the introduction of patents on pharmaceutical products to January 1, 2016.

The WTO-TRIPs Agreement heralds a fundamentally new era for developing countries. In the pharmaceutical sector a product patent refers to the chemical structure of a drug.[4] The final product (the actual drug) is protected, regardless of how it was manufactured and of the purpose it serves. Not surprisingly, a product patent is the most coveted form of protection. Process patents offer protection for the way in which the final product is made and for the way in which the product is used to reach certain goals (e.g. the treatment of specific diseases). A process patent offers a 'strong' form of protection only if there is no other (financially sound) way of producing the product in question, other than through the process covered by the patent. In the pharmaceutical sector, this is rarely the case.

Developing countries generally offer less substantial protection for patents than industrialised countries. Many developing countries have traditionally excluded pharmaceutical products from patent protection; only processes for the production of pharmaceuticals could be patented. The rationale of such a policy is to guarantee that the local industry can play a significant role in the manufacturing of pharmaceuticals. With the same objective in mind, most developing countries have traditionally quasi-automatically imposed a regime of so-called compulsory licences on patented inventions in the pharmaceutical domain. In almost every country that has a patent system, mechanisms exist to remedy or prevent abuses of patent rights. A very important instrument used to that effect is the compulsory licence.[5] The granting of compulsory licences implies that – after an administrative or judicial procedure – the government forces a patent holder to grant a licence to one or more third party/ies for the use of his patented product or process. The patent holder receives a royalty. In the context of the patent system, compulsory licences have a double aim: on the one hand to force the patent owner to allow society to benefit from

[4] P. Grubb. 1999. *Patents for Chemicals, Pharmaceuticals and Biotechnology*. Oxford. Clarendon Press.

[5] J-M. Salamolard. 1978. *La licence obligatoire en matière de brevets d'invention. Etude de droit comparé*. Genève. Librairie Droz.

his invention, and on the other hand to boost the industrialisation of the country in question. The basic principle of the system of compulsory licences is that they are only granted in the public interest. The rights ensuing from the possession of a compulsory licence are similar to those ensuing from the possession of a patent, except that compulsory licences have to be granted predominantly to supply the domestic market of the country that grants them.[6]

As a result of the implementation of the TRIPs Agreement, it becomes increasingly difficult – and probably even impossible – for developing countries to pursue a 'selective' patent granting policy, certainly as far as pharmaceuticals are concerned. Drugs cannot be excluded from patentability under TRIPs. For many developing countries the implementation of TRIPs in their national laws represents a major upheaval. This may have a profoundly negative impact on the access to drugs of people in these countries, while hundreds of millions of people already have no access to drugs.

What could possibly justify the quasi-worldwide introduction of such strong patent protection standards?

III. ON WHICH GROUNDS CAN DRUG PATENTS BE MORALLY JUSTIFIED?

Attempts to construct a moral justification of the patent system have been based on three grounds: (1) natural rights; (2) distributive justice; and (3) utilitarian (economic) arguments. Each of these attempts involves many problems. After briefly discussing the general argument, we will, for each of the three, investigate its implications for the justifiability of drug patents.

Natural rights

Some people believe that man has a natural right to his ideas and consequently that society is obliged to enforce that right. Thus, the use of ideas without the authorisation of the owner must be considered as theft. Natural property rights take precedence over social institutions and should be respected whatever the consequences.

---

[6] See art. 31(f) TRIPs.

Discussions on the natural rights argument generally refer to John Locke's 'labour theory of property.'[7] Although Locke seems to identify property with land, various commentators have applied his theory to other types of goods, including 'intangible' objects. According to Locke, the appropriation of a thing occurs by man applying his labour to it, by 'mixing' the thing with his labour. By adding something of his own to the thing, he excludes others from having a right to it.

If we look at the implications of this theory for the justification of drug patents, the main question seems to be: how much 'labour' is really involved in the research and development (R&D) of drugs? The greater part of pharmaceutical R&D budgets is spent on 'me-too' drugs – the slightly altered versions of successful products manufactured by the competition. The *American Food and Drug Administration* (FDA), for example, classifies the applications it receives either as 'priority drugs' (considered a significant improvement in relation to the existing drugs) and 'standard drugs' (considered similar to existing products). Of all drugs approved by the FDA over the past six years, almost 80% belong to the standard drug category. As a large-scale survey by the *National Institute for Health Care Management Foundation* (May 2002) shows, the ratio between priority-rated drugs and standard-rated drugs within this group of approved drugs is constantly shifting towards less priority-rated drugs and more standard-rated drugs.[8] The development of such drugs is not 'labour-intensive' (if 'labour' is understood as creative intellectual labour). Also, in view of the patentability requirement of inventiveness, the granting of patents for such drugs seems hard to justify.

Locke stipulated two conditions or 'provisos' which must be met in order for an appropriation (i.e. establishment of a property right) to be justifiable. Firstly, there must be 'enough, and as good left in common for others.'[9] Secondly, man is not allowed to appropriate more than he can use (even if he is the 'maker' of the things in question); there should be no waste.[10]

Robert Nozick has applied Locke's first proviso to the rights granted by a patent. For him, 'The crucial point is whether

[7] Which he formulated in his *Second Treatise on Government* (1690). See: P. Laslett, ed. 1988. *Locke, Two Treatises of Government*. Cambridge. Cambridge University Press: 285–302.

[8] Available at: http://www.nihcm.org/innovations.pdf.

[9] Laslett, *op. cit.* note 7, § 27.

[10] Laslett, *op. cit.* note 7, § 31.

appropriation . . . worsens the situation of others.'[11] He thinks this is not necessarily so, and provides the following example:

> If I appropriate a grain of sand from Coney Island, no one else may now do as they will with *that* grain of sand. But there are plenty of other grains of sand left for them to do the same with. Or if not grains of sand, then other things.[12]

In the case of patents, Nozick's arguments may not be tenable, *inter alia* for the following two reasons. As to the statement that enough objects will remain for others to use, this is clearly not valid for any thing protected by a patent. Any product or process that fits what is described in the patent's claims is also covered by the patent, including 'equivalent' (as opposed to identical) products or processes. With regard to Nozick's proposition that, if not enough samples of an appropriated object remain for others to use plenty of other objects will be available to them, this is irrelevant if they need that specific object, as is often the case with drugs.

As to Locke's second condition – the 'non-waste' condition – one aspect of the patent system which can induce waste is the fact that, in its present form, the system does not oblige patent holders to exploit their invention. If something is left unused by the one who appropriated it, while others need it – and drugs are examples of things that are often truly needed by a whole lot of people – the waste is all the greater. (Of course, in a system based on natural rights, the essence of the patent right exists in the patent proprietor determining what happens with the object of the patent. Thus, he cannot be forced to exploit his invention.) But even if a patent *is* exploited, waste is likely to occur. Indeed, the main consequence of issuing a patent is that the patent holder can limit the use of the invention. The extent of the waste depends on the utility of the invention for those who are excluded from using it. The utility of drugs, particularly essential drugs,[13] is often very high.

---

[11] R. Nozick. 1974. *Anarchy, State, and Utopia*. Oxford. Basil Blackwell: 175.

[12] Ibid.

[13] I do not understand the concept of 'essential drugs' as 'drugs that appear on the World Health Organization's essential drug list.' As some defenders of strong drug patents like to note, more than 95% of the drugs on that list are off-patent. However, the reason for this seems to be that a drug must be 'affordable' in order to get on the list, and patented drugs are usually expensive. But of course the fact that a drug is expensive does not necessarily prevent it from being 'essential' (in the sense of badly needed by a group of patients).

Distributive justice

According to the distributive justice argument, fairness requires that inventors be rewarded because they render a service to society. It would be unfair to allow people a 'free ride' at the expense of others who apply themselves to the act of inventing. Free riders – people who did not invest time or money in the development of an invention – should not be allowed to compete with the inventor under normal market conditions. Therefore society should grant exclusive rights to inventors.

When examined in the context of the justification of drug patents, this argument, too, seems problematic. First, the question arises whether fairness does not also require an equal access to drugs, which is prevented by the working of the patent system.[14]

Another question at issue here is: does justice require that inventors be rewarded with patents, allowing them to decide who may legally use the invention? Put differently: does it follow from the proposition that justice requires the rewarding of inventors that inventors must be granted exclusive rights of ownership on their inventions? Hettinger rightly observes that it does not:

> The mistake is to conflate the created object which makes a person deserving of a reward with what that reward should be. Property rights in the created object are not the only possible reward. Alternatives include fees, awards, acknowledgements, gratitude, praise, security, power, status, and public financial support.[15]

Thirdly: what about the fairness of granting private property rights to the results of R&D, which is, in great part, publicly funded? In the US, for example, the National Institutes of Health (NIH) (subsidised by the federal government) are great benefactors of the pharmaceutical industry. This year, the NIH will be spending $23 billion on research, and of course there are other public institutes investing in health-related research. Much of this research is directly beneficial to the industry. According to the NIH, 55% of the research projects leading to the discovery and development of the 5 best-selling drugs in 1995 was performed by researchers whose

---

[14] In a utilitarian framework, as discussed below, the unequal access is said to be justified by the incentive-to-invent it creates. However, in a framework of distributive justice such an argument cannot be decisive.

[15] E. Hettinger. Justifying Intellectual Property. *Philosophy & Public Affairs* 1989; 18: 41.

work had been financed with taxpayers' money.[16] As Bernadine Healy, former senior executive of the NIH, puts it:

There's no other industry in which you have so much public investment in the fundamental knowledge that enables . . . the development of the commercial industry itself.[17]

This seems to strengthen the case for allowing maximum access to the products of that knowledge – *inter alia* drugs.

Another problem with the justification of drug patents on fairness grounds is whether it is fair to grant inventors rewards that are excessive. Many manufacturers of brand-name pharmaceuticals relentlessly try to obtain extensions of the protection term of their patents, and they often succeed. This phenomenon, known as 'patent evergreening', hinders producers of generic drugs (products equivalent to brand drugs, which can be put on the market after the patent expires). Generic drugs are generally much cheaper than brand products. Even in the US, according to the *Kaiser Foundation*, the (retail) price of a prescription brand-name drug is 3.4 times higher than the price of a generic drug. In developing countries, the price difference is often even more striking. The public, of course, pays twice: people have to keep on paying artificially high prices for drugs, as well as the costs of a legal system used by the companies to delay competition.

Even supposing that the patent system, as we know it, could be justified on fairness grounds, the justification of the quasi-world-wide introduction of *drug* patents on such grounds would remain problematical. As Dan Brock justly remarks:

It can quite plausibly be argued that in not respecting patents developing countries are free riding on the research and development efforts of drug companies that are supported by the prices of drugs in countries in which patents are respected. But that free riding and resulting unfairness may not be enough to make it, all things considered, morally wrong for developing countries not to respect product patents . . . When developing countries choose

[16] National Institutes of Health. 2000. NIH Contributions to Pharmaceutical Development (administrative document). Cited in: Public Citizen. 2002. *America's Other Drug Problem: A Briefing Book on the Rx Drug Debate*. Washington, DC. Public Citizen: 51.
[17] Cited in: ABC News. 30 May, 2002. *Peter Jennings Reporting – Bitter Medicine: Pills, Profit and the Public's Health*. Available at: http://abcnews.go.com/onair/ABCNEWSSpecials/pharmaceuticals_020529_pjr_feature.html

not to respect product patents as their only effective means of making available pharmaceuticals necessary to save lives and protect the health of their citizens, doing so is arguably a step towards greater justice between the developed and developing world . . .[18]

Indeed, the health crisis in many developing countries has reached proportions beyond the imaginable. More than a third of the world's population has no access to essential drugs. In several countries life expectancy is dropping incredibly fast. And it is getting worse. The urgency of ensuring access to the necessary drugs cannot be ignored any longer. Rethinking the global patent regime is one of the keys to a solution.

A utilitarian justification

The utilitarian justification, which is considered by many as the most convincing, is essentially based on the following two arguments:

(a) The so-called 'incentive-to-invent-and-innovate' argument: in the absence of patents, inventions can be copied by competitors. Consequently, the price must be reduced and the investor does not have the opportunity to regain his investments, let alone make a profit. Thus, the incentive to invent and innovate is eroded. A 'special' incentive is required so that enough people should be prepared to invest in R&D. According to this argument, the patent system provides the necessary encouragement.

(b) The so-called 'incentive-to-disclose' argument: the patent system encourages inventors to disclose their inventions instead of keeping them secret. One of the patentability requirements is that the applicant must disclose the invention in sufficient detail in the application forms. Thanks to the patent system, it is said, technological information is spread – making technological progress possible, which in turn induces economic growth.

Several commentators claim that both these arguments are nowhere more valid than in the pharmaceutical sector, as this is the most research-intensive sector. However, both aforementioned arguments are problematic. We will only look at some of the problems

---

[18] D.W. Brock. Some Questions about the Moral Responsibilities of Drug Companies in Developing Countries. *Developing World Bioethics* 2001; 1: 36–37.

with the first argument, as the second one is less relevant with regard to the topic that concerns us here.

Of course, the availability of patents does result in more inventions of drugs; we do not wish to question this fact – but this positive effect may well be cancelled out by the limitation of the use of patented drugs. The patent system allows the price of patented items to be kept artificially high. The introduction in developing countries – mandated by TRIPs – of product patents in the field of pharmaceuticals will almost certainly lead to a price increase of 200–300%.[19] Moreover, as we noted earlier, pharmaceutical companies frequently take legal action to postpone the introduction of generic alternatives. This hinders the access to drugs even more.

The utilitarian (economic) arguments used to justify the patent system in industrialised countries do not necessarily apply to developing countries. Many commentators, nevertheless, automatically assume that they do. The advocates of strong drug patents claim that the implementation of the WTO-TRIPs Agreement will offer the following advantages: (1) the encouragement of local drug research, through which new drugs would become available catering to the country's specific needs (e.g. drugs for tropical diseases); (2) industrialised countries making important new drugs available in developing countries; and (3) the attraction of foreign investments in the pharmaceutical sector. Each of these arguments is susceptible to criticism.

More local R&D of drugs?

Hardly any drugs for diseases occurring primarily or exclusively in developing countries are being developed. Of the 1223 molecules that were sold worldwide between 1975 and 1996, less than 1% was intended for tropical diseases.[20] R&D of drugs for these diseases is desperately needed. According to some commentators, if

---

[19] J. Watal. 2000. *Access to Essential Medicines in Developing Countries: Does the WTO TRIPS Agreement hinder it? (Science, Technology and Innovation Discussion Paper No. 8).* Cambridge, MA. Center for International Development, Harvard University: 5.

[20] See: B. Pécoul, P. Chirac, P. Trouiller & J. Pinel. Access to Essential Drugs in Poor Countries – A Lost Battle? *JAMA* 1999; 281: 365 (Table 2). See also the recent survey by experts of the Harvard School of Public Health and an international group of experts, the *Drugs for Neglected Diseases Working Group*, available at: www.accessmed-msf.org. See also another recent survey which the umbrella organisation of the American pharmaceutical industry (*Pharmaceutical Research and Manufacturers of America*) held among its members, *New Medicines in Development*, available at: www.phrma.org.

developing countries were to grant strong patents for drugs, this would stimulate local research. Not granting strong patent protection may well yield short-term advantages, but it would be harmful in the long run, they say, because such a situation can never bring about drugs that meet the specific needs of the country in question.

The introduction and the application of new technologies are indeed important instruments to help developing countries improve their standard of living. However, the fact that in developing countries few new technologies are being developed has more to do with fundamental economical problems (e.g. a lack of skilled workers and the absence of infrastructures capable of absorbing new technologies) than with patent protection standards.

Moreover, the economic purpose of patents is to enable patentees to recoup their investments and, if possible, make a profit. In the pharmaceutical sector, they are used to achieve high profits: the pharmaceutical industry is eight times more profitable than the average of all industries represented in the Fortune 500 list.[21] It is highly unlikely that the recent strengthening of the patent system will incite pharmaceutical companies to invest in R&D of drugs for diseases occurring primarily or exclusively in developing countries, as the majority of the stricken patients have little or no purchasing power, which makes the market totally uneconomical. Indeed, while health spending per capita in the developing countries amounts to 11 dollars (of which 6 are 'public' dollars), rich countries spend 1907 dollars per capita (of which 1356 are 'public' dollars).[22] The pharmaceutical industry develops profitable drugs for the wealthy regions of the world, and makes its biggest profits from hair tonics, anti-impotency drugs, drugs for cholesterol, ulcers, depressions, allergies and high blood pressure. More money is invested in research of drugs against baldness than in research of all tropical diseases combined . . . strengthening drug patents in developing countries is not likely to change that. The diseases of patients with little or no purchasing power are simply neglected in the pharmaceutical market.

---

[21] See: Fortune 500. *Fortune Magazine* 2002; April. In 2001, the profits of America's 10 largest pharmaceutical companies went up by 33% – from 28 to 37,3 billion dollars! – despite the bad economic situation. Profits are also growing much faster than the volume of R&D investments. According to the 2001 Fortune 500 ranking, the pharmaceutical industry was the most profitable industry for the tenth time in a row.

[22] Keynote presentation on the occasion of the 'Forum 5' gathering organised by the *Global Forum for Health Research* (www.globalforumhealth.org), October 2001.

Increased transfer of (pharmaceutical) technology and increased foreign investment in the pharmaceutical domain?

The classical argument in this context is that those who possess technology are not too keen on transferring their technological knowledge to countries with a 'weak' patent system, for risks involving 'piracy.' If a developing country were to strengthen its patent system, so the argument goes, the industrialised countries will make new medicines available in that country. This prediction, however, does not sound very credible. Drugs that can be produced via conventional processes are already being brought onto the market by local production plants in numerous developing countries. Those drugs of which the production requires sophisticated technologies are generally not copied in developing countries, as the required manufacturing capacities are only available in industrialised countries. Moreover, such drugs are very expensive and therefore accessible only to the rich segment of the population in developing countries. It is therefore highly unlikely that the strengthening of patent protection in developing countries will bring in technology previously unavailable.

As far as the role of patents in the encouragement of foreign investments is concerned, various commentators claim that the absence or the availability of adequate protection of intellectual property rights constitutes a factor which plays an increasingly important part in the investment-related decisions of companies. An important element in this debate is, however, that under the TRIPs regime patentees are no longer under the obligation to manufacture their inventions in the (developing) country that issued the patent. Art. 27(1) of TRIPs stipulates that:

> . . . patents [can] be granted for any inventions, whether products or processes, in all fields of technology . . . [and] patent rights are enjoyable *without discrimination* as to the place of invention, the field of technology and *whether products are imported or locally produced.*[23]

Hence, lack of local exploitation of a patented invention can no longer be invoked as a ground for granting a compulsory licence. Patentees can freely choose to supply the market from their own country. This will lead to foreign companies investing in branches

---

[23] Emphasis added.

in developing countries only if the available human and/or infra-structural capacity offers them exceptional cost-reducing possibilities. As far as the pharmaceutical industry is concerned, such a situation is not very likely to occur.

Furthermore, research has shown that investment decisions are influenced by a whole series of diverse factors, one of which is the level of patent protection in the country in question – but this is by no means the most important one.[24]

IV. IN SEARCH OF A FAIRER BALANCE BETWEEN THE RIGHTS AND OBLIGATIONS OF PATENT HOLDERS AND BETWEEN PATIENTS' INTERESTS AND COMMERCIAL INTERESTS: THE DOHA DECLARATION ON THE TRIPS AGREEMENT AND PUBLIC HEALTH

The WTO Ministerial Conference in Doha (Qatar) in November 2001 produced, among other things, the landmark Doha Declaration on the TRIPs Agreement and Public Health.[25] The essence of the Declaration is worded in Paragraph 4. It stipulates that the TRIPs Agreement does not and should not prevent WTO member states from taking measures to protect public health, and that it can and should be interpreted and implemented in a manner supportive of member states' rights to protect public health and, in particular, to promote access to medicines for all. It declares the right of member states to use, to the full, the provisions in TRIPs that provide flexibility for this purpose. This is somewhat fleshed out in the fifth paragraph, which recognises that these flexibilities include *inter alia* that:

(b) Each Member has the right to grant compulsory licenses and the freedom to determine the grounds upon which such licenses are granted.

(c) Each Member has the right to determine what constitutes a national emergency or other circumstances of extreme urgency, it being understood that public health crises, including those relating to HIV/AIDS, tuberculosis, malaria and

---

[24] See e.g.: C.A.P. Braga et al. 1999. *Intellectual Property Rights and Economic Development (Background paper for the World Development Report 1999)*. Washington, DC. World Bank.
[25] WTO Ministerial Conference. Fourth Session. Doha, 9–14 November 2001. WT/MIN(01)/DEC/2, 20 November 2001.

other epidemics, can represent a national emergency or other circumstances of extreme urgency.

Subparagraph (b) is important because developing countries that intend to grant compulsory licences are sometimes put under great pressure (e.g. via threats to redraw investments), primarily by the US, not to do so. However, the system of compulsory licences enables a country to factor national interests into its patent system and allows it to achieve a better balance between the rights and the obligations of patent holders. Therefore it should be used to the full, especially in 'vital' sectors such as drugs. Unfortunately the developing countries did not take advantage of the Doha negotiations to obtain a reversal of the burden of proof when it comes to decisions on whether to grant a compulsory license. It would seem fairer to place the burden of proof on the side of the patent holder – in other words, to force the patent holder to prove that granting a compulsory licence is not necessary, instead of forcing the applicant to demonstrate that the patent holder has abused his monopoly.

Subparagraph (c) is important in that it stresses that every member state has the sovereign power of decision to proclaim a (national) state of emergency.

The sixth paragraph of the Declaration runs:

We recognize that WTO Members with insufficient or no manufacturing capacities in the pharmaceutical sector could face difficulties in making effective use of compulsory licensing under the TRIPs Agreement. We instruct the Council for TRIPs to find an expeditious solution to this problem and to report to the General Council before the end of 2002.

As foreseen, this provision has lead to negotiations in the TRIPs Council. In 2002, the TRIPs Council convened on several occasions to reach a concrete proposal on this issue.

Pursuant to Article 31(f) of TRIPs, compulsory licences must be used predominantly for the supply of the domestic market of the member state that issued the compulsory licence and can, therefore, only be used to a limited extent for export. However, it would seem to be necessary that, if a country has insufficient or no manufacturing capacities and the drugs offered by foreign manufacturers are too expensive, the country should be allowed to look elsewhere for a suitable supplier. Until 2005, this will not really pose a serious problem because a number of developing countries – with India as the most prominent example – have a good production capacity and are still legally allowed to export their drugs, even when these are patented in other countries.

As noted earlier, the so-called 'least developed countries' have been granted a postponement until 2016 to conform their drug-related patent provisions to the WTO-TRIPs Agreement, but once the developing countries that can export drugs to them (e.g. India) must acknowledge drug patents – already in 2005 as foreseen in TRIPs – the least developed countries are sure to encounter even more serious problems in obtaining affordable drugs. In this context, compulsory licences will become increasingly vital.

The discussions in the TRIPs Council concerning export strategies went off the rails during a debate about the question for which diseases the export of drugs under compulsory licence should be allowed. When the president of the TRIPS Council proposed a draft in December 2002 stating that the Doha Declaration was not limited to HIV/AIDS, malaria and tuberculosis, the US (as the only among the then 145 WTO members) refused to accept this draft and negotiations were broken off.[26] In the meanwhile they have been reopened, but there is still no consensus.

Numerous countries are opposed to a limitation of diseases for which medicines can be exported under compulsory licences and feel that this cannot be the subject of negotiations. They justly observe that the Doha Declaration states that the TRIPs Agreement has to be implemented in such a way as to give *everyone* access to medicines.

The US, however, fears that an interpretation of Doha that does not limit the diseases, for which drugs can be exported under compulsory licence, to HIV/AIDS, tuberculosis and malaria, will erode incentives for the development of new drugs. In a letter addressed to the trade ministers of all WTO members, US Trade Representative Robert Zoellick stated that:

[I]t became clear to us that some WTO members and advocacy organizations sought to expand the scope of disease beyond that

---

[26] As noted by several NGOs, the position of poor countries would have been significantly worsened had this draft been adopted. MSF (Médecins Sans Frontières) rightly observes that: '[I]t would have made generic production almost economically unfeasible after 2005 . . . At the end of the day, the supply of affordable versions of new medicines would have slowed to a trickle, with developing countries left with very few alternatives to the high process and long-term monopolies of originator companies.' See: MSF. 2003. *One Step Forward, Two Steps Back? Issues for the 5th WTO Ministerial Conference (Briefing Note)*. Cancún.

intended at Doha to allow countries to override drug patents to treat a wide range of public health concerns, including obesity, asthma, cancer, diabetes, among others – even including the use of Viagra. We were seriously concerned that this approach would undermine the WTO rules on patents that provide incentives for the development of new pharmaceutical products.[27]

Given the fact that North America, Europe and Japan together represent 80% of the global pharmaceutical market, and that of the remaining 20%, Africa represents only 1%,[28] Zoellick's concern about an 'undermining' of incentives for drug development is without foundation. The continuation of pharmaceutical R&D is not dependent on the markets of developing countries.

Another argument that the US has repeatedly referred to involves the risk of cheap medicines intended for the South being illegally diverted to the North. Brook Baker of the NGO Health GAP rightly remarks that this objection is untruthful:

> there are billions of generic pills being produced each year around the globe that have not been diverted into the US and Europe. Not only do US and Europe outlaw such diversion, but they also guard their borders with remarkable efficiency. As a matter of law and of practicality, the US and Europe are in total control of the diversion risk. Rich consumers in London, Paris, and New York are not going to buy black market, smuggled heart medicines out of the trunk of a Chevy.[29]

Indeed, the Doha Declaration should be implemented to the fullest extent without delay, in order to establish a fairer balance between the rights and obligations of patent holders and between the interests of patients and those of patent owners. Given the basic nature of health needs, patent rules should not prevent countries from adopting policies that protect public health and promote access to drugs.

However, after the adoption of the Doha Declaration, the US, the EU, Canada, Switzerland and Japan have constantly tried to undermine the Declaration through their attempts to limit its scope.

---

[27] InsideHealthPolicy.com. Daily Updates. 17 January, 2003.
[28] See: IMS Health Market Report: Five Year Forecast of the Global Pharmaceutical Markets (available at http://www.ims-global.com/insight/report/global/report.htm), quoted in: MSF. 2001. *Fatal Imbalance*. Available at: www.msf.org.
[29] Ip-health mailing list. 23 December, 2002.

In addition, the US has negotiated regional trade agreements such as the Free Trade Area of the Americas (FTAA) Agreement – and is continuously negotiating others – that threaten to erode or even abandon the Doha Declaration.

V. CONCLUSION

Drug patents, particularly the strong kind of drug patents granted today, are hard to justify on natural rights, fairness or utilitarian grounds. Many drugs are of vital importance for very large groups of people. This vital importance should be reflected in the debate about the justification of drug patents.

The proposition that in the absence of strong patents no R&D of drugs can be expected is typically presented as universally valid – whereas it may well be that the advisable level of patent protection (or even the decision whether or not to grant protection) has to be determined in relation to the level of economic development of a country. Unfortunately, since the forum for decision making with regard to intellectual property shifted from WIPO to WTO, a 'one size fits all' view of patents has been firmly established.

As Jagdish Bhagwati rightly notes, the inclusion of intellectual property has turned WTO into a royalty collection agency.[30] The unwillingness of the major industrialised countries to accept a full implementation of the Doha Declaration seems to threaten the legitimacy of the WTO-TRIPs Agreement.

It seems that the reason why pharmaceutical lobbies are such zealous advocates of strong patents in developing countries is that it would allow them to hinder competition from local drug manufacturers. There is no credible evidence that the new global patent regime will promote the development of new medicines for diseases occurring primarily or exclusively in developing countries. Instead, this regime severely limits these countries' possibilities to implement a public health policy that addresses the health crises they are confronted with, and it is one of the main factors that hinders access to existing (patented) drugs – access which the lives of millions of people depend.

---

[30] J. Bhagwati. Patents and the Poor. *Financial Times* 16 September, 2002.

Chapter 10

JUSTICE AND EQUAL OPPORTUNITIES IN HEALTH CARE

*JOHN HARRIS**

The principle that each individual is entitled to an equal opportunity to benefit from any public health care system, and that this entitlement is proportionate neither to the size of their chance of benefitting, nor to the quality of the benefit, nor to the length of lifetime remaining in which that benefit may be enjoyed, runs counter to most current thinking about the allocation of resources for health care. It is my contention that any system of prioritisation of the resources available for health care or for rationing such resources must be governed by this principle.

This principle can lead to apparently paradoxical conclusions in that, for example, it can seem wasteful to give someone with a very slim chance of a lifesaving treatment the same priority as someone with a much better chance. I set out the above ideas in this journal some time ago,[1] and in an important and thoughtful recent paper,[2] Julian Savulescu has concentrated on this apparent weakness and has argued for a particular conception of the good or benefit to be achieved by a health care system which purports to demonstrate the inadequacies of my approach and to replace it with an altogether better account.

Savulescu identifies my theory of the good of health care as providing each individual with an opportunity to live the best and longest life possible for him or her, and dubs this theory 'opportunism'. Savulescu notes that for the purposes of distribution of resources, I reject welfarism (the thesis that the good of health care is well-being) and that I have argued that utilitarianism in general

* Thanks are due to two anonymous referees for *Bioethics*.
[1] John Harris 'What Is the Good of Health Care?' *Bioethics* 10:4 1996 269–291. Justine Burley and Søren Holm have made helpful comments on an earlier draft of this paper. The author thanks the *European Commission* (DG XII) for a project grant, which made this work possible.
[2] Julian Savulescu, 'Consequentialism, Reasons, Value and Justice' *Bioethics* 12:3. 1998. 212–235.

may lead to *de facto* discrimination against groups of people needing health care. It is true that I do reject the thesis that the good of health care is well-being, but if welfare is defined in terms of *preference satisfaction* as it very often is, then what I have to say about equal opportunities in health may well be compatible with welfarism thus conceived.[3]

Savulescu argues that well-being is a superior theory of the good of health care to mine and that the weaknesses of utilitarian approaches that I have identified can be better addressed in two ways, by: (1) relating justice more closely to reasons for action and (2) by conceptualising the relationship between reasons for action and the value of the consequences of those actions as a plateau rather than as a scalar relationship. Justice, Savulescu suggests, can be understood as satisfying as many equally rational claims on resources as possible and that the rationality of a person's claim on health resources turns on the strength of that person's reasons to promote certain health-related states of affairs.

Savulescu's point is that 'the strength of that reason does not track the expected value of that state of affairs in a fully scalar fashion. Rather a person can have most reason to promote some state of affairs, even though he or she could promote other more valuable states of affairs. Thus there can be equal reason for a distributor of public resources to save either of two people, even though one will have a better and more valuable life.' Savulescu's claim is that this 'approach, while addressing many of Harris's concerns about utilitarianism, does not imply that doctors should give up prioritising patients according to prognosis altogether, but it does imply that patients with lower, but reasonable prognosis should share in public resources'.

The concentration on a reasons based solution to problems of allocation has many attractions and is worth pursuing. I shall first show that a rational 'reasons based consequentialism' is more in line with my 'equal opportunities for health' than with Savalescu's position. I shall then examine more closely the conception of equal opportunities in health care that is at issue between us and show that if we give weight to an individual's reasons, and to what is

---

[3] See for example Amartya Sen, 'Well-Being, Agency and Freedom', *Journal of Philosophy* 82, 1985. 187ff. See also G.A. Cohen 'On the Currency of Egalitarian Justice', *Ethics* 99. 1989 pp. 906–909.

expected to be good for them,[4] we will opt for exactly the equality based account of distributive justice that I have recommended.

REASONS BASED CONSEQUENTIALISM

What does a rational person have good reasons to promote?

If we ask what state of affairs I (or anyone) has most reason to promote, an obvious answer would be our own survival.[5] It surely must always be *rational* for someone who wants to live to choose a chance of continued survival over earlier death, even where the survival period will be relatively short or where the chances of survival are slim, so long as the life to be continued will likely be of acceptable quality. The *strength* of the agent's reason will be relative to the desire to live or to the fear of death, not to the chances of survival. If the chances of my survival are slim, I may be irrational to believe that I *will in fact* survive, but I surely am not irrational to take any chance of survival that offers, unless other costs to me (or to things I ought to value more, or would be irrational not to value more,) are greater. And here, of course, the strength of the desire to take a chance on life need not be proportional to the chances of that desire being realised.

We should note that while pursuing goals with scant chance of success is often an irrational activity, it is *so because there are better* (more rational) *uses of one's time.* So it would be irrational for a person to pursue a course of professional training if there were very little prospect of gaining anything useful from it. But if it is irrational, it is so because there are better (more likely successful) uses of that person's time, the course is literally time wasted. But where what is pursued is continued existence, which is the *sine qua non* of the pursuit of almost all other goals, it can hardly be irrational or unreasonable to pursue life however slim the chance. There are no more rational uses of that person's time for that person is pursuing time itself,[6] nor are there more rational goals he might pursue, for what he is pursuing is the condition of almost all other objectives

---

[4] Savulescu 1998 p. 235.
[5] We'll ignore cases in which our survival is incompatible with that of someone we care deeply about.
[6] With apologies to St. Augustine!

he may have. A slim chance of something[7] is always better (more objectively rational) than a certainty of nothingness.

Reasons and justice

Savulescu sets out a plausible account of reasons-based justice and applies it to health related claims. Savulescu outlines his position as follows, and I will quote in sufficient detail to make the subtlety of his argument clear:

> Justice is concerned with providing what there is good reason to provide for people. Let's say that a person has a rational claim to have some state of affairs, p, promoted if there is good reason to promote p. According to one version of consequentialism,
>
> > C1. The good of health care is satisfying a rational claim for some health-related state.
> > C2. The right distribution is that distribution which maximises the number of people whose equally rational health-related claims are fully satisfied.
>
> Call this view reasons-based maximising consequentialism for short. According to reasons based consequentialism the following claims are true:
>
> > C3. If a person (including a distributor of public resources) has equal reason to promote p, q or r, and that person can promote either p and q, or r, then he or she should promote p and q.
>
> C4. If a person, A, has the same strength reason to promote p as another person, B, has to promote q, there is as much reason to promote p as q. Thus, the distributor can have as much reason to provide A with the resources so that p is promoted as she can to provide resources to B to promote q. To use the preceding example . . .
>
> > A distributor of public resources can have the same strength reason to promote A in p (if that is what A most cares about) as to promote B in q (if that is what B most cares about), even if q is more valuable than p.

---

[7] If desired.

There are limits to this principle. When the expected value of one option greatly outweighs the expected value of another option, we are rationally required to choose the former . . . Consider . . . a related but slightly different example. Two 70 year old men have cancer and will die without treatment.

[Each loves his family dearly, the treatment is expensive and will leave each with little to bequeath]

Man A has a 1/50 chance of survival.
Man B has a 1/100 chance of survival.
[M]y intuition about this case is that there is as much reason for each man to choose a chance on life rather than his family's welfare . . .[8]

Compare these men to Man C. He has the same disease, the same assets and the same concern for his family. However, he has a 1/1000000 chance of survival. If Man C cares greatly about his family's welfare, he should not spend his money on the experimental treatment. The expected value of the operation is so small that the strength of his reason to have the operation is weaker . . .[9]

Savulescu says of man C who has only 1/1000000 chance of survival: 'The expected value of the operation is so small that the strength of his reason to have the operation is weaker'. But this is neither true nor plausible unless stipulated so to be. The value of the operation is as great as it could conceivably be, it is a life saving operation, it is C's only chance of continued life, just as for A and B who have a 1/50 and 1/100 chance respectively. On the view of what each stands to gain the value is equal, it is the value of a chance of survival versus the value of no chance of survival. True, C will not be rational if he believes that he has a *good chance* of survival, but then neither will A or B. True, also, C has a much worse chance of survival than A or B. I have suggested that in cases like this the value of the operation to A, B or C is the value of a chance of survival. The moral reason to afford any of them that chance is simply that equality demands it. The requirement that each person is shown the same concern, respect and protection as is shown to any, requires that the life of each person be equally

---

[8] This is an astonishing claim for someone sporting utilitarian credentials because *any* gain in utility is a gain in utility!

[9] Ibid. p. 232.

respected. In this sort of case, I have suggested, this means giving to each his or her chance,[10] whatever that chance may be.[11]

Perhaps Savulescu has a false analogy in mind here. If I am faced with a choice between rival therapies for the same condition, and one has a much greater chance of success than the other, I have a stronger reason to prefer the therapy that offers the best chance. But this case tells us nothing about 'stronger reasons' when we are comparing not a slim chance with a fat chance, but a slim chance with no chance at all; or when the slim and the fat chances fall to different people.

Savulescu, like many before him, is playing fast and loose with the meaning of the crucial phrase 'expected value'. He started by using the term 'expected value' to refer to the *magnitude or importance* of the benefit to be achieved by treatment, not to the *likelihood* of the benefit being realised. I agree with Savulescu when 'expected value' refers to magnitude and importance of the benefit. I have always maintained, as Savulescu concedes, that for example, life saving procedures are usually to be preferred to life enhancing procedures, precisely because of the magnitude of the benefit.[12] And I also agree with him that except where differences in magnitude are clear and sizeable it is better to respect a person's own preferences. Thus a distributor of public resources can have the same strength reason to promote what A most cares about as to promote what B most cares about, even if one is more valuable than the other.

I have argued that the value of someone's life either cannot, or should not, be proportional to their life expectancy, nor to their chances of achieving that expectancy.[13] There are many reasons for

[10] If that chance is wanted or claimed.

[11] Remember, although it may be hard to calculate, each claimant on health resources has, in fact, a different chance of benefit so any requirement to give all an equal chance cannot coherently refer to size of benefit or to the magnitude of the chance of obtaining that benefit unless equal just means 'proportional to size of benefit'.

[12] Savulescu, like several of my other critics, seems unable to distinguish between situations where life is at stake and situations where a person will survive with better or worse quality of life. In the former case it is always rational to take a very small chance on life, in the latter it may be rational to discount the value of the various outcomes with the probability of achieving them.

[13] See for example my 'More & Better Justice' in Sue Mendus and Martin Bell Eds. *Philosophy And Medical Welfare*, Cambridge, University Press, 1988. 75–97. 'QALYfyiing the value of life' in *The Journal of Medical Ethics* Vol.13 No 3. September 1987. p. 118. 'Could we hold people responsible for their own adverse health?' in *The Journal of Contemporary Health Law and Policy* Vol. 1 1996. 100–106. 'What the principal objective of the NHS should *really* be' in *The British Medical Journal* 314. 1st March 1997. And my *The Value of Life* Routledge & Kegan Paul 1985.

this and here I will mention two. Genome analysis will soon be able to reveal, at conception or birth, many reliable differences between individuals with respect to their life expectancy and their chances of continued existence when genetically predicted illnesses take hold. It would surely be invidious to distinguish between individuals on this basis, not least because it would amount to renunciation of the equality principle. If equality of consideration varies with life expectancy or chances of successful treatment and these are for everyone unique, then the value of each life is different, not equal.

Savulescu partly accepts this but believes that really slim chances change the game, a 1/1000000 compared with a 1/100 chance for example. There is some plausibility to this, but there are a number of problems too. First, I doubt there would be any consensus about how small a chance carries with it loss of equality of status.[14] Many would think 1/100 chance is far too small. What rational person would play 'Russian Roulette' where the chance is 1/6? The answer of course is it depends what is at stake. No rational person would play for a 1/6 chance of death, but when it is the only chance of life why not take even a 1/1000000 chance? It can't be irrational to take such a chance, although it may be selfish when costs to others are included in the calculation. In such a case, the argument must be about enforcing 'altruism' or about the objectivity of the size of the benefits, that is about the superiority of a maximising consequentialism.

But reasons based maximising consequentialism, of the sort espoused by Savulescu, cannot help here because it implies that the rationality of reasons for doing x is proportionate to the likelihood of achieving x; but this depends on what is at stake and what the alternatives are. When life is at stake and one alternative offers a chance of life (and there are no other alternatives which offer any chance of continued existence for the agent) then, arguably, any chance is worth having and therefore rational. This will be true unless the reasons the agent has to give others a chance of rescue are for some reason stronger than those she has to save her own life.

II. EQUAL OPPORTUNITIES AND DISTRIBUTIVE JUSTICE

Savulescu suggests that if I am saying 'something new and interesting, I think we should understand [Harris] literally as saying that

---

[14] For that's what it amounts to.

the good of health care *is* opportunity not welfare, and that opportunities are to be distributed among people, as utilitarians distributed welfare'.[15] He then identifies three ways in which opportunity as a good might be interpreted and finds fault with all of them. These are, crudely, that opportunity might be an intrinsic good, an instrumental good or what he calls a subjective intrinsic good. He points out, rightly, that each of the first two alternatives is flawed if strictly and exclusively interpreted. However, I am not claiming that equal opportunities for health care are either intrinsic or instrumental goods, they are *both and more*, like other accounts of the moral requirement for equal opportunities.

A denial of equal opportunities is a slap in the face; it is an existential rejection disproportionate to the value of the good or welfare that the opportunity might have afforded. So it is not the case that the opportunity is valuable only for what it is an opportunity to do or to be, nor is it merely valuable in itself. Equal opportunities recognise the existential or intrinsic value of people, they are neither simply intrinsic goods nor are they simply instrumental. Rather it is the case that the keeping open of opportunities is expressive of, and recognises that the person's objectives (whatever they are – however trivial or important) matter. When people champion equal opportunities in education, or to use public utilities (buses, for example, or lavatories) the liberty is not valuable in proportion to the importance of the particular object of the liberty (to make a journey by bus or wash your face). They are important because the denial of them is a rejection of equality and therefore an affront to human dignity.

Counting and discounting

Savulescu[16] attributes to me the suggestion that 'life *per se* is not of value, but of value to the extent that a person values it.' I stand by this remark so far as it goes. Savulescu goes on to claim that 'this strategy will not justify Harris' intuitions in the medical example because, even if every patient's life has value of 1, we must discount the value of operating on patients . . . by the probability that the operation will not achieve the valued outcome'.[17] Savulescu believes

---

[15] Savulescu 1998, pp. 217–218.
[16] Ibid. p. 219.
[17] Ibid. p. 220.

that the 'implication of these claims is that each person *values having the operation to the same degree*. On this view, opportunity is good to the extent that it is valued. Thus, if Tom, who has a brain tumour, wants the opportunity to live just as Alex, who has appendicitis, this grounds an equal moral claim, regardless of how great their chances are.' And Savulescu interprets this position as amounting to 'holding a ticket in a lottery not because of the money we might win, but simply for the chance to participate in the lottery'. But this is surely wrong. Tom has more than a chance of *participating*, and he wants more; he has and wants a chance of *winning*, winning the thing that matters most to him, his continued existence.

Of course, the opportunity of the operation is valued because it is seen as a means to continued existence. Tom and Alex each want *the same thing*, a chance of continued existence; although for each the chance is different and for each continued existence will be different (different length, different quality etc.). This no more shows that what each wants must be discounted for its peculiar value than does the fact that each human being is different show that the value of life is different for each and hence that there can be no such thing as a principle of equality.

To assert 'even if every patient's life has a value of 1, we must discount the value of operating on patients by the probability that the operation will not achieve the valued outcome' involves a fundamental fallacy. If every opportunity had to be discounted by the probability that it will achieve its objective there could be absolutely no claim to the equality of public provision of anything. Education is effective in proportion to the intelligence, ability to concentrate, application, capacity for hard work etc. of each and every student and these are different for each and every student. Access to education must be finely graded accordingly. The value of the provision of public lavatories is, on this view, proportionate to the strength of the bladder of individual users, in that the utility of the operation in question, how long before another, similar operation is required, is one obvious measure of the utility of restroom provision.

The fallacy of the principle of temporal neutrality

Savulescu also appeals to this principle of discounting when discussing the so called 'principle of temporal neutrality'. According to this principle if 'the value of a state of affairs is determined by our desires for that state, we should appeal not only to what people now desire, but also to what they will desire. And if we consider future preference satisfaction, we must discount the value of that satisfaction by the probability of it not occurring'.[18] Imagine a nation state 'Temporal Neutralitovia' (TN) that has two potential and very powerful enemies. One declares all out war reducing the chances of survival of all TN's inhabitants by 50%. The second enemy can now reason, correctly according to Savulescu, that if it also declares war the wrong it will do in waging war and probably killing many of TN's inhabitants is only half what it was previously, because the value of the lives of all the inhabitants of TN must be reduced by 50%, must, in short, be discounted by the probability of their survival.

To move from the cataclysm of war to more mundane and realistic policy choices: we can imagine two towns of exactly the same size in the European Union, one in the north of England, 'Ancient', and the other in the south of Italy, 'Vecchio'. Both towns are claimants for Community resources available to care for the elderly. As is well known, life expectancy is greater in southern Italy than in northern Europe, perhaps due to the famous 'Mediterranean diet' of olive oil and cooked tomatoes. The citizens of both towns want the security of better health provision in old age. They want it now and will still want it when they are old. However, although both towns have equal size populations, since life expectancy in Vecchio is much superior to that in Ancient, we must discount the value of devoting resources to the elderly the probability that the allocation will not achieve the valued outcome. That is, fewer elderly will benefit in Ancient than in Vecchio. Is it clear that the citizens of Vecchio have the better claim, and that the European Commission, for example, should allocate resources accordingly? Should Italy and Greece always win out over the United Kingdom and Denmark when such resources are available? I doubt this would (or should) strike the European Parliament, for example, as an equitable allocation of resources between member states.

The fallacy of the principle of temporal neutrality lies in attempting to extrapolate from decisions within particular lives to comparisons between lives where life itself is at stake. If the claim that 'if we consider future preference satisfaction, we must discount the value of that satisfaction by the probability of it not occurring' has

---

[18] Ibid. p. 221.

any validity this derives from its application within a particular life. I would be irrational to plan for future preferences I am unlikely to be able to satisfy. But this is entirely different, as the above examples show, to the false claim defended by Savulescu, that we must discount the existential value of a life by the probability of its not continuing.

In any event Savulescu has already conceded enough of the point. He allows that it is invidious to prefer a 1/50 chance of life to a 1/100 chance so it is clearly not true that in his view we *must* discount for probability of occurrence. However, if, as I have argued, the value lies in giving the person an equal chance of continued existence, and that doing so recognises their equal standing in the community, then *that* is the value of the opportunity. And we have already seen that the explanation of this exception cannot be simply a matter of the externally assessed rationality or of the strength of the agent's reasons for the choice.

Thresholds and plateaux

Savulescu's claim is not that it is simply a matter of the strength of the agent's reasons for choice, but of that strength *once a certain threshold or plateau is reached*. His suggestion is that 'the strength of reason to act increases as the value promoted by the action increases, until some plateau is reached where strength of reason no longer increases despite increments in value. Thus a person may have most reason to perform some act, even though other actions would promote more value, if the consequences of the chosen act are good enough'.[19] Savulescu makes clear that 'Distributors of public resources should not require that agent's change what matters most to them, provided that the object of that pattern of concern is worth achieving and good enough relative to other alternatives'.[20] The crucial point is that Savulescu believes that a slim chance of life is not a reason on the plateau, not something either worth achieving or good enough relative to other values.

I have argued that a chance of continued existence that is desired is always worth taking and that it is only other values of the same agent that can eclipse that chance. The object of the chance of life is not, as Savulescu sometimes implies, the particular percentage

[19] Ibid. p. 228.
[20] Ibid. p. 230.

chance, but the opportunity of life when the alternative is death. Thus the measure of the good to be achieved does not reside in the percentage chance of achieving it, but in the nature of what is to be achieved. Continued existence as opposed to immediate death is desired because it is everything as opposed to nothing. There could not be a more valuable objective or a more rational one. This must be on Savulescu's plateau if anything is.

What Savulescu must surely do is provide a principled account of when precisely differences in degree make for differences in quality, or in his terminology when scalarity breaks down. Without a principle for recognising the point of scalar shift, we have been given no account of anything, but merely a redescription of Savulescu's intuitions.

The value of life

The plateau or threshold is I concede attractive. Savulescu is certainly right to suggest that most people's intuitions suggest that really small chances of survival are not worth providing (as opposed to taking) when the same resources could be used to give better chances to others and hence save more lives. The same seems to be true where even good chances of continued life are available, but where the continuance will be only for very short periods, days or weeks for example. It may be that this is an objective matter in that a vast majority would see small chances or short periods of remission as obviously worthless or worth less. However, this paper has suggested that such plateaux are not supported by reasons based consequentialism, relying as it does on measures of the objective strength of reasons particular people have. There are various other ways such a rejection of small chances of life or small amounts of remaining life-span, might be supported. Such a plateau might, for example, be supported by some overarching theory of distributive justice. Such a theory might of course run into equally counterintuitive conclusions in other areas, as I have suggested is the case with Savulescu's version of reasons based consequentialism.

For these reasons I believe the paradoxical consequences of according equal concern and respect to claims to small chances of life, or small periods of continued existence, is more apparent than real. A reasons based consequentialism which is not burdened by the absurdities of the principle of temporal neutrality and is sensitive to the strength of reasons that particular individuals have to take their own chances on life, would probably be fully compatible with the position that I have defended. We must remember, however, that the crucial issue is that of distributive justice, of how public resources may be allocated to do justice to the equal claims of individual citizens. What matters therefore, is what a distributor of the public resources available for health care should do.

There is, I believe, no way to formalise at the level of public policy the information necessary to be fully sensitive to, and respectful of, individual reasons and circumstances. A distributor of public resources cannot (and perhaps should not) know or enquire into the detailed reasons why even a small chance of life or a short period of remission is wanted and needed. Such a distributor should be 'blind' to these individual differences, for to evaluate them violates the equality principle. This is why a distributor of public resources must afford equal opportunities for health care and not formalise principles that may accord different value to the lives of equals.

Chapter 11

CONSTRAINTS AND HEROES

CARL ELLIOTT

A story, perhaps apocryphal, is told about the United States surgical team which pioneered the first artificial heart procedure. It is said that the team received a number of telephone calls from people around the country who, worried about the ailing heart recipient, offered to donate to him their own hearts. When the surgical team, justifiably curious, sent psychiatrists to examine these donors, they found to their surprise that many of the donors were rational, competent, sincere, and fully aware that as a consequence of donating their hearts they would die.

Whether this story is true does not concern me here. I tell it only to make a factual point, which I believe few would disagree with, and to dramatize a still larger, moral point. The first, factual point is that even if it could be established that such potential donors were fully competent, virtually no surgeon would agree to perform the transplant. Though I have no data to demonstrate this, few people familiar with United States medicine would quarrel with me when I state that nearly all physicians would refuse to have anything to do with such a procedure.

The second, larger point is both morally important and paradoxical. The offer to give up one's life for another person clearly seems morally admirable. In fact, it seems more than that – heroic perhaps, beyond the limits of duty. However, if it is indeed a morally praiseworthy action, then the refusal of a physician to perform the transplant seems very puzzling.

This point would not, of course, be a puzzle for morality if the refusal of most physicians to perform such a transplant were merely a matter of custom, or avoidance of a malpractice suit, or just plain hard-headedness. Rather, I take it that the refusal of most physicians to participate would be based on moral grounds – that most physicians have the intuition that to participate in such a transplant would somehow be morally wrong. And the puzzle is why I, for instance, might have the dual intuitions that in this case it is morally praiseworthy for a person to offer to donate his heart, and that it would be morally wrong for me to assist him.

Though this case illustrates the puzzle clearly, we do not need to imagine a case as far removed from usual clinical practice as a heart transplant to find similar dilemmas. Such dilemmas come up, for instance, in any organ transplantation, and also in experiments on human subjects. The dilemma concerns how much harm to the donor a physician should risk in order to help others – how much harm is morally permissible, or, perhaps, how much benefit will make the procedure morally obligatory. We do not, of course, have to imagine a case where the donor's or the subject's life is at stake; the harm might be relatively minor, and the risk of incurring that harm small. The point is that most physicians feel some duty not to expose a patient to the risk of harm, even if the patient is perfectly willing to undergo that risk.

Many attempts to analyze cases such as this shift back and forth between two unpalatable alternatives. On the one hand, libertarians argue that there is nothing wrong with a physician exposing a person to harm, as long as the person is aware of the harm and consents to it. On the other hand we hear the physicians' refusals to undertake such procedures defended on grounds of conscience and professional ethics. Both alternatives, I believe, misrepresent the moral problem that this sort of case demonstrates.

My concerns here will be threefold. First, I want to add some substance to the widely-held intuition that there is something morally objectionable about a physician participating in procedures which put even a willing subject at risk. In so doing, I want to explore the larger question of why such a puzzle arises – why physicians, and many others, find it morally objectionable to help someone do something which all agree to be heroic. Finally, I will start by examining some ways of framing the issue, widely employed in medical ethics, which I believe are simply wrong. This sort of puzzle is much more interesting than proponents of these standard arguments would have us believe, and it illustrates some larger points about morality which are often overlooked.

PRIMUM NON NOCERE

One standard response in medical ethics to puzzles like the one just outlined is the injunction to do no harm. Sometimes dressed up as the 'principle of non-maleficence', this injunction appeals to the duties or obligations of physicans qua physicans. Being a physician, perhaps necessarily, and certainly historically involves taking on certain duties, one of which has traditionally been the duty not to harm patients. A heart transplant violates this duty if it necessarily involves taking the life of a patient.

However, despite the frequency with which the *primum non nocere* argument appears in medical ethics, and the force that it often justifiably carries, it does not do much to *explain* the pervasive intuition that there is something wrong with a physician taking part in a procedure like the one sketched out above. First, as a justification for refusing to participate in the transplant it will not do merely to say that physicians ought not to do harm, for physicians justifiably do harm routinely, as a means to some greater good – say, a course of chemotherapy for cancer. The problem is to justify applying the principle in a particular case, and in this case there is no immediately apparent reason why a physician ought not simply to view the willing death of a heart donor as a means to a greater good.

Often to sacrifice one person for the sake of a greater good would violate deeply held and widely shared values concerning personal autonomy. But in this case the patient actually wants to donate his heart and sacrifice his life, for rational, altruistic reasons. Perhaps he feels that his life is near its close, and that to donate to this potential recipient would be a worthy, noble way to finish his life. It is difficult to argue that it is violating a competent person's autonomy to participate in a transplant that he makes an autonomous choice to undergo.

Second, the *primum non nocere* argument fails in this case because we do not have to imagine a case where the physician actually *does* any harm. It may be that the patient agrees to commit suicide, on the condition that when he does the physician will transplant his heart. Here the physician does not actually do any harm; rather his agreement to perform the surgery forms part of the reason that the patient harms himself. But changing this condition does little to ease our discomfort with the physician's role. Thus this discomfort must be a result of something other than the harm that the physician actually *does*.

This point applies equally well to objections that a physician should not participate on the grounds that physicans must never kill. Our intuition that something is wrong with the physicians performing the transplant remains even if it is the case that the physician does not kill the patient.

Third, the *primum non nocere* argument shares a failing of most institutional or professional codes based on tradition, and that is: what is so special about tradition? To argue on the basis of a code of medical ethics requires some further justification other than the historical fact of that code; one must say why the code, or in this case a particular prohibition, is itself justified. One might in some cases appeal to a slippery slope – this sort of practice would lead to other morally reprehensible practices – but this does not explain our intuition about this particular case. It merely points to other harms which might result. Alternatively, one might argue that it would destroy trust in the medical profession, but this argument fails to say *why* trust would be destroyed. It is also circular: if trust is destroyed, it will be because there is something morally wrong with performing the procedure; one cannot then point to a destruction of trust as the feature which makes performing the procedure wrong.

Finally, any appeal to a professional code in this case misses the crux of the problem. For our intuition here is not merely that it is wrong for a physician to help a person perform such heroic actions, but that it would be wrong for *anyone* to help. This is not a puzzle only for medical ethics. One would have the same reservations about any person who helped another one perform such actions. We call a soldier a hero who throws himself on a grenade to save his battalion, but there is something ghoulish, for instance, about a man who throws a quadriplegic radio operator on a grenade, even if the radio operator begs him to do it.

AUTONOMY AND CONSCIENCE

Another way of casting the argument is in terms of respect for autonomy. Of course we ought to respect a person's autonomous choice to risk harm to herself, this argument goes, but are such choices truly autonomous? Such was the reasoning behind the chorus of wary voices at last year's landmark liver transplants from living donors at the University of Chicago. Many commentators expressed reservations about the Chicago transplant team's announced plan to transplant a hepatic lobe from a mother to her severely ill infant daughter.[1] The reasoning behind these reservations related to the mother's emotional ties and moral commitment to her daughter. These ties prevented the mother's decision from being free, and thus from being truly autonomous.

Plainly this is a misguided way of framing the issue. It seems to me an odd notion of autonomy indeed which would count emotional ties and moral commitments as constraints on autonomy. Moreover, the question is not whether the donor (or subject) should have the right to expose himself to harm; this right is little disputed, at least in the libertarian United States. The point at issue is the physican's role in exposing that donor to harm.

In debates over euthanasia and abortion, many physicians defend their refusal to participate on grounds of conscience. A patient may have the right to be euthanized or have an abortion, but this right has no claim on a physician, who may justifiably refuse to participate in a procedure which he conscientiously believes to be wrong. However, an attempt to cast the issue at hand in these terms merely sidesteps the real problem. The problem here is not whether a physician should have the right to obey his conscience; in the vast majority of cases he clearly will. The problem is how to justify one's conscientious choice – to say what accounts for the pervasive intuition that there is something wrong with a physician exposing a patient to such risk.

SAINTS AND HEROES

In his landmark essay "Saints and Heroes",[2] J.O. Urmson argued that traditional ways of evaluating moral worth classify actions into three sorts: first, actions that are duties, or that we ought to perform; second, actions that are not duties but are morally permissible; and third, actions that are morally wrong, that we ought not to do. Urmson thought that this classification ignored another sort

[1] For example, the popular press reported a number of these comments. B.D. Colen, *Los Angeles Times*, December 11 1989: 'Simply put, how can a parent be expected to make an informed, rational free choice when asked to consider donating an organ to his or her own dying child?' George Annas, *New York Times*, November 27, 1989: 'The parents basically can't say no'. Arthur Caplan, *Knight-Ridder Newspapers*, December 14 1989: 'Does anyone really think parents can say no when the option is certain death for their own son or daughter?'

[2] J.O. Urmson, 'Saints and Heroes', reprinted in *Moral Concepts*, ed. Joel Feinberg, Oxford: Oxford University Press, 1969, pp. 60–73.

of morally important action, actions which he called saintly or heroic. We reserve high moral praise for saintly and heroic actions, so we could not say that they are merely morally permissible. But they are not duties either. Such actions are, if anything, beyond the bounds of duty.

Urmson claims that there are several sorts of actions which we generally call saintly or heroic, and some of these actions may well fall within the traditional classification. A person may be called a saint if he does his duty in a situation where considerations of self-interest or desire might cause most people not to do it. A person might be called a hero if he does his duty in cases where fear or the drive to self-preservation would cause most people not to do it. In these cases the common element is self-control. But Urmson would still be willing to call a saint or a hero the person who does his duty effortlessly in cases where most of us would fail. The person who is virtuous in this Aristotelian sense may also be a saint or a hero.

However, the person who is most obviously saintly or heroic, Urmson says, is not the one who does his duty in extreme circumstances. Rather, saints or heroes *par excellence* do morally praiseworthy actions which are plainly not duties. The soldier who throws himself on a grenade to save his battalion has clearly done something of moral worth, but we could not say that the action was his duty. If he had not done it, no one could say to him that he ought to have thrown himself on the grenade. So the person whose actions Urmson believes to be most plainly heroic or saintly is the one who goes 'the second mile', whose actions 'exceed the demands of duty'.[3]

I will not discuss here the many objections to Urmson's argument which have been voiced over the years.[4] Rather I want to concentrate on what I think is an uncontroversial point, that of where saintly and heroic actions derive their moral worth. For whether or not one subscribes to Urmson's objections to the traditional way of classifying actions morally, it should be plain that one reason, among others, that we consider saintly and heroic action morally praiseworthy, is the fact that the saints and heroes voluntarily undergo self-sacrifice.

---

[3] Urmson, 'Saints and Heroes', 65.
[4] For a sampling of such objections, see Elizabeth Pybus, ' "Saints and Heroes" ', *Philosophy* 57, 1982, 193–199; Yogendra Chopra, 'Professor Urmson on Saints and Heroes', *Philosophy* 38, 1963, 160–166; Michael Clark, 'The Meritorious and the Mandatory', *Proceedings* of *the Aristotelian Society* LXXIX, 1978–9, 23–33. Joel Feinberg defends Urmson and takes his arguments still further in 'Supererogation and Rules', *Ethics*, 71, 1960–61, 276–88.

Now I do not wish to argue here that self-sacrifice itself confers moral worth on actions, for plainly a person might sacrifice himself for something morally bad, such as a terrorist might do on a suicide mission. And the element of self-sacrifice will be missing from the actions of some persons whom Urmson is willing to call saints or heroes: namely, the person who does his duty effortlessly in situations that would be too much for most of us. I merely want to argue that self-sacrifice is one reason, among others, that we consider some actions heroic or saintly, and that this is especially true for those actions that Urmson calls saintly or heroic *par excellence*.

When for any reason we are inclined to say that an action is morally praiseworthy, it will usually be the case that we consider it more morally praiseworthy if the agent has sacrificed his own interests to accomplish it. This might be a sacrifice in fulfilling one's duty, as in the case of a military officer who refuses to reveal state secrets even when faced with torture. But self-sacrifice may also incline us to think more highly of an action which is clearly outside the bounds of duty. If a billionaire gives away ten thousand dollars to feed the hungry, he has clearly done a good deed and we might think highly of him. But we would probably think even more highly of the person who gave away his last ten thousand dollars.

Those actions for which we reserve our highest praise are those where the agent has sacrificed his own interests for another good. The sacrifice may not be the sole reason that we call the action morally good, but it is usually the reason that we call the action heroic or saintly. The soldier who sacrifices his life to save his battalion, the nurse who devotes her life to taking care of lepers – these are the types of people whom we are most likely to call saints or heroes. Without self-sacrifice their actions might still be morally praiseworthy, but they will not be saintly or heroic.

The relationship of self-sacrifice to moral worth can help us to understand the intuition that there is something morally wrong with a physician exposing a willing patient to the risk of harm. We can agree that a person who offers to donate his heart to another person – or for that matter, to donate his kidney, his bone marrow or part of his liver – is doing something which is morally praiseworthy. And it is not only praiseworthy because it helps another person; it is praiseworthy because in helping that person the donor is sacrificing his own interests. And this element of self-sacrifice which is crucial the moral worth of the donor's action will be absent from the actions of the physician who performs the operation.

Conflicting intuitions created the puzzle that we saw with the heart transplant. On the one hand, we felt that the person who wanted to donate his heart to another person was acting in a morally praiseworthy, even heroic manner. On the other, we also felt that perhaps it would be wrong for a physician to perform such an operation; or, at least, we felt that a physician would be morally justified in refusing to participate. The role of sacrifice in the moral evaluation of actions makes sense of these conflicting intuitions. Self-sacrifice is precisely the element that inclines us to say that the donor's action is morally praiseworthy. And thus it is no wonder that we consider the physician's role less than praiseworthy, since in performing the operation he makes no sacrifice.

We would find morally abhorrent the soldier who threw a willing quadriplegic fellow soldier on a grenade to save the battalion. But what if to smother the grenade took two men, and the soldier threw himself on the grenade along with the willing quadriplegic? We would certainly not find such an action morally reprehensible; we might well call both the soldiers heroes. The fact that the soldier sacrificed himself seems to elevate him morally. Our moral evaluation of the physician who performed a heart transplant would also change if the physician underwent a sacrifice – say, if she risked catching a fatal infectious disease by operating. Plainly the fact that an agent sacrifices her own interests plays an important role in our moral evaluation of that agent's actions.

On the other hand, mere self-sacrifice does not morally justify actions. Though we might think better of the physician who risks her own life, we might still object to her performing the operation. We sometimes speak of people acting nobly, but wrongly: in the United States, Southerners often say this of their ancestors who fought to preserve the traditions of the South, including the enslavement of Blacks, in the War Between the States. While self-sacrifice may 'contribute positively to our assessment of a person's character, we may nevertheless judge that the sacrifice is being made in the service of an unjustified cause.

More importantly, the fact that, in assisting a saint or a hero, a physician has himself done nothing saintly or heroic does not mean that assistance is morally unjustifiable; it only means that the physician is not a saint or a hero. Thus to point out the absence of self-sacrifice in the physician's action only goes part of the way towards explaining our intuition that he ought to refrain from performing the operation. It explains how the physician's action differs from the patient's, and why this difference may mean that the physican's action is not as praiseworthy as the patient's, but it does not explain why we might feel that for the physician to help would be positively wrong.

Perhaps part of the reason why we feel that it would be wrong for the physician to remove the vital organs of one person to save another relates to familiar controversies about acts and omissions. By refusing to perform the operation, it might be argued, the physician merely allows the patient who needs the vital organs to die, but by performing the operation, he either kills the donor or endorses the donor's suicide, and in so doing he participates more actively in the donor's death. And since an 'act' is morally worse than an 'omission', the physician ought to choose the omission and refuse to perform the operation. Better to let a person die, and keep one's hands clean, than to save him with hands stained by the blood of another.

Or so the arguments goes. Like many other writers, I do not think that the distinction between acts and omissions is necessarily morally relevant, at least not in the way that those who bring up these distinctions intend. But here is not the place to rehearse such a well-worn and convoluted argument. I mention it here only because, whatever its faults, it demonstrates what I suspect is a widely-held intuition about this particular case: that refraining would play less of a causal role in the death of the patient than operating would play in the death of the donor.

A more important reason for our divided intuitions about this case is the fact that, morally, self-sacrifice is a double-edged sword. On the one hand, it is an aspect of actions which we generally judge to be morally admirable. Placing one's own interests above those of others is often the reason that we call an action morally wrong, and sacrificing one's interests for others is often a reason for calling an action morally praiseworthy. On the other hand, a sacrifice is still a sacrifice; that is, in making it a person has caused some harm to himself, and harm is certainly something that we want to minimize. Thus we might imagine problematic cases involving a person who has sacrificed his own interests for those of others, an aspect which we consider morally praiseworthy, but who has also caused more harm to himself than he has prevented – for instance, if he has undergone tremendous self-sacrifice in return for a relatively trivial benefit to another.

How the sacrifice is seen – whether it is a noble, praiseworthy aspect of an action, or whether it is a harm to be avoided – depends largely on the perspective of the moral agent. The donor, we think, should be praised for valuing his own interests less than those of the transplant recipient; at a minimum, he is justified in valuing his interests less. But not so for the physician: we usually think that he ought to value the interests of his patients equally. Thus while he may think that the donor's offer to sacrifice his life for that of another is morally admirable, he may also believe that he violates his duty to value the interests of both the potential donor and the potential recipient equally if he performs the operation. By performing the transplant, he is endorsing the donor's sacrifice, and thereby valuing the interests of the recipient more than those of the donor.

Finally, it is important not to leave out the one remaining player in the drama: the organ recipient. Assuming that the recipient is a competent adult, what are we to make of a person who would willingly accept a donor's vital organs, at the expense of the donor's life? Unless he had reasons besides those of self-interest – and perhaps even if he had such reasons – most of us would see his actions as selfish and cowardly. Understandable, perhaps, but certainly not the sort of actions we would commend. It is doubtful that anyone would see the recipient's behavior as admirable, even those who would argue that these transplants are morally acceptable.

And for this reason, the recipient also figures in our moral intuitions about this case. By agreeing to transplant vital organs into the recipient, the surgeon appears to be endorsing the recipient's willingness to accept the organs. Thus the surgeon not only seems to endorse the donor's willingness to do himself harm, he seems to endorse the recipient's willingness to take *advantage* of the donor's willingness to do himself harm. Now whether by performing the transplant he is in *fact* endorsing the actions of the recipient is a matter for debate; but even if he is not, he is helping the recipient to accomplish an action which few of us would find admirable.

CONCLUSION

How does it help us in this case, and like cases, to identify sacrifice as a point on which moral evaluation turns? It helps in three ways. First, it brings out a contrast between the proper response to an agent who is doing his duty, and to one who is going beyond his duty (who is acting heroically, or saintly, or supererogatorily). That is, we might well say that in general a person is at least morally justified, and perhaps obliged, to help a person who is trying to do his duty. It is a morally good thing for me to help a person provide food or medical care to his children, to help him keep his promises, tell the truth, and so on. But it does not follow that, in general, I am justified in helping him to go beyond his duty – to be a saint or a hero. If the reason that we reserve high praise for these sorts of actions is sacrifice by the person who is acting, then to help a person act heroically will not have the very element which is essential to that action's moral worth.

Second, we now have some fuel to rebut the libertarian argument that a physician ought to perform such operations. If we have a way of morally differentiating the actions of the physician and the donor – that is, by the element of self-sacrifice – we can defend the notion that the physician's role in the operation is substantially different morally than the donor's. It will be different not only because of the obvious facts that the physician's physical actions are different and that he is himself a moral agent with different moral beliefs, but also because a crucial factor in our moral evaluation of actions is the sacrifice of self-interest, which will be absent from the actions of anyone who merely assists the donor. Moreover, anyone who assists in the donor's sacrifice seems to be valuing the interests of the donor less than the interests of the recipient.

On the other hand, identifying self-sacrifice as a crucial difference does not show that the physician is not justified in transplanting the vital organs. It gives some backing to that point of view, and it shows the case to be more complicated than it first seems, but one might still argue, and not without some plausibility, that the physician ought to value the interests of the donor less than those of the recipient, on the grounds that the donor wants his interests to be valued less. And of course, the case would become still more complicated if there were more than one needy recipient – one who needed a heart, another who needed a liver, a third who needed a kidney – and if it were possible to transplant the organs of the willing donor into all three.

But finally, we do now have some substance to back the intuition that there is something wrong with helping or encouraging a person to do himself harm, no matter how heroic we think such an action might be. This is perhaps one reason for the resilience of medicine's injunction not to do harm, and for its particular rhetorical force. It is doubtful that most of us want a society in which physicians are unreflectively willing to endorse their patients' suicides. Because physicians are in a special position, with the capacity to do great harm to patients both willing and unwilling, *primum non nocere* gives voice to the widely-shared belief that physicians must exercise special care in practicing their art, and abstain from practices which harm patients, even if the patient, quite reasonably, wishes to be harmed.

Acknowledgements

I am grateful to Grant Gillett, Alastair Campbell, C.L. Ten and John Harris for their valuable comments, and to Alan Wertheimer for his helpful remarks while the paper was in its early stages. Part of the work for this paper was done while I was a Fellow at the University of Chicago Center for Clinical Medical Ethics, which is supported by grants from the Henry J. Kaiser Family Foundation, the Andrew W. Mellon Foundation and the Pew Memorial Trusts.

PART IV: PUBLIC HEALTH ETHICS

Chapter 12

THE GENESIS OF PUBLIC HEALTH ETHICS

RONALD BAYER AND AMY L. FAIRCHILD

In the beginning there was bioethics. The 1960s and 1970s witnessed extraordinary challenges to the broadly understood authority of medicine. Perhaps most strikingly, the paternalistic authority of physicians was brought into question by a new medical ethics that gave pride of place to the concept of autonomy.[1] Paralleling the challenges to medical practice were those that involved the research enterprise. Against a backdrop of scandal and abuse, and haunted by the experience of the violations of human dignity that had occurred under the aegis of medical research in Nazi Germany, a new ethics of research took hold.[2] Informing that moral world-view was the basic belief that no individual should be required to participate in research endeavours – no matter how important for the public good – without his or her informed consent.[3] Thus, the ethics of clinical research and the ethics of medical practice were conjoined by a commitment to autonomy and individual rights.

Remarkably, as bioethics emerged and began to have enormous impacts on the practice of medicine and research – fuelled, to be sure, by broad socio-political changes that gave rise to the struggle of women, African Americans, gay men and lesbians, and the anti-authoritarian impulse that characterised the New Left in democratic capitalist societies – little attention was given to the question of the ethics of public health. This was all the more striking since the core values and practices of public health, often entailing the subordination of the individual for the common good, seemed to stand as a rebuke to the ideological impulses of bioethics.

[1] David J. Rothman. 1991. *Strangers at the Bedside: A History of How Law and Bioethics Transformed Medical Decision Making*. New York, NY Basic Books.
[2] Ibid. pp. 96, 99, 185–197.
[3] Terrence H. Ackerman. 1996. Choosing Between Nuremberg and the National Commission: Balancing of Moral Principles in Clinical Research. In *The Ethics of Research Involving Human Subjects: Facing the 21st Century*. Harold Y. Vanderpool, ed. Baltimore, MD. Frederick Press: 83.

Just how vast a gulf existed between the ethos of public health and the individualistic and antipaternalistic values of bioethics is given historical referent in the person of Herman Biggs. Biggs – a highly influential New York City health official who implemented a new set of public health interventions targeting the individual in the late nineteenth and early twentieth centuries – gave full expression to the moral foundations of public health: 'The government of the United States is democratic, but the sanitary measures adopted are sometimes autocratic, and the functions performed by sanitary authorities paternal in character. We are prepared, when necessary, to introduce and enforce, and the people are ready to accept, measures which might seem radical and arbitrary, if they were not plainly designed for the public good, and evidently beneficent in their effects.'[4] It was the spirit of Biggs that informed thinking during the Progressive Era – the formative period of American public health.

When, at the beginning of the twenty-first century, a systematic effort to articulate an ethics of public health began, the deep differences between bioethics and public health would draw immediate attention.[5] In 'An Ethics Framework for Public Health', Nancy Kass thus writes, 'codes of medical and research ethics generally give high priority to individual autonomy, a priority that cannot be assumed to be appropriate for public health practice.'[6] Similarly, Daniel Callahan and Bruce Jennings, in their effort to begin a broad engagement on the ethics of public health, argued, 'In early bioethics, the good of the individual, and particularly his or her autonomy, was the dominant theme, not population health.'[7] That formative perspective, which retained its grip, compelled Callahan and Jennings to acknowledge that their own effort had to confront an epistemological 'obstacle': 'the difference between the individualistic orientation of bioethics and the population and societal focus

---

[4] Hermann M. Biggs. 1897. *Preventive Medicine in the City of New York*. New York, NY Health Department: 28, note 2.
[5] James F. Childress, Ruth R. Faden, Ruth D. Gaare, Lawrence O. Gostin, Jeffrey Kahn, Nancy E. Kass, Anna C. Mastroianni, Jonathan D. Moreno & Phillip Nieburg. Public Health Ethics: Mapping the Terrain. *Journal of Law, Medicine, and Ethics* 2002; 30: 170–178. Public Health Leadership Society. 2002. *Principles of the Ethical Practice of Public Health*. Version 2.2. Public Health Leadership Society.
[6] Nancy E. Kass. An Ethics Framework for Public Health. *American Journal of Public Health* 2001; 91: 11.
[7] Daniel Callahan & Bruce Jennings. Ethics and Public Health: Forging a Strong Relationship. *American Journal of Public Health* 2002; 92: 169.

of public health.'[8] These challenges echoed the trenchant arguments made by Renee Fox decades earlier.[9]

Of what relevance is autonomy-focused bioethics for public health, with its mix of justifications including those that are either implicitly or explicitly paternalistic or that seek to impose strictures on individuals and communities in the name of collective welfare? To examine the deep divide between the central commitments of bioethics and the values that animate the practice of public health, we focus on a series of controversies implicating the concepts of privacy, liberty, and paternalism.

FIRST ENCOUNTERS: EPIDEMIOLOGICAL RESEARCH AND THE LIMITS OF CONSENT

Epidemiology is the foundational science of public health. Regulations designed to protect the autonomy and privacy of research subjects would require modification in the face of public health-focused research, regardless of whether it was conducted by government agencies or academic entities. Beginning in the 1970s, a discussion began about whether the emerging rules and regulations for human subjects' research would apply to epidemiological studies. Was informed consent necessary when research involved the use of extant records? Would imposing consent requirements for the examination of data sets involving large numbers of people – many of whom would be difficult or impossible to locate – render epidemiological research virtually impossible?[10] 'The clash between the

[8] Ibid. p. 170.

[9] Renee C. Fox. Advanced Medical Technology – Social and Ethical Implications. *Annual Review of Sociology* 1976; 2: 231–268. Renee C. Fox & Judith P. Swazey. 1988. Medical Morality is Not Bioethics: Medical Ethics in China and the United States. In *Essays in Medical Sociology*. Renee C. Fox, ed. New Brunswick, NJ. Transaction Books: 645–670. Rothman, op. cit. note 1, pp. 242–243.

[10] L. Gordis, E. Gold & R. Seltzer. Privacy Protection in Epidemiologic and Medical Research: A Challenge and a Responsibility. *American Journal of Epidemiology* 1977; 105: 163–168. L. Gordis & E. Gold. Privacy, Confidentiality and the Use of Medical Records in Research. *Science* 1980; 207: 153–156. L. Gostin. Ethical Principles for the Conduct of Human Subject Research: Population-Based Research and Ethics. *Law, Medicine, and Health Care* 1991; 19: 191–201. A.M. Capron. Protection of Research Subjects: Do Special Rules Apply in Epidemiology. *Law, Medicine, and Health Care* 1991; 19: 184–190. C.I. Cann & K.J. Rothman. IRBs and Epidemiologic Research: How Inappropriate Restrictions Hamper Studies. IRB: *A Review of Human Subjects Research* 1984; July/August: 5–7. N. Hershey. JRB Jurisdiction and Limits on IRB Actions. IRB: *A Review of Human Subjects Research* 1985; March April: 7–9. K.J. Rothman. The Rise and Fall of Epidemiology, 1950–2000 A.D. *NEJM* 1981; 304: 600–602.

privacy rights of persons and the need for access to and disclosure of personal health-related information', noted one observer, 'is the most frequent ethical dilemma to confront epidemiologists.'[11] In 1981, the United States Department of Health and Human Services (DHHS) issued regulations for the protection of human subjects explicitly exempting epidemiological research involving already existing data from informed consent requirements provided the risk to subjects was minimal, the research did not record data in a way that was individually identifiable, and the research could not otherwise be conducted.[12] The concession represented a relaxation of the fundamental principle that individuals could not be conscripted into research without their consent, for it was clear that the benefits of records-based research were significant enough to trump the claims of the individual.

The tension between the claims of individual informed consent and the demands imposed by record-based epidemiological research was also confronted in other economically advanced democratic nations. How these tensions were resolved reflected the extent to which the rights of the individual were given priority, judgements about how significant a burden would be entailed by insisting upon consent, and the social value accorded to such retrospective record-based studies. The Australian National Health and Medical Research Council, for example, required ethical review of all epidemiological studies and the consent of subjects unless such a requirement would render it impossible to conduct the study. In 1991, the European Union likewise proposed that that all studies undergo ethical review.[13] However, the proposed directive gave such priority to privacy and consent that epidemiologists expressed alarm over the future of their efforts. In response to arguments that the directive would make epidemiological research unfeasible, a 1995 directive made provisions for research without consent in instances where confidentiality was adequately protected, obtaining consent was impracticable, and the research was of sufficient importance. France

---

[11] John Last. 1996. Professional Standards of Conduct for Epidemiologists. In *Ethics and Epidemiology*. Steven S. Coughlin & Tom L. Beauchamp, eds. New York, NY Oxford University Press: 57.

[12] Code of Federal Regulations, Title 45, Public Welfare, Department of Health and Human Services, National Institutes of Health, Office for Protection from Research Risks, Part 46, Protection of Human Subjects (45 CFR 46).

[13] Baruch A. Brody. 1998. *The Ethics of Biomedical Research: An International Perspective*. New York, NY. Oxford University Press: 57.

and Germany passed similar provisions a year before the European Union approved its final directive, though at the end of the 1990s, concerns remained, especially in Great Britain.[14]

The Council for International Organizations of Medical Sciences (CIOMS) also addressed the issues imposed by the use of existing clinical records as part of its broader analysis of the ethical issues posed by epidemiological studies. In its 1991 report, it acknowledged that prior efforts to provide ethical guidance for biomedical research focused on 'patients and individual subjects' were not sufficient for studies involving 'groups' of people. Thus, while emphasising the importance of the principles of research ethics first propounded in the Belmont Report, it recognised that their application in the epidemiological context would require flexibility. Most important, the CIOMS epidemiological guidelines, like those from nations that had addressed these issues before, noted that individual informed consent was not always practical in epidemiological studies, while asserting that individuals and their representatives should 'normally' be told that their medical records or stored tissue samples might be used for future epidemiological studies.[15] In the end it was the duty of researchers who sought to undertake such record-based studies 'to explain to an ethical review committee how the study would be ethical in [the absence of consent].'[16]

AIDS, PUBLIC HEALTH, AND ETHICS

The encounter over epidemiological research foreshadowed a more sustained and critical effort to enunciate an ethics of public health in the context of the AIDS epidemic, which began in the early 1980s. It is not surprising that when those schooled in bioethics first sought to address the ethical challenges posed by AIDS, they did so guided by the principles and values that had shaped the confrontation with medicine and the research enterprise.[17] Their efforts were informed by the intense concern of gay men about threats to

---

[14] Ibid. pp. 62–63.
[15] CIOMS. 1991. International. Guidelines for Ethical Review of Epidemiological Studies. Guideline 3.
[16] Ibid. Guideline 2.
[17] R. Bayer, C. Levine & S. Wolf. HIV Antibody Screening: An Ethical Framework for Evaluating Proposed Programs. *Journal of the American Medical Association* 1986; 256: 1768–1774.

privacy and civil liberties advocates fearful that AIDS would provide the occasion for the erosion of a set of substantive and procedural constitutional rights forged by the US Supreme Court. These concerns, in turn, were reflected in the posture adopted by public health officials in many cosmopolitan centres.[18]

Emerging from the complex mix of ideological, moral, and political forces was a commitment to treating AIDS differently from what the history of epidemic control might have suggested. In lieu of the compulsory tradition, that often involved mandatory case reporting by name, contact investigation, and where necessary the use of isolation, an 'exceptionalist' perspective took hold.[19] Focused on the centrality of education for mass behavioural change, the protection of the rights and privacy of people infected with HIV, and a rejection of coercive measures, the approach to AIDS was voluntarist at its core. A simple dictum emerged: no public health policy that violated the rights of individuals could be effective in controlling the spread of HIV. There was, therefore, no tension between public health and civil liberties. Indeed, the protection of civil liberties was critical to the public health.

This view informed decisions in virtually all advanced democratic nations and was reflected on an international level in the effort to forge a relationship between public health and human rights.[20] While recognising that, in principle, limits on rights could be justified by the claims of public health, the United Nations Office of the High Commissioner for Human Rights and the Joint United Nations Programme on AIDS concluded that coercive public health measures were counterproductive since they tended to 'drive away people most in need of services and failed to achieve their public health goal of prevention through behavioral change, care, and health support.'[21] It was thus possible to declare that 'public health interests do not conflict with human rights. On the contrary, it has

---

[18] R. Bayer. 1989. *Private Acts, Social Consequences: Aids and the Politics of Public Health.* New Brunswick, NJ. Rutgers University Press.

[19] R. Bayer. Public Health Policy and the AIDS Epidemic: an End to HIV Exceptionalism? NEJM 1991; 324: 1500–1504.

[20] David Kirp & Ronald Bayer, eds. 1991. AIDS in the Industrialized Democracies. New Brunswick, NJ. Rutgers University Press. Lawrence O. Gostin & Zita Lazzarini. 1997. *Human Rights and Public Health in the AIDS Pandemic.* New York, NY. Oxford University Press: xiv.

[21] Office of the United Nations High Commissioner for Human Rights and the Joint United Nations Programme on HIV/AIDS. 1998. *HIV/AIDS and Human Rights: International Guidelines.* New York & Geneva. United Nations: 37.

been recognized that when human rights are protected, fewer people become infected.'[22] Perhaps the most extreme formulation of this commitment to the protection of the rights of individuals was given voice by Jonathan Mann, who more than any other individual was responsible for seeking to embed public health in a human rights framework. He recognised the tension between public health and human rights, but in so doing, restated the conflict in a new way: 'For the present, it may be useful to adopt the maxim that health policies and programs should be considered discriminatory and burdensome on human rights until proven otherwise.'[23]

While AIDS provided the starting point, those committed to a health and human rights perspective saw the new articulation as having broad implications for public health more generally. If there were to be an ethics of public health, it would have to reflect in fundamental ways the values that gave birth to bioethics. Writing about the jurisprudential foundations of public health, George Annas challenged the relevance of *Jacobson v Massachusetts*, a 1905 case in which the US Supreme Court upheld mandatory smallpox vaccination, employing language that would serve as the basis for the broad exercise of public health powers in the twentieth century: 'Today, almost one hundred years after *Jacobson*, both medicine and constitutional law are radically different. We now take constitutional rights much more seriously, including the right of a competent adult to refuse any medical treatment, even if life-saving treatment.'[24]

SURVEILLANCE AND THE LIMITS OF PRIVACY

Since the end of the nineteenth century, surveillance has served as a critical element in the practice of public health. Central to the effort to monitor and intervene in the face of threats to the public health, surveillance has imposed on health care institutions and especially physicians the duty to report cases to confidential registries. Almost always such reports have included the names of the afflicted. Hence surveillance has represented a striking example of

---

[22] Ibid. p. 10.
[23] Jonathan M. Mann, Lawrence Gostin, Sofia Gruskin, Troyen Brennan, Zita Lazzarini & Harvey V. Fineberg. Health and Human Rights. *Health and Human Rights* 1994; 1: 16.
[24] George Annas. Blinded by Bioterrorism: Public Health and Liberty in the 21st Century. *Health Matrix* 2003; 13: 47.

the ways in which the claims of public health could intrude upon the privacy of the clinical relationship. For most of the twentieth century such practices, *once established*, went unchallenged. AIDS provided the context for an assault on the privacy-limiting features of surveillance activities.

Soon after the first cases of AIDS were reported by the Centers for Disease Control in June 1981, state health departments in the US began to require that physicians and hospitals report by name each newly diagnosed case.[25] Once the capacity to test for the presence of the antibody to HIV became possible in 1985, it was only a matter of time before some public health official would seek to extend to HIV infection the reporting requirements that were in place for AIDS. The rationale for such reporting drew upon the history of public health: reporting would alert public health officials to the presence of individuals infected with a lethal infection; would allow them to counsel infected individuals about what they needed to do to prevent further transmission; would permit the authorities to monitor the incidence and prevalence of infection. Alert to concerns about privacy and confidentiality, health officials underscored the existence of administrative, regulatory, and statutory protections for reported names. There was no reason to believe that state health departments would fail to protect the identities of those with HIV when they had protected those with AIDS, tuberculosis, and other reportable infections.[26]

To these propositions, gay community-based antagonists to name-based reporting and civil liberties advocates retorted that AIDS was different: social hostility and AIDS-related hysteria could lead to changes in policy, legislatively imposed, that would permit for breaches that would never occur with other conditions.[27] And then those in registries would lose their jobs, their housing, and perhaps their liberty. These were arguments that impressed many health officials in states with relatively large AIDS caseloads. Reporting, they came to believe, would be counterproductive; it would drive people away from testing and counselling – essential control measures in the public health campaign against AIDS in the United States and elsewhere. It did not matter that public health

[25] Bayer, *op. cit.* note 18, pp. 101–136.
[26] Ronald Bayer & Amy L. Fairchild. The Limits of Privacy: Surveillance and the Control of Disease. *Health Care Analysis* 2002; 10: 19–35.
[27] Bayer, *op. cit.* note 18.

departments had an exemplary record in protecting name-based reports.[28] If those most at risk for HIV had fears about what would happen to them, then that was all that mattered.

As therapeutic advances began to emerge in the late 1980s, fissures began to appear in the relatively broad and solid alliance against name-based reporting. The traditional values of public health began to reassert themselves against the privacy-based concerns that had prevailed during the epidemic's first decade. At the end of November 1990, the CDC declared its support for HIV reporting, which it asserted could 'enhance the ability of local, state and national agencies to project the level of required resources' for care and prevention services.[29] The House of Delegates of the American Medical Association endorsed the reporting of names as well, thus breaking with the traditional resistance of medical practitioners to such intrusions on the physician-patient relationship.[30] In 1991, New Jersey became the first high-prevalence state to require HIV-case reporting by name.[31] In the following years, the CDC continued to press for named reporting of HIV cases, an effort that assumed the dimensions of a campaign.

Although most, if not all, AIDS-service organisations as well as civil liberties advocates remained adamantly opposed to name reporting, arguing instead for the use of unique identifiers that could protect the privacy of people with HIV infection, the public health community, with the CDC in the lead, concluded that such an approach would simply impede the adoption of an effective system of surveillance. Nevertheless, marking the extent to which concerns for privacy continued to shape decision-making in public health, the CDC, in its 1999 recommendation for nationwide HIV case reporting, reluctantly opened the way to the use of unique identifiers in those states that preferred a reporting course that did not entail the use of names.

The debates that occurred over name-based reporting in the context of the AIDS epidemic would inevitably raise questions about the practice of surveillance itself as advocates of privacy, to the

[28] L.O. Gostin, J. Ward & C. Baker. National HIV Case Reporting for the United States: A Defining Moment in the History of the Epidemic. *NEJM* 1997; 337: 1166.

[29] Centers for Disease Control and Prevention. Update: Public Health Surveillance for HJV Infection – United States, 1989 and 1990. *MMWR* 1990; 39: 861.

[30] R. Bayer, *op. cit.* note 19: 1501.

[31] Intergovernmental Health Policy Project. Reporting in the States. *Intergovernmental AIDS Reports* 1989; November/December.

astonishment of public health practitioners, suggested that the warrant for the violation of privacy in the early twentieth century no longer deserved unquestioned obeisance.

CONFINEMENT AND THE LIMITS OF LIBERTY

Isolation and quarantine represent the most plenary exercise of the state's authority in the name of public health.[32] Historically, the imposition of isolation and quarantines to control infectious threats was bounded by few procedural protections. The rights of the individual were viewed as subservient to the judgements of those with public health authority. As the pattern of morbidity and mortality underwent an epidemiological transformation in the twentieth century, as chronic conditions replaced infectious diseases as the pre-eminent threat, the role of quarantine and isolation became marginal to the practice of public health in the United States. There were lingering threats that called forth the exercise of the power to confine – tuberculosis, for example – but they were relatively uncommon.

The worldwide threat of Severe Acute Respiratory Syndrome (SARS) in 2002 posed starkly the question of when, in the name of public health, individuals and communities could be deprived of their liberty. In several respects, SARS took society back to a pre-therapeutic era: no definitive diagnostic test, a non-specific case definition, and no effective vaccine or treatment.[33]

Countries used one of the oldest public health tools in response to the first outbreak of SARS: isolation and quarantine, underscoring the tension between liberty and the imperative to protect the public's health. During the first SARS outbreak, public health authorities implemented isolation and quarantine in countries with diverse socio-political and constitutional traditions, ranging from

[32] Although the terms are often used interchangeably, isolation is the separation of individuals known to be infectious. In contrast, quarantine is the restriction of the activities of healthy individuals or populations exposed to a communicable disease. A.S. Benenson, ed. 1995. *Control of Communicable Diseases Manual.* Washington, DC. American Public Health Association. J. Barbera, A. Macintyre, L. Gostin, T. Inglesbury, T. O'Toole, C. DeAtley, K. Tonat & M. Layton. Large-Scale Quarantine following Biological Terrorism in the United States: Scientific Examination, Logistic and Legal Limits, and Possible Consequences. JAMA 2001; 286: 2711–2717.

[33] J.L. Gerberding. Faster . . . but Fast Enough? Responding to the Epidemic of Severe Acute Respiratory Syndrome. *NEJM* 2003; 348: 2030.

China, Hong Kong, Vietnam and Singapore, to Canada and the United States.[34]

Confinement of individuals with disease and those exposed raised questions about the level of risk that justified loss of liberty. Frank cases needed to be isolated, but when a case was unconfirmed or when the individual had simply been exposed or was suspected of being exposed the justification for restricting liberty was problematical. Uncertainty about how wide to cast the net of quarantine for exposed, asymptomatic individuals was framed by the absence of a diagnostic assay that could rapidly distinguish between the infected and merely exposed with high specificity. But very broad quarantines were viewed as justifiable because of the uncertainties of risk.

Most jurisdictions confined patients in their homes or general hospitals, but others considered the construction of special infectious disease hospitals.[35] In Asia and Canada, authorities ordered mass quarantines or closures for schools, hospitals, factories, hotels, restaurants, places of entertainment, and residential buildings.[36] Some countries, particularly the United States, sought voluntary separation of exposed patients,[37] but others used more intrusive forms of enforcement. In Singapore, where thousands were subjected to quarantine, authorities used thermal scanners, web cameras, and electronic bracelets to enforce quarantine, supervised by a security agency.[38] In Hong Kong, the police department's electronic tracking system was used to enforce quarantine.[39] While recourse to compulsory measures posed few challenges to the underlying values of authoritarian regimes, officials underscored the extent to which the threat of SARS justified resort to coercive

[34] B.R. Bloom. Lessons from SARS. *Science* 2003; 300: 701.

[35] Hong Kong Economic and Trade Office Tokyo. Press release. Available at: http://www.hketotyo.or.jp/English/news_sars03060S_e.html (accessed 14 July, 2003).

[36] J.B. Kahn. Quarantine Set in Beijing Areas to Fight SARS. *New York Times* 25 April, 2003: A1. Centers for Disease Control and Prevention. Severe Acute Respiratory Syndrome – Singapore 2003. *MMWR* 2003; 52: 40–41. K. Bradsher. The SARS Epidemic: Economy; Outbreak of Disease brings Big Drop-off in China's Economy. *New York Times* 28 April, 2003: A1. A. Wayne. In Singapore, 1970s Law becomes Weapon Against SARS. *New York Times* 10 June, 2003: F4.

[37] M.H. Cooper. Fighting SARS. *CQ Researcher* 20 June, 2003.

[38] World Health Organization. Severe Acute Respiratory Syndrome – Singapore, 2003. *Weekly Epidemiogic. Record* 2003; 78: 161.

[39] World Health Organization. 2003. *Severe Acute Respiratory Syndrome (SARS): Status of the Outbreak and Lessons for the Immediate Future.* Geneva. World Health Organization.

measures even in liberal democratic societies. In Canada, a high school was closed and 1500 students ordered to home quarantine because of a single case involving a student with symptoms of SARS; Ontario's commissioner of public health warned those who violated the home quarantine that he had the authority to hospitalise those who failed to adhere to the order.[40]

In the fall of 2003, as the international community braced for the possibility of a resurgence of SARS, it became clear that the isolation procedures used during the initial outbreak had been far too stringent. The CDC reported that individuals quarantined after contact with an asymptomatic SARS patient 'had no detectable risk' of infection. Moreover, there were no cases in which an individual transmitted the disease to his or her contacts while under quarantine. Thus, the CDC concluded that 'Focusing only on persons who had contact with an actively ill SARS patient would have reduced the number of persons quarantined by approximately 66 percent, without compromising its effectiveness.'[41] The CDC then elaborated a finer range of surveillance and quarantine recommendations, these included: passive monitoring on the part of the individual with no activity restrictions; active monitoring by health care workers either by phone or in person (which might or might not include explicit quarantine restrictions); working quarantine (for people, such as health care workers, who provide essential services); focused measures (such as building closings or event cancellations) to increase the social distance among members of a group where transmission was believed to have occurred; and community-wide or regional measures (such as school closings and transportation system shut downs) to increase social distance in areas where extensive SARS transmission occurred, where there was a lack of clearly identifiable epidemiological links between cases, and where restrictions on known contacts was deemed insufficient.[42]

---

[40] D.L. Brown. Sick of Quarantine in Toronto; After School's SARS Scare, Teens Bored by Week in Isolation. *Washington Post* 3 June, 2003: A20.

[41] Centers for Disease Control and Prevention. Efficiency of Quarantine during an Epidemic of Severe Acute Respiratory Syndrome – Beijing, China, 2003. *MMWR* 2003; 52: 1039. See also: WHO. SARS – Epidemiological Findings, Clinical Picture, and Case Management. Available at: http://www.wpro.who.int/sars/docs/interimguidelines/part2.asp (accessed 9 February, 2004).

[42] Centers for Disease Control and Prevention. Public Health Guidance for Community-Level Preparedness and Response to Sever Acute Respiratory Syndrome (SARS). Version 2; Appendix Dl: Interventions for Community Containment. 8 January, 2004. Available at: http://www.cdc.gov/ncidod/sars/guidance/D/index.htm (accessed 9 February, 2004).

PATERNALISM AND THE LIMITS OF AUTONOMY

For government to impose restrictions on those who represent a risk to others falls clearly within the broadly accepted exercise of state power in liberal societies and in principle entails no fundamental problem for the autonomy-focused perspective of bioethics. Problems emerge where the risk to others is uncertain. It is here that an important divide emerges between the judgements of those committed to autonomy and those whose first priority is the public health. It is a divide characterised by complex questions of what moral weight to give to the *likelihood* and *severity* of harm. However these matters are resolved, they raise issues that are fundamentally different from those posed by behaviours that represent primarily a threat to individuals themselves. It is here that the spectre of paternalism emerges, and that the tension between public health perspectives and autonomy-focused bioethics is positioned in its boldest relief.

Tobacco consumption represents the single most important cause of morbidity and mortality in advanced industrialised societies. It thus serves as an object lesson in the ways in which the antagonism towards paternalism has both shaped and limited public health policy.

In 1964, when the Office of the US Surgeon General issued the first report on the hazards of tobacco use, 50% of men and 35% of women smoked cigarettes.[43] This meant there were millions of smoking adults whose health and lives were imperilled. But as the American campaign against tobacco took its first halting steps in the context of fierce resistance from the tobacco industry and its political allies, it avoided the taint of paternalism, the suggestion that the state was seeking to impose its preferences on those who smoked cigarettes.

Three broad sets of policies were adopted to confront the challenge posed by tobacco over the next four decades: restrictions on advertising; the imposition of taxes; and limits on public smoking. In each case, a public warrant for the measures adopted sought to demonstrate that it was third parties, innocent victims, or children that were the object of protective measures. Only insofar as

[43] US Department of Health and Human Services. 2000. *Reducing Tobacco Use: A Report of the Surgeon General*. Washington, DC. Government Printing Office.

warnings about tobacco, weak as they were, were posted on cigarette packages, did public health efforts direct themselves to those who bore the full burden of cigarette-related suffering, disease, and death.

Efforts to limit tobacco advertising, a complex matter in polities that accord protection to commercial speech, almost always focused on the claims of children. It was they who were vulnerable to the manipulations and seductions of advertising. If in order to protect them, it was necessary to limit advertising that could be viewed by adults – proposals in the US to ban outdoor advertising within 1000 feet of any school effectively meant a ban on all outdoor advertising in many communities – that was a price that had to be paid.

As public health officials came to recognise that cigarette consumption was price-responsive despite the addictive nature of nicotine, the possibility of facing the threat of tobacco-related disease by raising taxes became increasingly appealing. But the public justification of such taxes was almost always that either increasing the price of cigarettes would render them too costly for adolescents or that those who smoked cigarettes imposed health care costs on the non-smoking population.[44] Such externalities could be internalised by raising taxes on cigarettes. Indeed, fairness dictated the imposition of such burdens on smokers.[45] If such taxes also discouraged those who smoked from continuing their habit, that was simply an added advantage to a policy directed at the protection of non-smokers and those, who because of age, were an appropriate target of paternalistic interventions.

Finally, virtually from the dawn of the public health campaign against cigarette-related morbidity and mortality, the effort to restrict smoking in public settings has played a central role.[46] Such efforts *preceded* the first evidence that side-stream smoke posed a hazard – at least in enclosed environments – by more than a decade. By the end of the twentieth century, a radical transformation had occurred. Smoking, which was an integral dimension of the social

[44] Thomas A. Hodgson. Cigarette Smoking and Lifetime Medical Expenditure. *Milbank Quarterly* 1992; 70: 81–125.
[45] Kenneth E. Warner. Cigarette Taxation: Doing Good by Doing Well. *Journal of Public Health Policy* 1984; 5: 312–319.
[46] Ronald Bayer & James Colgrove. 2004. Children and Bystanders First: The Ethics and Politics of Tobacco Control in the United States. In *Unfiltered: Conflicts over Tobacco Policy and Public Health*. Eric Feldman & Ronald Bayer, eds. Cambridge, MA. Harvard University Press.

world, was increasingly relegated to the private domain.[47] Debate over how far to press such restrictions ultimately had to confront the question of whether bans on outdoor smoking could be justified in terms of annoyance abatement rather than disease prevention. An antismoking activist declared, 'Even if outdoor environmental tobacco smoke were no more hazardous than dog excrement stuck to the bottom of a shoe, in many places laws require dog owners to avoid fouling public areas. Is this too much to ask of smokers?'[48] Not all antismoking activists shared this view. Said the editor of *Tobacco Control*, 'We need to ask whether efforts to prevent people from smoking outdoors risks besmirching tobacco control advocates as the embodiment of intolerant, paternalistic busy-bodies, who, not content at protecting their own health, want to force smokers not to smoke.'[49]

Despite such concerns, by the end of the twentieth century, the willingness to embrace explicitly paternalistic justifications for antismoking policy was becoming more evident, no doubt facilitated by the emergence of a sharp social gradient in cigarette consumption – those who are educated smoke less and less, those at the bottom of the social ladder continue to smoke.

The most dramatic reflection of the willingness to embrace paternalism was to be found in measures seeking to 'denormalise' smoking. We typically do not think of health promotion campaigns as paternalistic. But when they go beyond the provision of information and systematically seek to transform the very desires and preferences of those to whom they are directed, they assume a fundamentally different character. Indeed, the use of social marketing techniques to undercut smoking behaviour must be viewed as paternalistic in impulse as well as practice. In a 1998 report, California's tobacco control programme openly advocated a social norm change designed to protect 'generations who have already reached adulthood.'[50] When New York City sharply increased tobacco taxes in

[47] Allan Brandt. 1998. Blow Some Smoke My Way: Passive Smoking, Risk, and American Culture. In *Ashes to Ashes: The History of Smoking and Health*. Stephen Lock, Lois Reynolds & E.M. Tansey, eds. Amsterdam. Rodopi Press.

[48] J. Repace. Banning Outdoor Smoking Is Scientifically Justifiable. *Tobacco Control* 2000; 9: 98.

[49] S. Chapman. Banning Smoking Outdoors Is Seldom Ethically Justifiable. *Tobacco Control* 2000; 9: 95–97.

[50] California Department of Health Services. 1998. *A Model for Change: The California Experience in Tobacco Control*. Sacramento, CA. California Department of Health Services: 4.

2002, the justification was not that smokers imposed costs on others, but rather that hefty prices might help force smokers to quit. The mayor of New York City saw this as an effort to save the lives of smokers themselves.[51]

TOWARD AN ETHICS OF PUBLIC HEALTH

What the foregoing discussion has demonstrated is that those involved in the practice of public health embrace a set of values that are often, if not always, in conflict with the autonomy-centred values of those who take an individualistic and anti-paternalistic stance. But ethos is not ethics. When bioethics first emerged it confronted a tradition of medical practice and research within which paternalism still commanded both loyalty and impassioned defence. It was that dominant world-view that bioethics sought to overturn. In the context of public health, the question that needs to be addressed is whether paternalism and subordination of the individual for the good of the commonwealth should serve as the foundation for an ethics of public health or whether the perspective derived from the dominant autonomy-focused and anti-paternalistic currents in bioethics should serve as a point of departure for a thoroughgoing challenge to the fundamental values and practices of public health.

We begin with the conviction that at the core of public health practice is the charge to protect the common good, to intervene for such ends even in the face of uncertainty. This stance may, we believe, necessitate limits on the choices of individuals on grounds of communal protection against both hazard and paternalism. It is in this regard that this article may be distinguished from other recent efforts to articulate a set of moral considerations for public health, which have commonly focused on the centrality of social justice for public health.

During the twentieth century, public health interventions were often justified by an explicit or implicit invocation of the harm principle. First enunciated by John Stuart Mill, that principle provides the standard for judging liberty-limiting acts of government.[52]

---

[51] Michael Cooper. Cigarettes Up to $7 a Pack with New Tax. *New York Times* 1 July, 2002: B1.
[52] John Stuart Mill. *On Liberty* quoted in: The *Philosophy of John Stuart Mills*. 1961. M. Cohen, ed. New York, NY. Modern Library: 185–319.

It would be hard to imagine a set of ethical arguments that could challenge this posture. Indeed, limitations on the rights of individuals in the face of public health threats are firmly supported by legal tradition and ethics.[53] All legal systems, as well as international human rights, permit governments to infringe on personal liberty to prevent a significant risk to the public.[54]

Nevertheless, there are limits to the application of even the most central of precepts. In recent decades, efforts to bind the harm principle have focused on employing the least restrictive or intrusive alternative that could protect the public health against significant risk. But what constitutes a least restrictive intrusive alternative and how the significance of risk is to be judged are only in part empirical matters. More important, moral judgements are involved. In fact, the tension between autonomy and public health perspectives is reflected in all such judgements. We believe that the standard appropriate to public health cannot be derived from the basic assumptions of a bioethics dominated by individualism.

The case of tuberculosis makes this clear. When individuals fail to complete the course of treatment they run the *risk* of reactivation and of developing multi-drug resistant strains of mycobacterium tuberculosis, which can be difficult and costly to treat, even deadly. The risk posed by any individual for such developments may not be judged 'significant.' But more important, when non-compliance characterises large numbers of individuals – as was the case in the US in the early 1990s – there is no question but that the threat to public health attains significance. It is therefore the *collective* hazard that provides the warrant for intervention even when the threat posed by any individual may not attain the standard of significance.[55] This is, of course, a point suggested by Geoffrey Rose in his now famous formulation of the ways in which small benefits to individuals from public health interventions may produce quite significant collective goods.[56]

[53] Lawrence O. Gostin. Public Health Law in an Age of Terrorism: Rethinking Individual Rights and Common Goods. *Health Affairs* 2002; 21: 79–93.
[54] United Nations Economic and Social Council (ECOSOC). The Siracusa Principles on the Limitations and Derogation Provisions in the International Covenant on Civil and Political Rights. UN Doc. E/CN.4/1985/4, Annex. Available at: http://www1.umn.edu/humanrts/instree/siracusaprinciples.html (accessed 7 July, 2003).
[55] Ronald Bayer & Laurence Dupuis. Tuberculosis, Public Health, and Civil Liberties. *Annual Review of Public Health* 1995; 16: 320–322.
[56] Geoffrey Rose. Sick Individuals and Sick Populations. *International Journal of Epidemiology* 2001; 30: 427–432.

The global outbreak of SARS discussed above provides an example of how in the face of grave threats a public health perspective may mandate interventions even when it is unclear whether such threats may become significant. The precautionary principle provides a starting point for the ethics of risk management. The principle stipulates an obligation to protect populations against reasonably foreseeable threats, even under conditions of uncertainty.[57] First articulated in the context of environmental hazards, the precautionary principle seeks to forestall disasters and guide decision-making in the context of in complete knowledge. Given the potential costs of inaction, it is the failure to implement preventive measures that requires justification. Proponents of the precautionary principle explicitly defend their position by noting that entities that threaten the environment are best able to bear the burdens of regulation. Opponents warn that the imposition of such burdens may stifle economic progress and scientific innovation.[58] In general, the principle has only recently been explicitly invoked in the context of epidemic threats where pre-emptive actions may burden individuals and impose limits on their freedoms. Nevertheless, the precautionary principle has implicitly guided public health interventions designed to limit or forestall epidemic outbreaks.

The challenge to the precautionary principle is illustrated by quarantine in the case of SARS. Health officials had to act without full scientific knowledge about the nature of disease transmission. To avoid catastrophe, they took action that proved unnecessarily extensive. The only safeguard against the misuse of authority is transparency and an open acknowledgement that new evidence may necessitate a reconsideration of policies.

In the end, a focus on population-based health requires a population-based analysis and a willingness to recognise that the ethics of collective health may require far more extensive limitations on privacy, as in the case of public health surveillance, and on liberty, as in the case of isolation and quarantine, than would be justified from the perspective of the autonomy-focused orientation of the dominant current in bioethics. Compulsion and, indeed, coercion – so anathema to this tradition of bioethics – are central to public

[57] J. Applegate. The Precautionary Preference: An American Perspective on the Precautionary Principle. *Human and Ecological Risk Assessment* 2000; 6: 413–443.
[58] J. Morris. 2000. *Defining the Precautionary Principle. Rethinking Risk and the Precautionary Principle.* New York, NY. Butterworth-Heinemann: 1–21.

health. Nevertheless, it is important to recognise that while mandatory measures and recourse to coercion may be necessary, efforts
designed to elicit the voluntary co-operation of those at risk for
acquiring or transmitting infectious diseases are preferable and,
indeed, may be more effective. From an ethical perspective, such
efforts are desirable because they enhance the public's health without gratuitously burdening privacy and liberty. From a pragmatic
perspective, such efforts reduce the necessity of invoking the coercive power of the state that may provoke resistance at a juncture
when co-operation is essential. Thus, while a public health perspective will not privilege liberty and privacy, it does not follow that it
should be insensitive to the importance of protecting individual
rights.

More challenging is the question of the role of paternalism in
public health. Mill's anti-paternalism has struck a powerful cord in
American political culture, as we noted in our discussion of tobacco
policy. Animated by a broad utilitarianism that seeks to maximise
communal well-being, public health has embraced measures that go
far beyond the very limited recognition of justifiable paternalism in
conventional bioethical accounts.

In a striking example of the effort to justify paternalism in the
context of occupational health regulations, Norman Daniels argued
that the protection of workers against hazardous workplace expo-
sures *that they themselves* might choose to risk could be justified
because of the 'quasi-coercive' economic context within which
workers were forced to choose.[59] But such a defence of paternalism
is too limited. The central commitment to collective well-being
requires a much more robust embrace of paternalism – one that
goes beyond interventions designed to protect those whose choices
are limited by lack of knowledge or understanding. We ought, for
example, to protect motorcyclists from the hazards of unhelmeted
riding not because they may impose costs on the community in the
event of accidents or because they are too young to appreciate the
hazards entailed, but because we are morally bound to prevent
avoidable suffering and death.

It is not surprising that among the most forthright defences of
public health paternalism has come from Robert Goodin, a utilitarian: 'We do not leave it to the discretion of consumers, however

[59] Normal Daniels. 1985. *Just Health Care*. New York, NY Oxford University Press: Chapter
7.

well informed, whether or not to drink grossly polluted water, ingest grossly contaminated foods, or inject grossly dangerous drugs. We simply prohibit such things on grounds of public health. That appeal is justified, in turn, most standardly by recourse to utilitarian calculations . . . To a very large extent . . . the justification of public health measures, in general, must be baldly paternalistic. Their fundamental point is to promote the wellbeing of people who might otherwise be inclined cavalierly to court certain sorts of diseases.'[60] The challenge, we believe, for public health ethics is to define those moments when public health paternalism is justified and to articulate a set of principles that would preserve a commitment to the realm of free choice.

The effort to shape public health policy in liberal societies will require a forthright acknowledgement of the tensions and tradeoffs that will inevitably arise when the claims of public welfare and well-being intrude on privacy, individual choice, and liberty. Recognising the role of moral values in decision-making was one of the signal contributions of bioethics in its formative period. To be sure, over the past three decades a broad array of perspectives has emerged under the rubric of bioethics. Dissatisfaction with the historically dominant commitments to individualism has been reflected in communitarian claims, feminist perspectives, and now even in explicitly politically conservative formulations. Nevertheless, individualism retains its hegemonic status. It is thus that bioethics cannot serve as a basis for thinking about the balances required in the defence of the public's health. As we commence the process of shaping an ethics of public health, it is clear that bioethics is the wrong place to start.

[60] Robert E. Goodin. 1989. *No Smoking: The Ethical Issues*. Chicago & London. The University of Chicago Press: 30–31.

Chapter 13

ETHICS AND INFECTIOUS DISEASE[1]

MICHAEL J. SELGELID

I. DISTRIBUTION OF RESEARCH RESOURCES

The '10/90 divide' is a phenomenon whereby 'less than 10 percent of [medical] research funds are spent on the diseases that account for 90% of the global burden of disease . . . [D]iseases affecting large proportions of humanity are given comparatively little attention.'[2] Because medical research so often aims at the promotion of profits rather than solutions to the world's most urgent medical problems, a majority of funds focus on the wants of a minority of the world's population – those who are relatively wealthy. As a result, health care is often unavailable to those who need it most.

A situation analogous to the 10/90 divide in medical research apparently holds true for research in bioethics. A quick flip through most bioethics texts and journals (or a visit to any number of websites) reveals attention on abortion, euthanasia, assisted reproduction, genetics, and doctor-patient relationships. To a large extent the issues examined one way or another involve advanced technologies or expensive interventions available primarily in wealthy developed nations. 'Distribution of resources' is a common topic; but discussion here often (at least implicitly) concerns domestic allocation rather than issues of *international* justice. Greatly lacking, in comparison, is discussion of ethical issues involving infectious disease and the (related) health care situation in the developing world. Infectious diseases (such as AIDS, tuberculosis, and a variety of other emerging and re-emerging pathogens) and the health care situation in developing countries pose some of the most serious problems of our times, but they have received relatively little attention from medical ethicists. In what follows I will (1)

---

[1] A version of this paper was presented at the VI World Congress of Bioethics, Brasilia, Brazil, October 2002.
[2] K. Lee & A. Mills. Strengthening Governance for Global Health Research. *British Medical Journal* 2000; 321: 775–776, at http://www.bmj.com/cgi/content/full/321/7264/775.

argue that the topic of infectious disease should be recognized as one of *the* most important topics for the discipline of bioethics, (2) briefly illustrate that it has received comparatively little attention from bioethicists,[3] and (3) attempt to explain why it has not received the attention it warrants.

II. THE ETHICAL IMPORTANCE OF INFECTIOUS DISEASE

The lack of bioethics discussion of infectious disease is both odd and unfortunate. Given that infectious disease was traditionally a – if not *the* – primary focus of medicine, for example, one would expect this to be obvious territory for a discipline concerned with 'medical ethics.'[4] More specific reasons why this should be recognized as one of the most relevant and important topics for bioethics are the following:

1 The historical and likely future consequences of infectious diseases are almost unrivalled,
2 Infectious diseases raise exceedingly difficult ethical questions of their own, and
3 The topic of infectious disease is closely connected to the topic of justice – which is a central concern of ethics.

1. Consequences

First, the paramount ethical importance of infectious diseases is illustrated by the fact that their consequences have been, and will likely continue to be, enormous. Epidemics have constituted some of the most catastrophic events in human history. The Black Death, for example, is famous for eliminating approximately one third of the European population between 1347 and 1350.[5] Another devastating

---

[3] Although I shall not in this article discuss this point at great length, others who have worked in this area, such as Margaret Battin and Solomon Benatar, have agreed that it is quite correct. A similar point is made by (especially Chapter 8 of) P. Farmer. 2003. *Pathologies of Power: Health, Human Rights, and the New War on the Poor*. Los Angeles. University of California Press.

[4] I shall use the expressions 'bioethics', 'biomedical ethics', and 'medical ethics', interchangeably.

[5] P. Ziegler. 1969. *The Black Death*. London. Penguin.

epidemic occurred in 1918 when a nasty strain of influenza killed somewhere between 20 and 100 million people. According to the historian Alfred Crosby, the 1918 flu undoubtedly 'killed more humans than any other disease in a period of similar duration in the history of the world.'[6] Gina Kolata writes that the 1918 flu killed 'more Americans in a single year than died in battle in World War I, World War II, the Korean War, and the Vietnam War.'[7] (According to the *New York Times*, '[J]ust about everyone who has studied the disease says [that] a new pandemic is inevitable.')[8]

A third major killer, which has received high-profile attention in American newspapers recently, is smallpox. Smallpox allegedly killed more people in history than any other infectious disease. In the 20th Century alone it killed somewhere between 300 and 540 million people – or 'more than all the wars and epidemics [of that century] combined.'[9] Michael Oldstone claims that smallpox killed three times more people during the 20th Century than were killed by all the wars of that period.[10] Although the disease was declared eradicated by the World Health Organization (WHO) in 1980, fears about smallpox have resurfaced. It has recently come to light that the Soviet Union, until its fall in the early 1990s, manufactured and froze tens of tons of smallpox for military purposes. Many are worried that stocks of the Soviet supply may have fallen into the hands of 'rogue nations' or terrorists. Experts claim that a smallpox bioterrorist attack could spark a catastrophic global epidemic now that the world population largely lacks immunity (because routine vaccination ended 20 or 30 years ago).[11] Modeling has shown that a smallpox attack could cause the devastation of (perhaps a series of) nuclear attack(s).

[6] A.W. Crosby. 1989. *America's Forgotten Epidemic: The Influenza of 1918.* Cambridge, UK. Cambridge University Press: 203.

[7] G. Kolata. 1999. *Flu.* London. Pan Books: xii.

[8] B. Gewen. 'The Great Influenza' and 'Microbial Threats to Health': Virus Alert. *The New York Times* March 14, 2004, available at: http://www.nytimes.com/2004/03/14/books/review/14GEWENT.html.

[9] J. Miller, S. Engelberg & W. Broad. 2001. *Germs: The Ultimate Weapon.* London. Simon and Schuster: 58.

[10] M.B.A. Oldstone. 1998. *Viruses, Plagues, and History.* New York. Oxford University Press: 3.

[11] For more on smallpox, see M.J. Selgelid. Smallpox Revisited? *American Journal of Bioethics* 2003; 3, 1, available at http://www.bioethics.net/journal/j_articles.php?aid=91, accessed 1 March 2005; and M.J. Selgelid. Bioterrorism and Smallpox Planning: Information and Voluntary Vaccination. *Journal of Medical Ethics* 2004; 30, 6: 558–560; available at http://jme.bmjjournals.com/cgi/reprint/30/6/558, accessed 1 March 2005.

Smallpox aside, it is important to recognize that the enormous impact of infectious diseases is not just a matter of history. Infectious diseases are currently the world's largest 'killer[s] of children and young adults. They account for more than 13 million deaths a year – one in two deaths in developing countries.'[12] The rapidly growing HIV/AIDS epidemic perhaps provides the clearest illustration that infectious diseases continue to have the power of their past. AIDS is arguably 'the greatest health disaster in history.'[13] In 24 years, it has killed 20 million people[14] (whereas the Black Death killed only 9 to 11 million people in Europe between 1346 and 1350).[15] HIV prevalence rates commonly exceed 30% (of adults) in sub-Saharan Africa, and similar scenarios may follow in parts of Asia and the former Soviet Union. As of 1999, anyway, only 5% of those infected could afford life-extending antiretroviral therapy.[16] In 2004, 3 million people died from AIDS, and 5 million people were newly infected with HIV. At the end of 2004, an estimated 39 million people were living with HIV.[17]

A related, but less well publicized, scenario involves the re-emergent spread of tuberculosis. Previously thought to be controlled, or at least considered controllable, TB was declared a global health emergency by the World Health Organization in 1993 and currently kills more people than ever before. 'Each year, 2 to 3 million people die from tuberculosis . . . despite the fact that the disease in its most common form is entirely preventable and treatable.'[18] One third of the world's population is infected with the latent form of the disease; and, a tenth of these are expected to develop active illness. 'It is estimated that between 2000 and 2020, nearly one billion people will be newly infected, 200 million people will get sick, and 35 million will die from TB – if control is not further strengthened.'[19]

---

[12] World Health Organization. 1999. Report on Infectious Diseases, Chapter 16, Removing Obstacles to Healthy Development, available at http://www.who.int/infectious-disease-report/pages/textonly.html, p. 2.

[13] C. Gilbert. AIDS Draws New Attention. *Milwaukee Journal Sentinel*, 15 April, 2002.

[14] See http://www.redribbon.co.za/.

[15] L. Garrett. 2000. *Betrayal of Trust: The Collapse of Global Public Health*. New York. Hyperion: 474.

[16] Ibid., p. 473.

[17] UNAIDS: AIDS Epidemic Update, 2004. Available at http://www.unaids.org.

[18] L.B. Reichman & J.H. Tanne. 2002. *Timebomb: The Global Epidemic of Multi-Drug-Resistant Tuberculosis*. New York. McGraw Hill: x–xi. See also P. Farmer. 1999. *Infections and Inequalities: The Modern Plagues*. Berkeley, CA. University of California Press.

[19] World Health Organization. Tuberculosis, Fact Sheet No. 104, revised April 2000, available at http://www.who.int/inf-fs/en/fact104.html, p. 1.

Of particular concern is the rise and spread of multi-drug resistant TB, resulting from the improper use of medication (in Russian prisons, for example).

The recent emergence and spread of SARS (Severe Acute Respiratory Syndrome) is, of course, the latest indicator that the impact of infectious diseases will continue to be severe. According to studies, the 'death rate from SARS may be . . . up to 55 percent in people 60 and older, and up to 13.2 percent in younger people . . . unless the numbers fall drastically, SARS would be among the infectious diseases with the highest death rates . . . By contrast, the influenza pandemic of 1918 . . . had an estimated mortality rate, overall, of 1 percent or less.'[20] In the meanwhile, there is no treatment, vaccine, or reliable diagnostic test for the SARS virus – which 'can survive on surfaces [such as doorknobs] for up to four days.'[21] Isolation, quarantine, travel advisories, travel restrictions, and related public health measures were put into effect; and the economic impact, alone, was staggering – '[j]ust a few weeks after SARS was identified, WHO [calculated] that the cost of the disease [was] already close to $30 billion.'[22]

It is now widely acknowledged that, in addition to posing global health and economic threats, AIDS and other infectious diseases threaten global security. Historical studies reveal that factors such as high infant mortality, low life expectancy, decreasing life expectancy, etc. – which are being severely affected in places like sub-Saharan Africa and the former Soviet Union – are among the most reliable indicators of major social upheaval. Given the serious historical and potential future consequences of infectious disease, it is no wonder that the CIA recently conducted (and published) a special investigation of '*The Global Infectious Disease Threat and Its Implications for the United States.*'[23] It is puzzling, on the other hand, that medical ethicists have not had more to say about infectious disease – compared to abortion, euthanasia, and genetics, for example, which have saturated the literature.

---

[20] L.K. Altman. Death Rate from SARS is Revised Upward. *International Herald Tribune* May 8, 2003.

[21] Ibid.

[22] I. Kickbusch. A Wake-Up Call for Global Health. *International Herald Tribune* April 29, 2003.

[23] Available at http://www.odci.gov/cia/publications/nie/report/nie9917d.html. One conclusion of the report is that we should perhaps worry most about new infectious diseases – more dangerous than AIDS – likely to emerge in the future.

2. Difficult ethical questions

A second reason why infectious diseases warrant more of bioethics' attention is that they raise serious, difficult philosophical/ethical questions of their own. Obvious examples arise from the fact that infectious diseases can be contagious. Depending on the disease in question, infected individuals can threaten the health of other individuals or society as a whole. The public health measures required to protect other individuals and society from contagion (again, depending on the disease) might sometimes involve surveillance, mandatory testing, mandatory vaccination or treatment, notification of authorities or third parties, isolation (of individuals), quarantine (of entire regions), or travel restrictions. Because such public health care measures could infringe upon widely accepted basic human rights and liberties, we are here confronted with conflicting values.

An extremely difficult ethical question asks how, in situations of conflict, the utilitarian aim to promote the greater good in the way of public health should be balanced against libertarian aims to protect privacy and individual rights and liberties such as freedom of movement, and so on. Most philosophers, policy makers, and ordinary citizens would (upon reflection, I imagine) deny that *either* liberty or aggregate utility should *always* be given *absolute* priority over the other regardless of the degree (in terms of likelihood and severity) to which the other is threatened. So the challenge is to find a principled way of striking a balance between these presumably legitimate, but apparently conflicting, social aims in contexts involving diseases that are – to varying degrees[24] – contagious, deadly, or otherwise dangerous.[25] I will later say more about the difficulty of ethical issues raised by infectious disease.

---

[24] I highlight variation in severity to suggest that there is likely no simple, obvious answer to this question. I should here point out the practical importance, in addition to theoretical difficulty, of this kind of question. It is now widely acknowledged, for example, that quarantine policy is outdated and in need of revision. Biodefense planning and the emergence of SARS provide the most recent illustrations of the immediate importance of this issue.

[25] This topic, of course, has not been altogether ignored. For discussion in the context of AIDS see U. Schuklenk. 1998. AIDS: Individual and 'Public' Interests, in *A Companion to Bioethics*, P. Singer & H. Kuhse. eds. Oxford, UK. Blackwell: 343–354. For recent discussion of quarantine policy in light of the smallpox bioterrorist threat, see G.J. Annas. Bioterrorism, Public Health, and Civil Liberties. *The New England Journal of Medicine* 2002; 346: 1337–1342.

3. Justice

Third, infectious disease should be recognized as a crucial topic for bioethics because the topic of infectious disease is closely connected to the topic of justice. Pathogens primarily prey upon the poor. Bad nutrition, dirty water, crowded living conditions, poor education, lack of access to basic medicines, disempowerment of women, and a complex host of other factors combine to make the populations of developing nations especially vulnerable to infectious diseases:

> Most deaths from infectious diseases occur in developing coun-
> tries – the countries with the least money to spend on health care.
> In developing countries, about one third of the population – 1.3
> billion people – live on incomes of less than $1 a day. Almost one
> in three children are malnourished. One in five are not immunized
> by their first birthday. And over one third of the world's popula-
> tion lack access to essential drugs.[26]

Today it is widely acknowledged that ailments called 'tropical diseases' are often not peculiar to tropical regions at all. To a large
extent 'tropical diseases' are those that afflict poor developing countries, rather than necessarily tropical ones.[27] Sanitation, hygiene,
vaccination, antibiotics, other drugs, and general improvements in
living conditions have, in recent decades anyway, left privileged
populations relatively sheltered from the scourges of the developing
world.

Relationships between poverty and disease are well illustrated by
the AIDS pandemic and the health care situation in Africa at the
beginning of the 21st Century. Of the (roughly) 40 million people
estimated to be living with HIV/AIDS in 2002, 28 million – or 70%
– lived in sub-Saharan Africa.[28]

> [A]nd 95% [in 2001] live[d] in developing nations. Most of the
> infected people who live in these countries have no access to new
> or existing drugs for HIV/AIDS. But the problem of access to
> medications goes far beyond the HIV/AIDS pandemic: people in
> developing nations also cannot afford medications used to treat
> or prevent malaria, tuberculosis, cholera, dysentery, meningitis,

---

[26] World Health Organization, *op. cit.* note 12.

[27] N.L. Stepan. 2001. *Picturing Tropical Nature*. Ithaca, NY. Cornell University Press; L. Garrett. 1994. *The Coming Plague: Newly Emerging Diseases in a World Out of Balance*. New York. Penguin.

[28] Gilbert, *op. cit.* note 13.

and typhoid fever. The affordability problem also extends beyond a lack of access to new drugs designed to treat devastating, infectious diseases: 50% of people in developing nations do not have access to even basic medications, such as antibiotics, analgesics, broncho-dilators, decongestants, anti-inflammatory agents, anti-coagulants, or diuretics.[29]

The fact that those who are already worse-off in virtue of their poverty thus have their misfortunes compounded – as they are more likely to fall victim to disease – will strike most of us as an injustice in itself.[30] It seems especially unjust when the ailments that cause the already unfortunate to suffer and die are – sometimes easily and inexpensively – treatable or preventable with existing medications (that have often been developed at least partly through public funding). Egalitarians and utilitarians should agree on this point.

Poverty and (consequent) illness in many cases can also be attributed to what should be considered injustices even by staunch libertarians. As (one of) the wealthiest African nation(s), for example, South Africa should have been better able than its sub-Saharan neighbors to stave off AIDS. It has, however, famously failed to do so. This country has more HIV positive persons than any other country in the world; and, its (increasing) prevalence rate is estimated (from antenatal clinic data) to be almost 25% of adults.

> About 5 [million] South Africans are living with HIV and, at the current rate of infection, about half the country's teenagers under 15 can expect to contract it. By 2005 South Africa is likely to have about 1 [million] orphans.[31]

A recent Medical Research Council (MRC) report estimates that AIDS, which is already the leading cause of death in the country, will kill between four and seven million South Africans within a decade.[32]

This situation is not merely *unfortunate*. We here suffer social and political *injustice*. The facts that the current South African

---

[29] D.B. Resnik. Developing Drugs for the Developing World: An Economic, Legal, Moral, and Political Dilemma. *Developing World Bioethics* 2001; 1: 11.

[30] Others, to the contrary, might claim that this situation is 'unfortunate' but not necessarily 'unfair' or 'unjust'.

[31] Fighting Back. *The Economist* May 11–17, 2002, 27.

[32] R. Dorrington, D. Bourne, D. Bradshaw, R. Laubscher & I.M. Timaeus. The Impact of HIV/AIDS on Adult Mortality in South Africa. Burden of Disease Research Unit, Medical Research Council of South Africa, available at: http://www.mrc.ac.za/bod/index.htm.

government (for mysterious reasons) consistently[33] but (apparently) illegitimately (1) challenged the causal link between HIV and AIDS (and perhaps even the very existence of HIV and AIDS), (2) challenged the safety and efficacy of antiretroviral therapy, (3) suppressed scientific research which cast doubt on its HIV/AIDS stance,[34] (4) failed to provide inexpensive (or, in some cases, free) antiretroviral treatment to reduce the risk of mother-to-child transmission of HIV, (5) refused to comply with court orders requiring it to do so, (6) forbid provision of prophylactic antiretroviral therapy to rape victims (some of which were *gang-raped babies*, less than a year old),[35] and (7) over-spent on the military (in an apparently scandalous fashion) while under-spending on health care are only a part of what I have in mind.

The current state of AIDS in South Africa – and the government's failure to effectively deal with the situation – should also be attributed to wrongs with longer histories. The etiology of the AIDS epidemic is extremely complex; its present state is the result of a wide variety of social, political, economic, and historical factors. The new South African government's failure to ameliorate the situation is at least partly forgivable – or, in any case, explainable – by virtue of the fact that it had so many other enormous tasks to accomplish in the aftermath of apartheid. In addition to overhauling the political apparatus of the country, provision of decent education, housing, sanitation, and water to those who were victims of systematic racial oppression for decades – i.e. the vast majority of the population – posed monumental challenges for the new South African government. The shambles in which apartheid left this country is thus at least partly to blame for the health care *status quo*.[36] The fact that urbanization, overcrowded living conditions, migrant working conditions, poor education, fatalistic behavior, prostitution, and other ravishes of poverty (including poor nutrition, widespread infection with worms, and lack of treatment for

---

[33] At the time of this writing the South African Government appears to finally be changing its stance on HIV/AIDS.

[34] This seemed to occur with regard to the above-mentioned MRC Report, for example.

[35] Note that points (4)–(6), at least, appear to conflict with the South African constitution by failing to respect what are recognized as human rights here. The same thing may be said about the failure to provide antiretrovirals to HIV-positive South Africans more generally speaking.

[36] See D. Webb. 1997. *HIV and AIDS in Africa*. London. Pluto Press; A. Whiteside & C. Sunter. 2000. *AIDS: The Challenge for South* Africa. Cape Town. Human & Rousseau; & H. Marais. 2000. *To the Edge: AIDS Review 2000*. Pretoria, South Africa. University of Pretoria, Centre for the Study of AIDS.

other STDS[37]) each contribute to the AIDS epidemic – and are each (at least partly) the result of exploitative racist colonial oppressive practices – corroborates the point that the South African AIDS epidemic should largely be blamed on social injustice.

Similar things can be said about other developing nations where health care is compromised because of impoverishment resulting from colonialization, oppression, exploitation, protectionist trade policies, domestic corruption, failure of democracy, and so on. According to Solomon R. Benatar, for example, the poverty and consequent poor health of many in the developing world should be attributed to (militarization and) exploitative global economic activities involving irresponsible business practices of multinational corporations in particular. The result is a widening of the gap – in terms of both wealth and human rights protection – between the haves and have-nots.[38]

Pulitzer Prize-winning journalist Laurie Garrett provides an extreme example of the link between disease and injustice. In her recent book *Betrayal of Trust: The Collapse of Global Public Health*, she blames the famous 1995 Ebola (hemorrhagic fever) epidemic in Zaire (now the Democratic Republic of the Congo) on the corruption of the leader Mobutu who stole billions of dollars from public coffers, leaving public hospitals (which were primary *sources* of infection) in complete disarray and lacking the most basic supplies.

> Two things are clear: Ebola spread in Kikwit because the most basic, essential elements of public health were nonexistent. And those exigencies were lacking in Kikwit – indeed, throughout Zaire – because Mobutu Sese Seko and his cronies had for three decades looted the national treasuries. Ebola haunted Zaire because of corruption and political repression . . . [Ebola's] emergence into human populations required the special assistance of humanity's greatest vices: greed, corruption, arrogance, tyranny, and callousness. What unfolded in Zaire in 1995 was not so much the rain forest terror widely depicted then in popular media worldwide as an inevitable outcome of disgraceful disconcern – even disdain – for the health of the Zairois public.[39]

---

[37] Increased risk of HIV infection results, for example, in the presence of other untreated STDs or when immune systems are weakened from poor nutrition or infection with worms.
[38] S.R. Benatar. Global Disparities in Health and Human Rights: A Critical Commentary. *American Journal of Public Health* 1998; 88: 295–300.
[39] Garrett, *op. cit.* note 15, p. 59.

Garrett implicates American meddling in the affair, insofar as the U.S. government backed Mobutu and propped him into power. She insinuates CIA involvement with the murder of his predecessor Patrice Lumumba, unfavored because of supposedly socialist sympathies. In her earlier book *The Coming Plague: Newly Emerging Diseases in a World Out of Balance*, Garrett suggests that the AIDS epidemic in Africa was at least partly fueled by the fact that under-equipped hospitals in places like Congo sometimes had no choice but to use the same unsterilized syringes over and over and over again.

III. WHY THE NEGLECT?

Based on what I have said so far, one would expect that infectious disease would already be a typical topic of dedicated discussion in a discipline called 'medical ethics.' One would expect that there would be books on ethics and infectious disease and that articles and sections specifically devoted to ethical aspects of infectious diseases would be regular fare in bioethics journals and anthologies. In reality, however, 'infectious disease' is hardly found even in indexes of standard bioethics texts; and I have never seen a book on this general topic. An October 2002 *Google* (internet) search of the phrase 'ethics and infectious disease' yielded only 11 entries.[40] Six of these referred to a single project (of Margaret Battin), and some of the others were false positives. In March 2005 a similar search yielded 35 entries[41] – while a search of 'ethics and genetics' led to 5,100 entries.

---

[40] Search conducted on October 30, 2002 at http://www.google.com.

[41] Many of these referred to a more recent work of Ronald Bayer. There have of course been books and anthology sections on ethical issues associated with AIDS in particular. And internet searches of 'Ethics and AIDS', as was pointed out by Peter Singer in discussion, will yield more results – i.e. 408 results on 1 March 2005. The fact remains, however, that discussion of infectious diseases in general (which would likely inform discussion of particular diseases such as AIDS) is lacking. In my opinion even AIDS – with the exception of doctor-patient relationship issues (especially the 'duty to treat') and AIDS-related international research ethics (especially the debate over 'standards of care') – has not received adequate attention in mainstream bioethics literature, given the magnitude of the problem. On 1 March 2005, in any case, a Google search of 'ethics and tuberculosis' yielded only 42 results (though tuberculosis kills two or three million persons per year) and 'ethics and malaria' yielded zero (though malaria kills one million per year). On the same date, 'ethics and stem cells' yielded 440 results – despite the newness of stem cell research (in comparison with AIDS).

1. High tech medicine

Why, then, has the topic been neglected by bioethics? It is likely that part of the explanation relates to the origins of the discipline of medical ethics itself. Although the roots of bioethics extend twenty-five hundred years back to the world of Hippocrates, bioethics' birth as an autonomous discipline is a relatively recent phenomenon. Medical ethics really came into its own during the last four or five decades, largely as a result of advancements in biological science and technology. With revolutionary developments in medical technology came unprecedented moral and policy dilemmas, and hence an academic discipline was born.[42] If this rough sketch of the birth of bioethics captures much truth, then there should be less surprise that there has been a high-tech, wealthy-world slant to discussion within the discipline.

2. Optimism in medicine

A second probable reason why infectious disease has not received more attention of medical ethicists similarly relates to the timing of the birth of the discipline. The rise of bioethics coincided with a period of tremendous optimism in medicine. The development of antibiotics in the 1940's and the hugely successful Salk Polio vaccination program in the 1950's, and other developments such as the discovery of DDT, led the medical community to believe that infectious disease would soon be defeated through medical progress.[43] As early as

> 1948 U.S. Secretary of State George C. Marshall declared at the Washington, D.C., gathering of the Fourth International Congress on Tropical Medicine and Malaria that the conquest of all infectious diseases was imminent. Through a combination of enhanced crop yields to provide adequate food for humanity and scientific breakthroughs in microbe control, Marshall predicted, all the earth's microscopic scourges would be eliminated.[44]

---

[42] The development of elaborate life-sustaining technologies made the question of euthanasia, for example, more urgent. I should note that – in addition to technological advance – the birth of bioethics was also importantly related to the civil rights movement of the 1960s. See H. Kuhse & P. Singer. 1998. What is Bioethics? A Historical Introduction, in *A Companion to Bioethics*, P. Singer and H. Kuhse eds. Oxford, UK. Blackwell: 3–11.

[43] See Garrett, *op. cit.* note 27, pp. 30–52, esp. pp. 30–31.

[44] Ibid., pp. 30–31.

In 1955 the World Health Organization decided to 'eliminate all malaria on the planet' via the eradication of mosquitoes with DDT. 'Few doubted that such a lofty goal was possible: nobody at the time could imagine a trend of worsening disease conditions; the arrow of history always pointed towards progress.'[45] 'By 1965, more than 25,000 different antibiotic products had been developed; physicians and scientists felt that bacterial diseases, and the microbes responsible, were no longer of great concern or of research interest.'[46] In 1967 U.S. Surgeon General William H. Stewart was so convinced of success that he told a White House gathering of health officers 'that it was time to close the book on infectious diseases and shift all national attention (and dollars) to what he termed "the New Dimensions" of health: chronic diseases.'[47] 'In 1972, the Nobel laureate Macfarlane Burnet concluded that "the most likely forecast about the future of infectious disease is that it will be very dull." '[48] Fields such as bacteriology and parasitology appeared less important and subsequently fell out of vogue in the medical scientific community. The rise of medical ethics thus occurred at a time when it was popular – though perhaps hubristic – to think that infectious disease would no longer be a central concern of medicine. This presumably explains at least part of the neglect on the part of those concerned with medical ethics.

3. 'The other'

AIDS, of course, has been on the scene for more than twenty years already – and thus overlaps with roughly half the lifespan of bioethics proper. And it has been clear for quite some time that malaria, TB, and other infectious diseases would not just disappear as planned. To the contrary, plenty of pathogens have developed more dangerous drug-resistant strains. And many morbid microbes – such as SARS and Ebola – have newly emerged during the last few decades.

---

[45] Ibid., p. 31. Not only did it fail, but this program was somewhat counterproductive. DDT-resistant mosquitoes returned in higher numbers than before; and misuse of medication promoted drug-resistant strains of malaria. By '1975 the worldwide incidence of malaria was about 2.5 times what it had been in 1961 . . . A new global iatrogenic form of malaria was emerging – "iatrogenic" meaning created as a result of medical treatment. In its well-meaning zeal to treat the world's malaria scourge, humanity had created a new epidemic' (p. 52).

[46] Ibid., p. 36.

[47] Ibid., p. 33.

[48] Gewen, *op. cit.* note 8.

A third reason why infectious diseases receive sparse discussion by academic ethicists is that they have likely been relegated as problems of 'the other.'[49] AIDS, for example, for a long time was, and perhaps still is, considered a problem for homosexuals, IV drug users, and poor black people in Africa. AIDS and other infectious diseases are, as has already been said, by far more prevalent in the developing world. Given that the vast majority of professional medical ethicists are straight, non-drug-injecting, relatively well-to-do whites who reside and work in wealthy developed nations, it should not be entirely unexpected that they have focused most on matters of more obvious central domestic concern, rather than problems of 'strangers' on the fringe of society and foreigners in faraway places. This third explanation involves both psychological and practical elements. Regarding the latter, (relatively conservative) university employers (and research funders) likely expect academic ethicists to focus most on pressing local issues rather than (radically) concentrating on international justice.[50] This has *explanatory* power, but I doubt it makes the failure of medical ethicists to further discuss one of world's most consequential topics *excusable*. Ethics and morality essentially involve elements of impartiality; and, *tenured* professors, in any case, have substantial freedom to choose their topics.

4. Complexity

A fourth explanation of neglect by bioethicists relates to the complexity of the issues in question.[51] Traditional topics in medical ethics already require difficult interdisciplinary study. Expertise in both ethics and science are required to do bioethics well. Though many scholars have expertise in the discipline of ethics and many scholars expertise in scientific and technological aspects of biology and medicine, it is rare to find both kinds of expertise embodied in single individuals. One result is the relatively weak reputation of medical ethics within philosophical circles. Philosophers commonly complain about a 'low level' of discussion in medical ethics. This is attributed to the fact that (1) contributors with philosophical

---

[49] See H. Joffe. 1999. *Risk and the Other*. Cambridge, U.K. Cambridge University Press; & N.L. Stepan, *op. cit.* note. 27, for discussions of how AIDS and tropical diseases, respectively, are regularly understood and portrayed as problems of others.

[50] Udo Schuklenk suggested this point in conversation.

[51] This was (independently) suggested by Mary Tjiattas. Peter Singer concurred in conversation.

mastery in ethics often fail to get the science right and are thus unrealistic while (2) contributors with scientific backgrounds too often lack sufficient training in rigorous philosophical argumentation to get the ethics right, and (3) too few contributors are skilled enough in both areas to generate a consistently high level of discussion.

I have been discussing the challenging nature of the interdisciplinarity of medical ethics scholarship because I believe this difficulty is greatly exacerbated with discussion of infectious disease and the health care situation in the developing world. In addition to grounding in ethics and science/medicine (the latter of which is itself complicated by entry into the realm of epidemiology and drug-resistant pathogen emergence), we here need a greater grip on complex social, political, historic, and economic dynamics in order to *explain* – and thus comment upon the justice of – the current global health care situation.[52] A similarly broadened understanding is needed to realistically assess – and base moral/policy prescriptions upon – *predictions of impact*. Exploring the issues I have in mind requires more *empirical* work than most (medical) ethicists are likely to be trained for or accustomed to.[53] With regard to distribution of resource questions, confrontation with issues of international (rather than merely domestic) justice is an additional obvious way in which *theoretical* discussion is complicated.[54] The fact that infectious diseases do not respect international borders is just one of the ways in which the topic is inherently international. My fourth explanation, thus, is that questions concerning infectious disease and the health care situation in the developing world have been neglected by biomedical ethicists at least partly because of the *difficulty* of working on them.

5. *Apparent ease*

My fifth explanation, ironically, is that this area has been ignored because of a *misperception* that the questions raised are all-too-easy. The injustice of the situation, which has received substantial *media*

---

[52] I do not mean to imply that other issues in bioethics do not require appreciation of social, political, historical, and economic phenomena. My point is one of degree: assessment of the health care situation in the developing world *often* requires substantially *more* contact with these other disciplines. Others who have worked in this area will agree.

[53] For further illustration of what I here have in mind see M.J. Selgelid. Ethics, Economics, and AIDS in Africa. *Developing World Bioethics* 2004; 4, 1: 96–105.

[54] See D. Moellendorf. 2002. *Cosmopolitan Justice*. Boulder, Colorado. West-view Press.

attention at least, whereby AIDS medications are unavailable because they are unaffordable – at least partly because of prices set by profit-driven pharmaceutical companies – to populations in sub-Saharan Africa where they are by far needed most will strike many as a clear and blatant injustice. 'Of course this is wrong. Of course more should be done to make medication available to AIDS victims in Africa,' many might say, 'and you don't need to be a philosopher – or priest – to figure that out.' Questions about the justice of the health care situation in the developing world, where the innocent poor are sick and suffering, at first glance anyway, *appear* to lack the deep philosophical significance of questions upon which medical ethicists usually focus their attention.[55] Topics such as euthanasia and abortion, for example, raise what might look like deeper and more intellectually challenging issues: When is it morally permissible to kill another human being? What is a person? Upon what is the moral status of human beings based? What does quality of life consist in? Notice that emerging bioethical debates surrounding genetics and embryo/stem cell research often revolve around these same sorts of questions. In comparison with these more theoretical (or perhaps *metaphysical*) questions, the injustice of a situation where tens of millions of (relatively innocent) people will soon suffer and die because they are too poor to buy medications might look like a no-brainer.

6. *Religious hijacking*

My final explanation of why infectious disease has not received more attention from bioethicists refers to the fact that bioethicists have been kept so occupied by discussion of *religious objections* to things like abortion, euthanasia, cloning, stem cell research, and so on. Contrary to Paul Farmer,[56] my own belief is that most bioethicists *are* (at heart, anyway) genuinely concerned about issues of justice. Liberal-minded bioethicists presumably would have focused much more attention on the topic of infectious disease and the injustice of the health care situation in the developing world if they hadn't been kept so busy battling the illiberal policy agenda (regarding abortion, euthanasia, cloning, stem cell research, etc.)

---

[55] This objection was (independently) raised by Julian Savulescu in discussion.
[56] In discussion.

advocated by the church.[57] Debate in bioethics has thus, to a large extent, been hijacked by religion.

CONCLUSION

I have offered six explanations of why ethical issues associated with infectious disease (and the related health care situation in the developing world) have not been more prominent in medical ethics literature. I have suggested that this is the case roughly because (1) bioethics was born (as an autonomous discipline) with advances in medical technology and thus has largely focused on these, (2) bioethics' birth and initial development (as an autonomous discipline) came at a time when it was believed that infectious disease would be conquered by medicine, (3) infectious diseases are often seen as problems of others, (4) bioethical research on infectious disease in the developing world is especially difficult because so empirical and interdisciplinary, (5) ethical questions about infectious disease (in the developing world) might not *appear* to pose the kinds of deep philosophical questions that academic ethicists are interested in, and (6) bioethics debate has been hijacked by the church. These are just suggestions; and this list is not meant to be exhaustive. Rather than choosing between these alternative explanations, I believe that they each likely capture *parts* of the story we are after. In any case, as argued above, it would be entirely wrong to explain the lack of discussion of infectious diseases by denying their central importance and/or relevance to the discipline of bioethics.

---

[57] James William Ley, philosophy Ph.D. student at the University of Sydney, encouraged explicit inclusion of this point.

Chapter 14

VACCINATION AND THE PREVENTION PROBLEM

ANGUS DAWSON

INTRODUCTION

This paper seeks to critically review a traditional objection to preventive medicine (which I call here the 'prevention problem'). The prevention problem is a concern about the supposedly inequitable distribution of benefits and risks of harm resulting from preventive medicine's focus on population-based interventions. This objection is potentially applicable to preventive vaccination programmes and could be used to argue that such programmes are unethical. Most discussion of ethical issues in relation to vaccination has focused on vaccines as agents for preventing disease.[1] However, there is increasing interest in the scientific literature in the idea of using vaccines as agents to treat diseases as well as prevent them. I focus on these two different types of vaccination (therapeutic vaccination and preventive vaccination) as a means of exploring the prevention problem. I argue that the 'prevention problem' cannot be fairly applied to the case of preventive vaccination because such programmes do not just focus upon benefits at the level of populations (as is claimed by the prevention problem). Most such preventive vaccination programmes explicitly seek to create and maintain herd protection. I argue that herd protection is an important public good which is a benefit shared by all individuals in the relevant population. This fact can then be used to block the prevention problem argument in relation to preventive vaccination programmes. The case of the likely future development and use of therapeutic vaccines is used to offer a contrasting case to that of preventive vaccination as a means of exploring the structure of the prevention problem.

---

[1] See T. Dare. Mass Immunisation Programmes: Some Philosophical Issues. *Bioethics* 1998; 12: 125–149; and J.B. Ulmer & M.A. Liu. Ethical Issues for Vaccines and Immunization. *Nature Reviews: Immunology.* 2002; 2: 291–296, for good discussions of these ethical issues in relation to preventive vaccination programmes.

I. VACCINES: PREVENTIVE AND THERAPEUTIC

A vaccine can be defined as any substance consisting of 'dead or attenuated living infectious material introduced into the body with the object of increasing its [the body's] power to resist or to get rid of a disease.'[2] Such a definition does not specify that vaccines are solely preventive in nature. However, it is true to say that the common understanding of the term 'vaccine' is of a substance (usually administered by injection) used to prevent infection. Such preventive or prophylactic vaccines are standardly used to induce immunity to a particular disease by way of stimulating the immune system. The idea is that such immunity prevents the relevant disease affecting the vaccinated individual. In addition, the vaccination of the individual will contribute towards herd protection when the preventive programme is designed to vaccinate for contagious diseases.[3] Herd protection is established once enough individuals are vaccinated for the disease in question to mean that unvaccinated individuals are likely to be protected from the disease if it enters the population. Both types of benefit can be seen as important reasons in favour of carrying out vaccination programmes.[4]

Therapeutic vaccines will work in the same way, to the extent that the primary aim is to stimulate the immune system to respond to the infectious agent or disease. However, in the therapeutic case the aim is to act to affect the immune system to the extent that it, hopefully, 'gets rid of' or cures the disease in question when the individual is already infected rather than merely seeking to prevent the infection. In both the preventive and the therapeutic cases the focus is on generating the immune reaction. However, how this end is attained might differ between the two cases. For example, where two vaccines are available, one to prevent and the other to cure a particular disease, the different vaccines may target different antigens (as is the case with Hepatitis B vaccines).[5] In other cases,

---

[2] G. Macpherson, ed. 1995. *Black's Medical Dictionary*. 38th edition. London. A & C Black: 542.

[3] I use the phrase 'herd protection' rather than 'herd immunity' following the distinction made by Y. Paul. Letter: Herd Immunity and Herd Protection. *Vaccine* 2004; 22: 301–302.

[4] I will ignore the special issues about individuals consenting to the vaccination of third-parties (such as parents agreeing or objecting to vaccination for their children) in this paper. However, for some discussion of this issue see my paper: The Determination of 'Best Interests' in Relation to Childhood Vaccinations. *Bioethics* 2005; 19: 188–204.

[5] See G.A. Poland, D. Murray & R. Bonilla-Guerrero. New Vaccine Development. *BMJ* 2002; 324: 1315–1319 for discussion of this case.

therapeutic vaccines focus on producing an immune response through the introduction of DNA into the infected cells bringing about the subsequent generation of proteins, which in turn create the required immune response.[6] Recent developments in the area of therapeutic vaccination have been rapid and significant. There has been much work on the use of vaccines as a method of treating many different types of cancer, autoimmune diseases, as well as many different types of infectious disease such as HIV, tuberculosis and hepatitis.

These developments open up the prospect of new ways of tackling these potentially devastating diseases.[7] This can only be welcomed. As Moingeon et al. make clear, therapeutic vaccines may be particularly useful in relation to infectious disease where existing drug interventions are ineffective or less than optimally effective. Examples of such situations might include the use of such vaccinations to provide a break in HAART therapy for individuals with HIV or as an aid to providing more effective treatment for TB due to the growth in drug resistant forms of this disease.[8]

For the purposes of this paper we don't need to know too much about the workings of the different vaccines. The important issue is that the intentions behind these two uses are different. Prophylactic vaccination is given to a large population with the intention of preventing a particular, usually contagious, disease. Therapeutic vaccination is given to already infected individuals as part of a treatment regime for that particular disease.[9] However, let's employ a modest science fiction scenario or a thought experiment and suppose that therapeutic vaccine development has moved on to the point where we have therapeutic vaccine treatments for such common infectious diseases as diphtheria, pertussis, measles and polio. If this were the case, and the vaccines were as effective as the existing

---

[6] Of course, there are other possible avenues for future development, such as the creation of a therapeutic vaccine leading on to the development of a related preventive one. Vaccines for HIV might be one area where this may occur in the future.

[7] See Poland et al., *op. cit.* note 5; and P. Moingeon, J. Almond & M. de Wilde. Therapeutic Vaccines against Infectious Diseases. *Current Opinion in Microbiology* 2003; 6: 1–10, for discussion of these developments.

[8] Moingeon, ibid.

[9] So this situation ends up being rather more like immunotherapy. This is a type of immunisation used for those already infected with a disease rather than being like preventive vaccination. Such immunotherapy is used for many diseases in such a context – e.g. Hepatitis B. See D. Salisbury & N. Begg, eds. 1996. *Immunisation Against Infectious Diseases.* London. HMSO: 109.

prophylactic vaccines with no additional risks, then it is possible to argue that we should move from continuing with the existing preventive programmes for these diseases to thinking about basing our vaccination policies upon therapeutic vaccination instead. The latter would have the benefit of only being given when an individual was already infected.[10] One possible reason to think this might be a good thing is that it provides a way to avoid a traditional objection to preventive interventions. I will call this objection the 'prevention problem' and will discuss it in the next section.

II. THE PREVENTION PROBLEM STATED

The 'prevention problem' as I will state it here is held by its supporters to be a general problem for preventive public health measures. It can be seen in such public health interventions as health promotion through lifestyle/dietary advice and cancer screening programmes. It is not very clearly articulated by identifiable individuals but elements of the view are outlined and discussed by Skrabanek and Rose.[11] I will provide a sketch of the argument in a general form and then apply it to the preventive vaccination case.

The key elements of the 'prevention problem' are that:

(a) Preventive public health measures are performed upon asymptomatic individuals;
(b) Every such public health intervention will carry some risk of harm;
(c) The benefits of such interventions lie at the level of populations, whilst any risks of harm are borne by the individual participants in the programme.

Conclusion: such preventive programmes are unethical (given the distribution of risk and benefits).

---

[10] Of course, it might still make sense to continue to provide preventive vaccination for some diseases, for example, if progression of the disease is particularly rapid (e.g. meningitis). Thanks to one of the anonymous referees for this point.

[11] See P. Skrabanek. Why is Preventive Medicine Exempted from Ethical Constraints? *Journal of Medical Ethics.* 1990; 16: 187–190; and G. Rose. 1992. *The Strategy of Preventive Medicine.* Oxford. Oxford University Press. Note that whilst Skrabanek is explicitly opposed to much preventive medicine, Rose is, rather, a concerned supporter and advocate of much preventive medicine.

The first concern is that preventive programmes focus on interventions that are performed upon asymptomatic individuals. The worry here is that where such an intervention carries *any* risk of harm it is harder to justify the exposure of individuals to such risk when they do not have the disease itself. On the other hand, symptomatic individuals clearly have something to gain from the intervention, and as a result they and their physicians can do a rough cost-benefits calculation to determine what sort of risks are appropriate (given the particular condition). In the preventive situation it may look as though individuals are subject to a potential cost in terms of risk of harm with very little chance of an individual benefit. In addition, there is a further concern that preventive programmes entail that in all likelihood the relevant individuals will have been sought out by health care professionals and asked to participate in the programme, rather than those individuals seeking out help for a particular problem themselves. One concern here is that such programmes might result in potential or actual coercion of individuals to participate in the programme for 'their own good', even though it is not apparent that they will be individually better off as a result.[12]

Secondly, the argument focuses upon the fact that any intervention will carry some risk of harm, although the amount of harm will of course vary in terms of likelihood and magnitude depending upon the type of intervention we are talking about. The reason why this might be thought to be a worry for preventive programmes is that such risks of harm are carried by all of the asymptomatic participants. There might also be a secondary concern that the information about potential risks of harm are unlikely to be presented fairly to the potential participants because the focus of such a programme will be, overwhelmingly, upon the supposed benefits of the prevention programme, rather than a sober assessment of both potential risks and benefits. Skrabanek can be seen to hold such a view.[13]

On the third point, the impact of risks and burdens of such preventive programmes might be highlighted through an application of Rose's formulation of what he terms the 'prevention paradox' as follows:

---

[12] This might well mean that not even welfare-based justifications of strong paternalism can be used here, as the justification for the action is on the creation of a public good or population benefit rather than the individual's good or benefit.

[13] Skrabanek, *op. cit.* note 11.

a preventive measure that brings large benefits to the community offers little to each participating individual.[14]

There are a number of elements of this point that are worth exploring. The first is that because the whole purpose of preventive interventions is to seek to ensure that certain events do not occur, it is difficult to measure the success of such programmes. This is because it is always possible to ask whether any such 'non-events' are the result of the programme or whether they would have occurred anyway. This is one reason for the appeal of measuring public health preventive interventions at the population level, as it should be easier to detect any changes produced through such population-level surveillance. The other related aspect that is interesting is that we can never tell which particular individuals will benefit from the prevention programme, and this is why the intervention is aimed at, and measured in terms of, the whole population. If the intervention carries any risk of harm (or perhaps just inconvenience) then all are subject to this, and any of the individuals may potentially be harmed, whilst only a few unidentifiable individuals will benefit. The concern might then be raised that individuals are being 'sacrificed' for the good of the population.[15] The implication of Rose's 'paradox' is that if potential participants are clearly informed of the relevant facts, then it is unlikely that they will consider it worth participating as the benefits for them as individuals are unclear: at best any such benefits are likely to be distant and small, but more likely they are probably non-existent (whilst any potential harms will clearly exist).

If we now consider the application of these three general features of the prevention problem to preventive vaccination programmes we can note the following results:

(a) The population is asymptomatic;
(b) The vaccination will carry some risk;
(c) Risks are carried by individuals and benefits lie at the level of populations.

Conclusion: This means that the prevention problem applies to preventive vaccinations.

---

[14] Rose, *op. cit.* note 11, p. 12.

[15] This argument would be a parallel one to the worry some people have about an individual's interests potentially being overridden by the interests of the population in medical research. Skrabanek, *op. cit.* note 11, explicitly draws this parallel.

There are a number of issues to explore here. Firstly, such vaccination programmes, by definition, focus on asymptomatic individuals, as the purpose of the intervention is to prevent infection. Secondly, it is significant to this argument that even the safest vaccinations will carry *some* risk of harm, even if it is a very small risk of an adverse reaction. These first two points might be combined to argue that even if the possible harm is a very small amount to each individual, its relevance is magnified by the numbers exposed to such a risk.[16] Thirdly, in relation to the balance of benefits and risk of harm it should not be forgotten that such preventive programmes aim to vaccinate many individuals so that the whole of a population can be protected from harm. This point relates to point (c) above, as the benefits might all be seen to be at the population level because we can never tell which individuals have actually, in fact, been saved from exposure to a risk of harm from the contagious disease. Arguably, individuals are put at risk of harm from the vaccinations without knowing whether they as individuals will derive any personal benefit. This is because they cannot know whether they will ever in fact be protected by the *vaccination* from the disease, rather than, say, just being lucky enough not to come into contact with the relevant virus or bacteria etc. The public health prevention focus is made all the more explicit in the case of traditional preventive vaccination programmes for contagious diseases because they are focused on creating and maintaining herd protection within a population. In such situations, although each vaccinated individual also gains some individual benefit, arguably, the benefit for any actual individual is unknown.[17]

The prevention problem might well look like a powerful argument against the use of prophylactic vaccination for contagious disease. Its apparent power as an argument might grow as a result of many factors, such as any increased risk of harm from the vaccination, a low frequency of the disease, and a low severity of the harm likely to result from the disease. It might also be thought that this argument can be further strengthened where we can identify a lack of confidence by the public in a particular vaccine (such as can be seen in the recent problem with the combined Measles-Mumps-Rubella vaccination in the UK and other places, as well as with

[16] Assuming such magnification or multiplication of risks is legitimate. If judgements are made at the population level, such calculations will be important.

[17] This is not true of all vaccines, of course. For example, given the mode of transmission tetanus vaccination will only directly benefit the vaccinated individual.

pertussis vaccination in the 1970s). However, it should be noted that while these factors might look as though they strengthen this argument, and they might indeed give added rhetorical weight to it in particular cases, these issues are all strictly irrelevant to the prevention problem, as that argument is about the disproportionate balance of benefits and harms between the individual and the population level, rather than about the supposed risks of harm attached to individual vaccines as such.

III. THE PREVENTION PROBLEM AVOIDED?

Let's assume for the sake of argument that the prevention problem is a reasonable argument. How might the introduction of therapeutic vaccines for diseases currently the target of preventive vaccination programmes allow us to side-step the prevention problem? The answer lies in the difference in the aims behind the applications of the two different types of vaccines and the difference that this makes to the ethical issues. If we perform the thought experiment suggesting that therapeutic vaccination was possible for contagious diseases such as measles, pertussis, polio and diphtheria, and these vaccines cured each disease, then we would have to accept that such therapeutic vaccine use is a clinical rather than a public health intervention. This is because a therapeutic vaccine will only be given to someone with a particular disease, rather than given 'unnecessarily' to the whole population with the aim of preventing a disease, as is the case with prophylactic vaccines. If this is true, and I will assume so here, it will mean that we can potentially side-step one of the traditionally controversial features of preventive medicine in general, at least as it applies to preventive vaccinations for contagious diseases.

If we now return to the three elements of the prevention problem as outlined above we can identify why therapeutic vaccine use makes the difference that it does to the ethical arguments. These issues can be summarised as follows:

(a) Individuals are symptomatic;
(b) The intervention will certainly carry a risk of harm;
(c) Any risks and benefits are run by the same individuals (i.e. those individuals who are vaccinated).

Conclusion: the prevention problem does not apply.

This can be explored in a little more detail. Firstly, therapeutic vaccination will only occur where someone already has a disease; so even if the individual has no symptoms, and so is strictly 'asymptomatic', the important issue is that they in fact have the disease in question. They are, of course, almost certain to be symptomatic, otherwise no one would know they are ill, and so no treatment would be contemplated. The important point is that vaccination in this context is a potential cure for an existing disease rather than being aimed at preventing infection. Secondly, just as in the preventive vaccination case, the intervention will carry some risk of harm. However, and this is central to the third issue, such risks are clearly run by the vaccinated individual but they also, importantly, derive all of the benefits from the intervention. This is because a therapeutic vaccination is given to the individual only after the disease is detected. In such a case, the argument might go, the prevention problem is clearly avoided and any risks synonymous with vaccine use will only be run when most appropriate; that is, when an individual is directly threatened by the disease already present within the body. So far I have outlined the general prevention problem, and suggested that it does apply to preventive vaccination but not to therapeutic vaccination. In the next section I move on to present an argument that can be used to undermine the application of the prevention problem to the case of preventive vaccination.

IV. THE PREVENTION PROBLEM REBUTTED

In this section I will propose an argument for dismissing the prevention problem (at least in relation to preventive vaccination for contagious diseases). If we return to the earlier discussion of the application of the three general features of the prevention problem to preventive vaccination programmes, we can recall the following results:

(a)   The population is asymptomatic;
(b)   The vaccination will carry some risk;
(c)   Risks are carried by individuals and benefits lie at the level of populations.

Conclusion: this means that the prevention problem applies to preventive vaccinations.

I wish to argue that the principle in (c) is incorrect, for two reasons. The first is that at least some individuals do benefit as individuals from the programme. The individual beneficiaries are the ones who otherwise would have become infected with the relevant disease. Whilst it is true that such individuals are only likely to be a subgroup in the vaccinated population, and that it is impossible to identify them in advance, we can be sure that at least some individuals will certainly benefit. However, far more importantly, and decisively for the prevention problem, I will argue that *all* individuals in fact benefit from such programmes (at least once herd protection exists in the relevant population).[18] This benefit is related to the share that each person has in the existence of herd protection as a public good.[19]

Such a view can be seen in the following modified application of the three general features of the prevention problem applied to preventive vaccination programmes as follows:

(a)   The population is asymptomatic;
(b)   The vaccination will carry some risk;
(c)   Risks are carried by individuals but both individuals and populations benefit where herd protection exists in the relevant population.

Conclusion: this means that the prevention problem does not apply to preventive vaccinations (at least for contagious diseases, where herd protection exists).

Aspect (c) in this summary is modified because individuals will benefit from participation in the public good that herd protection affords within suitably vaccinated communities. This issue can be explained as follows: vaccination for a contagious disease can be seen as an act that not only has potential benefits for the individual themselves, but as also making a contribution towards a collective benefit as everyone profits where herd protection exists in the population, including those that are not vaccinated (for whatever reason)

---

[18] In fact, there is another way that all benefit, as each vaccinated individual derives a real benefit through gaining some protection from the disease as a result of his or her vaccination. However, I do not discuss this point here as it might be argued that such a benefit attaches to each vaccinated individual *qua* individual. In this paper I focus on herd protection as a means of exploring benefits at the population level as a way to undermine the prevention problem. Thanks to one of the anonymous referees for reminding me of this point.

[19] I discuss the issue of public goods, herd protection and vaccination in more detail in: Herd Protection as a Public Good: Vaccination and our Obligations to Others. (Manuscript.)

and those who do not show sufficient immune response despite vaccination (for example, because they were ill when they were vaccinated). One way to think of these two positive outcomes is as being both a private (or individual) and a public (or collective) good. A private good is a good affecting only the individual concerned and a public good jointly affects the members of a group or population. It is because of such a shared population benefit from the existence of herd protection that we might think of the existence of such a state as being a public good. We can think of public goods in general, following Klosko, as being characterised by two main properties: nonexcludability, and dependence upon co-operation by a large number of people.[20] 'Nonexcludable goods' are those where no one can be excluded from the benefits of the existence of the relevant good, even when they have not contributed towards bringing it about.[21] This is the case where herd protection exists: the non-vaccinated benefit from the high immunity levels in the population. In addition, herd protection can only be generated through collaborative endeavour, as it cannot be obtained by any individual acting alone. In addition to these two aspects suggested by Klosko, I would add another proposed by Rawls when he suggests that public goods must also be indivisible. That is, public goods cannot be broken down or divided up into individual or private goods.[22] This is true of herd protection in the sense that the equal individual benefit can only come about as a result of collective action. Herd protection, where it exists, can therefore be seen to be a public good as it is indivisible, nonexcludable and dependent upon the co-operative actions of a group.[23]

An appeal to herd protection as a public good, then, provides a means of undermining the third aspect of the prevention problem argument in relation to prophylactic vaccination. Herd protection in such a context is a public good that benefits all in the population, not just those who are vaccinated who otherwise would have

[20] G. Klosko. Presumptive Benefit, Fairness and Political Obligation. *Philosophy and Public Affairs* 1987; 16: 241–259, at 242–243.

[21] An excludable good would be one created jointly where the benefits are only enjoyed by the participants themselves. Examples of excludable goods might include a library created by subscription or a private health insurance scheme. In such cases, contributing members control who benefits from their actions.

[22] J. Rawls. 1971. *A Theory of Justice*. Oxford. Oxford University Press.

[23] The characterisation given here is sufficient for the needs of this paper. However, a more substantive list of features of public goods is given by many authors such as G. Cullity. Moral Free Riding. *Philosophy and Public Affairs* 1995; 24: 3–34.

become infected with the relevant disease. The existence of herd protection as both a public good and a consequence of the preventive vaccination programme means that we can sidestep the prevention problem objection as individuals do benefit in a significant way from such a preventive programme. However, it is certainly the case that success for many preventive interventions is measured in terms of the level of certain factors across populations, even though individuals receive only marginal benefits (at best). Whilst the 'prevention problem' might have some weight in relation to such preventive programmes as those relating to diet modification or screening programmes, it is far from clear that they do so in the case of preventive vaccinations.[24] Whilst we might measure the impact of a preventive programme (be it preventive vaccination or screening) at the level of the population, it does not follow that the participant individuals do not all derive individual benefits from such participation. This is certainly the case in relation to preventive vaccination as I have argued above.

In addition to the argument above about herd protection being a public good, there are some other ethical and pragmatic reasons why we must continue with prophylactic vaccination even if therapeutic vaccination for all of the contagious diseases that we currently seek to prevent through preventive measures were to become available. The first such reason relates to the issue of access to health care. For example, even if it was the case that in developed countries we could cease prophylactic vaccination and move to therapeutic vaccination for contagious diseases, there is little likelihood of this happening in the developing world. In these regions it is hard enough to carry out preventive vaccinations for such major causes of death as measles. The lack of affordable and accessible health care is likely to mean that if we chose to end preventive vaccination, the main consequence would most likely be that the populations in developing countries would just get no access to vaccinations at all. Even in the developed world, if the relevant therapeutic vaccines did exist, there would still be a strong pragmatic argument in favour of retaining preventive vaccination for a long time to come. Indeed, even if therapeutic vaccinations were available and affordable it might still be better to concentrate on prevention rather than cure,

---

[24] A general discussion of prevention is beyond the scope of this paper. However, see M. Verweij. 2000. *Preventive Medicine Between Obligation and Aspiration.* Dordrecht. Kluwer, for excellent discussion of this topic.

given the way that contagious disease is spread.[25] In such circumstances it would seem little short of cruel to argue that we must wait until someone is infected before we do anything, even though we could easily do something in advance to prevent that event from occurring.[26]

I suggest that the relevant issue in deciding whether or not a preventive vaccination programme for contagious disease is ethical is not whether it is preventive in nature, but what the relative harms and benefits of vaccination versus non-vaccination might be. These will differ depending upon the disease and the particular vaccination in question. Where the risks of harm from the disease are high it might be worth running a greater risk of harm from the vaccine. Where the risks of harm from the disease are low, it might not be worth vaccinating at all. Ideally, we want to have as low a risk as possible and good effectiveness from each vaccine. What's wrong with prevention? Arguably, nothing: especially if the risk of harm from the disease you are seeking to prevent is great enough. In attempting to decide policy in this area and consider the ethical arguments we should concentrate on such risk assessments, not upon whether something is to be characterised either as a preventive or as a clinical intervention.

V. ADDITIONAL ETHICAL ISSUES IN RELATION TO THERAPEUTIC VACCINES

The potential benefits from therapeutic vaccination are immense and I do not want to suggest in any way that there is anything wrong with the development and use of therapeutic vaccination. My purpose has been, rather, to suggest that a potential ethical objection to preventive vaccination cannot be side-stepped in the future by appealing to the use of therapeutic vaccinations for contagious

---

[25] It might help to think of an actual example to illustrate this point, such as vaccination for Hepatitis B. Therapeutic vaccines have been developed for this disease, but given the nature of the disease and modes of transmission, it still makes sense to focus policy on preventive vaccination.

[26] The argument here is a little reminiscent of that about acts and omissions – although here the difference is between two different acts: acting now to prevent x or waiting until x occurs and then seeking to cure it. The supporters of the prevention problem clearly see the latter as being morally preferable.

diseases should they become available. This paper is an attempt to explore the structure of the prevention problem by casting a discussion of vaccination in terms of the contrasting intentions behind the two types of vaccinations. So far there has not been much discussion in the published literature of the ethical issues that might arise in relation to the use of therapeutic vaccination, at least partly because they have not had any sort of profile in the media or public consciousness. However, I think it is worthwhile to end this discussion by very quickly reviewing whether there are any potential ethical issues that might be raised by the development and use of therapeutic vaccines.

There are no doubt many biological issues that remain to be worked out with therapeutic vaccines, but there is no reason to think that given the possible benefits from their use that this work will not be done over the next few years. For example, some concerns have been raised about the possibility of mutant strains of the relevant viruses escaping, or the possibility of exacerbation of a viral infection as a result of vaccination (particularly where an individual had an impaired immune system).[27] In such circumstances, it might be that other therapies would be preferable for already-infected individuals (such as immunotherapy). Such issues relate to the balance between the risk of harms and the benefits consequent to treatment, both to the individual and to wider society. Given the nature of contagious disease, and the potential danger to third-parties, it might well be that a degree of caution is necessary in relation to such interventions beyond that normally accorded new drug interventions. However, given the potential benefits, these concerns do not provide a strong enough reason not to continue development of these potentially life saving treatments. Such issues do not raise any qualitatively different issues from those relating to the introduction of any other new clinical treatment. Whether therapeutic vaccines are used as well as or instead of preventive vaccines in the future, they are likely to become an increasingly important aspect of future medical care.[28]

---

[27] See Moingeon et al., *op. cit.* note 7, for discussion of these concerns.

[28] Of course there will be other relevant ethical issues relating to the development of research trials for such therapeutic vaccines. For example, if these were to be randomised controlled trials, would it be acceptable to trial a new therapeutic vaccine against the existing treatment where one existed? There will also be health economic issues about the relative costs of the different forms of vaccination. These issues will have to be discussed elsewhere.

CONCLUSIONS

The prevention problem argument does not work in relation to preventive vaccination for contagious disease because it fails to take seriously the view that herd protection is a public good and that this means that all individuals in the population derive benefit from the existence of a preventive vaccination programme (where herd protection exists). If, despite my argument, the prevention problem is held to be a serious objection to the prophylactic use of vaccines, then we need to face this fact. However, I do not believe it is, and have argued this in this paper. Therapeutic vaccines represent a welcome new way to combat disease. They are likely to raise some new ethical issues in relation to their use and development, but any concerns can be worked out in detail within the context of normal clinical usage. It is highly unlikely that therapeutic vaccinations will provide an adequate substitute for preventive vaccinations, given the reasons explored above and the advantages to using preventive vaccines in combating contagious disease. Therapeutic vaccination is always likely to be a supplement to preventive vaccination rather than a medically or ethically superior alternative. Any ethical objections to prophylactic vaccination on the basis of the 'prevention problem' will not be overcome through the substitution of therapeutic vaccines for preventive vaccines; indeed, the 'prevention problem' fails on its own terms in relation to preventive vaccination programmes.

Acknowledgements

Thanks to Marcel Verweij and my colleagues at Keele University for conversations on the issues discussed in this paper.

PART V: RESEARCH ETHICS

Chapter 15

INTERNATIONAL RESEARCH ETHICS[1]

UDO SCHÜKLENK AND RICHARD ASHCROFT

INTRODUCTION

Research ethics features currently prominently on the international bioethics agenda. There are good reasons for the prominence given to research ethics. Nazi doctors conducted some of the most gruesome medical experiments in German concentration camps during the Third Reich. Dr Mengele, for instance, killed Gypsy twin teenagers because he was interested in the fact that they had differently coloured eyes. Their eyes and other organs were removed after Mengele had killed them, and they were shipped to a laboratory for further analysis. Unfortunately, unethical research is not confined to Nazi doctors' research agendas. Lasagna reports that the ancient Persian kings and the Egyptian pharaohs have treated prisoners 'as expendable experimental material, much as modern laboratory researchers might order a supply of rats or rabbits.'[2] In the early 1970s the Tuskegee syphilis study came to light. Approximately 400 poor black men from rural areas in the south of the USA who were diagnosed with syphilis, had been left untreated as part of a study designed to observe the natural course of untreated syphilis. Breaches of research ethics have often resulted in irreversible damage to research subjects and sometimes even to death.

The international community responded to these events and to other crimes committed by medical researchers against research subjects with a variety of codes and other regulatory frameworks, such as the Nuremberg Code. This Code constituted the first international normative framework regulating the standards of

[1] We are grateful to Leslie London, University of Capetown, South Africa Richard Nicholson, *Bulletin of Medical Ethics,* United Kingdom, and John D. Arras, University of Virginia, USA for valuable support in our research for this article. Some of the arguments in this article have been presented by one of us during the 1999 5th International Conference on AIDS in Asia and the Pacific in Kuala Lumpur.
[2] L. Lasagna. 1972. 'Special Subjects in Human Experimentation.' In: P.A. Freund (Ed). *Experimentation with Human Subjects.* London: George Allen & Unwin: 262–275.

research clinical trials. This document was in many ways superseded by the Declaration of Helsinki, a code for research and experimentation the WMA (World Medical Association) issued in 1964 and revised several times thereafter.[3] This document constituted a watered down version of the stringent requirements set and the high standards demanded by the Nuremberg Code. Alongside the strict requirements on voluntary consent in the Nuremberg Code, the Helsinki Declaration introduced 'best interests' criteria, supposed to apply to incompetent research subjects, but in fact also raising question marks over the scope and applicability of the informed consent standard to *competent* subjects too. It eventually became the most influential international ethics document regulating medical research. In 1993 it was supplemented by international research ethics guidelines produced by the CIOMS (Council of Medical Organisations of Medical Sciences) in collaboration with the WHO (World Health Organisation).[4] This set of documents contains a series of important protections of people participating as research subjects in developing countries.

Research ethics guidelines on a variety of topics have been released by organisations such as the Australian National Health and Medical Research Council,[5] the US National Bioethics Advisory Commission, and by many other national bodies in both developed and developing countries.[6] This Background Briefing on International Research Ethics is not attempting to provide an all-encompassing overview of the various national research ethics guidelines which have come out or are in the making. Rather, this

---

[3] WMA. 'Declaration of Helsinki.' In: A. R. Jonsen, R. M. Veatch, L. Walters (Eds). 1998. *Source Book in Bioethics.* Georgetown UP: Washington DC: 13–15.

[4] CIOMS. 1993. *International Ethical Guidelines for Biomedical Research Involving Human Subjects.* WHO, Geneva.

[5] NH&MRC. 1999. *National Statement on Ethical Conduct in Research Involving Humans.* Canberra: Commonwealth of Australia. See for critical review and commentary M. Spriggs. 'Human Subjects Research: Review of the NH&MRC National Statement on Ethical Conduct in Research Involving Humans.' *Monash Bioethics Review* 1999; 18(4): 5–13 (suppl.). R. E. Ashcroft. 'The New National Statement on Ethical Conduct in Research Involving Humans: A Social Theoretic Perspective.' *Monash Bioethics Review* 1999; 18(4): 14–17 (suppl.).

[6] NABC. 1998. *Research Involving Persons with Mental Disorders that may Affect Decisionmaking Capacity.* NABC: Rockville, MD. See for critical review and commentary A. Capron. 'Ethical and Human Rights Issues in Research on Mental Disorders that may Affect Decisionmaking Capacity.' *New England Journal of Medicine* 1999; 340: 1430–1434. R. Michaels. 'Are Research Ethics Bad for our Mental Health?' *New England Journal of Medicine* 1999; 340: 1427–1430.

Briefing will provide a critical overview of the main issues currently debated internationally on international research ethics. The 5th World Congress of the International Association of Bioethics features various plenary and main sessions addressing problems to do with international research ethics. Intensive professional debate continues on research ethics guidelines and standards.[7] Pivotal international research ethics guidelines such as the World Medical Association's Declaration of Helsinki and the Council for International Organisations of Medical Sciences International Guidelines for Biomedical Research Involving Human Subjects are undergoing extensive revisions. Particular interest and controversy surrounds the question of ethically appropriate standard of collaborative international clinical research relying on research subjects in developing countries.[8]

THE ISSUES

The international discussions have focused on a number of issues, most notably on questions pertaining to the content of the

---

[7] Among the more important *recent* contributions to this debate are B.A. Brody. 1998. *The Ethics of Biomedical Research: An International Perspective.* Oxford UP: New York. N.M.P. King, G.E. Henderson, J. Stein (eds). 1999. *Beyond Regulations: Ethics in Human Subjects Research.* University of North Carolina Press: Chapel Hill & London. R. Macklin. 1999. *Against Relativism: Cultural Diversity and the Search for Ethical Universals in Medicine.* Oxford UP: New York. B.M. Dickens. 'Vulnerable Persons in Biomedical Research.' *Journal International de Bioéthique* 1999; 10(1–2): 13–23. US National Bioethics Advisory Commission. 1998. *Research Involving Persons with Mental Disorders that may Affect Decisionmaking Capacity.* NABC: Rockville, MD. T. Smith *Ethics in Medical Research.* Cambridge UP: Cambridge, UK. See also the articles published in the special issue of the *Bulletin of Medical Ethics* 1999; 150: 9–44.

[8] Among the more important *recent* contributions to this debate are P. Lurie, S. M. Wolfe. 'Unethical Trials of Interventions to Reduce Perinatal Transmission of the Human Immunodeficiency Virus in Developing Countries.' *New England Journal of Medicine* 1997; 337: 853–856. R.J. Levine. 'The Need to Revise the Declaration of Helsinki.' *New England Journal of Medicine* 1999; 341: 531–534. Nuffield Council on Bioethics. 1999. *The Ethics of Clinical Research in Developing Countries.* Nuffield Foundation: London. Two major symposia on ethical problems in collaborative clinical research in developing countries were published in *Bioethics* 1998; 12: 286–333 and the *Hastings Center Report* 1998; 28(6): 25–48. These issues were also debated in medical journals published in developing countries, such as the *South African Medical Journal.* L. London, J. de Gruchy, L. Baldwin-Ragaven. 'Revision of the Helsinki Declaration – Ethical Standards at Risk?' *South African Medical Journal* 1999; 89: 812–813. A MedLine database search should allow the interested reader and researcher to find literature pertaining to this subject. A summary of one of the more important *public* meetings on this issue can be found in R. Nicholson, F. P. Crawley. Revising the *Declaration of Helsinki:* A Fresh Start.' *Bulletin of Medical Ethics* 1999; 151: 13–17.

Declaration of Helsinki, its status, and the current *modus operandi* interpreting the document as a consensus based statement.
Of particular interest are

1. the question of whether the distinction between therapeutic and non-therapeutic research should be upheld;
2. the questions of whether the currently demanded best proven diagnostic and therapeutic method of treatment for all research subjects is feasible both in developed and in developing countries, and whether it should be upheld;
3. the question of who owns the Declaration and other international research ethics documents, the individual sponsoring organisations or the international community of clinical researchers, biomedical ethicists and other stakeholders such as non-governmental organisations; and the question of how decisions about changes to such international guidelines can possibly be achieved, given that it seems to be the case that genuine disagreement about issues of content is possible and likely.

THERAPEUTIC AND NON-THERAPEUTIC RESEARCH

The Declaration draws a fundamental distinction between therapeutic and non-therapeutic research, which reads: 'In the field of biomedical research a fundamental distinction must be recognised between medical research in which the aim is essentially diagnostic or therapeutic for a patient, and medical research, the essential object of which is purely scientific and without implying direct diagnostic or therapeutic value to the person subjected to the research.' The ethical justification for this distinction is more implied than explicated in this document. Therapeutic research is seen as justifiable because it is designed to benefit patients, while the latter has the overall well-being of society in mind.

Article II.4[9] of the Declaration limits risks to research subjects that this formulation might result in. It states that 'In research on

[9] The following and all subsequent quotes from the Declaration of Helsinki are taken from WMA. Declaration of Helsinki. In: A.R. Jonsen, R.M. Veatch, L. Walters (eds). 1998. *Source Book in Bioethics*. Georgetown UP: Washington DC: 13–15. The Declaration has been reprinted in many standard bioethics anthologies, such as J.D. Arras, B. Steinbock (eds). 1999. *Ethical Issues in Modern Medicine* (5th Edition). Mayfield: Mountainview, CA. It is also available on a large number of internet websites. A search on any of the major internet search engines should allow the interested reader to get hold of a copy of this document.

man, the interest of science and society should never take precedence over considerations related to the well-being of subjects.' Kantian inspired medical professionals such as the University of Chicago oncologist Samuel Hellman continue to defend this credo until today.[10]

Robert J. Levine has quite succinctly criticised the problems which would occur should the current wording of the Declaration of Helsinki be taken seriously by clinical researchers.[11] Articles II.6 and III.2 of the Declaration read as follows:

> II.6 The doctor can combine medical research with professional care, the objective being the acquisition of new medical knowledge, only to the extent that medical research is justified by its potential diagnostic or therapeutic value for the patient. III.2 The subjects should be volunteers – either healthy persons or patients for whom the experimental design is not related to the patient's illness.

Levine argues that the conjunction of these two articles leads to an absurdity:

> This pair of articles rules out all rational research on the causes of disease or on their pathogenesis or pathophysiology. Consider for example research designed to explore the role of neurotransmitters in the pathogenesis of depression. Since this research cannot be justified on the basis of its therapeutic benefit for the patient, as required by article II.6, it must be considered nontherapeutic. Therefore, as required by article III.2, the subjects of the research must be either normal volunteers or patients who have diseases other than depression.[12]

Of course, in the light of the Nuremberg doctors' trial, it is clear that research into pathogenesis is precisely the sort of research that posed most problems. So this sort of error is hardly 'unintended', if error it be.

---

[10] S. Hellman. 'The Patient and the Public Good.' *Nature Medicine* 1995; 1: 400–402. S. Hellman, D.S. Hellman. 'Of Mice but Not Men: Problems of the Randomised Clinical Trial.' *New England Journal of Medicine* 1991; 324: 1589–1592.
[11] R.J. Levine. 'The Need to Revise the Declaration of Helsinki.' *New England Journal of Medicine* 1999; 341: 531–534.
[12] R.J. Levine. 'The Need to Revise the Declaration of Helsinki.' *New England Journal of Medicine* 1999; 341: 531–534, at 531.

One could also question Levine's reading of 'potential', as its sense in the current Declaration is indeed quite ambiguous. His argument is not the knock-down argument he presents it as being because he trades on this ambiguity. However, Levine's broader quarrel is with the ambiguity and lack of definition given to the therapeutic/non-therapeutic distinction in the current Declaration. He proposes to give up the distinction as irreparable. This does not follow from his argument as stated. All he shows (if that) is that the current statement has difficulties, not that even with suitable conceptual clarification no equivalent statement can be produced.

Suppose the Declaration is reworked, as Levine suggests, in terms of therapeutic and non-therapeutic procedures. Do we gain clarity and precision, and avoid 'errors' of the type specified above? It seems not. Levine's argument rests at several key points on 'intended' benefit, whereas framers of guidelines are normally keen to avoid unobservable mental states like intentions in favour of public criteria such as consent and acceptance by peer and ethics committee review. He claims that non-therapeutic procedures can only be justified by reference to social benefit, without allowing volunteer's consent to override such considerations, and without allowing that volunteers can have perfectly good, non-moral reasons for taking part in research (curiosity, financial gain).[13] 'Health benefits' are not transparent criteria, either, such that they can pick out neatly therapeutic procedures any more than they did therapeutic research. If the way to pick out the non-therapeutic is the end in view, we are not on safe ground; nor are we if we try to pick out the therapeutic by examining the appropriate kind of justification (which could be volunteers' preferences rather than objective ends).

Levine seems to make life difficult for himself as he does for proponents of the 'therapeutic/non-therapeutic research' distinction. Given this problem, it is worth asking what he, and the WMA originally, want the distinction to do (and what he thinks it fails to do), such that precision is so important.

---

[13] See M. Wilkinson, A. Moore. 'Inducement in Research.' *Bioethics* 1997; 11: 5, 373–389. P. McNeill. 'Paying People to Participate in Research: Why Not?' *Bioethics* 1997; 11: 5, 390–396.

Firstly, the distinction sits alongside another equally problematic distinction, that between research and treatment.[14] More importantly, the distinction is meant to distinguish between those things done for the good of the patient and those done for the good of persons other than the patient or society. On one level, this presumes that this distinction applies in all cases, whereas it obviously does not always do so. On another, it is a way of formulating the concern that subjects shall be exploited in research, and it tries to pick out those safe cases where they are not exploited. On another level, it tries to apply standards of dignity, justice and beneficence to the treatment of research subjects (while leaving autonomy out of the picture at this stage). The practice of Research Ethics Committees to date underlines the priority of non-maleficence over autonomy in research review. Levine argues that the current Declaration ensures that this is so, but his distinction does nothing to change this. And finally, on a very trivial level, it suggests that we should look in a different way at non-therapeutic research to the way we look at therapeutic research.

The aim of avoiding exploitation is of huge importance (as will be discussed in the next section). But the nature of exploitation is not easily stated, and not amenable to being turned into general, once-for-all guidelines. Moreover, the anti-exploitation, protective stance is often at odds with the pro-autonomy stance. So, one could argue that for the reasons given Levine's critique is mistaken in its search for precision. The Declaration is a statement of principles, not a cookbook of guidelines. It could not be otherwise. The meaning is in the use. The distinction exists to prompt users of these principles to a particular way of thinking about 'non-therapeutic' research, with the emphasis on thinking. Clearly, Levine's error example is an absurdity, as he says, which is why no one thinks seriously that the Declaration should be applied in this way.

TRIAL STANDARDS IN DEVELOPING COUNTRIES

A number of authors have suggested that a requirement embedded in the wording of the current Declaration, that is that all

---

[14] I. Chalmers & R. Lindley. 'Double Standards on Informed Consent to Treatment: Ignored for a Quarter of a Century by Most Professional Medical Ethicists', in L. Doyal, J.S. Tobias (eds.). *Informed Consent in Medical Research.* BMJ Publications: London, 2001.

participants in a given trial receive the best proven diagnostic and therapeutic method of treatment, is difficult to meet, and often meeting it would make trials unfeasible in developing countries.

This argument asserts that if all participants in a given clinical trial in a developing country had to receive the best proven treatment it would be impossible to develop cheaper (innovative, new) drug regimens for people living in such countries. For instance the use of a placebo control would then be impossible.[15] As an example of the arguments put forward in this context shall serve the international controversy over the standards in perinatal HIV transmission prevention trials in developing countries. In 1994 officials of the WHO, UNAIDS, the US NIH, and the US CDC designed placebo controlled studies to answer the question of whether a course of the drug zidovudine, when given to HIV infected pregnant women is more effective in preventing HIV infections of the newborns than doing nothing. In the same year another collaborative trial, undertaken only in developed countries, discovered that 25% of HIV positive pregnant women who do not use zidovudine give birth to an infected baby, while less than 8% of those using zidovudine do. This trial protocol, known as ACTG 076, led in Western countries to the provision of zidovudine as a matter of course to HIV infected pregnant women. It is the standard of care in the developed world. However, the implementation of the ACTG 076 protocol requires at 1998 prices about US$ 800 per pregnancy. That is far more than the per capita health care allocation in many developing nations.

The trials criticised by Lurie and Wolfe in the *New England Journal of Medicine*[16] sought to test whether it is possible to develop a drug regimen that is substantially cheaper yet still efficient with regard to the mother-child transmission of HIV. This objective meets a demand set out in the CIOMS guidelines, that is that it should be 'responsive to the health needs and the priorities of the

---

[15] See ie D. B. Resnik. 'The Ethics of HIV Research in Developing Countries.' *Bioethics* 1998; 12: 4, 286–306. H. Varmus, D. Satcher. Ethical Complexities of Conducting Research in Developing Countries. *New England Journal of Medicine* 1997; 337: 1003–1005. These authors' point of view is more fully developed on a NIH website: http://www.nih.gov/new/mathiv/mathiv.htm.

[16] P. Lurie & S.M. Wolfe. 'Unethical Trials of Interventions Reduce Perinatal Transmission of the Human Immunodeficiency Virus in Developing Countries.' *New England Journal of Medicine* 1997; 337: 853–856.

community in which it is carried out.'[17] This is supposed to ensure that studies are done for the sake of the participants in the host community, rather than merely to benefit future patients elsewhere. So, for instance, research in Malawi should be designed to benefit Malawians, rather than future Americans. The studies under consideration required that all research subjects give first person informed consent. The HIV infected pregnant women were informed that they would be randomly assigned to receive either a placebo or zidovudine. This was designed to meet an important ethical standard requirement of any clinical trial involving competent subjects, that is that the trial subjects give first person voluntary informed consent.

Critics of the trials charged that the trial design was unethical, because it involved a placebo control, even though historical controls would have sufficed, thereby reducing the number of participants subjected knowingly to an inferior form of treatment. Lurie et al. argued that the results of ACTG 076 should have led to a research design asking the question of whether a shorter (and therefore cheaper) regimen of AZT is just as effective as the ACTG 076 regimen, and not to a placebo controlled study. They argued for the implementation of equivalency studies rather than placebo controlled studies.

Those who undertook the trial countered that the placebo controls led faster to statistically predictive results, and that, equally as important, no woman participating in this study was any worse off than she would have been had she not participated. The rationale here is that the standard of care locally was such that women would not have been able to afford an AZT intervention in any case, hence those in the placebo arm were not worse off, while those in the AZT arm were better off. Some have questioned this local standard of care concept (this idea has recently reincarnated, in another formulation, as the 'highest attainable and sustainable standard of care'). It is arguably doubtful that there exists a readily identifiable local standard of care anywhere. Rather, the local standard of care in, for instance Ivory Coast, is a standard of care determined crucially by the prices set by Western pharmaceutical multinationals. The main reason why the trials Lurie and Wolfe criticised took place was the pricing schedule set by the manufacturer of that drug.

[17] CIOMS. 1993. *International Ethical Guidelines for Biomedical Research Involving Human Subjects.* WHO: Geneva, at 25.

Glaxo-Wellcome therefore more than anything else determines the local standard of care. The South African government tried to improve this situation by proposing to compulsory license essential, life-saving drug. In a society with about 25% of the population HIV infected, and in excess of 40% of all newborns, this could be an ethically justifiable solution. After all, as Unger would argue, the survival interests of human beings must have priority over the profit-related interests of the shareholders of a pharmaceutical company.[18] Reportedly, the US government responded to this by threatening South Africa with a trade war. The South African government shelved its plan subsequently, even though this means further avoidable deaths and suffering in this country.

Depending on one's philosophical worldview one can both condemn these trials or deem them ethically justifiable.[19] One can consistently hold a view such as that expressed by casuist philosophers Crouch and Arras, who doubt that 'even taking past injustice (people in developed nations committed against people developing nations) into account (this) would yield a moral entitlement to expensive antiretroviral treatment.'[20] On this background, clinical trials undertaken to develop an affordable drug could be legitimate, because these authors do not question the economic context that gives rise to the purported necessity to develop cheaper drugs for people living in developing countries. Consequentialists could hold against this conclusion that the maximisation of human well-being requires the availability of essential (ie life-saving) medication. They might well conclude that trials such as the perinatal HIV transmission prevention trial are unethical, because a working drug regimen does exist and should be made available (ie affordable) to those who need them.

Preventive HIV vaccine trials: a special case

Preventive HIV vaccine trials raise a few additional important ethical issues. Currently a UNAIDS supported placebo controlled preventive HIV vaccine trial takes place in Thailand. Healthy

---

[18] P. Unger. 1996. *Living High and Letting Die: Our Illusion of Innocence.* Oxford UP, New York.

[19] See, for instance, the special issue of *The Journal of Medicine and Philosophy* 1999; 24(3), which was devoted to the question of whether health care is a commodity.

[20] R.A. Crouch & J.D. Arras. 'AZT Trials and Tribulations.' *Hastings Center Report* 1998; 28(6); 26–34, at 28.

volunteers in this trial who become infected during the course of the trial, will subsequently receive only whatever the local standard of care amounts to. Here the argument that none of the trial participants is worse off than they would have been had they not participated in the trial does not work. The reason for this is that in all trials, be they in developed or developing countries, some participants have a therapeutic misconception which entails that they believe strongly that they have received a successfully working drug.[21] This will inevitably result into a number of newly HIV infected trial participants who became infected because of their therapeutic misconception of the trial. Such infected research subjects' baseline has clearly worsened as a result of their trial participation. The 'local standard of care' idea means here that these people will not receive the best proven therapeutic means of treatment but only those available to other Thai people with HIV infection. This means no less then that some of these volunteers will die as a consequence of their participation in the trial. If the research subjects get sick, unlike people in developed countries, their subsequent care will be limited to the extent of non-existence. For any commercial organisation conducting such trials this constitutes a significant saving when compared to trials in developed countries.[22]

Universal ethical standards are ultimately undermined if they receive a context specific interpretation, as Kerin pointed out.[23] The UK based Nuffield Council sought to confront this problem by proposing to re-interpret the wording of the Declaration of Helsinki as really indicating that trial participants must be provided with 'the best proven diagnostic and therapeutic method available in the country where the trial is conducted.'[24] The problem for the authors of the Nuffield report is that the Declaration's actual wording leaves no room for this interpretation. It is unequivocal in its requirement

[21] This phenomenon is discussed in P.S. Appelbaum, L.H. Roth, C. Lidz, P. Benson, W. Winslade. 'False Hopes and Best Data: Consent to Research and the Therapeutic Misconception.' *Hastings Center Report* 1987; 17(2): 20–24. With regard to preventive HIV vaccine trials some preliminary empirical evidence is provided in O. Q. de Fonseca Filho, R. K. Lie. 'Informed Consent to Preventive AIDS Vaccine Trials in Brazil: A Pilot Study.' *AIDS and Public Policy Journal* 1995; 10: 22–26.

[22] This is stressed in a recent publication of a pharmaceutical industry publication. I Haydock. 'Asian clinical trials are gaining international credibility.' *Scrib Magazine* October 1999: 17–18. The author stresses the point that per patient trial costs in Asian clinical trials are 25% lower than in the US and Europe.

[23] J. Kerin. 'Double Standards: Principled or Arbitrary?' *Bioethics* 1998; 12: 4, i–vii.

[24] Nuffield Council on Bioethics. 1999. *The Ethics of Clinical Research in Developing Countries.* Nuffield Foundation: London, at 21.

that every research subject receive the 'best proven diagnostic and therapeutic method.' There is no qualification made that would allow us to slip in the word *available*, and to change thereby the meaning of this sentence.

It is worth noting that while some Western researchers and bio-ethicists are sympathetic to the ethical arguments in support of the perinatal HIV transmission prevention trials, most political treatment access activists, as well as many scientists and research ethics committees in developing countries reject the idea of a 'local standards of care' or 'the highest attainable and sustainable standard of care', and with it the proposed changes to the current minimum requirements of the Declaration of Helsinki.[25] South African doctors, for instance, express their worry about the negative effects of the proposed changes to the Declaration of Helsinki for African research subjects in these words:

> Through these proposed amendments, the universality of human subject protection is at risk, thus making it conceivable that companies will choose to conduct their research in locations where standards of care are lower, knowing that different regulations will apply.[26]

OWNERSHIP, STATUS OF AND HOW TO NEGOTIATE CHANGES TO INTERNATIONAL RESEARCH ETHICS GUIDELINES

Given the absence of a consensus among knowledgeable, well-intentioned bioethicists, scientists and political activists over the

[25] See for instance the debates on treatment access on one of the largest electronic international AIDS discussion fora http://www.hivnet.ch:8000/topics/treatment-access or D. B. Greco. Clinical Trials in 'Developing' Countries: The Fallacy of Urgency or Ethics vs. Economics. *Bulletin of Medical Ethics* 1999; 150: 33–34, P. A. Allotey. Clinical Trials in Developing Countries: Bringing People Into the Debate. *Monash Bioethics Review* 1999; 18(4): 18–23 (suppl.), 2nd National Meeting of Ethics Committee Representatives on Ethical Standards for Clinical Research in Thailand. Executive Summary July 16th, 1999. Faculty of Medicine, Chulalongkorn University, Bangkok, Thailand. Published in *Programme: International Workshop – Revising the Declaration of Helsinki: A Fresh Start*. Royal Society of Medicine, London, September 3rd–4th, 1999, L. London, J. de Gruchy, L. Baldwin-Ragaven. 'Revision of the Helsinki Declaration – Ethical Standards at Risk?' *South African Medical Journal* 1999; 89: 812–813.

[26] L. Baldwin-Ragaven, J. de Gruchy & L. London. 1999. *An Ambulance of the Wrong Colour: Health Professionals, Human Rights and Ethics in South Africa*. Capetown: University of Capetown Press, at 140.

central issue of research ethics standards, it cannot surprise us that the issue of the ownership of the various influential international research ethics guidelines resurfaced. The WMA as the current owner of the Declaration of Helsinki and CIOMS as the owner of its international research ethics guidelines have both been blamed for not consulting widely enough and for not asking all relevant stakeholders about their respective opinions. Indeed, a look at the participants lists of virtually all major meetings which discussed proposed changes to the Declaration shows a marked absence of patient representatives and political treatment access activists from developing countries. Often developing country delegates to such meetings were actually Western researchers working in such countries or they were developing country government representatives with no known expertise relating to clinical trials or research ethics. This raises the important question of whether a small self-selecting group of individuals should exclusively be in control of the content of documents such as the Declaration of Helsinki and the CIOMS guidelines. The point of this critique is not to question the professional standing or integrity of individuals belonging to this group, or the quality of their own contributions to this debate, but merely to highlight the continuing lack of a serious consultation with the relevant stakeholders.

This links into a related issue, given the absence of a consensus over the actual content of the Declaration and its status, how should the international community go about negotiating changes to the Declaration or the CIOMS guidelines. An international meeting in London concluded that 'consensus cannot continue to function as the modus operandi for the production support, and legitimation of international guidelines in biomedical research ethics.'[27] Unfortunately this and other meetings failed to suggest and defend a viable alternative modus operandi to tackle the crucial question of who should be in charge of organising and financing international debate over research ethics guidelines, and who should be considered (on the basis of which criteria) a relevant stakeholder in the debate.

There is a case for saying that the guidelines of any given organisation are its own to write; so the Declaration of Helsinki is a

---

[27] R.H. Nicholson, F.P. Crawley (with J. Bryant, R. Eiss, S. Fluss, D. Greco, V.I. Mathan and D. Shapiro). 'Revising the Declaration of Helsinki: A Fresh Start.' *Bulletin of Medical Ethics* 1999; 151: 13–17.

Declaration of the WMA, and thus is owned by it alone. It stands as a declaration of policy about how the WMA wishes itself (and its members and member associations) to implement commonly agreed ethical principles and international law. As such, it is not itself international law, although it would stand as a statement of what 'responsible medical opinion' believes, and so departure from that opinion, while not necessarily immoral, corrupt or illegal, would require justification. Perhaps the WMA could regard departure from its guidelines as professional misconduct, and apply its sanctions as a professional or trade organisation.

No one reads the Declaration this way. It is as near international law as makes no difference. Moreover, unlike, say the World Trade Organisation's protocols, but like the UN's Universal Declaration of Human Rights, a nation or professional organisation cannot simply secede from the world community, saying that it does not recognise these principles on pragmatic grounds. A group would have to argue that the principles of the Declaration were false, inconsistent or 'culturally inapplicable for us'. One step forward might be for this special status of the Declaration to be recognised by taking it out of the hands of the WMA and transferring ownership to the UN (or one of its associated organisations, for instance the WHO or UNESCO). This would, of course, have various pragmatic drawbacks, not least the fact that doctors and other health professionals tend to want to own 'their' guidelines and write them themselves. But in the current debate, not many seem to be arguing that the Declaration should be revised for medical reasons; the debate is about the conflicting needs of commerce and patient care. Indeed, it might be fair to say that the debate is not really a debate within ethics, but one between ethics and economic prudence, which certainly overlap but equally obviously do not coincide.

If, as all parties want to say, that the revision of the Declaration is about ethics, then there is a second problem to solve beyond that of ownership. Ethicists tend to say that as ethics is a rational business, it should have as little as possible to do with politics on the one side, and public opinion on the other (taken Platonically as the opposite of enlightened rationality). Yet the nature of the debate to date shows that this is not a viable stance to take up. While philosophers can try and straighten out statements of human rights, the political reality is that the interpretation and application of rights arguments, and the adjudication of rights claims, is a matter of law, policy and politics. Clearly, in the debate over the new Declaration, different interests are in conflict, and they must be adjudicated among. This is the task of politics, although a politics informed by evidence and by rational argument. Part of the task of the bioethics community must therefore be to account for whose interests should, all things considered, be accorded priority.

If we allow that ownership and content of the Declaration is a matter of global politics as much as of ethics and medicine, then we must ensure that the relevant stakeholders have the right and ability to speak in the political forum. And so there must be found ways of educating and facilitating the contribution of the currently excluded stakeholders, the patient groups and developing countries' publics.

CONCLUSION

The proposed revision of the Declaration has so far not been successful. Some of the reasons for this lack of success are due to doubts over the necessity for some of the revisions; most are due to public and professional suspicions over the meaning and purpose of proposed changes. This situation is unlikely to change much, although the debate will of necessity reach closure somehow. What would be a unfortunate would be for the Declaration to be seen as a rather vague and politically suspect sort of 'Good Clinical Practice' guideline, rather than as a clear statement of ethical principle. The Declaration cannot be or be seen to be the property of any particular interest group. Nor can ethics itself become seen as simply the ideology of some particular interest group. At present this is being risked, largely through the exclusion of the people most affected, the patients themselves. Conflict will remain, and indeed perhaps will grow. But we should distinguish conflict by debate, which most of us consider to be a good thing, from the conflict by armed or economic force, which most of us consider bad. It is possible that by promoting the former we avoid the latter; it is unlikely that by avoiding the former we avoid the latter.

Chapter 16

EQUIPOISE AND INTERNATIONAL HUMAN-SUBJECTS RESEARCH

ALEX JOHN LONDON

The question of how to formulate the equipoise requirement in the context of international human-subjects research touches on some of the most fundamental issues in research ethics, yet it has received surprisingly little explicit and systematic discussion. For instance, in the recent controversy over international trials of a short-course of zidovudine (AZT) for the prevention of maternal-infant HIV transmission, the earliest and most vocal critics argued that the use of a placebo controlled design was unethical because it violated the equipoise requirement. They then argued that the short-course regimen should be tested against the current standard of care in the developed world, known as the Aids Clinical Trial Group 076 protocol.[1] In the relatively acrimonious debate that ensued, defenders of the placebo controlled design vigorously challenged the second of these claims, namely, that research conducted in a developing country should be governed by the same standard of care that prevails in the developed world.[2] Surprisingly, however, relatively little explicit attention was paid to the more fundamental point from which it was derived: that as proposed the short course trials would violate the equipoise requirement. Without a careful elucidation of the role of equipoise in evaluating international research it has been difficult to locate the crux of several important disputes and I have argued elsewhere that the disagreement over the interpretation of the standard of care for international research is a case in point.[3]

On a more fundamental level, however, the absence of a careful and sustained analysis of equipoise in this context has given rise to

---

[1] M. Angell. The Ethics of Clinical Research in the Third World. *NEJM* 1997; 337: 487–489 and P Lurie, SM Wolf. Unethical trials of interventions to reduce perinatal transmission of the human immunodeficiency virus in developing countries. *NEJM* 1997; 337: 853–856.

[2] R.J. Levine. The 'Best Proven Therapeutic Method' Standard in Clinical Trials in Technologically Developing Countries. *IRB* 1998; 20: 5–9.

[3] A.J. London. The Ambiguity and the Exigency: Clarifying 'Standard of Care' Arguments in International Research. *Journal of Medicine and Philosophy* 2000; 25: 379–397.

the uncritical acceptance of a particular way of applying the requirement to international research. In what follows, I will argue that the received position suffers from a number of problems. I will also argue that there is an alternative way of formulating the equipoise requirement that licenses very different evaluations of some research proposals. In particular, the received interpretation of the equipoise requirement results in restrictions on international research that are either much more stringent or much more permissive than either side of these recent debates may recognize. Furthermore, it frames the question of equipoise in a way that exaggerates the appearance of intransigent conflict and the need for making 'tragic choices' between important moral values.

The alternative conception of the equipoise argument that I sketch below avoids these problems. I will show that the difficulties that remain are either not unique to this interpretation alone, or that they are less problematic than they first appear. In the end, I hope that articulating these competing conceptions of equipoise and discussing their respective strengths and weaknesses will provide a framework in which the relationships between a cluster of important values can be more clearly charted.

THE BASICS OF EQUIPOISE AND A CAVEAT

In its most basic formulation equipoise represents a state of genuine and credible doubt about the relative therapeutic merits of some set of interventions that target a specific medical condition. The requirement that equipoise exist as a necessary condition for the moral acceptability of a clinical trial comparing these interventions is motivated by two interlocking ideas. First, when equipoise obtains it is morally permissible to allow an individual's medical treatment to be assigned by a random process because there is no sufficiently credible evidence to warrant a judgment that one intervention is superior to the other(s). Second, clinical trials that are designed to break or disturb equipoise provide information that will enable the medical community to improve its existing clinical practices.[4] The requirement is thus seen as a way to reconcile the need

[4] B. Freedman. 'Placebo-Controlled Trials and the Logic of Clinical Purpose' *IRB* 1990; 12 (Nov/Dec): 1–6.

to improve the state of medical knowledge and clinical practice with the duty to ensure that the welfare of individual subjects is not knowingly sacrificed for the welfare of future patients or greater scientific understanding.

The equipoise requirement is thus a normative standard that articulates important scientific objectives, relating to the value of the data such trials should produce, as well as ethical boundaries that constrain the way this data may be obtained. In this latter respect, equipoise links together several important moral concepts. First, it stipulates that medical research must not violate what is called the 'duty of personal care,'[5] or the 'therapeutic obligation.'[6] Second, the concept of equipoise underscores an important epistemological aspect of this duty, namely, that the content of the obligation – what is required of a physician or researcher in some instance – depends in part on our ability to predict or foresee possible outcomes with an appropriate degree of certainty. For there to be a positive duty to provide a subject with a specific intervention there must be evidence of sufficient weight to license the judgment that it is likely to advance that person's interests. Finally, these considerations help to ensure that a clinical trial is just or fair by mandating that the interests of individual subjects are valued equally. A trial that begins in equipoise gives equal consideration to the interests of all subjects, even though that trial may ultimately show that one treatment option is superior to another.

Within the US and other technologically and economically developed nations the equipoise requirement continues to play an important role in the evaluation of human-subjects research, even though it remains the subject of searching philosophical criticism.[7] In particular, there is considerable debate over different interpretations or specifications of the concept of equipoise itself, as well as a debate over whether or not any of these interpretations succeed in reconciling the goal of advancing clinical knowledge with the duty to protect the interests of individual trial participants. Different interpretations of equipoise are individuated by the way they specify a range of interlocking variables that determine how the concept will

---

[5] C. Fried. 1974. *Medical Experimentation: Personal Integrity and Social Policy*. Amsterdam. North-Holland Publishing.

[6] D. Marquis. Leaving Therapy to Chance. *Hastings Center Report* 1983; 13: 40–47.

[7] For very clear and current review of several of these controversies, see F. Gifford. Freedman's 'Clinical Equipoise' and 'Sliding-Scale All-Dimensions-Considered Equipoise.' *Journal of Medicine and Philosophy* 2000; 25: 399–426.

be employed in practical decision making. So, for instance, we need to specify *who* is to weigh the relevant evidence in order to decide whether or not equipoise exists. Is this a judgment that is up to individual physicians, individual patients, the medical community as a whole, or some larger community that includes patients and possibly others? Likewise, we need to specify the kind of evidence that will warrant a judgment that equipoise has been achieved or disturbed. Here, possible answers can range from evidence as thin as an individual's personal hunch to as strict as data from double-blind randomized clinical trials.

These are but two in a range of important disagreements. For the purposes of the present discussion, however, I am going to focus on a facet of equipoise that has special relevance to the international context. To the extent that different stances on the issues mentioned above add an additional degree of complexity to this issue, it strengthens, rather than detracts from, the point that the equipoise requirement in international research deserves more careful consideration than it has currently received. Although I do in fact believe that there are good, independent reasons to think that these broader issues are more tractable than they are sometimes made out to be, this is a subject that will have to be dealt with on another occasion.

THE RECEIVED CONCEPTION OF EQUIPOISE

Perhaps the most prominent reference to the concept of equipoise in the recent debate over international research was made by Marcia Angell in her provocative critique of the short-course AZT trials. Angell's editorial in the *New England Journal of Medicine* begins by recounting the importance of equipoise for both the scientific and ethical acceptability of a clinical trial. She notes that there should not be solid evidence that one proposed intervention will be superior to the other and that:

> [1] If there is, not only would the trial be scientifically redundant, but the investigators would be guilty of knowingly giving inferior treatment to some participants in the trial. The necessity for investigators to be in the state of equipoise applies to placebo-controlled trials as well. [2] Only when there is no known effective treatment is it ethical to compare a potential new treatment with a placebo. [3] When effective treatment exists, a placebo may not

be used. Instead, subjects in the control group of the study must receive the best known treatment.

[4] All except one of the trials employ placebo-control groups, despite the fact that zidovudine has already been clearly shown to cut the rate of vertical transmission greatly and is now recommended in the United States for all HIV-infected pregnant women.[8]

Here Angell spells out in some detail a position that is frequently espoused more tersely by subsequent commentators. For example, one writes: 'The only way that these placebo-controlled trials should be allowed [in the developing world] is if there is a genuine doubt about the benefits of AZT. No such doubt exists in the United States.'[9]

In a moment I will question the validity of Angell's argument on the grounds that her understanding of its conclusion [3] is inconsistent with her understanding of the equipoise requirement itself, as expressed in [1] and [2]. In order to demonstrate this inconsistency, however, it will be necessary to investigate one facet of Angell's conception of the equipoise requirement in a bit more detail.

Consider the claim that it is unethical to compare a short-course of AZT to a placebo in the context of the developing world because researchers in developed countries have shown that the 076 protocol can substantially reduce the rate of perinatal HIV transmission in the context of the developed world. If this claim could be established then let us grant, for the sake of the argument, that researchers conducting such a trial would indeed be guilty of knowingly allowing one group of subjects (members of the control group) to suffer foreseeable and (practical limitations aside) preventable harms. What needs to be considered, however, is what it takes to show that the results of research and clinical practice conducted in the context of the developed world are relevant to the context of the developing world.

Put in its most general terms, in order for the fact that no doubt exists in the US concerning the benefits of AZT to be relevant to the design of a trial in the developing world, we must assume that

---

[8] M. Angell. The Ethics of Clinical Research in the Third World. *NEJM* 1997; 337: 487–489 at 487. The numbers in brackets do not appear in the original.
[9] P.A. Clark. The Ethics of Placebo-Controlled Trials for Perinatal Transmission of HIV in Developing Countries. *The Journal of Clinical Ethics* 1998; 9: 156–166 at 162.

the context of treatment in the developing world is *relevantly similar to* the context of treatment in the developed nations in which the 076 protocol demonstrated its effectiveness. This is because differences in the context of treatment bear on our ability to reliably project the knowledge of causal relationships from the one context into the other. Whether or not this is a controversial assumption, however, will depend on how we understand the criteria by which relevant contexts of treatment should be compared.

There are, however, narrow and broad interpretations of the criterion for similarity between the relevant contexts of treatment in the above argument. According to the narrow interpretation, the context of treatment in the US and Uganda, for example, is relevantly similar just in case we have no credible reason to doubt that AZT, as successfully administered in the 076 protocol, would have the same biological effects in both populations. On this interpretation, the relevant criterion of similarity is the physiological equivalency of the two populations. So understood, the only way that equipoise would exist between a placebo and the short-course of AZT in Uganda, when equipoise does not exist between them in the US, is if there were physiological differences between these populations of sufficient significance to generate a credible uncertainty as to whether AZT would behave the same way in the bodies of Ugandans as it does in Americans. In the absence of such physiological differences, proponents of this position argue that the short-course regimen should be compared against the 076 protocol rather than a placebo.

Angell appears to embrace this narrow interpretation of the context of treatment when she dismisses as subterfuge the idea that information gained in the industrialized world may not be relevant to developing countries because 'diseases and their treatments are very different in the Third World'. Instead, she argues, 'unless there are specific indications to the contrary, the safest and most reasonable position is that people everywhere are likely to respond similarly to the same treatment'.[10] These remarks are aimed at countering claims that there were in fact important physiological differences between treatment populations in industrialized nations and test populations in the developing world. In particular, it was argued that the 076 protocol was tested in a well-nourished population with a low incidence of anemia whereas populations of the

---

[10] Angell, *op. cit.* p. 848.

developing world are frequently malnourished and anemic. Given that AZT can exacerbate anemia, it was argued that a placebo group was necessary to ascertain the relative safety of AZT in such populations.[11] This is probably the clearest instance of a straight-forward clash over the question of equipoise in the debate over the short-course AZT trials and it is carried out against the backdrop of the narrow interpretation of the context of treatment. Both Angell and her critics accept the narrow interpretation of the clinical context; they simply disagree over the empirical issue of whether or not we have sufficient warrant for doubts about the effects of AZT in the bodies of malnourished populations of the developing world.

In the sections that follow I challenge the narrow interpretation of the clinical context on several grounds.

One implication of the narrow interpretation is that it undercuts the alternative approach to research in the developing world that Angell herself supports. Angell argued that equipoise did not exist between the short course and a placebo because there were strong indications that even a short course of AZT would be better than nothing at all. From this premise she then argued that unless members of the control group received the 076 protocol, researchers would be guilty of sacrificing the welfare of one group of subjects for the sake of medical knowledge. Yet, if we consider the design that Angell recommends it is unclear how this second point is supposed to follow from the first. Based on the available data, it was reasonable to believe that the short course of AZT would be better than nothing. But it was just as reasonable to believe that the short course would not be as effective as the full 076 protocol.[12] So it looks as though Angell's own argument applies to the trial design that she herself recommends, only here it is the welfare of members of the short-course arm whose welfare is being sacrificed for the sake of knowledge.

---

[11] H. Varmus, D. Satcher. Ethical Complexities of Conducting Research in Developing Countries. *NEJM* 1997; 337: 1003–1005 at 1004; M.H. Merson. Ethics of Placebo-Controlled Trials of Zidovudine to Prevent the Perinatal Transmission of HIV in the Third World (editorial). *NEJM* 1998; 338: 836; R.J. Simonds, M.F. Rogers, T.J. Dondero. Ethics of Placebo-Controlled Trials of Zidovudine to Prevent the Perinatal Transmission of HIV in the Third World (editorial). *NEJM* 1998; 338: 836–837.

[12] This suspicion appears to have been confirmed by an equivalence study recently completed in Thailand: M. Lallemant, G. Jourdain, S. Le Coeur, et al. A trial of shortened zidovudine regimens to prevent mother-to-child transmission of human immunodeficiency virus type 1. *NEJM* 2000; 343: 982–991.

On what grounds would it be permissible to conduct the sort of trial Angell recommends? Both the placebo controlled design and Angell's alternative seem to violate the equipoise requirement as Angell articulates it and if the sheer need to find an effective intervention for developing world populations justifies her preferred trial design then it also justifies the placebo controlled design that she criticizes. Alternatively, if we are to take the requirements of equipoise seriously, and if we embrace her interpretation of them, then it becomes unclear how we could *ever* justify searching for less expensive, less cumbersome, more portable alternative interventions that might provide some significant but less than optimal degree of relief to populations of the developing world.[13] Consider the following dilemma. Either we think that a proposed intervention may be as good as or better than the existing alternatives, or we do not. If we do, there would be no reason to place additional burdens on developing world populations by locating the research there since the trial could be ethically conducted in the developed world. If we do not have reason to think that the proposed intervention will be equivalent to or better than the current alternatives then equipoise would not exist and it would be unethical to conduct the trial anywhere in the world.

Neither side of this debate seems to recognize the importance of this dilemma. In particular, it seems to undermine the compatibility of two claims that each side seems to embrace, namely, that (1) equipoise should play an important role in evaluating international clinical trials and (2) that there are a range of cases in which conducting clinical trials aimed at finding interventions that can be widely utilized in the developing world can be a legitimate and morally permissible means of addressing certain distinctive and pressing health care needs of those populations. It is reasonable to believe that a more sophisticated conception of equipoise should help to identify some of these cases.

It is difficult to see how those claims can be reconciled if we adopt biological equivalency as the relevant criterion of similarity between research populations. To amplify this point, consider how the narrow interpretation construes the relationship between the question

---

[13] One implication of the present paper is that ethical international research is *not* premised on finding sub-optimal but affordable interventions for the developing world. Rather, ethical international research is premised on locating *optimal* interventions where these are the most effective interventions that can be implemented and maintained over time within a treatment context that is practically attainable in a population.

of equipoise and important, practical considerations that pertain to our ability to implement a protocol in a particular place.

THE ROLE OF BROADER, PRACTICAL CONSIDERATIONS

A narrow view of equipoise focuses on physiological equivalency as the criterion for similarity between the research context in countries such as the US and Uganda. This means that in the absence of credible doubts about the physiological similarity of these two research populations, it cannot be the case that equipoise exists for a research protocol in one country and fails to exist for the same protocol in the other. If we return to the case of the short-course AZT trials, proponents of the placebo design frequently pointed to a variety of important, practical obstacles to implementing the 076 protocol in the host nations, not only on a large-scale basis, but perhaps also within the context of a clinical trial. The most obvious and important obstacle was the sheer poverty of the developing nations in which the short-course trials were proposed. At approximately $800 per mother, the 076 protocol was far beyond the reach of the $8 average per-capita health care expenditures of these developing countries. Even if the AZT for clinical trials was donated by pharmaceutical companies, it was generally recognized that the developing nations in question could not afford the staggering cost of fully implementing the 076 protocol on a widespread basis. In fact, it was the recognition of this fact in conjunction with the high incidence of HIV in the developing world that motivated researchers to look for an alternative intervention in the first place.

The cost of the 076 protocol was not its only drawback, however. It was also pointed out that the 076 protocol requires mothers to stop breast feeding, since this is a known pathway of HIV transmission. In many of the developing nations in question, however, this requirement would be practically unachievable in part because of the scarcity of clean water. Additionally, the burden of having to purchase infant formula would add to the cost of an already expensive intervention.[14] Similar objections were raised with respect to the availability of the kind and quality of staff and facilities that the

[14] R.A. Crouch & J.D. Arras. AZT Trials and Tribulations. *Hastings Center Report* 1988; 28: 26–34 at 26.

076 protocol requires. Most of the nations in question lack the sort of well established health care infrastructure that has become the norm in the developed world. This generated doubts about the ability of researchers to implement effective screening programs at a sufficiently early stage of pregnancy for the 076 protocol to be implemented, especially in light of the fact that most pregnant women in these countries do not appear in a clinical setting until fairly late in pregnancy.[15]

These sorts of practical concerns do not bear directly on the permissibility of clinical trials if we adopt the narrow interpretation of equipoise.[16] If they are relevant at all, it is because they generate a set of additional, practical problems, that have to be weighed alongside of, and possibly against, the independent question of equipoise. On this view, Angell's interpretation of the equipoise requirement is accepted and, if she is right about the biological similarity of the two populations, then we are left with two basic options. First, if these various practical concerns are in fact insurmountable and it would thus be practically impossible to implement the 076 protocol in these countries, then it might be that the question of equipoise simply becomes irrelevant. That is, one might admit that Angell's narrow interpretation of equipoise is correct but argue that since we cannot be obligated to do what is practically impossible (or perhaps so difficult as to become supererogatory), her objections lose their normative force. Alternatively, however, given the same facts, one might take the opposite view and argue that the equipoise requirement cannot be set aside because of practical obstacles that bar people in the developed world from access to top-flight medical care. In this case, one might argue that it is not permissible to conduct clinical trials in the developed world until the conditions for equipoise can be achieved. The time and resources of western researchers, agencies, and governments should therefore be spent trying to ameliorate the very basic conditions that make effective therapies unattainable in those countries rather than conducting clinical trials in which they knowingly allow some members of the trial to suffer foreseeable and preventable harms.

[15] Varmus and Satcher, p. 1004.

[16] It has been pointed out, for example, that in the disputes over the short-course trials, 'the vehement emphasis on the 'best proven drugs' eclipsed considerations of whether the drug regimen could be safely applied in different settings.' S.R. Benatar, P.A. Singer. A new look at international research ethics. *BMJ* 2000; 321: 824–826 at 824. One purpose of the present paper is to give an account of equipoise that directly links issues of implementation and effectiveness.

Neither of these options is easy to accept because each appears unable to account for important moral intuitions about the case at issue. On the one hand, the view according to which the question of equipoise becomes irrelevant to international research fails to do justice to the considerations that underwrite the equipoise requirement in the first place. It allows research to proceed without articulating moral boundaries that require, among other things, that those who design and carry out such trials prevent foreseeable harms from befalling an identifiable group of people. On the other hand, the alternative view – which prevents research from going forward on the grounds that equipoise does not exist – seems content to sacrifice the welfare of the literally thousands of people who might benefit from the results of such research to the glacial pace of international justice and social change.

These alternatives, neither of which is satisfactory, characterize the present state of the debate about the standards that should govern international research. It is important to stress, however, that they are predicated on the narrow interpretation of the criterion of similarity between clinical contexts. That is, they presuppose that the question of whether or not equipoise exists between two proposed interventions in a specific population can be settled independently of the practical considerations that bear on the degree to which those interventions can be implemented within a population. The possibility that such practical concerns might be relevant to the question of equipoise itself has been left largely unexplored. To a certain degree this may be because they look like two different, and possibly incommensurate, sets of concerns: equipoise deals with what we know (e.g., that the 076 protocol has proven highly effective in the developed world) whereas practical considerations deal with what we can, or cannot, do (e.g., whether we can effectively implement the 076 protocol in the context of a developing nation). To see the way in which these questions are intimately connected with one another, we must explore some of the virtues of the broad interpretation of the criterion for similarity between contexts of treatment.

A BROADER CONCEPTION OF EQUIPOISE

From a clinical standpoint, the practical considerations that bear on our ability to successfully implement a treatment protocol in a particular population are of fundamental importance when evaluating the impact that such a protocol might have on the health of individuals in that population. This point was recognized by Freedman when he argued that equipoise should be a '*portmanteau* measure including all the elements that contribute to the acceptance of a drug within clinical practice.'[17] Among other things, Freedman argued that the question of equipoise should be framed around an intervention's 'net therapeutic advantage' where this is 'a compendious measure of a treatment's attractiveness.' This measure includes physiological considerations such as an intervention's direct impact on disease reduction, symptomatology, and ability to function, discounted by its particular side effect profile. However, it also includes broader, more practical considerations relating to differences in mode of delivery and ease of administration.

Factors that are ancillary to the brute biological characteristics of an intervention are important for several reasons. For Freedman, to weigh the attractiveness of competing interventions requires a comparison of the 'dynamic balance' created by a host of factors that are relevant to their clinical profile. For instance, he suggests that an antibiotic that is attractive because of its specific microbial action may have a lower net therapeutic advantage than alternatives that have fewer toxic side effects *or* that do not require intravenous delivery and constant medical monitoring. This example is particularly interesting in the present context because it reveals one way in which an intervention's net therapeutic advantage is influenced by the nature of the context in which the intervention is to be implemented.

In order to answer the question of how effective a particular intervention is likely to be relative to some alternative in a particular setting, we must first answer a host of practical questions about the nature of the context in which those treatments can be effectively administered and our ability to create and sustain such a context in a particular place or community. For this reason, a more robust conception of equipoise adopts a broader and more flexible criterion for similarity between treatment contexts, what I will call the criterion of 'clinical comparability.' This conception of equipoise can be stated formally as follows. Let an intervention I represent a treatment for a problem P and a protocol for its implementation.

---

[17] B. Freedman. Placebo-Controlled Trials and the Logic of Clinical Purpose. *IRB* 1990; 12: 1–6 at p. 5. The following quote is from p. 2.

Let a treatment setting S represent an identifiable population and the set of background conditions within which that population lives and receives medical care. Such background conditions may include unique physiological characteristics of that population, certain social and cultural norms operative within the population, material resources available in that population including infrastructure and other social resources, and other conditions that may be relevant as well.

> **Principle of Equipoise**: Equipoise exists between interventions I_1 and I_2 relative to problem P in a treatment setting S, just in case credible doubts exist about the relative net therapeutic advantage of I_1 and I_2 for treating P in S and there is no intervention I_3 that is preferable to either or both I_1 and I_2 for treating P in S.

> Credible doubt about the relative net therapeutic advantage of I_1 and I_2 for P in S exist just in case there is no treatment setting S* such that both (1) S and S* are clinically comparable and (2) good evidence exists for the superiority of I_1 or I_2 or some I_3 for P in S*.

> **Clinical comparability**: S and S* are clinically comparable with respect to an intervention I for a problem P just in case both (1) for the set of identifiable conditions C* that are judged to be necessary for realizing the effectiveness of I as a treatment for P in S*, a functionally equivalent counterpart C can be practically attained in S and (2) the functional equivalency of C in S can be practically sustained over time.

This formulation of equipoise is much more explicit about possible sources from which credible doubts about the effectiveness of an intervention may arise. For example, they may exist because its net therapeutic advantage over a placebo has yet to be demonstrated or effectively measured. Additionally, however, even if an intervention I is known to be an effective treatment for P in one treatment setting (S*), the reliability of our judgments about its likely net therapeutic advantage over alternatives in another treatment setting (S) depends crucially on whether the conditions under which I is known to be effective in the first setting (S*) can be replicated in the second (S). This is true regardless of whether S* is the context of treatment in the US and S is the context of treatment in a developing world population or S* is the context of treatment established in clinical trials of I (in the US, say) and S is the context of treatment in which I will be used in clinical practice (in the US or elsewhere). As the degree of clinical comparability that can be achieved between these contexts of treatment increases or decreases, so does the reliability of our judgments about the likely net therapeutic advantage of I in the new treatment setting.

Even within developed nations, clinicians may have difficulty achieving in clinical practice results that can be attained within the context of well run clinical trials. In fact, this is a general problem that experimental research of any kind must grapple with: ensuring that the conditions under which something is known to be effective can be replicated in its use outside of that context. This is an especially important point for international research, however, where a wide variety of differences between treatment contexts can affect the calculation of an intervention's net therapeutic advantage.

Differences between treatment settings are only counted as relevant to the extent that they may foreseeably influence the measure of an intervention's net therapeutic advantage. Nevertheless, the likely net therapeutic advantage of an intervention may vary significantly across treatment settings. Some of the reasons for these variations are rooted to different degrees in economic differences between developed and developing nations. It would be a mistake, however, to construe all economic issues in this context as questions of a people's ability to purchase expensive interventions.[18] In addition to the costs of procurement, the economic profile of health care interventions includes the level of infrastructure required for their implementation including requirements relating to technology, availability of facilities and staff of a certain quality in appropriate quantities. The fact that an intervention requires intensive staff supervision, or a particularly high degree of skill to implement, may be a substantial problem for populations in which relatively few medical personnel must strive to meet the needs of comparatively large numbers of people. Furthermore, the economic profile of an intervention also includes the burdens that patients incur from possible opportunity costs related to the treatment. The fact that one population of people is nomadic and highly migratory while

---

[18] For instance in, U. Schüklenk, R. Ashcroft. International research ethics. *Bioethics* 2000; 14: 158–172 at 167. It is pointed out that in many cases, what we can achieve in a particular population may hinge on the kind of reductions we can carve out of the pricing structures of extremely profitable international pharmaceutical companies. The equation of availability and affordability is then put into the mouth of a possible consequentialist position at 168.

another is highly immobile and agrarian may not bear on the question of equipoise if the intervention in question has a benign side effect profile and can be made sufficiently portable. But it may be relevant if the intervention in question requires prolonged hospitalization, frequent and lengthy treatment visits, or has a side effect profile that would prevent travel for long periods of time.

For these reasons, even treatments with relatively low procurement costs may have significantly different economic profiles and the net therapeutic advantage of such interventions may vary widely relative to different contexts of treatment. This means that in some cases, to make an intervention 'available' in a community will not (only) require lowering its procurement cost, but increasing or otherwise modifying the surrounding infrastructure so that it can support its effective implementation.

Although some of the relevant differences between contexts of treatment will have an important economic aspect to them, this need not always be the case. Differences in the convenience of long term treatments may affect their relative net therapeutic advantage, especially if they generate significant differences in compliance. Such factors can also be magnified by differences in social or cultural norms. In agrarian populations where people must work away from their homes and the careful measurement of time is not as important as in urban or developed world settings, potent but complicated drug regimens that must be taken on a strict schedule throughout the day may be less attractive than less potent, single dose options. Or again, even within the developed world, certain identifiable groups may maintain deeply held religious convictions that prevent them from accepting certain forms of medical intervention. The net therapeutic advantage of artificial blood products relative to transfusion may differ significantly between the general American population, say, and the population of Jehovah's Witnesses. This is due not to some unique physiological constitution of the Witnesses but to their beliefs about the religious significance of blood products. These beliefs are clinically relevant to the extent that they dispose Witnesses to reject blood transfusions and to accept artificial alternatives. This may be an exceptional case, but it illustrates another possible way in which a population's beliefs or cultural norms may themselves be relevant to the question of equipoise.

With these points in mind, it is particularly important to emphasize that the central issue for the broad interpretation is not the degree of clinical comparability that *already exists* between two treatment settings, but the degree of clinical comparability *that is practically attainable and sustainable*. This is because the latter question links up directly with the epistemological aspect of the duty of personal care. Regardless of whether I is currently available in a population, if we know that the clinical context in which I can be effectively implemented in a population *is practically attainable* then it would violate the duty of personal care to conduct a clinical trial in which an alternative to I is tested against a placebo there.[19] To do so would be to knowingly give unequal consideration to the equal interests of the participants in such a trial. It would violate the same duty of care to conduct a clinical trial of any alternative to I in a population unless there are credible doubts about the net therapeutic superiority of I to such an alternative in a treatment setting that is practically attainable in the population in question.

This point is of particular importance because it provides a safeguard against exploiting the mere fact that some population does not currently have access to needed health care interventions. Economically disadvantaged, socially isolated or oppressed groups may lack access to a host of inexpensive, easily administered interventions for a variety of health care conditions precisely because they are disadvantaged, isolated, or oppressed.[20] By focusing on the

---

[19] It is an innovation of the present paper that it links this emphasis on practical attainability with the epistemological requirements of equipoise. Recently, some researchers have begun to adopt the language of the 'highest practically attainable' standard of care in the context of international research. For instance, one recent consensus statement repeatedly emphasizes that in the developing world participants in clinical trials, 'should be assured the highest standard of care practically attainable in the country in which the trial is being carried out' (Science, ethics, and the future of research into maternal infant transmission of HIV-1. *The Lancet* 1999; 353: 832–835 at 833.) A few lines later, however, the same statement argues that:

> Where there is no antiretroviral therapy currently available in the host country, and no reasonable expectation of its availability during the time frame of the planned trial, it is imperative to test and identify rapidly a regimen that is more effective than no anti-HIV-1 intervention and more affordable and implementable than the proven ZDV regimens. A no intervention controlled design may be ethically justified in host countries where there is no antiretroviral therapy currently available and no reasonable expectation of its availability during the time frame of the planned trial (p. 834).

This suggestion seems to violate the epistemological aspect of the duty of personal care. I would also suggest that this position can only be seen as a viable alternative if the notion of a 'standard of care' is separated from the requirements of equipoise. For problems with this general move, see London.

[20] See important examples in George J. Annas, Michael A. Grodin. Human Rights and Maternal-Fetal HIV Transmission Prevention Trials in Africa. *American Journal of Public Health* 1998; 88: 560–563.

degree of clinical comparability that can be practically achieved between two clinical contexts, we provide a greater degree of protection than if we require only that the level of care provided to members of the control group not fall below the level of care that they would otherwise receive within their community.[21] The latter standard licenses clinical research in any situation where social or economic deprivation results in lack of access to basic medical care. The former standard only licenses clinical research when the circumstances of a particular population are such that a reasonable effort would not be able to achieve the relevant degree of clinical comparability between their clinical situation with respect to a particular intervention, and the context in which that intervention has proven to be effective.[22] Since it is likely that this degree of clinical comparability already exists, or can easily be achieved, in most developing world populations with respect to basic health care interventions, this standard will only license clinical research in cases that are 'unique' in some identifiable, clinically relevant way.

Whether it appears this way on the surface or not, both conceptions of equipoise outlined in this paper are committed to certain views of the role of economic considerations in formulating the equipoise requirement. By focusing on biological equivalence the narrow interpretation frames the question of equipoise in a way that most closely resembles clinical contexts in which sufficient economic resources are available to overcome the myriad obstacles that may hinder the effective implementation of an intervention. Wealthy nations with robust health care infrastructures and socio-political mechanisms that attempt to provide fair access to well established health care systems can *act as if* economic considerations are transparent to the question of equipoise because it is only in fairly exceptional circumstances that such nations would be unable to maintain the appropriate clinical context to support an intervention. This does not explain, however, why nations with significantly less developed health care infrastructures, whose health care systems must operate within much tighter resource constraints, should be required to act as if this is the case for them as well.

By requiring that clinical comparability be practically sustainable over time, this standard also provides a check against a second kind of exploitation, namely, the use of developing world populations

---

[21] For criticism of this standard, see London.

[22] I will return to the question of what constitutes a 'reasonable effort' at the end of the paper.

solely for the purpose of gaining knowledge to be used for the benefit of citizens of the developed world. As a result, it provides a greater degree of protection than the narrow interpretation defended by commentators such as Angell. For example, as some critics have recently pointed out, by insisting that the short-course of AZT be compared against the 076 protocol, Angell is in effect insisting that the alternative intervention be compared against a baseline clinical context that is widely available in the developed world and that, if it is practically attainable at all, is nevertheless practically unsustainable in the developing world.[23] The results of such a trial would be more immediately relevant to the clinical context of populations in the US and Europe rather than Africa and South East Asia so that even if it is not conducted with the intent of using developing world populations to answer questions that are most relevant to developed world populations, it may nevertheless have this effect.

This last problem with the narrow interpretation simply reiterates in a more concrete fashion the dilemma that I posed earlier. While physiological equivalence may seem on its face like an elegantly simple and clear interpretation of equipoise, it provides no moral guidance on how to conduct the very research that would be most relevant to populations of the developing world.

By focusing on clinical comparability, rather than biological equivalence, the broader conception of equipoise requires trials to address questions that are specific to the needs of the target population. It does so, however, precisely because it recognizes that the health care needs of developing world populations are intimately bound up with a network of complex social and economic issues. Furthermore, by factoring those issues into the question of equipoise it ensures that they are not neatly swept under the moral rug. By having to articulate the limits to what can be done to improve the baseline situation of a particular people with respect to some proposed intervention, we are forced to confront difficult issues in a way that is public, and makes clear the decisions for which we are accountable. These decisions may not be popular, but public controversy and earnest deliberations are surely preferable to a procedure that also confronts these issues, but in a way that leaves their role unarticulated and hidden from public scrutiny.

[23] R.J. Levine. The Need to Revise the Declaration of Helsinki. *NEJM* 1999; 341: 531–534 at 533.

The broad interpretation of equipoise thus has a number of important features to recommend it. Focusing on the specific needs of a particular population increases the likelihood of producing actual benefits for that population and decreases the likelihood that research will be conducted in developing world populations solely for the benefit of populations of the developed world. At the same time, however, because it focuses on the degree of clinical comparability that can be achieved between the relevant treatment contexts, it ensures that research targets only problems that cannot be addressed by means that could reasonably be implemented within that population. As a result, it licenses only research that targets those needs of a population that would remain after a reasonable effort has been made to improve clinically relevant aspects of their baseline situation. Finally, by requiring that clinical comparability can be practically sustained over time, this standard ensures that research is designed to address these problems in ways that the nations in question – perhaps with the continued support of third party funding, negotiated discounts on expensive equipment and supplies, or some combination of these – can reasonably be expected to maintain and continue to implement once the research in question has been completed. This will ensure that clinical research is designed in a way that it can be reasonably expected to make a lasting contribution to the medical needs of the populations in which the trial is carried out.

These considerations should make it clear that the broad interpretation of equipoise – unlike its alternative – is not a double standard for clinical research. It is, rather, the same standard applied the same way to substantively different clinical contexts in order to set the same ethical limits on a single end: finding health care interventions that can be implemented within conditions that are practically attainable in a treatment population. As a result, it offers an important middle way between two equally unacceptable alternatives. On the one hand, the fact that economically and technologically developed nations can achieve a very high level of care for the overwhelming majority of their populations should not in itself preclude developing nations from undertaking the very programs of research that would facilitate their ability to better meet the health care needs of their own populations. On the other hand, the absence of effective health care interventions within developing world populations should not by itself justify using those populations as subjects of clinical research. The broad interpretation of equipoise alone articulates terms for navigating these extremes in a way that is both scientifically sound and ethically responsible.

DIRECTIONS FOR FURTHER INQUIRY

The arguments of the previous section have been directed at two ends. First, they have outlined significant deficiencies in the narrow conception of equipoise. Second, they have described a broader conception of equipoise that avoids these difficulties and holds out the promise of reconciling the need to find interventions that can be employed in developing world contexts with the requirements of substantive moral constraints that must set ethical boundaries on such research. If the debate over international research standards is to go forward in a way that is coherent and fruitful, much more careful and concerted attention will have to be paid to the details of the broader conception of equipoise outlined here.

In particular, a number of important issues require more detailed treatment than I have been able to provide here. Some are practical and involve our ability to implement this standard in a way that is coherent and principled. For instance, what are the standards that should be used to determine when some set of conditions is practically achievable in a treatment population and when they are not? At what point in the lobbying industry, international organizations, and governments can researchers or their sponsors claim to have made a sufficient effort to bring about possible improvements in the baseline situation of a population such that they may then initiate clinical research? Furthermore, what kind of assurances are necessary to establish the 'reasonable likelihood' that the benefits of international research will be implemented effectively over time in the host population, before that research may proceed? The debate over some of these issues has already begun and against the background of the present discussion their resolution takes on increased importance.

Prior to these more pragmatic issues, however, the broader conception of equipoise requires additional conceptual and technical clarification. In particular, as the number of variables relevant to the effective deployment of an intervention increases, so does the difficulty in reliably projecting our knowledge of the relevant causal relationships from a developed world context, into a developing world context. Overestimating these difficulties, or adopting an overly fastidious standard of proof, would inappropriately expand the boundaries of permissible international research. Underestimating them, however, or adopting an overly permissive epistemic stance, would restrict the boundaries of ethically acceptable research and perhaps result in the deployment of interventions that, although effective in developed world settings, do not actually improve the condition of those who receive them in the developing world. As a result, it is particularly important to find an epistemic standard that strikes an appropriate balance between these two possibilities.

Finally, although I cannot justify this assertion here, a possible implication of this conception of equipoise is that morally acceptable international research cannot take place in a vacuum. That is, to pass the equipoise requirement international research initiatives will have to be coordinated with, or at least responsive to, a nation's larger public health initiatives and political needs. This is an aspect of the broad interpretation that needs to be explored in much greater detail, in part, because it may provide a natural bridge between requirements for the ethical design of international clinical trials, and larger political issues relating to the value of international research as a non-paternalist means of assisting developing nations.[24]

[24] Acknowledgment: I would like to thank Tracy E. London and Richard Schemes for their very helpful comments on this manuscript.

Chapter 17

DEVELOPING DRUGS FOR THE DEVELOPING WORLD: AN ECONOMIC, LEGAL, MORAL, AND POLITICAL DILEMMA

DAVID B. RESNIK

INTRODUCTION: THE PHARMACEUTICAL INDUSTRY AND ACCESS TO MEDICATIONS

Providing people with affordable prescription drugs is probably the important health care issue for the developing world as we begin the 21st century.[1] In the last few years, the media has raised public awareness of the developing world's need for medications to treat or prevent HIV/AIDS. The numbers in Africa speak for themselves: of the 36 million people worldwide infected with HIV, 67% live in sub-Saharan Africa and 95% live in developing nations. Most of the infected people who live in these countries have no access to new or existing drugs for HIV/AIDS. But the problem of access to medications goes far beyond the HIV/AIDS pandemic: people in developing nations also cannot afford medications used to treat or prevent malaria, tuberculosis, cholera, dysentery, meningitis, and typhoid fever. The affordability problem also extends beyond a lack of access to new drugs designed to treat devastating, infectious diseases: 50% of people in developing nations do not have access to even basic medications, such as antibiotics, analgesics, bronchodilators, decongestants, anti-inflammatory agents, anti-coagulants, or diuretics.[2]

The high cost of HIV/AIDS medications has helped to focus attention on the lack of access to drugs in developing nations. For example, fluconazole, a drug produced by Pfizer, Inc., which is used to treat AIDS complications, costs $18 per pill. An AIDS patient that needs this medication would have to spend over $500 a month for fluconazole, which exceeds the per capita income of most people

---

[1] S. Benatar. Avoiding Exploitation in Clinical Research. *Cambridge Quarterly of Healthcare Ethics* 2000; 9: 562–565.

[2] M. Reich. The Global Drug Gap. *Science* 2000; 287: 1979–1981.

in Kenya.[3] Nevirapine, a drug used to prevent perinatal HIV transmission, costs $874 for 100 units in Kenya.[4] The high cost of zidovudine (AZT) has played a large role in making it difficult to prevent the perinatal transmission of HIV.[5] Since the governments of developing nations have very low health care budgets, often less than $10 per person per year, many people who need these HIV medications must pay for them out-of-pocket. This means that only the very wealthy citizens in developing nations can afford most of these expensive HIV medications; most people receive no medication for HIV at all.

Many people blame the pharmaceutical companies for the problem of access to medications: medicines are unaffordable because drug companies are only concerned about maximizing profits and they have no sense of social responsibility. Companies charge outrageously high prices for their products and gouge consumers whenever they can. According to some critics, drug prices result from greed with no concern for fairness of equity.[6,7] It is no secret that the pharmaceutical industry is one of the most profitable businesses in the world. In 1999, the top ten pharmaceutical companies had an average profit margin of 30%, and the pharmaceutical industry averaged an 18.6% return on revenues.[8] (As an aside, a 10% profit margin is considered to be excellent in most industries. Many industries, such food service or textiles, operate at profit margins that are 5% or lower). In the United States (US), prices of prescription drugs have risen at a rate far greater than the inflation rate: the average cost of filling a drug prescription rose from $34 in 1990 to

---

[3] D. McNeil. As Devastating Epidemics Increase, Nations Take on Drug Companies. *New York Times.* 9 July 2000: A1.

[4] D. McNeil. Prices for Medicine are Exorbitant in Africa, Study Says. *New York Times.* 17 June 2000: A1.

[5] D. Resnik. The Ethics of HIV Research in Developing Nations. *Bioethics* 1999; 12, 4: 287–306. The cost of AZT for the 076 protocol used to prevent perinatal transmission of HIV is $800, which far exceeds the per capita income of most developing nations. To develop a less expensive treatment, researchers tested a regimen that uses less than 10% of the AZT used in the 076 protocol. Many people objected to this study because it used placebo control groups even though the 076 protocol was recognized as effective in preventing the perinatal transmission of HIV.

[6] A. Chetley. 1990. *A Healthy Business? World Health and the Pharmaceutical Industry.* London. Zed Books.

[7] M. Angell. The Pharmaceutical Industry – To Whom is It Accountable?. *New England Journal of Medicine* 2000; 342: 1902–1904.

[8] J. Gerth & S. Stolberg. 'Drug Firms Reap Profits on Tax-Backed Research. *New York Times.* 23 April 2000: A1, A20–21.

$61.33 in 1999. Pharmaceutical sales in the US rose from $59 billion in 1990 to $91.8 billion in 1999.[9]

On the other hand pharmaceutical companies also spend over $6 billion per year on clinical trials, and they sponsor 70% of the clinical trials conducted in the US.[10] According to industry estimates, pharmaceutical companies spent $26.4 billion on research and development (R&D) in the US in the year 2000, or more than 60% of total biomedical R&D funding. According to industry estimates, pharmaceutical companies spent $14 billion on marketing in 2000.[11] The percentage of biomedical R&D funded by the industry has risen dramatically in the last two decades.[12] Although many writers have pointed out that companies spend too much money on marketing and not enough on R&D, there is no denying the fact that the world now depends heavily on drug companies to fund biomedical research. While many people regard the drug companies as villains, the plain truth is that a great deal of research would simply not be done without money from this industry.

Thus, the pharmaceutical industry is a highly visible and obvious target for anger and criticism as well as hope or even praise. Many governments in developing nations have taken or are considering taking steps to combat the industry. Some governments, such as India, Bangladesh, Thailand, and Brazil do not honor pharmaceutical product patents. India honors patents on manufacturing processes but not patents on products, which allows generic drug companies to reverse engineer and manufacture drugs without paying royalties to the companies who own patents on those drugs.[13] As a result, the price of drugs is much cheaper in these countries. For example, the wholesale price of fluconazole is $6.38 per pill in South Africa, $8.52 in Kenya, $9.78 in the US, but $0.41 per pill in Bangladesh. Madawa Pharmaceuticals manufactures the drug in Bangladesh and pays no royalties to Pfizer.[14] According to

[9] Ibid.
[10] T. Bodenheimer. Uneasy Alliance: Clinical Investigators and the Pharmaceutical Industry. *The New England Journal of Medicine* 2000; 342: 1539–1544.
[11] Pharmaceutical Research and Manufacturing Association (PHRMA). 2000. The Pharmaceutical Industry's R&D Investment. Washington, DC. PHRMA.
[12] A. Jaffe. Trends and Patterns in Research and Development Expenses in the United States. *Proceedings of the National Academy of Sciences* 1996; 93: 12658–12663.
[13] McNeil, note 3.
[14] D. McNeil. Selling Cheap Generic Drugs, India's Copycats Irk Industry. *New York Times*. 1 December 2000: F1.

pharmaceutical industry estimates, the industry loses about $100 million per year in India. Most of the large companies have abandoned efforts to obtain or enforce patents in India.[15]

Other tactics for making drugs more affordable include importation of 'generic' drugs and compulsory licensing. A country might honor pharmaceutical patents but allow drug distributors to import drugs from countries that do not honor those patents, thereby insuring a lower price. For example, Kenya's parliament debated a law that would allow the health minister to declare a public health crisis and void drug patents or allow importation of cheaper, 'generic' drugs.[16] Compulsory licensing is a strategy a country might use to force a drug company to license another company to manufacture a drug. Although the company would still have to pay royalties to the company that owns the patent, it could offer the drug at a cheaper price. A global trade treaty signed in 1994 allows countries to use compulsory licensing to deal with a public health crisis. South Africa has considered compulsory licensing as a way of making drugs more affordable for its citizens.[17]

Although each of these potential responses to the problem of making drugs more affordable for people in the developing world have some merit, they can establish an atmosphere that is combative rather than cooperative. As one might expect, pharmaceutical companies have objected to some of these tactics on the grounds that they violate intellectual property rights.[18] If developing nations do not honor pharmaceutical patents, companies may decide that it is not worth the trouble of developing drugs for the developing world. Indeed, it has only been recently that pharmaceutical companies have considered taking major steps to expand their markets into developing nations. From the pharmaceutical industry's perspective, developing drugs for the developing world is not a lucrative business proposition, since these nations lack buying-power. Why bother with developing drugs for the third world if those countries that need those medications cannot afford them? Why do business with a country that refuses to honor your drug patents? It would be more profitable to develop a drug designed to enhance sexual performance for Anglo-American males than to develop a medicine

---

[15] Ibid.
[16] McNeil, note 3.
[17] Ibid.
[18] Ibid.

designed to treat or prevent malaria. There is more money to be made in developing a slightly improved lipid-lowering drug than in developing a vaccine for dysentery. One startling piece of data speaks of itself: 90% of the money spent of health R&D focuses on medical conditions responsible for only 10% of the world's burden of disease.[19]

Should developing nations just ignore the pharmaceutical companies and develop their own drugs? This is probably not a realistic option, since most of these nations lack sufficient funds to invest in pharmaceutical R&D. According to pharmaceutical industry estimates, it costs on average of $500 million to develop and test a single drug that will be sold in the US.[20] Since it often takes several different drugs to treat or prevent an infectious disease, it could cost well over a billion dollars to develop drugs to treat one disease. Developing nations are too poor to pay this price. For better or worse, the people of developing nations need help from the pharmaceutical industry. If Pfizer, Merck, Glaxo-Wellcome, and other pharmaceutical companies do not develop drugs to combat the infectious diseases that plague developing nations, then who will? There is a real danger that people in developing nations will become 'therapeutic orphans' if the pharmaceutical companies lack the proper incentives to develop drugs for the developing world.[21]

Thus, developing drugs for the developing world is an economic, legal, political, and moral dilemma for both pharmaceutical companies and for the governments of developing nations. Pharmaceutical companies must decide 1) whether and how to invest R&D money for medications designed to treat disease epidemics that plague the developing world, and 2) how to address the problems of affordability and accessibility of medications for the developing world. Developing nations, on the other hand, must decide how best to respond to pharmaceutical companies and whether to use any of the tactics described above. I cannot hope to solve all these problems, as they involve many different political, cultural, legal, medical, and economic factors and conditions that are beyond the scope of a short essay. However, I will offer an analysis of these dilemmas that may provide some insights for industry leaders and policymakers. I will argue that large, global pharmaceutical companies have

---

[19] Benatar, note 1.
[20] Angell, note 6.
[21] Reich, note 2.

a moral obligation to develop affordable drugs for the developing world and to make these drugs accessible, and that developing nations should cooperate with these companies in achieving these goals. Pharmaceutical companies and developing nations should negotiate agreements where these countries promise strong patent protection and a productive business environment in exchange for a commitment to develop medicines that are affordable and accessible.

THE PHARMACEUTICAL INDUSTRY AND SOCIAL RESPONSIBILITY

Let us begin our analysis by considering the pharmaceutical industry's obligations to developing nations. One popular conception of private businesses is that they are either immoral or amoral, operating outside the bounds of morality and barely within scope of the law.[22] Without a doubt, many business practices have contributed to this attitude, such as the use of sweatshops in the textile industry, the production of vehicles that are known to be unsafe in the automotive industry, or the use of exploitative marketing in the tobacco industry. During the 20th century, many business professors and economists provided a theoretical basis for this idea by arguing that companies have one primary obligation, to make profit. By pursuing profit, companies manage their resources effectively and produce goods and services that benefit society. Laws can be useful in regulating corporate conduct, but corporations have no moral obligations over and above the requirement to comply with the law.[23] I suspect that many people regard pharmaceutical companies in the same light: pharmaceutical companies are pariahs.

Although it is undoubtedly the case that many companies frequently ignore or violate moral standards, many scholars hold that businesses do have moral responsibilities. All businesses are shaped by and depend upon social values, such as honesty, integrity, fidelity, diligence, and fairness. These values provide a social infrastructure for contractual arrangements, employer-employee relations, marketing, investing, trading, and so on. Values play a key role in

---

[22] R. DeGeorge. 1995. *Business Ethics*, 4th ed. Englewood Cliffs, NJ. Prentice-Hall.

[23] M. Friedman. The Social Responsibility of Business is to Increase its Profits. *New York Times Magazine.* 13 September 1970: 1.

creating a climate within and among companies for conducting business. Without these values in place, corruption, theft, fraud, disloyalty, and other ethical problems would make it impossible to do business. Thus, most businesses today recognize the importance of ethical conduct in business and many adopt and enforce codes of conduct.[24]

Many people would accept the idea that moral values play an important role within business, but they might argue that they play no role in the interaction between businesses and society at large. A business could adopt and enforce a code of ethics that applies to its dealings with employees, customers, stockholders, and associates yet show absolutely no respect for other social values not directly related to business. Although it is also probably the case that many businesses ignore these other values, many writers argue that businesses have social responsibilities. Businesses have these responsibilities because they exist within societies where people care about the environment, public safety, public health, and other goods. There are at least two reasons why businesses have social responsibilities. First, businesses that ignore their social responsibilities may face the public's wrath. A company that wantonly pollutes, for example, will one day have to deal with additional pollution regulations. Companies that make unsafe products may have to deal with expensive lawsuits or consumer boycotts. Thus, social responsibility makes good business sense.[25]

Second, corporations are like moral agents in that they make decisions that have important effects on human beings. In making these decisions, corporations can decide to either accept or ignore social values, such as respect for the environment, public safety, and so on. Although corporate decision-making differs from individual decision-making in many ways, e.g. corporations do not have a conscious mind that deliberates about decisions, corporations can still be held legally and morally responsible for their decisions and actions. If corporations are like moral agents, then they have some of the same duties that apply to other moral agents. In particular, corporations have obligations to avoid causing harm and to promote social welfare and justice. That is, they have social responsibilities.[26]

---

[24] P. Murphy. 1998. *Eighty Exemplary Ethics Statements.* Notre Dame, Indiana. University of Notre Dame Press.
[25] DeGeorge, note 22.
[26] Ibid.

Since pharmaceutical companies are corporations, they also have social responsibilities. Consider two kinds of duties that apply to pharmaceutical companies:

1. *Beneficence.* Pharmaceutical companies should promote the greatest balance of benefits harms for society. They should avoid doing harm and try to do good.
2. *Justice.* Pharmaceutical companies should distribute benefits and burdens equitably.

The rationale for a duty of beneficence is fairly straightforward and uncontroversial. Indeed, most countries have a variety of laws designed to regulate drug testing, manufacturing, and sales in order to prevent harms to the public and promote the development of effective drugs. In the US, the Food and Drug Administration (FDA) regulates drug testing, manufacturing, and sales.[27] Although this duty is fairly obvious, its application is usually complex and controversial, as societies must weigh benefits, harms as well as justice and basic liberties in deciding questions about approving the sale of new drugs. For example, many medications that offer some chance of a cure for patients with advanced cancer or HIV also involve many harmful side effects and one must balance benefits and harms in deciding whether to make the medications available to patients.[28]

The rationale for the duty of justice is not as obvious or straightforward, but there is a growing recognition that pharmaceutical companies should promote access to medications. For example, Brody has argued that pharmaceutical prices should not be so high that they make important medications inaccessible.[29] Spinello applies egalitarian principles to pharmaceutical pricing and argues that medication prices should promote social justice.[30] However, both authors acknowledge that the duty of justice must be balanced against the practical need to make a reasonable return on investment. A 'reasonable price' is therefore a price that allows the

---

[27] B. Brody. 1995. *Ethical Issues in Drug Testing, Approval, and Pricing.* New York. Oxford University Press.
[28] U. Schüklenk. 1998. *Access to Experimental Drugs in Terminal Illness.* New York. Pharmaceutical Products Press.
[29] B. Brody. Public Good and Fair Prices: Balancing Technological Innovation with Social Well Being. *Hastings Center Report* 1996; 26, 2: 5–11.
[30] R. Spinello. Ethics, Pricing, and the Pharmaceutical Industry. *Journal of Business Ethics* 1992; 11: 617–626.

company to earn its money but also promotes accessibility and equity.[31]

Other writers have argued that companies should distribute the benefits and burdens of research participation equitably. For example, if a company sponsors a study using a specific population, then members of the population that participate in the study should derive some benefits from their participation. In particular, the drug should be made available to members of the population at a reasonable price. It is not fair to place members of the population at risk without a reasonable expectation of a benefit. Research protocols that recruit subjects from a population without a reasonable expectation of some benefit to that population are exploitative.[32]

How do the above considerations apply to developing drugs for the developing world? In general, these considerations imply that pharmaceutical companies have moral responsibilities to develop drugs that benefit society and to make those drugs available to participant populations at a reasonable price. These responsibilities apply to new, existing, and prospective drugs. Some pharmaceutical companies, such as Bayer Corporation, have adopted ethics and values statements that mention responsibilities to the community, customers, and the environment. Ciba-Geigy, a chemical company that merged with Sandoz (a pharmaceutical company) in 1997, adopted a vision and values statement that includes responsibilities to the environment and society.[33] However, merely recognizing that pharmaceutical companies should be socially responsible provides little guidance in determining how companies should exercise that responsibility. It does not provide specific guidance as to what a company should do, how much is should do, how many resources it should devote to a project, or even where it should focus its attention.

To get some insight into these questions consider how an individual might decide how to act socially responsible. Most major

[31] Brody, note 29; Spinello, note 30.

[32] This issue of exploitation has come up many times in research involving the developing world. One of the criticisms of the HW trials (mentioned in note 4) is that these studies would not make the new treatment reasonably available to the population. See Crouch, R. and Arras, J. AZT Trials and Tribulations. *Hastings Center Report* 1998; 28, 6: 26–34. Some writers have argued that the Human Genome Diversity Project will not offer participant populations a reasonable benefit. See Resnik, D. The Human Genome Diversity Project: Ethical Problems and Solutions. *Politics and the Life Sciences* 1999; 18, 1: 15–24. See also Benatar, note 1.

[33] Murphy, note 24.

moral theories, including Kantianism, utilitarianism, and virtue ethics, hold that individuals have duties relating to beneficence and justice. However, there is also strong theoretical support that for the idea many moral duties, including the duty of beneficence, are not absolute: there are morally acceptable and desirable limits on the amount of good one may do for others. Although we should all do our part for society, we are not required to be moral saints. The conduct exemplified by Mother Theresa deserves great praise, but it is above and beyond the call of duty. Since most individuals cannot completely sacrifice themselves for the good of society, they must weigh and consider other moral obligations and commitments in light of their circumstances and conditions in order to decide how to be socially responsible. To use Kantian terminology, social responsibilities, such as the duty of beneficence, are 'imperfect duties.'[34]

For example, consider a person, let's call her Joan, who struggles with meeting her social responsibilities. She gives money to charity, provided that it fits within her budget. She will do volunteer work, provided that she has the time, talent and interests. She decides to work for Habitat for Humanity, an organization that builds houses for economically disadvantaged people, because she is good at carpentry and likes working with her hands. However, Joan decides that she can only work one weekend a month, due to her other commitments to family and work: she works during the week and takes her children to soccer games on other weekends. One of her friends asks her to work for the Red Cross during a blood drive during a Wednesday evening, so she decides to help out because she can fit it in her schedule. Several charities call her on the phone asking for money, but she refuses their request since she has already

---

[34] See L. Pojman. 1995. *Ethics.* Belmont, CA. Wadsworth. Although most people would agree that beneficence is an imperfect duty, I would also maintain that justice is an imperfect duty if we understand the duty as including a duty to follow specific material principles of justice, such as the obligation to distribute benefits and burdens equitably. First, it is impossible for a person to follow these principles perfectly. As any parent can testify, it is impossible to distribute benefits and burdens to different children in a perfectly equitable fashion, no matter how hard one tries. Second, these principles must be weighed against one another and against other values or commitments. For example, when faced with a scarce resource in health care, such as a shortage of influenza vaccinations, it is morally acceptable to emphasize utility while de-emphasizing equity. If there is a shortage of influenza vaccines, then public health officials are justified in offering these vaccines to the patients who need them the most. For further discussion, see Beachamp, T. and Childress, J. 1996. *Principles of Biomedical Ethics*, 4th edition. New York. Oxford University Press.

given all that she has budgeted for charity. A panhandler asks her for money but she decides not to give him any because she believes he will spend it on booze. However, she does give money to UNICEF when some children from her church come by to collect money for this organization. Is Joan callous or irresponsible? I would say not: Joan is probably a lot like other people who must decide how to meet social responsibilities. She must weigh and consider many different factors when deciding how to act responsibly.

I think the same points apply to social responsibility considered at a corporate level. Companies, like individuals, have obligations to be socially responsible, but these obligations are not absolute. Companies should not act like moral scoundrels, but they do not need to act like moral saints. To meet their social responsibilities, corporations must weigh and consider many factors, such as their talents, abilities, resources, interests, commitments, and obligations. As far as pharmaceutical companies are concerned, the goals of developing medications for populations and promoting access to those medications would seem to be a natural fit, given their interests, talents, and so on. But this still leaves open the question of how far a company should go in meeting this responsibility. Corporations, like Joan, must consider their resources, such as time and money, as well as other obligations and commitments, when deciding how to act responsibly. Most pharmaceutical companies will have little trouble fulfilling some minimal responsibilities if they develop drugs that benefit people and make those drugs accessible. But the harder question to answer is *how far* companies should go in exercising this responsibility. Companies also have commitments to their stockholders and employees. They have obligations to make a profit and to use their economic resources effectively. For example, Bayer's values statement also mentions duties to capital investment and resource allocation. Ciba-Geigy's statement mentions commitments to financial performance and improved market shares.[35] If one agrees that profit (and other financial factors) should play a key role in business decisions, then it is morally legitimate (and perhaps even morally responsible) for a company to weigh and consider these or other financial factors when making a decision to be socially responsible.[36]

[35] Murphy, note 24.
[36] DeGeorge, note 22.

Money is not the only factor in deciding how to exercise social responsibility. Companies may also consider social, economic, legal, or political conditions, since these factors may impact the effectiveness of a particular program aimed at meeting social responsibilities. These factors may provide significant barriers to implementing social responsibility. For example, a company might decide that it is not worth the effort to supply free medications to a country if that country is in such political turmoil that distribution is futile or impossible. A company might also decide that it is not worth selling a medication at a discounted price in a country if that country does not honor the company's pharmaceutical patents. On the other hand, a company might decide to initiate a research program aimed at developing a vaccine for an infectious disease, if the company obtains financial and political support from a country that would like to have such a vaccine.

Finally, companies also need to consider geography in deciding how to exercise their social responsibility. A corporation could consider all the factors we have just discussed yet conclude that it should provide free medications in the US and Europe but ignore the developing world. Would it be acceptable (or even consistent) for a pharmaceutical company to ignore the developing world while claiming to be socially responsible?

I think there are several reasons why pharmaceutical companies have social responsibilities to the developing world. First, if a company conducts business in a country, then it has duties to act responsibly in that country. This type of social responsibility can be justified in terms of reciprocity and should not be especially controversial: if you make money in a country, you have an obligation to give something back to that country over and above taxes, goods and services. But companies can avoid this responsibility by simply not doing business in developing nations. A pharmaceutical company could market its products in the developed world in order to avoid the economic, social, political, and legal challenges of conducting business in the developing world. This brings us to a second, perhaps more important reason why pharmaceutical companies have social obligations to the developing world: companies should promote the welfare of humankind. This implies duties of beneficence and justice to all people, not just to people living in the US or Europe. Obviously, it may be difficult for small, local corporations to promote the welfare of humankind, but large, global corporations, such as Merck, Glaxo-Wellcome, or Pfizer, should be concerned with the welfare of humankind and they should therefore conduct business in developing nations and attempt to meet social responsibilities to developing nations.[37] However, even global companies may decide to avoid doing business in some countries in the developing world due to adverse financial, political, legal, or other conditions: companies do not have to expand their markets to developing nations no matter what the costs. I will return to this point later.

Many pharmaceutical companies have taken important steps to act on their social responsibilities to the developing world. First, companies are now sponsoring research on diseases that affect people in the developing world, such as tuberculosis, HIV/AIDS, and malaria. Second, some companies have decided to provide free medications to people in developing nations. For example, Merck and the Gates Foundation have pledged to give $100 million worth of medicine and money to Botswana. Bristol-Myers Squibb is providing $100 million over five years to train doctors and develop community outreach programs in sub-Saharan Africa.[38] Pfizer recently agreed to donate $50 million worth of fluconazole to be distributed in South Africa, a nation where 20% of adults are infected with HIV.[39] Although these offers have been met with a degree of skepticism and cynicism, they do represent a step on the path of social responsibility.

Thus, I conclude that global pharmaceutical companies have social responsibilities to developing nations. But how far should they go to meet these obligations? How much should they do to help? These are complex issues that depend, in part, on how developing nations respond to pharmaceutical companies. If we think of exercising social responsibility as an attempt to make a gift to a society (or societies), and we understand giving as a relationship (or agreement) between the giver and recipient, then we need to say a bit more about the recipient of the gift. Exercising social responsibility in the developing world depends, in part, on social, economic, political, and legal conditions in the developing world, since these conditions can either assist or impede a company's attempt to

---

[37] J. Simpson. Ethics and Multinational Corporations vis-à-vis Developing Nations. *Journal of Business Ethics* 1982; 1, 4: 227–237.

[38] S. Steinberg. AIDS Activists Discount Big Drugmakers' Gifts. *USA Today.* 11 July 2000: 9D.

[39] R. Swains. South Africa to Distribute $50 Million in Donated AIDS Drugs. *New York Times.* 2 December 2000: D1.

exercise social responsibility in its business practices. Most companies, I believe, will resist doing business in the developing world if (1) they have no guarantee of a reasonable profit; (2) they must overcome or adapt to an unproductive (bad or adverse) business climate. But what is a reasonable profit and what is an unproductive business climate? We need to address these issues before returning to the topic of social responsibility.

REASONABLE PROFITS, DRUG PRICES, AND PATENTS

As mentioned earlier, the pharmaceutical industry is very profitable, with profit margins as high as 30% in some companies. Determining what counts as 'reasonable' profit is a complex issue in business ethics. According to some commentators, there should be no limits on profit other than the free market. If a company can make a 30% profit, then this is 'fair' in the market sense of 'fairness.' Moreover, profits are morally justifiable in that they contribute to the overall social welfare. Businesses that make profits can use those funds to compensate employees or stockholders or make investments in new equipment, buildings, or other resources.[40] Furthermore, according to this argument, attempts to control or regulate profit margins could have drastic economic consequences for businesses that would restrict their ability to contribute to society. First, investors might avoid an industry where the government regulates profits. Second, companies will have a more difficult time with financial planning and resource allocation if there are some legal limits on profits. Third, since profits depend, in part, on prices, profit regulation must involve some form of price regulation which could lead to market inefficiencies because prices need to change quickly in response to market demands but government agencies often act slowly. Fourth, if companies face limitations on profits or prices, they may cut back on their investments in R&D and focus more on marketing.

For these as well as many other reasons, government regulation of profits under normal, free market conditions is morally questionable. However, when free markets cannot set fair prices due to

[40] R. Jacobsen. Economic Efficiency and the Quality of Life. *Journal of Business Ethics* 1991; 10, 3: 201–209.

monopolies, exclusive dealing, price discrimination, or collusion, then the government may regulate or scrutinize prices in order to buffer or counteract these restrictions on trade. For example, there are good reasons to regulate the prices charged by public utilities and other corporations that have a monopoly. There may also be good reasons to investigate pricing practices when one suspects that different companies have adopted agreements designed to inflate prices.[41]

On the other hand, one might accept the thrust of this argument yet maintain that companies that make healthy profits have strong moral obligations to return more of those profits to society because they are better equipped to meet obligations of beneficence and justice. Consider the analogy with an individual. A person making a high salary, one might argue, has an obligation to give more money to charity than a person making a low salary because he can afford to give more to charity. When the hat is passed in church, the wealthy businessman should make a proportionally higher tithe than the not so wealthy teacher. There is nothing inherently wrong with being wealthy (or having a high profit margin) but greater wealth implies greater responsibility.

Now there are many ways that a profitable company could return some wealth to society. The company could offer price discounts, it could give away some of its products, it could invest funds in developing drugs to treat 'orphan' diseases, or it could invest in other social programs. Regardless of how wealthy companies choose to exercise their social responsibilities, it should be clear that their decisions affect their overall profit margins because these choices will incur additional costs or expenses. Thus, a morally reasonable profit (the profit a company should be allowed to realize) might be lower than an economically reasonable profit (the profit a company can realize). If a company decides to return some wealth to society through pricing practices, then its 'morally reasonable' prices (the prices it ought to charge) could be lower than its 'economically reasonable' prices (the prices it can charge).

How does all of this apply to the pharmaceutical industry? The argument implies that companies with high profit margins should consider taking additional steps to be socially responsible, such as discounts on prices, product giveaways, etc. If a company decides to fulfill its social responsibilities through pricing policies, then the

---

[41] O. Ferrell & J. Fraedrick. 1991. *Business Ethics.* Boston: Houghton Mifflin.

company should be willing to lower its drug prices (and therefore perhaps lower its profits) in order to make those drugs more accessible. Since it is probably not very efficient to lower the prices of all drugs in all markets, a company should probably be selective in its socially responsible pricing policies, focusing its discounts on specific drugs in specific markets. If we focus our attention on the developing world, this argument implies that global companies with high profit margins, such as Pfizer, Merck, and Glaxo-Wellcome, should be willing to forego some profits in the developing world in order to fulfill social responsibilities to the developing world. They can accomplish this task in many different ways, including price discounts or drug giveaways.

But how much money should a pharmaceutical company devote toward socially responsible projects? The answer to this question depends in part on the company's current and projected profits. By almost any standard, most large, global pharmaceutical companies are highly profitable. Global pharmaceutical companies can (and should) be able to devote hundreds of millions of dollars toward projects designed to benefit developing nations without losing a great deal of profit. However, their ability to continue realizing these profits depends on strong patent protection. Patents play a key role in profitability in the pharmaceutical industry since patents allow companies to obtain returns on their R&D investments.[42] Without this protection, companies would not make these risky investments. Pharmaceutical R&D investing is a high-risk proposition for several reasons. First, the new drug may not prove to be safe and effective and the company may decide to abandon the drug in the middle of clinical testing. Second, if the company completes its clinical trials, there is no guarantee that the FDA (or other relevant agency) will approve the new drug. Third, if the agency approves the new drug, it may not have a strong market due to competition from other drugs or lack of consumer demand. Fourth, once the drug is on the market, the agency could take it off the market to protect public health and safety. Finally, there is always the possibility that the company will face lawsuits from consumers that are harmed by the drug. Without adequate patent protection, a company might take these risks and develop its product only to have a competing company manufacture the product at a lower price.

---

[42] Pharmaceutical Research and Manufacturing Association (PhRMA). 2000. PhRMA Policy Paper: Strong Patent Protection is Essential. Washington, DC. PhRMA.

According to the pharmaceutical industry, only 30% of new drugs are profitable.[43]

Although patents offer pharmaceutical companies control over their inventions, this control is not absolute or unlimited. First, in the US (and most other countries), a patent lasts 20 years from the time of the application, which gives a drug company an approximately 10-year window to make a return on its R&D investment.[44] Once the patent expires, anyone can make the drug without infringing the patent. Second, most patent laws allow for some degree of 'copycat' inventions. A copycat invention is an invention that is very similar to a previous invention but represents a useful innovation or improvement. In the United States, companies can produce legally sanctioned generic drugs by making slight changes to the original patented drugs. (An illegal copycat would be an exact copy of the drug.) The possibility of copycat drugs creates a potential limit on a company's ability to control the market for a drug. For example, the company could invent a new blood pressure medication and dominate the market for this product until other companies develop copycat versions of the medication.[45] However, it is important to realize that the US Patent and Trade Office (PTO) does not accept all copycat drugs; it only accept those drugs that are useful improvements.

We should also note that patents only provide legal protection in the country in which they are issued: a US patent provides no legal protection in Britain. Thus, when a drug company develops a new drug, it usually applies for patent protection in the countries where it plans to sell the drug. If a country does not provide the company with patent protection, then it may lose business in that country and perhaps others. If we think of the whole world as a potential market, a company that invents a new drug and patents it in many countries may still lose a significant portion of its potential market volume if several countries do not honor the patent and export the drug around the world. This is why the pharmaceutical companies find India's patent policies so troubling: they lose the market in India as well as in other countries that import drugs from India. Drug companies can still make a profit when their patents are not

---

[43] Ibid.

[44] PTO. 2000. General Information Regarding Patents. Washington, DC. PTO.

[45] G. Stolberg & J. Gerth. Medicine Merchants: Holding Down the Competition. *New York Times.* 23 April 2000: A1.

honored around the world, but they have to make their profits in countries that honor those patents. It is hard to say exactly how much money pharmaceutical companies lose as a result of the failure to recognize patents globally. Industry representatives say they lose as much as 10% of their profits this way, and it likely that drug prices would be lower if the companies could take advantage of a larger market.[46]

So what does pharmaceutical patenting have to do with reasonable profits, prices, and social responsibility? A great deal, I think. Briefly, companies can afford to do business in a country and exercise social responsibility insofar as they have a guarantee of reasonable profits. But obtaining these profits depends, in large part, on patent laws. When companies have strong patent protection, they can expect to profit from their R&D investments, and they can afford to devote more resources to socially responsible programs. If they fail to realize profits, they have less money to devote to programs designed to enhance social welfare. Thus, developing nations that fail to honor pharmaceutical patents may actually be harming themselves in the long run. In the short run, a developing country might obtain some benefit by not honoring pharmaceutical patents because it could acquire inexpensive drugs or attract 'generic' drug companies or distributors. This strategy could backfire in the long run, however, since larger, global pharmaceutical companies may decide not to do business in countries that do not honor their patents and they may decide not to invest money in R&D to develop drugs for the developing world. Why invest several billion dollars in developing a malaria vaccine if 'generic' drug companies will reverse engineer the vaccine and sell it at a very low price? If companies lack sufficient patent protection in the developing world, many patients in the developing world will remain therapeutic orphans.

PRODUCTIVE BUSINESS ENVIRONMENT

In this section I would like to address briefly another important factor in conducting business in the developing world and exercising social responsibility, the business environment. There are many

---

[46] Reich, note 2.

different social, economic, political, and legal characteristics that contribute to a good business environment. A few of these are:[47]

(1) A coherent and effective legal system.
(2) Ethical business practices.
(3) A stable currency.
(4) A reliable banking system.
(5) Free and open markets.
(6) A well-educated public.
(7) A middle class or consumer class.
(8) A physical and social infrastructure.
(9) Democratic institutions.

These characteristics played a key role in the rise of capitalism, and they can be found, to a great degree, in the developed nations, such as the US, Germany, and Britain. Very often, developing nations lack the characteristics that define a good business environment. Moreover, it may take many years for developing nations to develop some of these characteristics, such as a well-educated public, a physical and social infrastructure, or democratic institutions. It simply takes time to build bridges, roads, power lines, and telephone networks, acquire education, develop a middle class, establish democracy; to and so on. A company that refused to do business in the developing world because its business environment is less than ideal would be acting foolishly and unfairly: in order to expand their markets and their influence, companies need to take some risks and conduct business in undeveloped nations.

On the other hand, there are some acceptable limits on what a company should be willing to do to expand into a developing nation. Some business environments can be so adverse that doing business in that country is impossible or highly inefficient. Consider the difficulties involved in selling products in a society that uses the barter system, investing funds in a society where the banks do not insure savings or checking accounts, hiring employees in a society where employee theft is common, or signing contracts in a society where bribery is expected. In order to do business in the developing world and exercise their social responsibility, companies need to have a reasonable expectation that those nations are taking steps to promote the rule of law, ethical business practices, a stable currency and banking system, free and open markets, etc. Doing business in

---

[47] P. Samuelson. 1980. *Economics.* New York. McGraw-Hill.

a country with an extremely poor business climate is going above and beyond the call of corporate duty. Developing nations can attract businesses by demonstrating that they are making progress toward developing a good business environment. (As an aside, even a developed nation can have a poor business environment. Many global companies have faced a variety of problems, such as corruption and an unreliable banking system, in trying to conduct business in Russia and other former Soviet Republics.)

CONCLUSION: RECIPROCITY

Let's retrace the steps of my argument. In the second section, I argued that large, global pharmaceutical companies have social responsibilities (or duties of beneficence and justice) to the developing world. There are a variety of ways that companies can exercise these responsibilities, including investing in R&D related to diseases that affect developing nations, offering discounts on drug prices, and initiating drug giveaways. However, I also argued that these social responsibilities are not absolute requirements and may be balanced against other obligations and commitments in light of economic, social, legal, and other conditions. In the third and fourth sections, I argued that the degree to which a company may exercise social responsibility in a society depends on two major factors, (1) the prospects for a reasonable profit and (2) the prospects for a good business environment. Developing nations can either help or hinder the pharmaceutical industry's efforts to exercise social responsibility through various policies and practices. To insure that companies can make a reasonable profit, developing nations should honor pharmaceutical patents. If they do not honor those patents, this will lower the industry's profits and take away money that could be devoted to projects designed to promote access to medications. To insure that companies have a good business environment, developing nations should try to promote the rule of law, ethical business practices, stable currencies, reliable banking systems, free and open markets, democracy, and other social, economic, legal, and political conditions conducive to business.

Overall, I hold that reciprocity and cooperation are the keys to developing drugs for the developing world. Pharmaceutical companies and developing nations need to work together in order to develop and market drugs to treat or prevent diseases that affect the developing world. Companies can do their part by investing in R&D for the developing world's diseases, offering drug discounts, or establishing drug giveaway programs. In return, they should expect developing nations to provide strong patent protection and to take steps to establish productive business environments. Developing nations should adhere to international agreements on intellectual property, such as the Trade-Related Aspects of Intellectual Property Rights (TRIPS) agreement. Nations that abide by TRIPS honor pharmaceutical product patents and do not allow importation of inventions from countries that violate TRIPS. TRIPS allows for some compulsory licensing to address public safety or public health crises. Developing nations should also take steps to promote a sound legal, ethical, financial, and social environment for business.

In pursuing this cooperative approach, developing nations may use a variety of other strategies to encourage pharmaceutical companies to act responsibility. For example, a nation could help reduce the cost of R&D and marketing by subsidizing R&D funding and by providing a company with a guaranteed market. If developing nations lower these costs to the company, the company will be able to develop a drug, sell it at a low price, and still make a reasonable profit. A developing nation could also help a drug company design research protocols and help the company with recruitment of subjects, informed consent, data monitoring, and other important aspects of humans subjects research. A nation could also help a company develop a drug giveaway program by providing an efficient, reliable, and fair system for distributing these medications. Finally, developing nations can also buy drugs in large quantities directly from pharmaceutical companies in order to take advantage of bulk buying. Nations could sell these drugs at a discounted price or give them away. Many countries have already pursued some of these strategies and there are many more constructive solutions than those mentioned in this essay.[48]

Although I believe strongly in the importance of reciprocal arrangements between pharmaceutical companies and developing nations, I also recognize that these agreements may not always work and that an atmosphere of animosity can easily develop. If a developing nation starts making concessions to the pharmaceutical

---

[48] Reich, note 2.

industry and the industry does not respond through socially responsible policies and programs, then it would be reasonable for that nation to take retaliatory measures, such as compulsory licensing or importing drugs from countries that do not honor pharmaceutical patents. On the other hand, if a pharmaceutical company offers to aid a developing nation and that nation does not respond in kind, then that company would also have reasons to not make good on its commitment to that nation. I can foresee that these situations will arise and I would not admonish either side for retaliatory conduct. However, I would still strongly urge developing nations and pharmaceutical companies to work together in addressing the urgent economic, legal, moral and political dilemma of developing drugs for the developing world.

Chapter 18

SOME QUESTIONS ABOUT THE MORAL RESPONSIBILITIES OF DRUG COMPANIES IN DEVELOPING COUNTRIES

DAN W. BROCK

David Resnik begins his paper with the claim that 'Providing people with affordable prescription drugs is probably the most important health care issue for the developing world as we begin the 21st century.'[1] I believe he is correct. He goes on to argue that drug companies have social responsibilities, including moral obligations based in beneficence and justice, to help meet this need by such practices as drug giveaways, discount pricing, and special licensing arrangements. However, this responsibility is contingent, he believes, in part on developing countries establishing a business climate in which drug companies can expect to make reasonable profits, which includes in particular respecting the product patents of drug companies.

While I am in full sympathy with Resnik's desire to increase the availability of prescription drugs in developing countries, I want to raise two concerns about his argument in the paper. The first concern is the nature of drug companies' moral obligations to develop affordable drugs for the developing world and to make these drugs accessible. The second concern is whether drug companies fulfilling this social responsibility would be at all adequate to meet the developing world's needs, and what implications this has for the responsibilities Resnik argues developing countries have to establish a profitable business climate.

First, some worries about his argument for the social responsibilities of drug companies. Resnik offers two reasons why drug companies have social responsibilities. The first is that if they ignore these responsibilities they may face the public's wrath, but this is no reason why they have any moral responsibilities in the first place;

[1] D. Resnik. Developing Drugs for the Developing World: an Economic Legal, Moral and Political Dilemma, *Developing World Bioethics* 2001; 1, 1: 11–32.

and it can only show at most that it is in their self-interest, not a moral obligation, to carry out some social responsibilities. The second reason is that corporations are like individual moral agents and as such have moral obligations of beneficence – 'to promote the greatest balance of benefits/harms for society' – and justice – 'to distribute benefits and burdens equitably.' There are two sorts of problems here that need more argument than Resnik provides. The first is that while corporations are like individual moral agents in some respects, they are unlike them in many other respects, as he himself notes. In particular, we have a variety of social institutions that are established for specific purposes and functions, which make them unlike persons and affect their responsibilities; many of course believe that corporations' responsibilities are to their shareholders and that they do not have moral responsibilities of beneficence and justice comparable to those of individuals. Resnik too quickly assumes that corporations have the moral obligations of individuals.

The second worry concerns his account of the moral obligations of beneficence and justice of individuals. Few people believe and few moral theories hold that individuals have a moral obligation to promote the greatest balance of benefits/harms for society. Individuals may have some obligation to benefit others, although even that is controversial as a moral requirement, but it is widely held that our moral obligations to benefit others in the absence of any special relations are sharply limited. Moreover, as Resnik acknowledges, these are understood to be imperfect obligations, meaning individuals have substantial discretion in deciding whom to help, opening the possibility of drug companies restricting their beneficence to the developed world. However, he argues that this duty is owed 'to all people' – it requires companies to 'promote the welfare of humankind' – and so drug companies are morally required to do business in the developing world, not to restrict their activities to the more profitable developed world, and to carry out their duties of beneficence and justice in the developed world. But even if we do have obligations of beneficence 'to all people' or to 'humankind' generally, since we cannot in fact help all, it is generally accepted that we have discretion about whom among the needy to help. More argument is needed to establish a moral obligation to do business in, and exercise social responsibilities in, the developing world.

Similar worries concern Resnik's claims about justice. It is not clear to me what it means to claim that individuals have an obligation to distribute benefits and burdens equitably. What benefits and burdens must I distribute equitably – my time, efforts, assets, etc. – and what is an equitable distribution of them? Setting these questions aside, principles of justice at the most fundamental level apply not to the actions of individuals, but rather to the design of basic social institutions. Individuals, as Rawls has argued, have obligations to help establish and to support just institutions, but it is quite another thing to claim they have moral obligations to 'distribute benefits and burdens equitably.' Meeting other basic needs such as for food and shelter is commonly taken to be, even among those who regard them as human rights, a governmental responsibility, not a special responsibility of the food or real estate industries. Securing coverage of prescription drugs for the elderly is a major political issue in the United States today, but no side in the controversy argues that it is the drug companies' social responsibility of beneficence and justice to meet the need.

To establish the social responsibility of drug companies that Resnik supports then, we need a more detailed analysis of how corporations both differ from as well as resemble individual moral agents, a more developed account of obligations of beneficence and justice of corporations that better reflects these similarities and differences, and finally an integration of these analyses of the social responsibilities of corporations into a broader account of the obligations of national and multinational institutions to establish social justice.

Set aside these worries and suppose that Resnik is correct that drug companies do have social responsibilities based in moral obligations of beneficence and justice to develop affordable drugs needed in developing countries and to make those drugs accessible. How adequate would carrying out that responsibility be in meeting the needs of the developing world for prescription drugs? This is of course extremely difficult to know with any precision. The answer depends both on an estimate of the resources that the drug companies are morally obligated to expend to meet their social responsibilities, which would of course be extremely controversial, and on an estimate of the pharmaceutical needs of citizens of developing countries and the costs of meeting them; the marginal costs of producing the additional drugs would be much less than the developed world price of those drugs. But let me just use a figure that Resnik cites to illustrate the scale of the problem. He notes that worldwide there are 36 million people infected with the HIV/AIDS virus and that 90% of them, or over 32 million, live in developing countries. Suppose that the costs of pharmaceuticals for each person infected with the virus would be $500 per year – of course in the developed world the costs are many times this, although that is on the basis of arguably inflated charges for these drugs in the developed world. That means the costs of supplying these drugs to HIV+ persons in the developing world would be over $16 billion per year, a substantial portion of the net earnings of the pharmaceutical industry in 1999. AIDS is of course only one of many diseases generating pharmaceutical needs in the developing world, although a relatively expensive one.

Resnik grants that pharmaceutical companies' principal responsibility is to earn profits for their stockholders and so I believe it is clear that no reasonable account of their social responsibility to make drugs accessible in the developing world would come anywhere near meeting the needs for pharmaceuticals there, quite apart from the pragmatic likelihood of the companies meeting that responsibility. In these circumstances is it morally wrong for countries to reject the cooperative strategy that Resnik supports, which involves respecting product patents, and instead to ignore patents in order to produce or purchase drugs necessary to save lives at a small fraction of their patent protected costs? Resnik suggests that even in terms of self interest not respecting product patents may purchase short term benefits at the cost of greater long term losses because pharmaceutical companies are unlikely to work cooperatively with countries that do so. But this prudential judgment is certainly arguable, so is there sufficient moral reason not to ignore patents if countries judge that doing so is necessary to save the lives and health of their citizens?

Certainly, some patent system is important to enabling companies to earn back the large development costs of new drugs, though as Resnik notes the current patent system has made the pharmaceutical industry the most profitable major industrial sector in the world for many years. But the vast majority of pharmaceutical industry profits are derived from the developed world in which product patents are respected, and so whether or not developing countries respect product patents will not significantly restrict research and new product development, though it will encourage continuing to focus those efforts on developed world health needs. It can quite plausibly be argued that in not respecting patents developing countries are free riding on the research and development efforts of drug companies that are supported by the prices of drugs in countries in which patents are respected. But that free riding and resulting unfairness may not be enough to make it, all things considered, morally wrong for developing countries not to respect product patents.

The enormous income inequalities between developed and poorer developing countries, which make it impossible for the latter to afford the prices of patent protected pharmaceuticals, are in my view, though there is not space to argue it here, one of the most serious injustices in the world today. If that is correct, then pharmaceuticals are unaffordable in the developing world largely because of unjust global inequalities in income and wealth. When developing countries choose not to respect product patents as their only effective means of making available pharmaceuticals necessary to save lives and protect the health of their citizens, doing so is arguably a step towards greater justice between the developed and developing world; this may be a case where two wrongs do make a right, that is where existing global injustices make not respecting product patents, which in the absence of those injustices would be wrong, all things considered, morally justified. This may have a greater impact in making pharmaceuticals accessible in the developing world than voluntary efforts from the pharmaceutical firms, and the threat of ignoring product patents may have a greater effect on the 'voluntary' efforts of pharmaceutical companies than arguments about their social responsibility.

I want to make clear that I am in full agreement with Resnik that it would be a significant step in the direction of justice for pharmaceutical companies to accept a social responsibility to do substantially more to make drugs accessible in the developing world, and I would welcome their doing so, but I believe an adequate and convincing case delineating the moral obligations of pharmaceutical companies in this regard has to be more carefully made than he has done. Nevertheless, his paper is to be welcomed in helping give these issues the attention they deserve.

Chapter 19

SOCIAL RESPONSIBILITY AND GLOBAL PHARMACEUTICAL COMPANIES

NORMAN DANIELS

David Resnik accurately describes the problem faced by developing countries in securing affordable drugs aimed at their particular disease burden.[1] I am, however, skeptical of the solution he describes, which appeals to the respective 'social responsibilities' of global pharmaceutical companies and developing countries. I am not persuaded we can derive his claims about such responsibilities in the way he does or that appealing to them solves the problems of commitment and enforcement that must be addressed in any realistic solution. I offer some reasons for that skepticism, realizing full well that my brief remarks cannot do justice to his view.

Global pharmaceutical companies, he argues, have 'social responsibilities' – presumably moral, not legal responsibilities – to the developing world. These responsibilities can be exercised by investing in research and development for diseases affecting developing countries or by offering drug discounts and drug giveaways that make necessary drugs more affordable. In return, developing countries have a 'social responsibility' to respect pharmaceutical property rights, especially those recognized in international treaties. Of course, if they have signed such treaties, their responsibilities are legal; if they have not (though Resnik is claiming they should), then these social responsibilities presumably are just moral.

Where does Resnik believe such moral responsibilities come from? Intent on showing that private businesses do not operate 'outside the bounds of morality,' Resnik argues that social values like 'honesty, integrity, fidelity, diligence, and fairness' create the climate within which business is conducted. Without commitment to these values, business would be undermined by 'corruption, theft, fraud, and disloyalty.' This argument proves too little, however, for

[1] D. Resnik. Developing Drugs for the Developing World: an Economic, Legal, Moral, and Political Dilemma. *Developing World Bioethics* 2001; 1, 1: 11–32.

the specific obligations or responsibilities ascribed to global pharmaceutical companies cannot be derived from the list of values Resnik offers.

Resnik then says that businesses have other social responsibilities because they 'exist within societies where people care about the environment, public safety, public health, and other goods.' Ignoring what society cares about risks public wrath and ultimately regulation. It is important to see, however, that the specific responsibilities or obligations ascribed to businesses within a society are the result of a societal negotiation in which the protection of business incentives and productivity are weighed against the consequences to the public of failing to impose specific – legal and administrative – duties and obligations.

Perhaps we should, as Resnik does, posit moral responsibilities that correspond to and perhaps justify the legal duties and obligations that result from such a negotiation. My complaint is that the specific nature of any of these duties or responsibilities is the result of a kind of social contract that establishes them. They do not simply 'derive' from what society cares about or what it threatens. Internationally, the duties and obligations we may impose on global corporations are also the result of both domestic and international negotiation. I think we can be clear and specific about what social responsibilities are assigned to corporations in either the domestic or international case only when we have undertaken the appropriate negotiation in the context of the appropriate social or inter-societal contract.

Resnik's second reason for claiming businesses have social responsibilities is that they are 'like' moral agents in that their decisions have important consequences for people affected by them. In one sense he is surely correct: we all engage in moral condemnation of some of these consequences and some of these actions. Just what responsibilities follow from the fact that corporate decisions have effects on people outside the corporations is not, however, clear. Nor does Resnik provide adequate details about the derivation. Within nation-states, and internationally, societies and their legal institutions take these effects into consideration, engage in the weighing of benefits against consequences, including the effects of corporate decisions on the rights of other parties, and establish a legal (and arguably moral) framework for talking about social responsibilities. The specifics, however, do not follow from the nature of agency but from the kind of deliberation I have noted.

I turn now to some skepticism about Resnik's reliance on appeals to social (moral) responsibilities as a solution to the problem of affordable, appropriate drugs. Consider the point of view of the developing country that has long faced a world in which global pharmaceutical companies have rarely exercised the social responsibilities that Resnik ascribes to them. Arguably, such countries do a better job of meeting the needs of their populations by taking drug production into their own hands, ignoring intellectual property rights, even if doing so makes them parasitic on the rest of the global system. Resnik says that this act deprives corporations of profits they need to remain competitive, but this cannot be argued from the existing facts, since Resnik himself points to the high profitability of these corporations despite the presence of such renegade states.

Resnik also argues that, in the long run, the corporate system would better meet the needs of these states if both corporations and countries met their respective social responsibilities. He may be right, but that is no *assurance* to the developing countries that such corporations will consistently meet their social responsibilities – and there is everywhere evidence they act on other commitments. Without solving the assurance problem through some mechanism of enforcement of those responsibilities, there is no way to counter the behavior of countries desperate to solve the problem of affordable drugs by making their own. Indeed, the very treaties that establish international property rights fail to enforce the social responsibilities of corporations and focus only on the responsibilities of countries to respect property rights. Without the quid pro quo, there is no solution to the assurance problem and so no basis for appealing to moral commitment to solve the problem of public goods lurking in the background.

The assurance problem also arises among corporations and not just among developing countries. The 'socially responsible' corporation may calculate that it is doing its fair share by undertaking certain measures to help developing countries. If competition becomes stiffer, say because more developed countries rely on large scale purchasing or price regulation, then some previously 'responsible' corporations will recalculate what they are willing to do for developing countries. Corporations more willing to sacrifice profits will then be at a competitive disadvantage. The unremitting pressure of competition moves all parties toward reneging on social responsibilities, perhaps even arguing they no longer exist. Since no regulation is in place to collectivize the contribution of global corporations – say through an internationally administered research and development fund derived from a levy on them or through a fund to support discounts and giveaways – the appeal to social responsibility may be whistling in the capitalist wind.

In short, I believe the solution to the problem of affordable, appropriate drugs for developing countries lies in domestic and international action to regulate global pharmaceutical companies and to regularize their contributions toward meeting the needs of developing countries. With the institutionalization of such responsibilities in place, we would then have addressed the assurance problem that will keep some countries from respecting intellectual property rights, and the institutionalization will have embodied a balance – preferably more rather than less reasonable – between incentives, profits, and public benefits, especially for developing countries. If we then want to say that we have 'recognized' (rather than created) social responsibilities, so be it. Whatever we have recognized, however, is not visible to us in the form of a clear, determinate moral realm of responsibilities absent our deliberation and social negotiation about the design of that institution.

PART VI: GENETICS

Chapter 20

DO HUMAN CELLS HAVE RIGHTS?*

MARY WARNOCK

The British Government's Committee of Inquiry into Human Fertilization and Embryology, of which I was Chairman, recommended that research using human embryos should be allowed to continue, under certain conditions.[1] The question is, were we right so to decide? Or, on the other hand, is it the case that the collection of cells that is the embryo during the fourteen days after fertilisation has *rights* which must be protected, a right, for example, to the life it has, and a right not to be used as research material, but to be implanted in the uterus where it may develop?

Some people have sought to answer this question by raising a further question, namely whether the early embryo is a *person* or not. The presumption is that if it can be shown that the embryo *is* a person, then it will follow that it has rights, for certainly all persons have rights, and, it is sometimes held, only persons have them. For example, it can be argued that, in the case of children, the law recognises them as in one sense persons, since they have a right to live, and a right not to be used as research material. Not even parents have any right to permit research to be carried out on their children. The rights of the child are, in this respect, absolute. If the human embryo can also be held to be a person in the way a child can, then its rights will be the same.

I would like, however, to attempt to approach the question of the embryo's rights without reference to the question whether or not it is a person. Personhood is a notoriously difficult and ambiguous concept, and if we can get on without it in this matter, so much the better. To take one example: John Harris of Manchester University in an article in *The Philosophical Quarterly*,[2] argued that to ask

---

* This article is the text of a lecture given by Baroness Warnock as George Scott Visiting Fellow at Ormond College, Melbourne, in July 1986.

[1] *Report of the Committee of Inquiry into Human Fertilisation and Embryology*, 1984, London, HMSO.

[2] Harris, John. 1983. 'In Vitro Fertilization: The Ethical Issues'. *The Philosophical Quarterly*, 33, 217–237.

whether research using human embryos should be permitted or not, and for how long, is to ask *when human life begins to have moral significance*. With this I would completely agree. But he goes on to say that this question is the *same* as the question when does an embryo become a person? And here I think confusion is likely to set in. For the question about *moral significance*, the question, that is, *when do embryos morally matter*, is quite obviously one that must be answered by judgment and decision, according to a particular moral standpoint. It is not a question of fact but a question of value. How much *should* we value a human life in its very early stages? But to translate this into a question about whether or not in the early stages an embryo *is a person* looks like translating this question into a question of fact. It looks as if by inspecting the embryo and finding out what features it has, we could discover a non-controversial answer. That personhood, its possession or non-possession, is as much a question of value as is the question when human life begins to matter, is hard for people to grasp. And yet it is manifestly the case. The philosopher John Locke understood that, as he put it, the word 'person' (which he distinguished from the word 'man') is not a biological but a *forensic* term. That is as much as to say that whether or not someone, or some corporate body, is to be deemed a person is something that must be *decided*. To settle it, we need to know the criteria that have been established for settling such cases, or else we must establish new criteria for ourselves.

Of course, there may be good or bad criteria for making such designations. Some will result in morally acceptable, some in morally unacceptable, consequences. If among the criteria for personhood were that the human in question should not be a war captive, for example, it would result in the consequence, acceptable to the ancient Romans but not to us, that humans captured in war could be owned by their captors and would have no rights. To take another example, there is a school of paediatricians who, wanting to know whether to strive to keep a neonate alive, try to determine whether he is a person, and in order to decide this, they try to find out whether his parents *want him to live*.[3] This somewhat bizarre criterion, if more widely applied, would have consequences that

[3] W.A. Silverman. 1981. 'Mismatched Attitudes about Neonatal Death' *Hastings Center Report*, 11: 6, 12–16.

almost everyone would think immoral. For why should the criterion of 'wantedness' apply only to neonates? Why should it not apply to other children, or indeed grownups? If, on this criterion, there was someone who was wanted by no-one, he would not be a person, and therefore would have no rights. It is easy to imagine how senile and dependent adults might fall into such a category. To raise this objection to the criterion is, of course, to use a 'slippery slope' form of rebuttal. And, on the whole, I am not greatly impressed with such arguments. For it seems to me that one can generally put up a barrier somewhere on the slope; anywhere that looks essential. There is no need to slither to the bottom; and indeed the Inquiry's proposals to prohibit the use of embryos for research after 14 days is precisely such a barrier, erected to prevent sliding down a different slope. Nevertheless, I think that if a criterion of Personhood is suggested, it must be allowed to hold generally; and this particular criterion of being wanted must be rejected for its general consequences.

The commonest form of criterion for personhood, however, is different from Silverman's. The criteria are usually set out in terms of certain characteristics which a creature *must possess in himself*, if he is to count. The characteristics demanded are various. Rut they almost always include rationality, whatever is meant by this, and the ability of the creature to 'value his own life'. This last criterion, included by John Harris, among others, in the definition of a person seems to me either to exclude, or to include, too many creatures. For instance, those humans who are suicidal, or who wish to lay down their lives for a cause might fail to meet the criterion. Or else the criterion fails through uncertainty. How do we know whether a creature fulfils it or not? If the creature shows that it values its life by displaying a will to survive, then most animals, most of the time, would have to count as persons. If, on the other hand, a creature has to *say* that it values its life in order to be held to do so, then once again too many humans will be left out. The same kind of difficulties arise whatever the criteria proposed for personhood may be. I believe that the only way out of the difficulty is the short one: to bypass the concept of the person altogether. After all, the notion was introduced only on the grounds that persons are the bearers of rights. Since there seems no separately satisfactory way of distinguishing a person from a non-person, apart from their supposedly having rights, it seems better to take the direct route forward and ask whether or not human embryos have rights.

Once again, the question so posed looks like a question of fact. It seems to be a question to which the answer will be either true or false, in form like the question whether an embryo has legs. But, of course, this is not so. You cannot look at an embryo in a test-tube and discern whether or not it has rights. It is more complicated than that. There are circumstances where I may claim a right, and may assert as a matter of fact that I possess this right. For instance, if I have reserved a seat on the train to Edinburgh, and I find someone else occupying it, I may claim a right, and prove my right by producing the ticket, itself an evidence of a contract completed. Equally, if I am refused entry to some bar in a pub, on the grounds that I am female, I may claim a right to enter, and appeal in this case to the sex discrimination Act. If it is true that I am supported by the Act, that the circumstances are those envisaged by the Act, then I have shown that I do indeed have the right I claim. If I accuse you of trespassing on my land, you may reply that it is a right of way, and the issue can be settled one way or another by consulting the local bye-laws. Wherever a law exists conferring a right, permitting someone to do something or forbidding someone from hindering him, then it is a *fact* that a right exists, created by the law.

Suppose now that I claim a right in an area where the law does not operate. Let us suppose that my parents left me a mere pittance in their will, far less than the generous provision they made for my brothers and sisters. If I now claim a right to an equal share to the inheritance, I must base my claim on something other than my parents' will. Under that I am *not* entitled. I have been cut off with a shilling. And so I must fall back on the claim that I am *morally* entitled; it is a case of Natural Justice. I have a moral right; I may even try to invoke the law to uphold it, and it is possible that I may succeed.

But quite often when people claim moral rights, they know that the law will not support their claim, as things are, but believe that it should. They are asserting that there is a moral principle in accordance with which they have a right, and that the law ought to, though it does not yet, reflect that principle. Imagine, for example, someone with a severely handicapped child who in the 1960s was in dispute with his local education authority over the question of the education of the child. The local authority has said that there is no school suitable for the child to attend. The parent claims that the child has a right to education. In those days, in the U.K. at least, the parent was wrong, as far as the law went. If a child was held to be ineducable, that child became the responsibility of the Department of Health and Social Security, not the Department of Education. All that the parent could do, in those days, was to say that, since the child *ought* to be educated, had indeed a *moral right* to education, the *law ought to be changed*. And, of course, in the early 1970s, the law was changed, and the child acquired the right which before had been only a moral right.

Let us apply this example, then, to the case of embryos. How are we to answer the question *does an embryo have rights?* First we should perhaps look at what rights are claimed. Earlier, I suggested that those who thought embryos had rights in virtue of being persons would claim that their rights were the right to life, and consequentially the right not to be used for research. But the 'right to life' is perhaps not quite accurate. For if an embryo, fertilised *in vitro*, is inserted into a woman's uterus, but fails to implant, it will not develop into a baby, and, indeed, will not live. But no-one would, presumably, argue that its rights had been infringed. The right seems rather to be a right to be placed in a uterus; to be given, that is, the *chance* of life rather than life itself.

There is something rather odd here which I must call attention to, though it need not detain us long. From the point of view of the embryo, and in the present context, (that is, given the present relatively low success-rate of I.V.F.), the likelihood of achieving life is pretty small, even if the embryo is not to be used for research, It is rather like the chance of actually getting to University in the UK if you are a member of a sixth form. In that case, in the past, all that was demanded was equality of opportunity . . . the right to compete. Only later did people recognise that the right to compete was, in itself, worth very little if you were sure to lose. And so then, educationally, equality of outcome, not just of opportunity, began to be demanded as a right. Today, embryos are said by some to have a right to a chance of implanting. Perhaps in a few years it will be thought that, for embryos, what is important is the right to develop, not just to have a *chance* of developing, if it is certain that some that are returned to the uterus will not succeed.

But, that aside, at present the right is thought to be a right to a chance of life; and consequentially, the right to be protected from research which would put an end to even the remotest chance to survive, to become first a foetus and then a baby. *So does the embryo at the 2 or 4 cell stage have these rights?* One thing is certain. As the law stands, in Britain as in most other countries, it does not. There is no law whatever protecting the rights of embryos *in vitro*; no law permitting or not permitting any treatment of embryos in the laboratory, whatever kinds of treatment are envisaged. The right of the embryo, therefore, cannot be an *actual* right, underpinned by *actual* law. It must, at best, be a *moral right*, claimed on behalf of the embryo, and perhaps suggesting a law that *ought* to exist, though at present it does not. Anyone who now says that embryos have rights is saying that there *ought* to be an Act of Parliament which would protect them. And, as we have seen, any such claim must rest not on law but on moral principles . . . the principles which perhaps *ought* to be incorporated and expressed by a new law.

But if the argument for the rights of embryos depends on certain moral principles, in accordance with which, if things were as they should be, the law would be enacted, and not on the present state of the law, what is the value of talking about *rights*? Why not talk instead about what *ought* to be the case, about how we *ought* to treat embryos, about the moral principles involved? If we were content to talk in terms of what ought to be, we would be quite explicitly talking in terms of value, not fact; and this, in my opinion, would be a great advantage. The moral, *essentially* moral, foundations of the argument would be explicit and clear.

A similar case could be made with respect to the so-called rights of animals; and indeed it has been made, by R.G. Frey, in his book *Interests and Rights: the case against animals*,[4] and in *Rights, Killing and Suffering*.[5] Briefly, the point he makes is that, since a right which is not dependent on a law is dependent instead on a moral principle, there is much to be said for eliminating the vocabulary of rights in such cases altogether, and going straight for the moral principle on which, if there were a law, it would be founded, and which would confer or create a right.

And so, having argued for bypassing the concept of the person, introduced only to serve as an introduction to the concept of the rights of the embryo, I am now suggesting that we also bypass the notion of the right itself, and talk instead about the way that embryos ought to be treated . . . a discussion that will be quite explicitly moral in force.

---

[4] R.G. Frey. 1980. *Interests and Rights: the case against animals*. Oxford, Clarendon Press.
[5] R.G. Frey. 1983. *Rights, killing and suffering*. Oxford, Basil Blackwell.

And so at last we come to the punch-line: Not *what are the rights of human embryos*, but *how ought we to treat them*? What. protection ought they to be offered by the law, so that, in the end, they may have some rights created for them by new laws, if this is what we want?

Since we are now quite openly in the field of moral principles, not matters of fact, and in a sphere which is to be incorporated in legislation, it is natural that our first appeal for help in determining what *should be done*, what public policy *should be*, should be to Utilitarianism. For of all moral philosophies, it was utilitarianism above all, in its original form under James Mill, Jeremy Bentham and J.S. Mill, that was explicitly aimed towards *directing public policy*, determining the course of legislation with a view to the greatest good of the greatest number. Now there are those, among them the illustrious Dr. Robert Edwards of Bourne Hall, one of the founding fathers of the *in Vitro* fertilisation programme, who are quite explicit utilitarians in the matter of determining how human embryos should be treated. He argues that, since the sole criterion of what is morally right is the balance of pleasure over pain, happiness over unhappiness, if the results of research using embryos is beneficial to the infertile, and to those whose interest is in reducing crippling genetic disease, or to those whose aim is simply to increase our knowledge of the earliest stages of embryonic development; and if, on the other side, there is no pain caused to the subjects of research, the embryos themselves, then there can be no possible doubt about where *right* lies. It is *right* to treat human embryos, provided it is certain that they experience no pain, in any way which is conducive to the benefit of the rest of the human race. There are innumerable medical and therapeutic gains from present and future research using human embryos. It is certain that the embryos suffer, themselves, no pain, since at this stage they have no central nervous system, and no brain. Therefore the balance of good over harm, pleasure over pain, is completely on the side of research.

Nevertheless, even on utilitarian grounds, some questions remain to be answered. In particular, there remains the question how far, in the calculus of pleasures and pains, one ought to take into account, not, doubtless, the pains of the embryos (for they will not experience any) but the feelings of outrage suffered by those who think it simply morally wrong to use human embryos for research at all. If someone is a utilitarian, and therefore committed to the view that right action is that which gives rise to more benefit than harm, is he or she obliged to weigh in the balance the moral outrage or distress caused to people, where a practice they deeply and sincerely believe to be wrong is permitted, or perhaps even encouraged?

An embryo which is spare, which could not be implanted because it was one of a set of embryos some but not all of which are needed for an attempted pregnancy, could not be harmed by being used for research purposes and then destroyed. For it would die anyway if not implanted. It could not, being a number of cells without a nervous system, suffer pain. So no harm could come to *it* by its being destroyed, only to someone else. But the harm to someone else could take no other form than *an offence to moral feelings*. If outrage to moral feelings is not to count in the calculus of pleasures and pains, the state could not be justified in intervening to stop or even to control, research using human embryos. All such research could be permitted just so long as it is beneficial. This I believe is the argument, carried to its conclusion, of many utilitarians today, including, perhaps, Dr. Edwards.

But, as I have suggested already, in *fact*, theory apart, most scientists are quite ready, indeed anxious, for controls to be exercised over research, in order at least partly to accommodate the *moral feelings* of a large number of the general public, and some of the scientific community itself. And, at this point, I am inclined to think that utilitarianism breaks down. For as soon as the criterion of right and wrong moves from a plain calculation of benefits and harms, and begins to take into account people's *moral sentiments*, then I believe it becomes a different theory. It is no longer in the business of working out exactly what is right and what is wrong, nor even of working out with precision what outcome is better than what other. It is in the much messier, less tidy, business of compromise . . . of attempting to come up with a moral solution to problems which, while retaining as many of the calculated benefits to society as possible, will nevertheless offend and horrify people as little as possible. What is the morally best foundation for law must be something which is practical, reasonably beneficial as far as can be foreseen; and yet will not be seen as a total sell-out as far as ideals or ideology are concerned.

For in trying to identify a public policy which is morally the best possible, one cannot overlook the strong and deeply held moral feelings of large numbers of the population. Laws must be made with a view to the public good: and broadly this means that they must be based on the utilitarian principle of the greatest happiness of the greatest number, or at least the greatest welfare. Laws cannot express feelings. Yet such is the relation between law and morality that feelings cannot be disregarded in the drafting of legislation. For morality, as Hume said, 'is more properly felt than judg'd of', and to pay no attention to people's moral sentiments is to abdicate from morality altogether. And this the law cannot do. No-one's morality consists of nothing but a calculation of benefits and harms, even though such calculations have their place. If morality is to exist at all, either privately or publicly, there must be some things which, regardless of consequences *should not be done*, some barriers which should not be passed.

What marks one of these barriers is often a sense of outrage, if something is done; a feeling that to permit some practice would be indecent or part of the collapse of civilisation. Someone who feels that, for example, to shovel the dead into the ground without ceremony is wrong, may be able to say no more than that he regards such practices as unfitting or unseemly or uncivilised. But these very sentiments give rise to imperatives: one *must* treat the dead with respect. Similarly, to move nearer home, those who object on moral grounds to commercial agencies for the supply of surrogate mothers may feel simply that they would be ashamed to live in a society where such agencies were permitted. To have such a feeling of shame must lie at the root of any moral principle.

I should perhaps say a word here about religion. There are many who say that their religion teaches them that there must be no research using human embryos. Most of those who say this will go on to justify this teaching by some such proposition as that all human life, being God's gift, is equally sacred, and that this is the teaching of the Church, or other religious authority. But although believers may properly base their moral beliefs on authority, of church or bible, legislators cannot do so. Their base, and their justification, must be the moral sense of those for whom they are legislating. Only a proportion of these people are believers, and, of those who are, only some hold that their religion must supply the ultimate authority for their moral principles. Many, even among the religious, hold that people must consult their own consciences in trying to decide what is morally right or wrong. Religious belief may influence such decisions but not dictate them.

Those who believe that religion demands an absolute and total protection of embryos under the law will not, of course, be moved by any argument, utilitarian or other. But they cannot claim the right to impose on the country at large a law that would ultimately be based on dogma. It is perhaps relevant to say that some of the Roman Catholic members of the House of Lords who were at first convinced that their religion demanded a law to prohibit all research using human embryos, have now changed their views, after visiting laboratories at which such research is at present conducted. These self-educating peers now argue that the pre-fourteen day embryo ought not to be fully protected by the law. They have seen for themselves what a four-cell embryo actually is, and they prefer to call it not an embryo but a 'pre-embryo'.

The difficulty, obviously, in trying to recommend legislation which will be properly founded on moral principle is that, especially in a pluralistic society like our own, there do not exist uniform or universal moral sentiments. Having rejected the view that human embryos have a *right* to life or to the chance of life (for there is at present no law which affords them such rights), the Inquiry was faced, as I have suggested, with the stark and overtly non-factual question how *ought* human embryos to be treated? How far *ought* they to be protected by law? And although we tried with our utmost endeavour to listen to each other, to avoid hasty or ill-thought-out judgments, to express our moral convictions openly and without rancour or exaggeration, yet we could not agree.

We agreed in some important respects. Most important, we agreed that an embryo's being human placed it in a different category with regard to research from any other creature, embryonic or full-grown. Simply in virtue of being human, and consisting of human cells, even a two-cell embryo was subject to considerations different from those that would apply to a perfectly formed specimen of any other species. Such preference for the human is sometimes held to be irrational, even arbitrary. It is thought by some to be a groundless and unjustifiable prejudice, like racism or sexism, and is referred to, indeed, as 'speciesism'. We all believed, on the contrary, that it would require justification *not* to prefer one's own species to another. Those who thought that an argument was needed to explain why they would save a human rather than a dog or a fly would themselves be guilty of prejudice. We none of us had any doubt that the human embryo in the laboratory, fertilised from human egg and human semen was a *special* entity, deserving of special legal protection. The only question was the nature and extent of this protection. It was on this that we could not reach an agreed conclusion.

Let me quote from the minority report, signed by three members of the Inquiry who held that a human embryo must be afforded complete protection from use for research. The minority wrote as follows: 'The special status of the human embryo and the protection to be afforded to it by law do not, in our view, depend upon the decision as to when it becomes a person.' (And I would add, do not, therefore, depend either on the decision as to whether or not it is the bearer of rights). 'Clearly, once that status (that of a person) has been accorded, all moral principles and legal enactments which relate to persons and their rights will apply. But before that point has been reached, the embryo has a special status *because of its potential for development* to a stage at which everyone would accord it the status of a human person. It is, in our view, wrong to create something with the potential for becoming a human person and then deliberately to destroy it. We therefore recommend that nothing should be done that would reduce the chance of successful implantation of the embryo.' And this recommendation, of the minority of the committee, would, of course, rule out any use of the embryo for research, after which it could not be implanted and would have lost its chance to develop.

The majority of the committee, on the other hand, recommended that research should be permitted for fourteen days after fertilisation. Up to fourteen days, that is, we regarded the human embryo, though definitely human and definitely alive, as so far from a full human being, that it could be treated as a subject for research, unlike a child or adult, provided that the research was warranted, and not frivolously undertaken. We, like the noble lords aforementioned, might prefer to call it a 'pre-embryo'.

It could, I suppose, be said that any human being, child or adult, was 'nothing but a collection of cells'. But of humans in general (or indeed other animals) such a description would be paradoxically reductionist. Of the immediately post-fertilisation embryo, however, such a description would be justified. It is a collection of special, that is, of human, cells, but a collection of cells nevertheless. I will not attempt to enter in detail into the complicated story of the very early development of the embryo after fertilisation, as far as it is now understood. I will only say that very soon after fertilisation the collection of cells, multiplied now from two to sixteen or more, are hanging together in a loose configuration, and divide themselves into an inner and outer group. Within the inner group, the embryo proper begins to form, by means of the accumulation of a plate of cells called the embryonic disc. It is within this disc that the first recognisable features of the embryo proper will form. The first of such features is called the Primitive Streak which appears as a further heaping up of cells within the embryonic disc. This heaping up occurs on the fourteenth or fifteenth day after fertilisation. A single embryonic disc may produce two primitive streaks, and this is the last moment at which identical twins may form. From the fourteenth day onwards, several identifiable features form, in and around the embryonic disc, and this is a period of rapid change. And then, on the seventeenth day, the neural groove appears which, after six days more, begins to form into the beginnings of the spinal cord. We, the majority of the Inquiry, recommend that research on the human embryo should be brought to an end on the fourteenth day because of the development then of the primitive streak. Up to that time, it is difficult to think of the embryo as an individual, because it might still become two individuals. None of the criteria of identity that apply to me, or Tom or Dick or Harry, and distinguish one of us from the others, are satisfied by the embryo at this very early stage. The collection of cells, though loosely strung together, is hardly yet one thing, nor is it several. It is not yet determined to be either one or several. But from the fourteenth or fifteenth day onwards, there is no doubt that it is Tom or Dick or Harry that is developing, or all three of them, but as three individuals. At this stage, then, the embryo proper has become distinct from those cells which will become its protective cover in the uterus, the placenta. Up to this time as I have said the whole collection of cells may be thought of, not as an embryo, but as a pre-embryo.

We did not, of course, differ among ourselves as to the facts of the case. We differed only in one thing: if this collection of cells is to be thought of as 'potentially' an individual human being, what follows from that? Or, if this is still a misleading question, we could ask another question: what does being 'potentially' something or other entail? If we agree that the pre-embryo *is* potentially a human being (or two human beings), does this necessarily entail *that this potentiality must not be frustrated*? I do not think that it does. If a child is a potential scholar, it may mean that the child will be a scholar *if* certain conditions are fulfilled, such as that the child is well taught or encouraged. But the child may, nevertheless, not turn out to be a scholar, and no blame may attach to anyone for not fulfilling the required conditions. If x is potentially y, this means that x may be y in certain circumstances. But to give precise weight to the importance of this condition is not at all easy, nor can it be done by rule of thumb or in general terms. If I say that my garden is potentially fertile, I have not said very much. Who knows how many conditions need to be satisfied before it will grow things? Do I mean that it will be fertile if the weather is right? If it rains as much as it did three years ago? If I change all the soil? The value we attach to my garden will *vary* according to what has to be done to render it fertile. Of course, there may be gardens that are not even potentially fertile, and these are the least valuable. But the scale of value for potential fertility is enormous. Similarly, it seems to me, with potential humans. Human semen is potential human material, *if* it fertilises an egg and is implanted. Human ova are likewise potential human beings *if* they are fertilised by semen, and implanted. Yet no-one supposes that sperm and egg are in themselves to be protected, although they are plainly of *value*, and are not to be thought of as just like anything else.

To say that eggs and sperm cannot by themselves become human, but only if bound together, does not seem to me to differentiate them from the early embryo which by itself will not become human either, but will die unless it is implanted. In short, I do not think that the concept of *potentiality* has any precise sense which will necessitate the treatment of early embryos as requiring the full protection of the law. The question whether or not they may be used in research must be answered, not with regard to their potentiality, but with regard to what they are . . . how far they are along the long road to becoming fully human. And the majority of the Inquiry thought that they were so far from being full humans that the protection of the law need not be absolute. But the protection should be limited only *given* the advantages that would come to the rest of the human race, (not potential, but actual humans) from using them for research.

And *so* we come to the compromise . . . the attempt to balance utilitarian consideration of beneficial outcome against moral feelings that human cells, though not identical with human beings, yet need to be treated differently from any other living matter; against the belief that though these cells are not the bearers of rights, yet there are limits to what should be done with them. They are not to be used frivolously, or for no good end. The Committee of Inquiry recommended that research using human embryos should be carried out *only subject to licence*. Each research project would require a separate licence; and the licence would be issued subject to conditions, for example, that the research was scientifically valid and that it could not be pursued *without* the use of embryos. A licensing body should be set up which would consist not only of scientists and medical practitioners but also of lay people; and there should be an inspectorate to ensure that research workers were not violating the terms of the licence. In addition we recommended that no licence would be issued for the use of embryos of more than fourteen days; and that anyone keeping an embryo alive in the laboratory for longer than fourteen days should be guilty not only of a breach of the licence regulations, but also of a separate criminal offence. These, then, were some of our recommendations.

Before concluding, I should like to deal with one objection to our recommendations, which is not a fundamental but a practical objection. People have frequently said that the proposed fourteen day limit will simply be disregarded by scientists. If they want to keep embryos alive in the laboratory for longer, they will go ahead and do so, regardless of licensing regulations, or even of the criminal law. I do not believe this. I am certain that the system of monitoring research can, and will, be effective. The Inquiry relied here on the analogy of research using live animals. Licences have been issued for more than a hundred years for the use of animals in laboratories; and there is a new Act, which has recently gone through all its Parliamentary stages, which institutes a revised Home Office Advisory committee to issue licences and to monitor research yet more strictly. The inspectorate for animal experiments is well-established and well-respected. Scientists seldom go beyond the terms of their licences, realising that if they did, they would be unable to publish the results of their research. They would forfeit the respect of their peers, and at the same time be liable, if their activities were discovered, to lose their licence and be refused any other licence on a new project. The system actually works for the protection of animals, given that their experimental use is necessary. And there are cases where the sanctions are used. Both academic research, mainly funded by the Research Councils, and commercial research are covered by the Act.

I believe, then, that in the same way a statutory body to advise control and monitor research in the case of the experimental use of human embryos could be effective. The scientific world recognises the need for strict controls, if only to allay public suspicion and anxiety. If the number of embryos used in the laboratories is published each year, and there is public assurance that no embryo is kept alive for more than fourteen days, then gradually public confidence may be built up. The fear of nameless and horrible experiments or of the creation of Frankenstein monsters in the laboratory may gradually fade, and scientists will be able to get on with their work, even though subject to considerable controls and restrictions, in a relatively peaceful and undramatic atmosphere. In short I believe that the system will work; and also that it is of the utmost importance that it should.

Scientists themselves wish to be seen to be behaving morally well. They do not wish to commit offences or to cause moral revulsion. It is for this reason that our compromise is, usually, morally acceptable to them. And I hope it may eventually be acceptable to parliament and to the public at large. I hope at least to have said enough to show how we came to the conclusion we did. We know, and knew all along, that the compromise would not seem right to everyone, and would, to some, seem exceedingly wrong. But matters of legislation must necessarily seek to find a balance between the individual and society; between the demands of public and of private morality.

Brave words about Rights will here only confuse the issue, seeming to clarify and make definite, in reality obscuring the moral questions to be asked. Rhetoric is totally out of place in such a context. We need thought, and the will to establish a successful balance, weighing one good against another. Such thought takes time and effort, but it is the only foundation of good law.

Chapter 21

GOING TO THE ROOTS OF THE STEM CELL CONTROVERSY

SØREN HOLM

INTRODUCTION

The ability to produce and culture human embryonic stem cells has raised hopes for a range of new cell based therapies, but has at the same time created intense national and international debate.

The purpose of this paper is to describe the scientific background to the current ethical and legislative debates about the generation and use of human stem cells, and to give an overview of the ethical issues that are central to these debates. Because the paper is intended to be reasonably comprehensive the presentation and analysis of each individual argument must necessarily be rather brief.[1]

THE SCIENTIFIC BACKGROUND TO THE STEM CELL CONTROVERSY

Three partially independent scientific developments underlie the current debates about stem cell research. These are 1) the discovery of methods to derive and culture human embryonic stem cells, 2) the discovery of nuclear replacement techniques, and 3) the discovery of new and previously unsuspected potentialities of stem cells in the adult human body.

A stem cell is a non-differentiated cell that can divide and multiply in its undifferentiated state, but which can also give rise to more specialised differentiated cells. It has been known for a long time that adult human tissues contain stem cells that can replenish cells lost through normal wear and tear or through trauma or disease.

---

[1] One major topic has been left out of this paper because of space constraints. That is the question of intellectual and actual property rights in human stem cell lines and the techniques by which they are produced. This is a huge topic on its own, actualising all the issues of ownership of the human body, body parts and human genetic material.

This fact has been utilised as a basis for a number of different treatments including bone marrow and skin transplants.

It has also been known that cells from the inner cell mass of the early embryo are stem cells (since we know that they must necessarily be able to become every cell in the body during the development from embryo to adult individual), but no method existed by which these embryonic stem cells could be grown in culture in the laboratory in a way that preserved their stem cell character.

In 1998 researchers at the University of Wisconsin published a method for deriving and culturing human embryonic stem cells indefinitely.[2] This development made it possible to create stable human stem cell lines and generate (in principle) unlimited quantities of any particular embiyonic stem cell, and thereby the possibility to 1) standardise research into human stem cells, and 2) create reproducible stem cell therapies.

Almost at the same time as the Wisconsin group developed the method for culturing human embryonic stem cells, a group at the Roslin Institute in Scotland developed methods for the cloning of adult mammals using nuclear replacement techniques.[3] The techniques basically work by removing a cell from an adult animal, and then taking the cell nucleus from the adult cell and placing it in an ovum from which the original nucleus has been removed. This procedure reprogrammes the adult nucleus to an embryonic state and creates a cell that is more than 99% genetically identical with the original adult cell from which the nucleus was taken.[4] It is, however, not the ability to reproduce a fully-grown mammal by nuclear replacement that is of main interest to the stem cell debate. It is the combination of nuclear replacement techniques and embryonic stem cell culture. When these two techniques are combined it becomes possible to produce embryonic stem cells that are almost genetically identical to any given adult human being.

Research into the potentialities of the remaining stem cells in the adult human body has also progressed apace in recent years. Stem

---

[2] J.A. Thomson, J. Itskovitz-Eldor, S.S. Shapiro, M.A. Waknitz, J.J. Swiergiel, V.S. Marshall & J.M. Jones. Embryonic stem cell lines derived from human blastocysts. *Science* 1998; 282: 1145–1147.

[3] I. Wilmut, A.E. Schnieke, J. McWhir, A.J. Kind & K.H. Campbell. Viable offspring derived from foetal and adult mammalian cells. *Nature* 1997; 385: 810–813.

[4] The mitochondria in this cell come from the ovum, and contain their own genetic material. It is thus only if both nucleus and ovum come from the same woman that 100% genetic identity is achieved.

cells have been found in a number of tissues in which it was previously 'common knowledge' that they did not exist (e.g. neuronal stem cells in the brain),[5] many kinds of adult stem cells[6] have been cultured, and adult stem cells have been shown to be capable of transdifferentiation into different kinds of cells than the cells of the tissues in which they originated.[7] These discoveries have opened the possibility that adult stem cells may be used in a range of stem cell therapies far beyond what was thought possible.[8]

At present there are thus three main research programmes that are pursued in stem cell research: 1) research on adult stem cells, 2) research on embryonic stem cells from embryos produced through IVF techniques, and 3) research on embryonic stem cells produced through nuclear replacement techniques.[9]

All three research programmes are directed at 1) increasing our knowledge about basic cell biology, 2) creating new therapies through stem cell culture and control of cell differentiation, and 3) producing commercially viable stem cell products either by the direct patenting of stem cell lines, or by combining stem cell technology with genetic engineering or other patentable interventions.

---

[5] C.B. Johanson, S. Momma, D.L. Clarke, M. Risling, U. Lendahl & J. Friesen. Identification of a neural stem cell in the adult mammalian central nervous system. *Cell* 1999; 96: 25–34.

[6] In this paper 'adult stem cell' will be used for any stem cell derived from a human being after birth.

[7] D.L. Clarke, C.B. Johansson, J. Wilbertz, B. Veress, E. Nilsson, H. Karlstrom, U. Lendahl & J. Friesen. Generalized potential of adult neural stem cells. *Science* 2000; 288: 1559–1561; P.A. Zuk, M. Zhu, H. Mizono, J. Huang, J.W. Futrell, A.J. Katz, P. Benhaim, H.P. Lorenz & M.H. Hedrick. Multilineage cells from human adipose tissue: implications for cell-based therapies. *Tissue Engineering* 2001; 7: 211–228.

[8] Two recent papers cast some doubt on these possibilities for transdifferentiation, but their validity and relevance is contested. N. Terada, T. Hamazaki, M. Oka, M. Hoki, D.M. Mastalerz, Y. Nakano, E.M. Meyer, L. Morel, B.E. Petersen & E.W. Scott. Bone marrow cells adopt the phenotype of other cells by spontaneous cell fusion. *Nature* 2002; 416: 542–545; Q-L. Ling, J. Nichols, E.P. Evans & A.G. Smith. Changing potency by spontaneous fusion. *Nature* 2002; 416: 545–548. N. Dewitt, J. Knight. Biologists question adult stem-cell versatility. *Nature* 2002; 416: 354.

[9] The term 'research programme' is here used in the sense given to it by Lakatos, i.e. a group of concrete research endeavours kept together by a common core of relatively stable assumptions about the goals of research, the proper research methodologies and the most fruitful research topics. What distinguishes the three stem cell research programmes from each other is primarily different beliefs about what kind of stem cell is going to be the basis for the most progressive (i.e. productive in terms of scientific and commercial results) research. I. Lakatos. 1974. Falsification and the methodology of scientific research programmes. In *Criticism and the Growth of Knowledge*. I. Lakatos and A. Musgrave, eds. Cambridge. Cambridge University Press: 91–196.

As we will see below, much of the discussion on stem cells is concerned with the ethical issues raised by each of these programmes, and with whether or not these ethical issues should influence decisions about regulation and/or funding of the research programmes.

THE EXPECTED BENEFITS FROM STEM CELL RESEARCH

Stem cell research is undoubtedly going to increase our knowledge about basic cell biology considerably, but this is not the benefit of stem cell research that excites most people. The really exciting thing about stem cell research is in the therapeutic potential of stem cells.

If we can develop methods to grow human stem cells in unlimited quantities, and if we can further learn how to control their differentiation, then a whole range of therapeutic possibilities becomes (theoretically) available.[10] The most immediate therapeutic gains are likely to be in the area of cell therapy. Many diseases are caused by, or accompanied by, loss of specific cell types. The lost cell types could be produced in the laboratory and later implanted to cure or alleviate the disease.

Further into the future it may become possible to grow whole organs from stem cells and use these for transplantation, removing the need for organ donation; and even further into the future we may be able to use stem cells for rejuvenating therapies leading to an increased life-span.

The therapeutic potential of stem cells spans such a wide range of diseases and conditions that it will constitute a major medical breakthrough if only even a small percentage of the most likely uses (e.g. in the area of cell therapy) become a reality. Even if stem cell therapy turned out only to be effective in myocardial infarction it would still alleviate huge amounts of human suffering.

These very large, and very likely benefits of stem cell research indicate that prohibition of certain kinds of stem cell research needs strong justification. The ethical and regulatory debates have therefore concentrated on whether such justification can be found.

---

[10] R.P. Lanza, J.P. Cibelli & M.D. West. Prospects for the use of nuclear transfer in human transplantation. *Nature Biotechnology* 1999; 17: 1171–1174; E. Fuchs & J.A. Segre. Stem Cells: A New Lease of Life. *Cell* 2000; 100: 143–155.

THE ETHICAL ISSUES

Stem cells and embryos

One of the main ethical issues discussed concerning stem cell research originates in the fact that embryonic stem cells have to be generated from embryos that are destroyed in the process. This means that stem cell research again raises the question of whether there are any ethical limits concerning the destruction of human embryos for research or therapeutic purposes, as well as the more fundamental question of the moral status of the human embryo. If human embryos have any moral status we need a good justification to destroy them, and the greater their moral status the more important or weighty the justification has to be.[11]

The question of the moral status of the embryo was not resolved during the abortion debate nor during the debates about various forms of assisted reproductive technologies. It is unlikely to be resolved during the current debates about stem cells, since no really new arguments seem to be forthcoming.[12]

If one looks at the legislation about abortion and assisted reproductive technologies it is evident that no jurisdiction has legislation which is compatible with the view that human embryos are just things with no moral status, and that no jurisdiction has legislation compatible with the view that embryos have the same moral status as born human beings. Most legislations implicitly or explicitly adopt some kind of middle position, although it is often unclear to what extent this represents a considered view or whether it is the result of a political compromise.

The important question with regard to regulation or legislation therefore becomes how the use of embryos for stem cell research and therapy can be fitted into a legislative structure that either relies on a view that embryos have some moral value, or is a direct result of political compromise. Giving some moral status to embryos does not automatically rule out embryonic stem cell research, since it can be argued that the likely benefits in terms of reduction of human

---

[11] R.M. Doerflinger. The ethics of funding embryonic stem cell research: a Catholic viewpoint. *Kennedy Institute of Ethics Journal* 1999; 9: 137–150.
[12] L.H. Harris. Ethics and politics of embryo and stem cell research: Reinscribing the abortion debate. *Women's Health Issues* 2000; 10: 146–151; D.C. Wertz. Embryo and stem cell research in the USA: a political history. *TRENDS in Molecular Medicine* 2002; 8: 143–146.

suffering and death in many cases outweigh the sacrifice of a (small?) number of human embryos.[13]

All of the ethical questions concerning the use of embryos would be by-passed if it became technically possible to produce cells equivalent to embryonic stem cells, without the creation of embryos. This could, for instance, be the case if other methods for reprogramming nuclei from adult cells became available.

PPL Therapeutics PLC has claimed to have done this using bovine cells and is working towards doing it with human cells, but very few details have been released because of commercial concerns.[14]

The spare embryo

In arguments about the use of embryos for stem cell research the distinction between embryos produced for research and spare embryos left over after IVF and other forms of assisted reproduction has also been invoked. It has been argued that the use of spare embryos is less problematic than the use of embryos produced for research, and that at present the use of specifically produced embryos for stem cell research should not be allowed.[15] No new arguments to support or refute this distinction have, however, been forthcoming in the stem cell debate.[16]

Women and the need for ova

If stem cells are to be produced from embryos that are not 'spare' after IVF, the ova for this production must come from women.[17] In the initial research phase the number of ova needed will be relatively

---

[13] G. McGee & A. Caplan. The ethics and politics of small sacrifices in stem cell research. *Kennedy Institute of Ethics Journal* 1999; 9:151–158.

[14] PPL Therapeutics PLC. 2001. *Interim Report 2001*. Edinburgh. PPL Therapeutics PLC.

[15] See for instance the report from the American National Bioethics Advisory Commission. National Bioethics Advisory Commission. 1999. *Ethical Issues in Human Stem Cell Research*. Rockville. NBAC. A number of jurisdictions have legislation concerning assisted reproductive technologies that allow research on spare embryos, but prohibit the creation of embryos for research purposes.

[16] On the cogency of the distinction see S. Holm. The spare embryo – A red herring in the embryo experimentation debate. *Health Care Analysis* 1993; 1: 63–66.

[17] Unless it is possible to use ova obtained from aborted foetuses, dead women, or ovaries removed as part of surgical interventions. The first two of these alternative sources of ova may in themselves raise ethical issues but these are beyond the scope of this paper.

small, but for stem cell therapy the number may become very large. If, for instance, a specific therapy is based on nuclear replacement from the intended recipient in order to ensure perfect immunological compatibility, at least one ovum will be needed for each patient (and probably more since the techniques for nuclear replacement are unlikely to become 100% effective any time soon).

This raises general problems concerning how we can ensure that the ova are obtained without coercion or exploitation of the ova donors, sellers or providers, but also more specific questions about how a new practice of non-reproduction related ova procurement would influence the status of women in society.

At an even more general level there is a connection to the debate about the rights and wrongs of the commodification of human body parts.[18]

Stem cells produced using ova from other species

One way of solving the problem of shortage of ova, and the potential ethical problems in using women as donors of ova for these purposes, is to use ova from other species (e.g. bovines) in the creation of stem cells by means of nuclear replacement techniques.

It is, as yet, unknown whether the use of ova from other species is technically possible, and if possible whether the stem cells produced would be functionally and immunologically equivalent to stem cells produced using human ova. The technique has been patented by the American firm Advanced Cell Technology, but there is still doubt in the scientific community whether it actually works.[19]

The additional ethical problems created by this different source of ova can, however, be argued to be small as long as the resulting

---

[18] L.S. Cahill. Genetics, Commodification, and Social Justice in the Globalization Era. *Kennedy Institute of Ethics Journal* 2001; 11: 221–238; S. Holland. Contested Commodities at Both Ends of Life: Buying and Selling Gametes, Embryos, and Body Tissues. *Kennedy Institute of Ethics Journal* 2001; 11: 263–284; L. Andrews & D. Nelkin. 2001. *Body Bazaar: The Market for Human Tissue in the Biotechnology Age*. New York. Crown Publishers; M.J. Radin. 1996. *Contested Commodities*. Cambridge, MA. Harvard University Press; R. Macklin. 1996. What is Wrong with Commodification? In *New Ways of Making Babies: The Case of Egg Donation*. C.B. Cohen, ed. Bloomington. Indiana University Press: 106–121.

[19] Advanced Cell Technology. *Advanced Cell Technology Announces Use of Nuclear Replacement Technology for Successful Generation of Human Embryonic Stem Cells*. Press Release November 12, 1998. Available at *http://www.advancedcell.com/pr_11-12-1998.html* E. Marshall. Claim of human-cow embryo greeted with scepticism. *Science* 1998; 282: 1390–1391.

embryos are only used for stem cell production and not for reproductive purposes.[20]

On some lines of argument the ethical problems may actually be
less than if human ova are used, since it could be argued that the
embryos produced are not really human embryos. If the moral
status of human embryos is based in their being human, then the
moral status of these 'less than human' embryos could be argued
to be less important.

Slippery slopes towards reproductive cloning

A classical slippery slope argument has been prominent in the
specific debate about whether the creation of stem cells by means
of cell nuclear replacement techniques should be allowed. Opponents of this technique have claimed that allowing this would put
us on a slippeiy slope towards reproductive cloning. The slope that
is imagined is of a technical nature. If all the technical problems in
the first steps of cell nuclear replacement techniques are solved
succesfully then it becomes both easier and more tempting (because
certain risks have been reduced) to try to use nuclear replacement
techniques for reproductive cloning.

This is clearly not a problem if reproductive cloning does not
raise any serious ethical problems because in that case there is no
slope, slippery or not.[21]

If reproductive cloning is ethically problematic the question then
becomes how to respond to the existence of the slope. The slope
has to be taken seriously by politicians as a policy problem. Whatever the analysis of bioethicists as to the cogency of the belief that
reproductive cloning is a serious ethical problem, there is no doubt
that this belief is shared by many people and by many politicians.

The political reaction to the perceived slippery slope depends on
whether it is seen as a possible threat to the positive development
of stem cell research (as it is perceived by the government in the
UK and a number of other European countries), or whether it is

---

[20] There are two lines of argument seeing major ethical problems in the use of non-human
ova. The first sees the technique in itself as a transgression of an important boundary line
between human and animal. The second points to a possible slippery slope from the use of
this technique for the production of stem cells, to a use for reproductive purposes.

[21] The literature on the ethics of reproductive cloning is extensive. A range of views can be
found in a thematic issue of the *Journal of Medical Ethics* 1999; 25(2), and in a thematic issue
of the *Cambridge Quarterly of Health Care Ethics* 1998; 7(2).

seen as a possible tool to justify the prohibition of stem cell research by nuclear replacement as part of a more comprehensive ban on all kinds of human cloning (as it is perceived by the government in the US).[22]

If the slope is seen as a possible threat to the acceptance of stem cell research the logical response is to legally prohibit human reproductive cloning, and to try to convince the public that such a prohibition will be effective.[23] Whether legal prohibition can be effective given the possibilities for international reproductive tourism to more permissive jurisdictions is, however, questionable.[24]

The presentation of stem cell research – Promising too much too early?

The public presentation of the benefits of stem cell research has often been characterised by the promise of huge and immediate benefits. Like with many other scientific breakthroughs the public has been promised real benefits within 5–10 years, i.e. in this case significant stem cell therapies in routine clinical use.[25] Several years have now elapsed of the 5–10 years and the promised therapies are still not anywhere close to routine clinical use.[26] There are similarities to the initial enthusiastic presentation of gene therapy in the late 1980s and the later problems encountered, and some reason to fear that stem cell therapies will have an equally long trajectory between theoretical possibility and clinical practice. It is likely that many of the current sufferers from some of the conditions for which stem cell therapies have been promised will be long dead before the therapies actually arrive.[27]

---

[22] E. Check. Call for cloning ban splits UN. *Nature* 2002; 416: 3.

[23] This is the approach chosen by the governments of the UK, Denmark and the Netherlands among others. For an overview of European policies in this area see: L. Matthiessen. 2001. *Survey on opinions from National Ethics Committees or similar bodies, public debate and national legislation in relation to human embryonic stem cell research and use*. Bruxelles. European Commission Research Directorate-General.

[24] P.G. Wood. To what extent can the law control human cloning? *Medicine, Science & the Law* 1999; 39: 5–10.

[25] Anon. Taking stock of spin science. *Nature Biotechnology* 1998; 16: 1291.

[26] Given the time needed for basic research, clinical research and regulatory approval it is unlikely that any therapy using biological materials, and based on a truly novel therapeutic approach could move from initial discovery to clinical use in 5–10 years. See also R. Lovell-Badge. The future for stem cell research. *Nature* 2001; 14: 88–91.

[27] B. Albert. *Presentation to the All-Party Disablement Group* – July 25th 2000. Unpublished manuscript.

It is clearly ethically problematic to raise false expectations in seriously ill people, and even more problematic if this is partly done from self-interest (e.g. to promote one's own research in the media). But the problem may go deeper because the optimistic predictions and the targeting of these predictions on certain groups of diseases also have a function in the political arena where public policy is decided. When gene therapy was initially promoted, and the public and political resistance overcome, gene therapy was promoted as a treatment for the unfortunate people suffering from genetic disorders. Gene therapy was put forward as their only hope of cure and alleviation. Today we do know however, that most gene therapy projects are not directed towards genetic disease, but towards the treatment of common diseases (partly for commercial reasons). The groups that were used as symbolic 'battering rams' to gain political and public acceptance of the gene therapy, have not yet benefited significantly from gene therapy, and many of the people having rarer forms of genetic disorders are unlikely ever to benefit.

Scientific uncertainty, ethical unease and the formulation of public policy

At the current point in time it is not known which (if any) of the three main lines of research described above is going to be most successful in terms of a) generating scientific knowledge about cell biology, and b) generating new stem cell based therapies for common diseases. That each is, at least at the moment, seen as a viable approach with regard to therapy is attested by the fact that many biotech firms have been founded aiming at exploiting each of the approaches.[28]

The question is important because it has been argued that there is no need to permit more ethically contentious ways of generating stem cells, if the same benefits can be realised using less contentious stem cells, either adult stem cells or stem cells from aborted foetuses.[29]

[28] N. Axelsen. 2001. Commercial interests in stem cells. In *Nordic Committee on Bioethics. The Ethical Issues in Stem Cell Research*. Copenhagen. Nordic Council of Ministers: 79–80.

[29] J.R. Meyer. Human embryonic stem cells and respect for life. *Journal of Medical Ethics* 2000; 26: 166–170; V. Branick & M.T. Lysaught. Stem cell research: licit or complicit? Is a medical breakthrough based on embryonic and foetal tissue compatible with Catholic teaching? *Health Progress* 1999; 80: 37–42. This kind of reasoning also seems to underlie the National Bioethics Advisory Committee report *op. cit.* note 15, although it draws the line of contentiousness between the spare embryo and the embryo produced for research.

What factors could we use to decide whether one line of research is more promising than another?[30] One possibility is to think about what characteristics a stem cell should have in order to be therapeutically useful and then try to decide which of the research programmes is most likely to be able to lead to the production of such cells, and if more than one can produce the required cells, which one will progress fastest to the goal.[31] We do know (some of) the characteristics that the therapeutically optimal stem cell should display:

1. No immunological rejection
2. Immediate availability
3. Availability in large numbers
4. Controlled differentiation to desired cells
5. Controlled integration into existing tissues and biological niches leading to normal function
6. No other biological risks

From a theoretical point of view embryonic stem cells created by nuclear replacement should be able to fulfil most of these requirements. We know that they can become all types of cells, and we know that they are immunologically perfectly compatible. We are, however, not yet able to control their differentiation into all desired cell types, and there may be situations of acute organ or cell failure where we do not have the necessary time to grow a sufficient number of cells to initiate therapy in time.

Embryonic stem cells derived in other ways have the disadvantage of not being immunologically perfectly compatible, but they do, on the other hand, offer the advantage of being potentially immediately available from a stem cell bank in the necessaiy quantities. Adult stem cells are immunologically compatible, but it is still uncertain whether we can derive all types of cells from adult stem cells, and they may also not be available in sufficient quantities in acute cases.

---

[30] Most of this debate has centred on the therapeutic uses of stem cells. With regard to the 'pure' scientific production of knowledge about cell biology it seems clear that each of the research programmes will produce at least some unique bits of knowledge, and that each of them must therefore be pursued if complete scientific knowledge is the goal.

[31] A difference in speed of development between two research programmes is important, even if they will both eventually lead to the same goal, since any delay in implementation of stem cell therapies entail costs in term of human suffering.

No type of stem cell therefore fulfils all the criteria for a thera-peutically optimal stem cell. How should we evaluate this evidence in order to decide what research programmes to pursue?

At approximately the same time, the American National Bioe-thics Advisory Commission and a British government expert group reviewed the evidence and came to two rather different conclusions. The National Bioethics Advisory Commission concluded that:

> Currently, we believe that cadaveric fetal tissue and embryos remaining after infertility treatments provide an adequate supply of research resources for federal research projects involving human embryos. Therefore, embryos created specifically for research purposes are not needed at the current time in order to conduct important research in this area.
>
> [. . .]
>
> We conclude that at this time, because other sources are likely to provide the cells needed for the preliminary stages of research, federal funding should not be provided to derive ES cells from SCNT. Nevertheless, the medical utility and scientific progress of this line of research should be monitored closely.[32]

Whereas the British Chief Medical Officer's Expert Group con-cluded that:

> For some people, particularly those suffering from the diseases likely to benefit from the treatments that could be developed, the fact that research to create embryos by cell nuclear replacement is a necessary step to understanding how to reprogramme adult cells to produce compatible tissue provides sufficient ethical jus-tification for allowing the research to proceed.[33]

What was a fact for one group of experts was clearly not a fact for the other. What is at play here is a different evaluation of the available scientific evidence, but possibly also a different approach to the decision of whether a line of research should be deemed 'necessary'. Is a particular line of research only necessary if it is the

---

[32] National Bioethics Advisory Commission, *op. cit.* note 15, pp. 71–72.

[33] Chief Medical Officer's Expert Group. 2001. *Stem Cell Research: Medical Progress with Responsibility – A Report from the Chief Medical Officer's Expert Group Reviewing the Potential of Developments in Stem Cell Research and Cell Nuclear Replacement to Benefit Human Health*. London. Department of Health. p. 40.

only way to get the knowledge we need for stem cell therapies, or is it necessary if scientific progress will otherwise be slowed down and will be much more costly, but will eventually lead to stem cell therapies any way even if this particular line of research is not pursued?[34]

The policy-maker is thus left with a very difficult problem. If we knew that adult stem cell research could deliver therapies for all the conditions where stem cell therapy seems to be a possibility, then there would be a straight forward policy argument for choosing only to support this ethically uncontentious research programme. If the same goal can be obtained in two ways, and if one of them is less contentious than the other it makes good political sense to choose the uncontentious one.[35] If on the other hand there was unequivocal certainty that research using embryonic stem cells was necessary for the development of stem cell therapies for one or more important diseases, a relatively strong consequentialist argument would offer itself based on a moral imperative to reduce human suffering, and this could be combined with appeals to consistency in those jurisdictions that already allow some kinds of embryo research.

Because there is scientific uncertainty each of these two lines of argument is, however, considerably weakened because an opponent can always point to uncertainty about the underlying empirical premises concerning whether embryonic stem cell research is necessary or not.

CONCLUSION

It should by now be evident that many of the most discussed ethical issues in connection with stem cell research are minor variants of issues that have been discussed in reproductive ethics since the beginning of modern bioethics in the late 1960s and early 1970s. Many arguments in the stem cell debate, for instance, merely re-iterate arguments for or against giving moral status to embryos, or

---

[34] S. Holm. 2001. European and American ethical debates about stem cells – common underlying themes and some significant differences. In *Nordic Committee on Bioethics. The Ethical Issues in Stem Cell Research*. Copenhagen. Nordic Council of Ministers: 35–45.

[35] This might be the proper policy response even if it would lead to some delay in the development of treatments.

arguments concerning the validity of the distinction between 'spare' embryos and embryos produced specifically for research. The underlying points of contention in these recycled arguments have not been resolved during the abortion debate, or during the debates about assisted reproductive technologies, and they are unlikely to be resolved now. Each side has arguments that it sees as compelling, but which the other side rejects utterly. It is probably this re-ignition of old debates that has added to the heat of the stem cell debates, because neither side can give ground without fearing a knock on effect on the political accommodations or compromises reached in the abortion and the assisted reproduction areas.

If we take all of these already well known debates into account it seems that there is a rough hierarchy of contentiousness ordering the different ways of producing human stem cells according to how many issues each raise. This would look something like the following (with the most contentious first):

Embryonic stem cells created by nuclear replacement
Embryonic stem cells from embryos created for research
Embryonic stem cells from spare embryos
Adult stem cells

This proposed hierarchy is not very illuminating for ethical analysis, but it may well influence public policy.

There are, however, also a few issues raised by the stem cell debate that are not as well worn. The most interesting of these are the questions surrounding how public policy should be formed in an area where there is 1) agreement about the value of the goal of a particular kind of research (i.e. the creation of effective stem cell therapies), 2) genuine scientific uncertainty about exactly what line of research is most likely to achieve this goal, and 3) disagreement about the ethical evaluation of some of these lines of research but not about others. This question is perhaps more a question of political or legal philosophy than a question of ethics, but it is nevertheless an issue that should be of interest to those bioethicists who want their elegant analyses transformed into public policy.

Chapter 22

DESIGNING BABIES: MORALLY PERMISSIBLE WAYS TO MODIFY THE HUMAN GENOME[1]

NICHOLAS AGAR

The Human Genome Project is revealing the genetic bases of diseases such as muscular dystrophy, cystic fibrosis, and various cancers. This knowledge brings with it the hope of treatment by appropriately modifying a person's DNA.[2] The problem, as many see it, is that genetic manipulation might not be limited to disorders like the above. Characters such as intelligence, physical prowess, sexual orientation and law abidingness are all genetically influenced. Considerably refined, the same techniques that might help eliminate the above diseases could be put to use building super intelligent people, exceptionally law abiding people, super capable production line workers, or a uniformly heterosexual population.

Most people want to draw a sharp dividing line between the two categories of genetic intervention. Genetic engineering which many would consider to be under some circumstances morally acceptable is called *therapeutic*. Roughly, this kind of engineering aims to remedy defects not present in normal humans. In the other category comes *eugenic* engineering. The goal of this kind of genetic manipulation is to produce individuals whose capacities go beyond the normal.[3] Many people think that eugenic engineering ought never to be permitted. In the first part of this paper I will examine and

[1] Thanks to Anthony Agar and Tony Fielding for many helpful criticisms and to an anonymous referee for this journal for correcting errors on the science involved.
[2] There is an important distinction here as to whether we are talking about the manipulation of Somatic or Germ-line DNA. Germ-line manipulation is potentially transmissible to future generations. By contrast, the effects of somatic cell manipulation end with the individual in question. Germ-line modification is considered more contentious. The arguments I raise can be taken to apply to this more problematic form. For a good discussion of the moral significance of the difference see John Harris, *Wonderwoman and Superman: The Ethics of Human Biotechnology*, New York: Oxford University Press 1993.
[3] Peter Singer and Deane Wells, *The Reproduction Revolution: New Ways of Making Babies*, New York: Oxford University Press, 1984 and Jonathan Glover, *What Sort of People Should There Be?* Harmondsworth: Pelican, 1984 argue convincingly that this distinction is far from absolute. As I do not intend to place moral significance on it, I will not consider their arguments here.

reject a few of recent attempts to distinguish morally between various kinds of genetic engineering. I will then seek to draw a line between morally permissible and impermissible forms of genetic manipulation in such a way that does not coincide with the therapeutic/eugenic distinction. If I am right many forms of intervention that we would intuitively see as eugenic will be permissible.

THE RELATIONSHIP BETWEEN GENE AND PHENOTYPE

Before I proceed it will be important to say something about the relationship between a gene and a phenotypic character. A gene contributes to the production of a certain feature by producing a specific protein. The sum of my genes produce a collection of proteins which combine with environmental input to produce my body and brain.

We need more than this holistic relation. Researchers into the human genome are interested in understanding how particular genes can be for particular phenotypic characters. There are a number of ways in which writers have proposed that the relationship between a phenotypic character and a gene be captured.[4] The analysis of genes for phenotypes I favour is the very liberal one pushed by Richard Dawkins and further elaborated by Kim Sterelny and Philip Kitcher.[5] Theirs is a causal account focusing on phenotypic changes that genetic modifications produce against constant genomic and extra genomic backgrounds.[6] According to them

> . . . we can speak of genes for X if substitutions on a chromosome would lead, in the relevant environments, to a difference in the X-ishness of the phenotype.[7]

This analysis is an extremely powerful one. For example, it enables Dawkins to justify his claim that there is a gene for reading.[8] I can

---

[4] See Elliott Sober, *The Philosophy of Biology*, Oxford: Oxford University Press, 1993, chapter 7.

[5] Richard Dawkins, *The Extended Phenotype*, Oxford: Oxford University Press, 1983 and Kim Sterelny and Phillip Kitcher, 'The Return of the Gene', *Journal of Philosophy*, 85, 1988, pp. 339–361 have more detail on this conception of 'gene for'.

[6] An organism's genome is the complete genetic complement of that organism.

[7] Sterelny and Kitcher, 'The Return of the Gene', p. 348.

[8] Dawkins, *The Extended Phenotype*, p. 23.

read. There are changes that could be made to a gene of mine in a counterfactual history that preserved all the rest of my DNA and environment which would result in an individual that could not read. This way of understanding the gene/phenotype relationship does not lay itself open to the charge of genetic determinism. Though we can identify certain genes as having played a specific causal role in accounting for my ability to read, we can acknowledge that there are also a variety of changes which could be made to the environment of my developing, genetically identical twin which would result in someone who could not read.

The fact that there are many normal environments in which the genes we have identified do not produce people who read would tend to indicate that most interesting generalisations about reading are to be made in terms of environmental input. Effects of genes which are expressed across a very wide range of normal environments will be those that are best investigated by the gene researcher. Instead she might investigate some much wider spread capacity that underlies reading. The relationship between a specific set of genes and this underlying capacity will, in likelihood, prove to be more robust.

Genetic diseases can result when DNA of a gene at a specific locus on the genome is scrambled or deleted, resulting in the correct protein not being produced.[9] In the past a defective gene was guessed at after discovering that a missing or abnormal protein was responsible for a certain inherited condition. Unfortunately, in many cases it is very hard to find the dysfunctional gene product for a condition which inheritance patterns seem to indicate is genetic. The Human Genome Project is built on the reversal of this process, allowing the gene to be targeted directly. The genetic deletion or scrambling that sufferers of a specific disease have is isolated, allowing the structure of the absent or aberrant protein to be determined. In the early years progress was unexpectedly rapid. Genes for Huntington disease, muscular dystrophy and cystic fibrosis, amongst others, were found. In these cases there seems a fairly straightforward correlation between a certain mutant gene and the disorder. However, despite much trumpeting in newspapers the quest for genes for such diseases as manic depression and alcoholism has been more troubled.[10] There are two reasons why this is the

---

[9] A locus is a gene's location on a chromosome.
[10] Richard Lewontin 'The Dream of the Human Genome', in *The New York Review of Books*, 28 May, 1992, pp. 31–39 is a good place to look for skepticism about the claimed achievements of the Human Genome Project.

case. First, unlike many of the monogenic, or single gene diseases, alcoholism and manic depression will be polygenic. Many genes will contribute to them. Further, the genetic component of these conditions appears multiply realisable. Conditions that current medical science groups together may have a number of very different genetic causes. Despite difficulties like these, progress has still been considerable. The recent production of an albeit hole-riddled map of the entire human genome in Paris promises to provide a framework against which genes for traits can be more easily located.[11]

The future promises a range of genetic cures for hitherto untreatable conditions. As the genome is lain bare and techniques for inserting DNA into human cells are refined, the hope is that doctors might one day routinely treat by replacing a defective gene with a healthy one.[12] As the Human Genome Project moves forward the genes which control characteristics such as intelligence may be exposed. If this is so, then less-than-Einsteinian intelligence might be treated in much the same way as cystic fibrosis. There seems a very big difference between the two cases. Can we find moral grounds for making a distinction?

There are some varieties of genetic manipulation that a broadly consequentialist approach will reveal are clearly impermissible.[13] Tampering with the DNA of a person in such a way as to cause cystic fibrosis or cancer will be straightforwardly ruled out. Intervention that has patently bad consequences for society, such as the creation of super intelligent, super strong, psychopathic individuals, or the attempt to do a Jurassic Park on genetic material extracted from fragments of Hitler's skull will be impermissible. Clearly we should also frown upon genetic tampering where we do not know all the implications for the body or phenotype with a high degree of certainty. This is complicated by the fact that genes are pleiotrophic; they have more than one effect on the phenotype. If a genetic engineer is only aware of a proper subset of the total effects of a gene then directed and controlled modification of one effect

---

[11] See *New Scientist*, 1 January 1994, p. 25. Jerry Bishop and Michael Waldholz, *Genome*, New York: Simon and Schuster, 1990 offers a very informative account of the discoveries that are part of the Genome Project.

[12] This treatment might be germ-line or somatic. See footnote one.

[13] I will not discuss concerns about the identity of the resulting person, which have been well covered in Jeffrey Kahn, 'Genetic Harm: Bitten by the Body that Keeps You?', *Bioethics*, 5:4, 1991, pp. 289–309 and Robert Elliot, 'Identity and the Ethics of Gene Therapy', *Bioethics*, 7:1, 1993, pp. 27–40.

will cause uncontrolled or random change to another of the gene's effects. Evolutionists have long known that the vast majority of random changes to DNA result in phenotypic changes which are deleterious to the organism.[14] Genetic engineers cannot afford to approach design with the same attitude to wastage as nature.[15]

AN ACROSS THE BOARD ARGUMENT AGAINST GENETIC THERAPY

Many predict dire consequences for society from almost any systematic eugenic modification. Early eugenic intervention is likely to be very expensive. This means it will only be available to the wealthy. One fairly representative example of this reasoning can be found in Jerry Bishop and Michael Waldholz. They say

> It wouldn't take many generations of this discriminatory genetic selection to produce an ever-widening gap between the upper and lower strata of society. [. . .] [A] society in which a butcher's son has little opportunity to be anything but a butcher and an executive's child is born to be an executive may not seem unreal as it might seem today.[16]

Given the analysis of genes 'for' appealed to above, being an executive or a butcher will be highly non robust effects of genes. There will be many normal environments in which what we might want to call the butcher gene or the executive gene will not have these effects. It seems more likely that some of the intellectual, emotional and physical capacities that permit one to become a butcher or executive will be more robust effects of genes.

The prospect that the benefits of eugenic genetic enhancement might be unfairly distributed is of concern. I don't think that the risk should provoke an across the board restriction. Richard Lewontin points to a common mistake amongst writers on the

---

[14] See Richard Dawkins, *The Blind Watchmaker*, New York: W.W. Norton, 1986 for a good account of this argument.

[15] The existence of pleiotrophy does not represent an in principle barrier to genetic engineering. Nature overcomes linked deleterious pleiotrophic effects by means of suppressor genes. (See Dawkins, *The Extended Phenotype*, chapter 2). Sufficiently sophisticated genetic engineers might also use such genes.

[16] Bishop and Waldholz, *Genome*, p. 322.

Human Genome Project.[17] Much of the language seems very genetic determinist. Some talk as if it is DNA *alone* that creates the phenotype. Genes alone produce nothing; only in combination with environmental input is an organism built. Understanding the nature of the impact of these two kinds of input on the phenotype has interesting consequences for many arguments which attempt to trade on the specialness of genetic manipulation.[18] Improving the genotype of a person might boost the quality of that person's phenotype. However, much systematic and socially divisive improving of the phenotype already occurs as a result of varying qualities of environmental input. Environmental input combines with genetic input in a fairly prescribed fashion to make a functioning heart. Boosting the quality of either kind of input might produce a better functioning heart. We see the effects of differing qualities of environmental input in the levels of function of all human organs everywhere. The differences in average life-spans between the nutritionally impoverished and the nutritionally wealthy are considerable. This is especially noticeable when we compare first and third world inhabitants; a fairly close correlation exists between average life expectancy and per capita GDP.[19] Differing levels of educational and medical input from socio-economic group to socio-economic group within the one society result in the kinds of gap opponents of eugenic engineering fear. These disparities are almost as heritable as genetic differences.

Genetic tampering might be considered to be more dangerous through producing disparities that are greater than those that could be produced through changing the quality of environmental input. Our basic genetic makeup limits us to a certain upper limit of intelligence and physical ability. The right modified genotype together with the right kinds of environmental input might produce an organism of almost unbounded intelligence and physical ability. This may, in principle, be true, but I think that the kinds of proposals for eugenic engineering that we may face in the near future will not pose these kinds of problems. A major obstacle relates to the

[17] Lewontin, 'The Dream of the Human Genome'.

[18] John Harris, *Wonderwoman and Superman*, chapter 7 and 'Is Gene Therapy a form of Eugenics?' *Bioethics*, 7:2/3, pp. 178–187 places modifications achieved by genetic manipulation along side those produced by environment modification and convincingly urges a parity of moral reasoning about them.

[19] See A.J. McMicheal, *Planetary Overload*, Cambridge: Cambridge University Press, 1993, chapter 3.

unpredictable pleiotrophic effects of an invented gene. We know about any additional effects of a gene that protects against cystic fibrosis because nature has 'tested' this gene in other humans. We could not say this for new super intelligence genes.

So, in regard to the generation social inequality, genetic engineering presents problems that are not different in kind to those posed by differing environmental influences. Adding the potential for genetically produced disparities to already existing environmentally produced disparities does promise to compound the problem. However, the same kinds of moral remedies that ought to apply when we work out how to share out familiar environmental resources can be assumed to apply when we come to resources required for the manipulation of DNA. Resources necessary for eugenic engineering will much less likely to be mistaken for limitless than those on the environmental side of the equation, requiring special attention that they not all be gobbled up by one group of people. Many moral theories might be wheeled in to do the work here. Some will permit me to show some kind of special regard for those who are close to me whilst demanding that I show some concern for those who are not.[20] Principles like this will apply equally in apportioning more familiar environmental resources and resources for genetic manipulation.[21]

SOME ATTEMPTS TO DRAW A DISTINCTION

Some writers are not tempted by across-the-board arguments. They allow that genetic therapy is permissible under some circumstances. Jeffrey Kahn argues that some genetic conditions can be seen as 'on-balance harmful', bringing with them a duty of treatment.

> If genetic disposition affects interests such that the state is on-balance harmful, gene therapy could be justified as avoiding the future harms genetic disposition holds, with reference to

---

[20] Allowing special consideration to those who are close to us is more familiar from deontological theories. However see Frank Jackson, 'Decision-theoretic Consequentialism and the Nearest and Dearest Objection', *Ethics*, 101:3, 1991, pp. 461–482 for a consequentialist argument in favour of special consideration.

[21] Singer and Wells, *The Reproduction Revolution* goes into detail on the kinds of measures which might be taken to ensure that the benefits of genetic engineering are relatively evenly spread.

obligations to avoid harm growing out of the principle of non-maleficence.[22]

Eugenic manipulation is not directed against conditions which are on-balance harmful. This means that no similar requirement for their treatment exists.

> If the determination is that genetic disposition adversely affects interests but that the state is *not* on-balance harmful, gene therapy would only be justifiable based not in avoiding harm but in providing benefit, growing out of the more tenuous moral arguments in support of obligations of positive beneficence.[23]

'Tenuous moral arguments in support of obligations of positive beneficence' may fail to show that genetic manipulation that does not seek to remedy harm to be morally required, but is this the same as showing that it is morally impermissible? Turn again to the parallel I drew between the moral significance of genetic and environmental input. There are clearly environmental influences which are on-balance harmful, and therefore must be avoided. Excessive use of pesticide in parts of what was once the Soviet Union has resulted in children with five times the morbidity of those living in relatively unaffected areas.[24] Efforts to reduce this level would be correcting an influence which is on-balance harmful. Some environmental influences such as after school Japanese lessons are not targeted at conditions which are on-balance harmful. No obligations of positive beneficence will show that they are morally required. Surely we shouldn't conclude that they are morally impermissible.

What feature would make genetic manipulation special in this regard, so that an act's not being morally required equates to that act's being morally impermissible? Parents certainly go further in apportioning environmental input than the mere avoidance of harm. Why shouldn't they, given the provisos I discuss above, do the same with genetic input?

Some fear that certain kinds of genetic engineering might debase the traits that we currently value. Patricia Greenspan puts an argument along these lines, focusing on genetic engineering targeted at

---

[22] Kahn, 'Genetic Harm', p. 306.

[23] *Ibid.*, pp. 306–307.

[24] See A.J. McMicheal, *Planetary Overload*, chapter 4.

psychological features such as self control. Even if no immediate threat to free will is posed, Greenspan thinks that genetic engineering diminishes 'the *value* we place on freedom as self control . . .'[25] She favours an Aristotelian picture of character formation according to which traits that make up the character are, in large parts, the results of rational evaluation and training by the agent. According to Greenspan genetic engineering of character traits stands to undermine Aristotelian character training in the same way that science fiction psycho-surgery might. We would value traits produced in such a way as we value weight control by shrinking of the stomach.

> The sort of temperance achieved thereby would not seem to have quite the same status as a virtue insofar as it would not involve genuine responsiveness to the dictates of reason. The connection between the deliberative processes the led the agent to submit to the operation and his later, more moderate appetite for food would be misdescribed as a case of 'listening to reason' . . .[26]

I think that genetic intervention has quite different consequences from psycho-surgery for character formation. Psycho-surgery on a person's character cuts in on the processes that constitute rational character formation. Any resulting self control need depend in no way on that person's earlier character forming processes. No similar hiatus is required by the genetic engineer. Consider an example pertinent to Greenspan's argument. Researchers suspect that an enhanced sensitivity to dopamine may be partially responsible for the lack of self control associated with some forms of alcoholism.[27] This heightened sensitivity is supposed to cause a greater feeling of reward on imbibing alcohol. The aim of genetic engineers might be to replace the, in utero, gene that predisposes a person to this enhanced sensitivity with the gene that non alcoholics possess. The individuals that resulted would be much more likely to exhibit self control in respect of alcohol. This self control would be, in large part, due to genetic engineering. It is important to note that someone who underwent this kind of genetic intervention would be no different in regard to rational

[25] Patricia Greenspan, 'Free Will and the Genome Project', *Philosophy and Public Affairs*, 22:1, 1993, p. 42.
[26] *Ibid.*, p. 42.
[27] See Bishop and Waldholz, *Genome*, chapter 7 for discussion.

character formation from those who started with the normal gene. The changes that are most likely to be proposed, the replacement one gene with another that is prevalent in the population, will result in a biasing of character development that is compatible with the Aristotelian picture. Even more extreme cases need not pose a threat to character formation. Genetic engineering is unlikely to be able to give a parent Tolstoys for children. It might give them children with the genetic makeup of Tolstoy. This is only the beginning of the story. A particular genetic makeup may be necessary for Tolstoy-like talent, but it will not be sufficient. As occurred in Tolstoy's case, there is plenty of scope for the right kind of character and personality formation.

IMPERMISSIBLE KINDS OF GENETIC MANIPULATION

Though many forms of manipulation of the genes that underlie personality may pose no threat to the self control, many will see a problem in the idea of another person's intentions lying behind the production of the mechanisms that generate my intentions. There doesn't seem to be much difference for me if a given psychological feature, be it good or bad, is the result of the random juggling of genes in the formation of my parents' sex cells which then come together to produce my genotype, or are the consequences of the intervention of another person. In the second set of circumstances I may have someone to blame, but that will not make any condition that ails me better or worse.

In what follows I will argue that a relative of this point might carry force in an argument for restricting certain kinds of genetic therapy. The argument will hinge on an asymmetry in the way a person's goals on the one hand, and that same person's capacities on the other, can be influenced by way of genetic engineering. My argument depends on a certain idealised picture of human psychology and the relationship between goals and capacities. I hope it is close enough to the truth in important respects for the conclusions I draw from it to be translatable to the real world.

A good life is had when a person's important or life-goals are matched by her capacities. There will obviously be some interaction between goals and capacities. Capacities can be shaped by goals. Certain goals will not survive long in a person who lacks the required raw capacities. Despite this, much input that goes into our capacities does not pass via our goals, and vice versa. Life-goals are often formed in relative ignorance about one's capacities. Often, even recognising that one has been born with a certain range of raw capacities will not suffice to produce an appropriate goal.

In a certain environment, there will no doubt be a genotype coding for the set of raw capacities which best enable a person to pursue a given goal. Most people will make do with only a small subset of this ideal package of raw capacities. It is significant that raw capacities appropriate for some goals will be incompatible with those required for other goals. The drive the ideal merchant banker requires will be incompatible with the reflection needed to be a great poet or the patience of the perfect file sorter. The best body build for a rugby player will not suit a basketballer. A set of genes necessary for rugged individualism valued in Western societies might work against a set of genes which predisposes a person to a high sense of community responsibility, more prized in Asian societies. In what follows I am going to suggest that a difference in the ability of genetic engineers to influence raw capacities and goals ought to rule out certain kinds of intervention.

I start with what I hope are a couple of fairly uncontroversial empirical claims. A moderate adaptationist holds that many, but certainly not all, traits of an organism are adaptations.[28] They exist now because they boosted the inclusive fitness of the organism's ancestors.[29] We recognise an adaptation by its complex design, its species typicality and its capacity to play some fitness enhancing role for an organism in the environments its ancestors have occupied. Natural selection works by harnessing genes for these traits, causing them to spread throughout the population. Why tell this relatively well known story about natural selection? I think that there is an interesting connection between phenotypic properties that might be targeted by genetic engineers, adaptations and the nature of genetic input.

Keeping the Sterelny/Kitcher analysis of genes for phenotypes in mind, we can distinguish between *fine-tuning* and *all-or-nothing* genes for a trait. First, we need to make a distinction. Changes to the genes that control heart development determine, with others,

---

[28] See Dawkins, *The Blind Watchmaker*, and Elliott Sober, *Philosophy of Biology*, Oxford: Oxford University Press, 1993 for discussions of adaptationism.

[29] Inclusive fitness is a measure of fitness which includes an organism's relatives to the degree which they are related.

whether or not there is a brain at all. They are all-or-nothing genes for the brain. These genes do not govern the fine tuning of a person's intellect. In order for a gene to be a fine-tuning gene there must be a fairly reliable correlation of specific small genetic modifications with phenotypic effects in a range of environments in which humans happen to find themselves. These fine-tuning genes for a trait will be important for what I say below.

I think that very many of the capacities that genetic engineers will seek to enhance will be adaptations. Many of the things that people would like to do better they already do quite well. They want to think better, run faster, jump higher and so on. This, 'doing quite well' is a sign of the complex design that is a hallmark of adaptation. A person might wish to have the ability to look into the future, or lift objects by telekinesis, but since these are things that we can't do at all, it would be exceedingly difficult to work out which genes to manipulate. Indeed, if they are physical impossibilities then no such genes could ever be found.

Of course, none of this means that the goals that natural selection had in designing these traits will be at the forefront of a genetic engineer's mind in enhancing them. As we saw, the boosting of the inclusive fitness of an organism is nature's goal. Intelligence presumably serves nature's ends by enabling the organism to find a mate with the optimal genetic makeup, and allowing the protection of offspring so that they can go on to reproduce. Intelligence enables us to pursue goals which may be irrelevant to our inclusive fitness; the selection of the right chess openings, the interpretation of Latin jokes, and so on. A person may well desire these traits at levels that are injurious to inclusive fitness. Genius in a particular skill may result in the obsessive pursuing of projects relating to it, to the exclusion of having or appropriately caring for offspring.

The fact that the traits that serve nature's goals also serve different human goals will help the genetic engineer. Assuming evolutionary gradualism we can guess that there will be a collection of fine-tuning genes originally used by nature to construct the trait in question. These genes will be the ones that will be modified in the careful and gradual enhancement of the trait.

I suggested above that our goals are very often not nature's goals. If this is so then human goals will often not be adaptations. There may be some doubt here. Sociobiologists talk about natural selection of mechanisms that have causal impact on the formation of a person's goals.[30] As in the case of capacity-adaptations, the biological goals these human goal producing mechanisms have is the promotion of the organism's inclusive fitness by ensuring that it finds mates of a certain kind, and is disposed to care for its offspring. We must distinguish what we half metaphorically call nature's goal in designing a piece of psychological machinery, from the human life-goals that it might play a role in generating. Modern people in modern environments acquire, partially with the help of these mechanisms, a wide range of aims. Many of these human goals contribute to our genes' goals; some do not. Amongst those that do not is the desire to become a nun. Even excluding these there is a very wide range amongst those that do. Becoming a lawyer, or a tennis player may both be ways of contributing to our inclusive fitness, produced by the same selected mechanisms. If sociobiologists are right, then it will be no accident that good lawyers and tennis players have high inclusive fitness. Yet, they are very different goals from our point of view, requiring very different combinations of capacities. Even human goals which seem very close to nature's targets are importantly different in so far as they involve capacities. Many humans desire to have and care for children. In doing so they do not view them exclusively as bearers of their genes. Much of what goes into caring for children may have no obvious direct impact on their reproductive fitness.

The fact that specific human goals are not themselves adaptations means that we cannot count on there being fine-tuning genes for them. Fine-tuning genes may account for the fact that a person typically chooses inclusive fitness enhancing life-goals. However, they probably will not account for the differences between the possibly equally inclusive fitness enhancing goals of being a good lawyer or tennis player. Clearly there will be a number of all-or-nothing genes for goals. There are many loci on the human genome, changes to which will result in creatures with no goals at all. Certain genetic modifications may even produce small changes to particular goals in specific environments. However, in this case, we have no reason to believe that there will be a reliable correlation between gene and fine phenotypic detail across normal human environments. If

---

[30] See E.O. Wilson, *Sociobiology: The New Synthesis*, Cambridge MA: Harvard University Press, 1975 for early sociobiological arguments. The articles in Jerome Barkow, Leda Cosmides, and John Tooby, eds., *The Adapted Mind*, New York: Oxford University Press, 1992 present more sophisticated 'Darwinian psychological' formulations.

sociobiologists are right about the pervasive influence of natural selection on our minds and behaviour then there may be very few environments which would produce large numbers of humans whose life-goals never boost their inclusive fitness. Despite this, it is very likely that a person's social environment does the fine-tuning work in deciding which of these, from our points of view very different fitness enhancing goals, we adopt. When we get to those, perhaps rare, life-goals which tend to decrease a person's fitness the role of the social environment in fine-tuning will be clearer.

If this is so, then prospects for directed modification of capacities are much better than for goals. I think that all of this will have important consequences for the kinds of genetic therapy directed at capacity enhancement that we should permit. There are two kinds of change we might make. We might enhance a person's capacities so as to expand the cone of possibilities for her. Here, we attempt to list the whole range of morally acceptable human goals and aim to provide capacities which better enable a person to pursue them in such a way that does not discriminate between them. I think that this kind of ecumenical enhancement is, given the provisos discussed earlier in this paper, permissible.

There is a second kind of intervention which is more choosy. Rather than broadly enhancing in a way that rules out nothing before hand, it aims to produce a collection of raw capacities that is the optimal set for a specific set of goals. In doing this, given the conflict of capacities relevant to different goals, we eliminate options. Of course, the elimination of options is an unavoidable part of settling on the goals that will rule our lives. If this occurs in a way that is sensitive to a person's goals there is no harm. The problem is that the fine tuning of goals will probably occur during a person's lifetime. So the elimination of options by genetic intervention will, very likely, not be accompanied by a corresponding directing of goals. In all likelihood we will end up with people whose capacities doom them to a life for which they have no passion.

What I say above can be applied to the complaint that eugenic engineering is likely to be culturally tainted. Will widespread genetic intervention result in the correcting of everyone's genotype to 'an ideal "white, Judeo-Christian, economically successful" genotype'?[31] No, because, even within Western culture there are morally

---

[31] Quoted in Bishop and Waldholz, *Genome*, p. 305.

acceptable goals which do not revolve around, and indeed would be harmed by, these qualities. I think that there are some kinds of genetic enhancements which are as clearly interculturally desirable as lack of cystic fibrosis and muscular dystrophy. Enhanced intelligence or physical agility are examples. By contrast, it is hard to imagine a worthwhile option for which an absolute prerequisite is being completely unintelligent and totally physically immobile. The restrictions I have argued for above would prevent the inscription of ideals peculiar to one culture in the genes of all. In taking the effort to screen off from my values those qualities that are peculiar to my way of life, I should also screen off those qualities that are peculiar to my culture. There are clearly morally acceptable options which are opened to a person through being enculturated in a different way. So, genetic barriers to a person's being differently enculturated will not be permissible. Further, an ability to be part of one community and able to understand another very different community may be central to many morally laudatory life-plans. This understanding is already made difficult by the contrasting environmental influences from culture to culture. People are already shaped to a considerable degree by their cultures. These projects would clearly be harmed if the boundaries between members of different cultures were made even greater through the inscription of cultural values into their genotypes.

Its newness and strangeness incline many to want to build an ethical bogey out of genetic engineering. We are much more familiar with attempts to modify people by modifying their environments. In this paper I have criticised arguments which have attempted to say about genetic manipulation what we have no disposition to say about environmental manipulation. The near causal parity ought to bring with it some kind of moral parity. If what I have said in the immediately preceding paragraphs is right, then concern about genetic enhancement of a certain type is a particularly dangerous manifestation of a more general concern about ways an individual can be shaped by others. The worry I have told about certain kinds of genetic tampering is a relative of more familiar concern about ways of modifying a child's environmental input. I am talking here about parents who attempt aggressively to shape a child's capacities in a way that is appropriate to their own life-goals. Parents can place children in environments in which certain of their raw capacities are likely to be shaped in certain ways. Not all the fine-tuning influences which feed into life-goals are in a parent's hands however. As in the case of certain forms of genetic engineering, the problem does not reside so much in the influencing of a person's capacities by another, but in their being influenced in such a way that narrows rather than widens the range of morally acceptable possibilities for that person.

Chapter 23

THE NON-IDENTITY PROBLEM AND GENETIC HARMS – THE CASE OF WRONGFUL HANDICAPS

DAN W. BROCK

The world-wide Human Genome Project (HGP) will produce information permitting genetic screening for an increasing number of genetic diseases and genetically based increased susceptibilities to diseases and other harmful conditions. In the foreseeable future, the capacities for preconception and prenatal screening for these diseases and conditions will almost certainly far outstrip our capacities for genetic therapy to correct for the harmful genes and their effects. The vast majority of decisions faced by prospective parents, consequently, will be whether to screen for particular genetic risks and/ or conditions and when they are found to be present, whether to avoid conception or to terminate a pregnancy. Moreover, the vast majority of genetic risks that will be subject to screening will not be for diseases or conditions incompatible with a life worth living – wrongful life cases – but rather for diseases and conditions sufficiently less severe or grave as to be compatible with having a life worth living. These genetic conditions and diseases will take different forms and many factors will affect the moral case for preventing them. But there is a systematic objection to all preconception wrongful handicap cases which must be resolved to clear the way for judgment about specific cases.

To fix attention on the general sort of case and problem in question, which is not restricted to the context of genetic disease, let us alter slightly a case of Derek Parfit's, call it case P1, in which a woman is told by her physician that she should not attempt to become pregnant now because she has a condition that would be highly likely to result in mild mental retardation in her child.[1] Her condition is easily and fully treatable by taking a quite safe medication for one month. If she takes the medication and delays

[1] Derek Parfit, *Reasons and Persons*, Oxford University Press, 1984, ch. 16.

becoming pregnant for two months there is every reason to expect that she will have a normal child. Because she is impatient to begin a family she refuses to wait, gets pregnant now, and gives birth to a child who is mildly retarded. In common sense moral views, the woman in case P1 acts wrongly, and in particular wrongs her child, by not preventing its handicap for such a morally trivial reason. Most people would likely say that her action in P1 is no different morally than if she failed to take the medicine in a case, P2, identical to P1 except that the condition is discovered, and so the medicine must be taken, after conception and when she is already pregnant, or if, in a case, P3, she failed to provide a similar medication to her born child, in each case necessary to prevent a comparable degree of mental retardation to her child. On what Derek Parfit has called the 'no difference' view, the view of common sense morality that he endorses, her failure to employ the medication to prevent her child's mental retardation would be equally and seriously wrong in each of the three cases. But her action in P1, which is analogous in relevant respects to genetic screening to prevent handicaps, has a special feature that makes it not so easily shown to be wrong as common sense morality might suppose.

In wrongful handicap cases such as this, the person's handicap leaves him with a worthwhile life, a life that is better than no life at all. The philosophical problem, as noted earlier, is how this judgment is compatible with the common view that it would be wrong not to prevent the handicap. The difficulty is that it would *not* be better for the person with the handicap to have had it prevented since that can only be done by preventing him from ever having existed at all; preventing the handicap would deny the individual a worthwhile, although handicapped, life. The handicap could be prevented either by conceiving at a different time and/or under different circumstances, in which case a different child would be conceived, or by terminating the pregancy, in which case this child never comes into existence and a different child may or may not be conceived instead. None of these possible means of preventing the handicap would be better for the child with the handicap – all would deny him or her a worthwhile life. But if the mother's failing to prevent the handicap has not made her child worse off, then failing to prevent the handicap does not harm her child. And if she does not harm her child by not preventing its handicap, then why does she wrong her child morally by failing to do so? How could making her child better off by giving it a life worth living, albeit a life with a significant handicap, wrong it? A wrong action must be bad for someone, but her choice to create her child with its handicap is bad for no one. So actions with effects for a child that would constitute seriously wrongful child abuse if done to an existing child are no harm, and so no wrong, if done to a child when they are inextricable from the choice to bring that child into existence with a worthwhile life. This argument threatens to undermine common and firmly held moral judgments, as well as public policy measures, concerning prevention of such handicaps to children.

Some philosphers accept the implications of this argument and hold that in choices of whether a particular individual will be brought into existence, only the interests of actual persons, not the interests of possible persons, which here means the individual whose existence is in question, are relevant to the choice.[2] So in case P1 above, the effects on the parents and the broader society, such as the greater childrearing costs and difficulties of having the mildly retarded child instead of taking the medication and having a normal child two months later are relevant to the decision; but the effects on and interests of the child itself who would be mildly retarded are not relevant. In P2 and P3, on the other hand, the fundamental reason the woman's action would be wrong is the easily preventable harm that she causes her child, or allows it to suffer.

I share with Parfit the no difference view that the woman's action would be equally wrong in P1, P2, and P3. As Parfit notes, the difficulty is identifying and formulating the moral principle on the basis of which the woman's actions in all three cases are equally wrong, and which therefore remedies the limits of traditional ethical theories and their principles of beneficence – doing good – and non-maleficence – not causing or preventing harm. Perhaps the most natural way of trying to account for the moral wrong in wrongful handicap cases is to abandon the feature of the moral principles we appealed to above that generates the difficulty when we move from standard cases of prevention of harm to already existing persons, as in P3 above, to harm prevention in what David Heyd has called genesis cases like P1. That feature is what philosophers have called the person-affecting property of principles of beneficence and non-maleficence, such as principle M:

---

[2] David Heyd, *Genethics: Moral Issues in the Creation of People*, Berkeley, CA: University of California Press, 1992.

M: Those individuals responsible for a child's, or other dependent person's, welfare are morally required not to let it suffer a serious harm or handicap that they could have prevented without imposing substantial burdens or costs on themselves or others.

Since harms to persons must always be harms to some person, it may seem that there is no alternative to principles that are person-affecting, but that is not so. The alternative is clearest if we follow Derek Parfit by distinguishing 'same person' from 'same number' choices. In same person choices, the same persons exist in each of the different alternative courses of action from which an agent chooses. Cases P2 and P3 above were same person choices; the harm of mild retardation prevented is *to* the woman's fetus or born child. In same number choices, the same number of persons exist in each of the alternative courses of action from which an agent chooses, but the identities of some of the persons who exist in those alternatives are affected by the choice. P1 is a same number, but not same person choice – the choice affects *who*, which child, will exist. If the woman does not take the medication nor wait to conceive, her child is born mildly retarded, whereas if she takes the medication and waits to conceive she gives birth to a different child who is not mildly retarded. Arguably, the concept of 'harm' is necessarily comparative, and so the concept of 'harm prevention' may seem necessarily person-affecting, which is why harm prevention principles seem not to apply to different person choices like P1. But it is a mistake to believe that non person-affecting principles, even harm prevention principles, are not possible. Suppose for simplicity that the harm in question in P1 from the mild retardation is suffering and limited opportunity. Then there would be suffering and limited opportunity in P1 if the woman were to choose to have the mildly retarded child which will not exist and so would be prevented if she made the other choice and took the medication while waiting to conceive a different normal child. An example of a non person-affecting principle that applies to P1 is:

N: Individuals are morally required not to let any possible child or other dependent person for whose welfare they are responsible experience serious suffering or limited opportunity if they can act so that, without imposing substantial burdens or costs on themselves or others, any alternative possible child or other dependent person for whose welfare they would be responsible will not experience serious suffering or limited opportunity.

Although, of course, suffering and limited opportunity must be experienced by some person – they cannot exist in disembodied form – and so in that sense N remains person-affecting, N does not require that the individuals who experience suffering and limited opportunity in one alternative exist without those effects in the other alternative; it is a same number, not same person principle. The non person-affecting nature of a moral principle concerning the evils of suffering and limited opportunity is clearer still in the following principle:

N′: It is morally good to act in a way that results in less suffering and less limited opportunity in the world.

On N′, the woman in P1 acts in a morally good way by taking the medication and waiting to conceive a normal child. In the genetic screening analog, a couple acts in a morally good way by taking steps not to have a child whom they learn from genetic screening will experience suffering and limited opportunity that another child they could have instead would not experience. On N′, it is morally good to act in a way that makes the suffering and limited opportunity 'avoidable by substitution', as Philip G. Peters, Jr. has put it.[3]

There is time to mention only one apparent difficulty with this way of avoiding the non identity problem. It is that it does not account for the apparent aspect of the commonsense moral judgment about P1 that the woman specifically wrongs *her child* by not preventing its handicap, that is, that her child is the victim of her wrong and so has a moral grievance against her. Her child is the person with the handicap which should have been prevented, but applying N or N′ the handicap should not have been prevented for the sake of that child since doing so would have made that child worse off (it would never have had its worthwhile life). Rather, applying N or N′, it should have been done only for the sake of less overall suffering and loss of opportunity.

This apparent difficulty with N and N′ is that they fail to identify a victim of the harm done who as victim has a special moral complaint against its mother. But when we appeal to non person-affecting principles to criticize the failure of the mother to prevent harm in P1, her child who suffers the harm is not a victim who is

---

[3] Philip G. Peters, 'Protecting the Unconceived: Nonexistence, Avoidability, and Reproductive Technology', *Arizona Law Review* 31, 1989, 487–548.

worse-off and so does not have a special moral complaint against her for her failure which must be accounted for. Unlike the typical cases of harm and rights violations, her child *cannot* claim that *he* has a special complaint against her because he is better, not worse, off as a result of her not meeting her obligation. It is therefore unclear that our moral principles must account for any special wrong done the woman's child, as opposed to a non person-affecting wrong done. This suggests that non person-affecting principles like N or N′ may not only be adequate for cases like P1, but that they are indeed preferable to person-affecting principles like M precisely because they do *not* direct us to the special standpoint and complaint of a victim who has been made worse-off; principles for P1 and other wrongful handicap cases should not direct us to a victim in that way because there is no victim who has been made worse-off and so has a special complaint.

Abandoning person-affecting principles of beneficence and non-maleficence to account for wrongful handicap cases may thus be a promising approach to those cases, especially if reflection on them leaves us confident of our judgment that the woman in P1 acts wrongly, but weakens our earlier confidence that she wrongs her child in letting it be born handicapped. The latter confidence that she wrongs her child may be further weakened by reflection on wrongful life, not wrongful handicap, cases. Wrongful life cases arise only when the child has a life that is overall not worth living, a life that is worse than no life at all. That is the correct threshold for the claim that the mother acted wrongly in conceiving and/or carrying the child to term knowing how bad its quality of life would be. But since her child's handicap in P1 could also be prevented only by not conceiving it, or by terminating her pregnancy after it had been conceived, she would not wrong it by allowing it to be born unless its life is not worth living, which by definition in wrongful handicap cases like P1 it is not. If she does act wrongly, then perhaps it is correct to insist that she nevertheless wrongs no one, as N and N′ imply, and that there is no wrong to her handicapped child for which our principles must account.

What principally explains resistance to this view, I believe, is the handicap that her child suffers, but if her child suffered a similar handicap as a result of an accident for which no one was at fault and which no one could have prevented, there would be no temptation to insist that it had been wronged. The difference, of course, is that she could, and I believe should, have prevented the handicap, but she could not have prevented *this child* from having the handicap except by never having conceived it, and so we should resist saying that she wrongs *this child*. In same number, but not same person, cases such as this, if anyone is wronged it is the class – her children – whom she permits without adequate reason or justification to be worse off than her children could have been.[4] But if this class – her children – has been wronged, it is in a sense from which it does not follow that any member of that class – that is, any one child – has been wronged. This is exactly the implication that N and N' have. I conclude that the apparent difficulty with abandoning person-affecting principles – that they fail to identify a victim of the wrong who has a special moral complaint – in favor of impersonal principles like N and N' in wrongful handicap cases is no difficulty after all.

It is worth pointing out one implication of my argument that any moral principle which best fits the features of wrongful handicap cases will be a non person-affecting principle. Others have attempted to solve Parfit's non-identity problem by seeking to show that person-affecting principles, such as appeal to moral rights, can be successfully applied to it.[5] But my argument has been that appeal to any person-affecting moral principles in cases of wrongful handicap like P1 will mischaracterize the wrong done. The very features of any appeal to person-affecting principles that are typically their advantage – that they make the wrong a wrong done *to the child* and the loss from the wrong a loss suffered *by the child* – are what I have argued mischaracterize wrongful handicap cases. Non person-affecting principles are correct for wrongful handicap cases because the non-identity problem at the heart of those cases makes the wrong that is done *not* done to the child and the handicap *not a loss* that is suffered by anyone. No person-affecting account of wrongful handicap cases will be correct. The general philosophical non-identity problem is not an obstacle to the position that a woman in cases like P1 is guilty of causing a wrongful handicap.

---

[4] Peters, *op cit.*; Michael D. Bayles, 'Harm to the Unconceived', *Philosophy & Public Affairs* 5, 1976, 292–304.

[5] James Woodward, 'The NonIdentity Problem', *Ethics* 96, July 1986, 804–31; see also, Derek Parfit, 'Comments', *Ethics* 96, July 1986, 854–62.

Chapter 24

CODING AND CONSENT: MORAL CHALLENGES OF THE DATABASE PROJECT IN ICELAND

VILHJÁLMUR ÁRNASON

INTRODUCTION

In the spring of 1998, a bill was introduced in the Icelandic parliament authorising the construction of a central database with medical information about the entire population.[1] In order to finance the construction of the database, the license to operate it would be open to competition.[2] In the following months this small nation (approximately 290 thousand inhabitants) was shaken with fierce debates about the project. The bill was passed in December 1998, and in January 2000 the genetic research company Íslensk erfdagreining (or deCODE genetics Inc. as it is called in English) was given an exclusive license to operate the database for 12 years.

In this paper I will attempt to map and analyse what I take to be the major moral components of this issue. After explaining what the database is, I will discuss the moral questions regarding privacy and consent. I critically evaluate the arguments that have been presented for the policy of presumed consent and find them unconvincing. I then focus on the question of whether the requirement of obtaining informed consent for participation in research is

---

[1] Much has been written about the history of this project and the controversial issues. See, for example: K. Stefánsson. 2000. The Icelandic Health Care Database: A Tool to Create Knowledge, a Social Debate, and a Bioethical and Privacy Challenge; T. Zoëga & B. Andersen. The Icelandic Health Sector Database: deCODE and the 'New' Ethics for Genetic Research; and S. Gudmundsson. The Icelandic Health Case – Current Status and Controversies. All in *Who Owns Our Genes?* Proceedings of an International Conference. Nordic Council of Ministers: 23–73. See also: R. Chadwick. The Icelandic Database – Do Modern Times need Modern Sagas? *BMJ* 1991; 319: 441–444; H.T. Greely. Iceland's Plan for Genomics Research: Facts and Implications. *Jurismetrics* 2000; 40: 153–191; and H. Rose. 2001. *The Commodification of Bioinformation: The Icelandic Health Sector Database*. The Wellcome Trust.

[2] This was a mere formality. The idea initially came from deCODE Genetics Inc. and there never was a serious contender.

applicable in this case. I will argue for a negative answer to this question and spell out an alternative way to obtain consent for participation in database research. This alternative, which I call an informed authorisation, is to strike a balance between protecting the interests of the participants in the database and paving the way for this new type of genetic research.

THE DATABASE

To start with, it is necessary to understand what the database is. Unclarity about this basic matter has made the issue opaque and confusing. In the law we find the following definition: 'Health sector database: A collection of data containing information on health and other related information, recorded in a standardised fashion on a single centralised database, intended for processing and as a source of information.'[3] In accordance with the law, I will refer to this 'centralised database of personally non-identifiable health data'[4] that will be processed from medical records, as the Health sector database or HSD. But the Act also authorises the licensee to connect data from the HSD to data from two other databases. The first is a database with genealogical data that have been processed from public genealogical records. The second is a database of genetic information that has been processed from biological samples obtained for research by physicians cooperating with deCODE. The genealogical database and the genetic database are not covered by the Health Sector Database Act but by other legislation.[5]

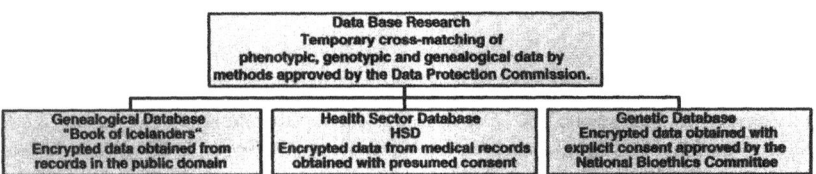

Figure 1. A Diagram of the Icelandic Central Database Complex

---

[3] Act on a Health Sector Database no. 139/1998, Art. 3.
[4] Act on a Health Sector Database no. 139/1998, Art. 1.
[5] The genetic database is covered by the Act on Biobanks no. 110/2000, the Patients' Rights Act no. 74/1997, the Data Protection Act no. 77/2000 and other legislation. The genealogical database is covered by the Data Protection Act.

In effect, therefore, the Icelandic central database is a cluster of three databases with information that can be (temporarily) inter-connected on certain conditions for research purposes. One of the confusing issues in the debate is that people mean different things when they mention the database. Often, 'the database' refers only to HSD,[6] but sometimes it refers to the complex of the three data-bases.[7] Sometimes, especially in the international press, the entire database is even reduced to a biobank or a genetic database, usually in relation to the remark that Icelanders have sold their genome to a private company.[8] This deceptive picture has been effectively used by critics to discredit this controversial project.

While it is correct, useful and important to distinguish between the three databases, it is clear that the threefold complex is regarded as of major research interest for the licensee: as two major spokes-men of deCODE write, 'One of the principal advantages of this data base is the ability to cross-reference phenotypic information with a large amount of genotypic and genealogical data.'[9]

---

[6] This is most obvious from the Act itself. A clear example of this use is a pamphlet put out by the Icelandic National Directorate of Health, and sent to every household in Iceland, intended to inform the population about the HSD. The question 'What is a centralised database?' is answered: 'A centralised database is a collection of selected health data, derived from medical records and stored in computerised form in one location. The data will be coded, and protection [sic!] by access limitations. They are not traceable to individuals (i.e., not personally identifiable), except by expending considerable funds and manpower, and subject to revocation of the operating licence, fines and imprisonment.' Centralised Health Sector Database. Questions and Answers. May 1999: 3. Later it is explained that 'the database may be linked to a database of genealogical data.' There is no mention of a database of genetic data. Instead, this doubly misleading clause: 'Genetic data derived from biological samples previously donated for purposes of scientific study will not be entered into the database, except with the consent of the individual concerned (informed consent).'

[7] This complex has no official name. The Act on a Health Sector Database no. 139/1998, Art. 10 simply states: 'The licensee shall develop methods and protocols that meet the requirements of the Data Protection Commission in order to insure confidentiality in con-necting data from the health-sector database, from a database of genealogical data, and from database of genetic data.' Moreover, the act permits that the HSD be connected 'with other databases than those specified here.' The Government regulation on a Health Sector Data-base No. 32/2000, Art. 32 states: 'The Licensee shall establish rules of procedure and work processes which meet the conditions of the Data Protection Commission in order to insure privacy protection in the cross-referencing of data from the Health Sector Database, a genealogical database, and a database containing genetic data.'

[8] To take only one typical example of this pervasive misunderstanding: R. Lewontin writes that the HSD project implies 'selling of Icelandic DNA.' People are not Commodities. *New York Times* 23 January, 1999. I have frequently heard scientists and politicians describe the Icelandic database in this way, for example at parliamentary hearings about biobanks in Uppsala 16 September, 1999, and in Copenhagen 2 October, 2002.

[9] J. Gulcher & K. Stefánsson. The Icelandic Healthcare Database and Informed Consent. *NEJM* 2000; 342: 1827.

THE ISSUE OF PRIVACY

The moral issue of privacy is closely related to respect for persons and their liberty: 'the right to privacy protects liberty by delineating a zone of private life within which the individual is free to choose and act.'[10] In this context, the right to privacy could be seen as the rightful control of individuals over access to information about themselves. In the debate about the Icelandic database project, however, the single issue that caught the most attention was the worry that individuals could be identified by the information in the HSD.[11] The emphasis has mainly been on two kinds of technical issues. The first is a legal technicality about personal identifiability. The HSD Act states that a person is identifiable 'if he can be identified, directly or indirectly.'[12] This clause has been interpreted in accordance with a Recommendation of the European Council of Ministers: 'An individual shall not be regarded as "identifiable" if identification requires an unreasonable amount of time and manpower.'[13] In light of this, data in the HSD have been regarded as unidentifiable because of the sophisticated coding techniques employed.[14] This stipulative definition of unidentifiability is debatable and relatively weak. Unidentifiable data in this sense must not be confused with anonymous and anonymised data that 'have been irreversibly stripped of all identifiers and are impossible to link to their sources.'[15] On this standard, information in the HSD is not anonymous; they are more correctly described as 'unidentified for research purposes, but can be linked to their sources through the use of a code.'[16] This is important because the unidentifiability of information has been used

---

[10] T.L. Beauchamp & J. Childress. 1989. *Principles of Biomedical Ethics*. Oxford. Oxford University Press: 318.

[11] This was the main concern of professionals and politicians; it is not clear whether the common Icelander was much concerned with this question.

[12] The Act on a Health Sector Database no. 139/1998, Art. 3: 'An individual shall be counted as personally identifiable if he can be identified, directly or indirectly, especially by reference to an identity number, or one or more factors specific to his physical, physiological, mental, economic, cultural or social identity.' This is in accordance with the European Data Protection Directive (95/46).

[13] Recommendation No. R (97) 5 (50).

[14] The Data Protection Commission's definitions of technology, security and organisation terms, which the Licensee must fulfil in relation to the preparation and operation of the HSD, is found at: http://www.personuvernd.is/English

[15] The American Society of Human Genetics Report. Statement on Informed Consent for Genetic Research. *Am. J. Hum. Genet.* 1996; 59: 472. Similar definition is in: E.W. Clayton et al. Informed Consent for Genetic Research on Stored Tissue Samples. *JAMA* 1995; 274: 1787.

[16] ASHG Report. *Am. J. Hum. Genet.* 1996; 59: 472.

as one of the main arguments for not obtaining explicit consent for entering information into the HSD. But unidentifiability in the sense used in the Act on a Health Sector Database is by itself not strong enough for waiving individual consent.

Secondly, it is relative to decoding techniques at each time how safe the coding devices are. Since there will never be an absolute protection of privacy of coded data, the risk of identification is always there. Moreover, it can be argued that when health care data are connected to genealogical and to genetic information, there is a considerable risk in a small society that individuals can be identified, even though the data obtainable for research and inquiries from the HSD will only be in statistical form and never about fewer than a group of ten.[17] There are also instances in the process where the data are not coded and the only protection is the confidentiality of the staff working with the information.

It is unrealistic to expect that disputes about the identifiability of health care data will be settled. Although the data are not unidentifiable in the strict sense,[18] it is not unreasonable to expect that they can be kept coded and confidential. Moreover, there are important arguments for retaining links to samples. Irreversibly unlinking them not only precludes the possibility of cross-referencing data, but also makes it impossible to contact the source of the sample in cases where that could be of benefit to him or her and possibly to relatives. Linkability can also increase individual control over data. It could be argued, therefore, that there is an ethical presumption in favour of linkability with emphasis on strong measures of confidentiality and privacy, coupled with means of obtaining individual consent.

Security of information of the kind that goes into the Icelandic database is a crucial issue. My criticism is aimed at the way in which the emphasis on coding has been used to exclude the question of consent. There is a tendency to focus either on coding or consent. An emphasis on consent should certainly not ignore the need for the security of the data,[19] and sophisticated coding is not always a

---

[17] Cf. E. Arnason. Personal Identifiability in the Icelandic Health Sector Database. *The Journal of Information, Law and Technology* 2002; 2. http://elj.warwick.ac.uk/jilt/02-2/arnason.html (accessed on 27 November, 2002).

[18] For discussion of this issue, see: A. Meyer & A.C. Zeller. The Icelandic Health Sector Database and the Right to Privacy. *Human Rights and Law Journal* 2000; 21: 404.

[19] Jane Kaye correctly emphasises this in: Genetic Research on the UK Population – Do new Principles need to be Developed? *Trends in Molecular Medicine* 2001; 7: 529.

good reason for waiving consent. If consent were obtained from individuals for entering the HSD, this would be one of the factors for their deliberation about whether to participate or not. Instead, they are told that because the information will be so well protected their consent will be presumed. Strong encryption has thus not only been used to protect the data but also to paternalistically override the autonomy of the Icelandic people.

Technical secrecy cannot, either, replace the trust between patients and professionals. It should be up to the individual participants to decide whether they trust researchers and other staff to deal with important medical information about themselves in a responsible way. It is also an important issue of trust for the individual to delegate decisions about storage and use of their personal data to ethical committees and other supervisory institutions. Due to the exclusive emphasis on the technical aspects of coding and secrecy in the HSD debate, the moral issue of privacy that is intimately linked with individual consent and trust has been neglected.

THE QUESTION OF CONSENT

It complicates the issue of consent for participation in the database that there are different requirements for the three databases explained above. For the HSD there is a blanket presumed consent for placing information from medical records on the database and an opt-out policy.[20] The law states that a patient may at any time request that any existing or future information about him or her will not be placed or stored in the database. According to a special agreement between deCODE and the Icelandic Medical Association, participants in the database will also have the right to withdraw their information when they so wish.[21] For the genealogical database, which is processed and encrypted (in computerised sequence codes) from a publicly accessible collection called the 'Book of Icelanders', there is no consent obtained or presumed and

[20] The initial proposal did not require any form of individual consent for the inclusion of medical information in the HSD, but this was later changed to the 'opt out' mechanism because of international and domestic pressure.

[21] This agreement, which was signed on 27 August, 2001, was part of an effort to settle deep disagreement between the two parties about the HSD. http://www.icemed.is/frettir/yfirlysingLI-IE.htm (accessed 15 November, 2002). But this important agreement has no legal standing.

no opting out policy either. And for the genetic database, which is being built up by deCODE, there is an explicit written consent. The consent policy for each of these databases is problematic. I will first briefly discuss the consent for the genealogical database and then focus on the consent for the genetic database and for the HSD.

To start with the genealogical base, which is the simplest case, people are not asked whether they would like to participate in this database since in Iceland genealogical records are public material. But this is by no means unproblematic. It is one thing to be presented in a family tree that is accessible to curious members of the public, and quite another thing to have these genealogical data be subjected to scientific research where they can be connected to health care information and genetic data. It could be argued that those individuals who do not opt out of the HSD are thereby also consenting to their presence in the genealogical database in a coded form. But then the reverse should also apply, that individuals who opt out of the HSD are thereby refusing to be in the genealogical database. Although it would be more of symbolic than substantial significance, they should have the right to be sheared from their family tree before the genealogical data are processed into the database.

As for the genetic database, I said that an explicit consent is obtained from participants in genetic research. In co-operation with contracted physicians, deCODE genetics has collected blood from thousands of people in relation to several research projects of diseases in families.[22] Participants in this research have been given options to sign either of two consent forms, '1A' and '1B.' The A option authorises the researchers to use the sample for a particular research that is described and then to destroy the sample. This 'restricted' option meets in principle the requirements of informed consent, but these samples will only be stored in a genetic databank as long as is necessary for the specified research. Consent form B authorises the researchers to use the sample for the particular research described in the protocol *and* to use it for further research of the same kind, provided that it will be permitted by the Data Protection Commission and the National Bioethics Committee. By signing the B form, participants also consent to having their DNA

---

[22] On the deCODE homepage, under the heading of 'Science and Research' / 'The deCODE Population Approach' / 'Unique Resources', it says that the company has collected 'DNA samples and detailed disease data from approximately 80.000 volunteer participants in more than 50 disease projects.' http://www.decode.com/ (accessed 9 December, 2002). These samples have been collected with either A or B consent.

extracted from the blood sample that will be coded and stored (presumably in a genetic databank). This genetic material may be used for any research that has been approved by the Data Protection Commission and the National Bioethics Committee.

The National Bioethics Committee decides in each case whether new consent shall be obtained.[23] According to their criteria, the committee will permit additional research without obtaining new consent from those who signed the B form, provided that the initial research has been adequately performed and the additional research:

- is scientifically/medically grounded;
- poses no risk to the participants;
- is such that it would not have affected the participants' decision to participate; and
- is a natural continuation of the initial research and/or deals with the same or related research question.[24]

It is questionable whether this 'wider' option B meets the requirements of informed consent in all cases. It depends on the information and understanding the participants have about this 'additional research' at the time the consent is obtained. But even granting that genetic information is collected on the genetic database with informed (B type) consent, that does *not* imply informed consent for the intended database research (i.e., the cross-matching of genetic, genealogical and disease information).[25] The B consent will not be sufficient for the new type of database research that could not be specified at the time of collection. In fact, database research of this type requires a still broader consent ('C'!) which would not meet the requirements of informed consent.[26] Such a policy is not,

[23] The criteria of the Icelandic National Bioethics Committee 'on informed consent for participation in genetics research and/or research which is based on the use of biosamples' were accepted by the committee in October 2000. They are published in Icelandic on the website: http://www.visindasidanefnd.is/ (accessed 18 November, 2002).

[24] My summary.

[25] This can be quite misleading. For example, G. Palsson and K. Hardardottir (in: For Whom the Cell Tolls. Debates about Biomedicine. *Current Anthropology* 2002; 43: 271–301, at 275) say that blood samples for the genetic database will be 'obtained with informed consent.' The reader is likely to wrongly assume that this implies informed consent for the use of genetic data in database research.

[26] This is acknowledged by J. Gulcher and K. Stefánsson (*op. cit.* note 9, p. 1828) who say that genetic data are obtained 'with individual consent': 'An unresolved issue is whether deCODE will be allowed to ask for broad consent from participants to correlate any information in the database with data on variance in their genomes (genotypic data). "Broad consent" as applied here indicates consent in which the potential subjects cannot be informed in the same detail required by informed consent.'

however, permitted by Icelandic law, which requires informed consent for participation in scientific research.[27] Moreover, database research that includes all three types of information cannot be performed except by permission from a separate Interdisciplinary Ethics Committee which regulates every inquiry from the HSD.[28]

It remains to be seen, therefore, what the actual consent policy for database research will be. It will mainly depend upon three things. The first is the regulations of the Data Protection Commission concerning conditions for the connections of the health-care data and genetic data.[29] These regulations are still in the works. Secondly, the Icelandic parliament will have to take up this issue again if the law on Patients' Rights needs to be changed before the use of genetic data for database research can be permitted. The third is the enactment of the Icelandic law on biological samples. This act permits research on biological samples that have been collected for clinical tests without obtaining explicit individual consent.[30] According to the law, deCODE genetics could negotiate an agreement with already existing biobanks to carry out research on biological samples which have been collected for clinical tests, provided that the Data Protection Commission and the National Bioethics Committee give their permission.[31] The only control for individuals over their biological samples is the right to restrict their

---

[27] The Patients' Rights Act (no. 74/1997), Art. 10.

[28] Act on a Health Sector Database no. 139/1998, Art. 12.

[29] It must be stressed that although deCODE has already constructed extensive genealogical and genetic databases, no central database has yet been constructed in Iceland and some crucial regulations are still in the works. The specifications for the database are attached to the license agreement which can be obtained at the Icelandic Ministry of Health homepage: http://www.ministryofhealth.is

[30] Act on Biobanks no. 110/2000. For a critical discussion of this Act, see: D.E. Winickoff. Biosamples, Genomics and Human Rights: Context and Content of Iceland's Biobanks Act. *Journal of BioLaw and Business* 2000; 4: 11–17.

[31] Act on Biobanks no. 110/2000, Art. 7, para. 3: 'If biological samples have been collected for the purpose of clinical tests or treatment, the consent of the patient may be assumed for the storage of the biological sample in a biobank for use as provided in art. 9. provided that general information on this is provided by a health care professional or health institution.' Art. 9 para. 3: 'The board of the biobank shall negotiate with scientists on access to biological samples. Access to biological samples for scientific studies may not, however, be granted until the permission of the Data Protection Authority has been granted on the basis of the Act on personal privacy and handling of personal data, and a research protocol has been approved by the National Bioethics Committee or the ethics committee of the relevant health institution, as provided in the Act on the Rights of Patients and of regulations issued on the basis of the Act.'

use for research or to withdraw from research.[32] This right is altogether ineffective, however, unless the population is well informed about the policy. The Icelandic population sorely stands in need of such education.

I will return to the question of consent for participation in genetic database research in the last two sections of the paper.

CONSENT FOR PARTICIPATION IN HSD

The health sector database provides for an interesting and controversial issue of consent. This is partly because the objectives of HSD have not been clearly explained and partly because its relation to the other databases is not entirely clear.

The presumed consent fleshed out in the opting out policy has been supported with four main arguments. The first argument has to do with the usefulness of the database. If explicit consent would be required, it would obstruct the gathering of information and the scientific quality of the database would be diminished. Although this might be correct, which I doubt, such an argument does not weigh heavily in the discourse of research ethics: 'There is legal and ethical presumption in favor of obtaining informed consent even though it means that much medical care is based on research that relies on biased samples because potential subjects could choose not to participate.'[33] The appeal to patients' benefit in the argument (the scientific quality of the database is presumably linked to its possible benefits for people) cannot be legitimately used to outweigh the requirement of respect for autonomy unless it is coupled with other important considerations.

The remaining arguments are meant to provide those other important considerations. We do not need to explicitly obtain individual consent, it is argued,[34] because the data are securely coded. Since there is no personally identifiable information in the database,

---

[32] Act on Biobanks no. 110/2000, Art. 7, para. 4.: 'A donor of a biological sample may at any time withdraw his/her assumed consent for his/her biological sample to be stored in a biobank for use as provided in art. 9, in which case it shall thereafter only be used in the interests of the donor of a biological sample or by his/her specific permission . . .'

[33] E.W. Clayton et al. Informed Consent for Genetic Research on Stored Tissue Samples. *JAMA* 1995; 274: 1789.

[34] Icelandic politicians have been particularly keen on this argument.

the requirement of respect for persons, their explicit consent can legitimately be waived. I have already tackled this argument in my discussion of the issue of privacy above where I argued (i) that the information in the database is identifiable, and (ii) that technical secrecy must not be confused with, and hence cannot replace, the requirement of consent. While technical secrecy protects important interests of individuals, obtaining consent shows respect for their moral status.

The third argument is based on the notion of 'community consent.'[35] The idea seems to be that because of the extensive debate that took place in Iceland about HSD and the overwhelming support for it shown in Gallup polls, it is fair to collect data under the presumption of consent.[36] This could be true under ideal dialogical conditions of fully competent and informed people. But members of marginalised groups (e.g., mentally ill, poor, illiterate, children), the protection of whom should be the primary concern of research regulation, are likely to be exactly those people who have not participated in or even followed the national debate over this issue, however intensive and extensive that debate may have been.

Moreover, quantitative facts about extensive debate and overwhelming majority opinion must not be confused with the qualitative notion of consent to participation in research, which implies an understanding of the issue consented to.[37] Community consent has to meet both procedural and substantive criteria. The procedural requirements have to do with the time allowed for the debate, the unhindered access of the public to relevant information about the case, and so on. The substantive requirements have to do with the subject matter of the debate, whether the public was well

[35] See, for example: Gulcher & Stefánsson, *op. cit.* note 9, pp. 1827–1830.

[36] Gulcher and Stefánsson even define presumed consent in this context as 'the consent of society to use health care information according to the norms of society'. Ibid. p. 1827. As G. Annas correctly points out, 'a community can approve a research project. It cannot legally or ethically require individual members of the community to participate' (Rules for Research on Human Genetic Variation – Lessons from Iceland. *NEJM* 2000; 342: 1831). And as R. Macklin writes: 'When a society's norms and customs diverge from the basic principles of research ethics, researchers are obligated to adhere to the research ethics and not to local or cultural customs' (1999. *Against Relativism*. Oxford. Oxford University Press: 203).

[37] G. Palsson and P. Rabinow state, for example, that the decision about HSD 'was clearly the product of informed democratic consent' (Iceland. The Case of a National Human Genome Project. *Anthropology Today* 1999; 15: 17). The same authors rightly point out, however, that by comparison Icelanders have done quite well and 'the construction of centralized medical databases has gone largely unnoticed' in some other countries: G. Palsson & P. Rabinow. The Icelandic Genome Debate. *TRENDS in Biotechnology* 2001; 19: 169.

informed about the relevant issues and the principles needed to assess them. It seems to me, if the debate would be scrutinised, that it would fail on both accounts. Much of the HSD debate was uninformed, misleading and prejudicial. The bill was rushed through parliament, informed criticism was largely ignored, and only 13% of the population claimed to have a good grasp of the issue, according to a Gallup poll conducted a month before the law was passed.[38] To a large extent the community debate took place after the bill was passed. Community consultation was minimal and conducted by the prospective licensee. A prior, free, reasoned and informed public dialogue, which alone can engender a community consent, never took place.[39]

It is interesting to note that the appeal to the overwhelming support for the HSD in the Icelandic population could clearly be used as an argument for obtaining explicit rather than presumed consent. The argument of substantially decreased coverage, as Henry Greely has pointed out, 'contradicts the premise of the opt-out form of consent, which presumes that people who do not return the opt-out form really do agree to be research subjects.'[40] It is only an educated guess, but I believe that the main reason why many people opted out is that they simply find it wrong not to seek explicit consent from participants in this unique project. If this is correct, participation in the HSD perhaps would have been even more extensive had explicit consent been sought.[41]

The core of the fourth argument for the practice of presumed consent is that since HSD consists of information from medical records, it will mainly be used for epidemiological research and statistical analysis of data useful for public health policy. Presumed consent is the rule in epidemiological research on non-identifiable data routinely collected in the health care services.[42] In fact, the

---

[38] The newspaper: *Morgunbladid* 18 November, 1998.

[39] Cf. V. Árnason & G. Árnason. Community Consent, Democracy and Public Dialogue: The Case of the Icelandic Health Sector Database. *Politeia. Rivista di Etica e Scelte Pubbliche* 2001; 63: 105–116.

[40] H.T. Greely. Iceland's Plan for Genomics Research: Facts and Implications. *Jurismetrics* 2000; 40: 182.

[41] As of 30 June, 2003, 20 426 had opted out of the HSD: http://www.mannvernd.is (accessed 6 September, 2003). An unfortunate effect of the opt-out policy is that a databank with the names of those who opt out is stored at the Icelandic National Director of Health!

[42] Cf. B. Brody. 1998. *The Ethics of Biomedical Research*. Oxford. Oxford University Press: 60.

argument goes, the opting out policy implies further recognition of individual autonomy than is strictly required for data collected for research of this kind. Even if they are wrongly assumed to be unidentifiable, they are probably more safely protected than any other information in the Icelandic health care system.

In response to this argument, I will sort out three points that I deem to be of major importance. The first is that the statement that HSD will be merely suited for standard epidemiological research presumes that it is an isolated base with no connections to the genealogical and the genetic information. This is misleading at best and diverts attention from the database complex that is the main asset of this project. Clearly, if health care data are cross-referenced with genealogical and/or genetic information, there is more than ordinary epidemiology at work.[43] There is something new, interesting and possibly risky going on in this research, which individuals should be explicitly informed about before they decide whether to take part or not.

Secondly, it has been argued that individual consent should be required 'because of the commercial nature of the data bank and its for-profit research agenda.'[44] This is an important point that deserves more attention than I have space for in this paper. The Act on HSD implies that health care information is handed over to a third party that is not involved in the patient's care.[45] Had the HSD been within the public domain of the Icelandic national health care system, a presumption of consent could have been substantiated by an appeal to reciprocity and common benefit. When the information has become a commodity to be exploited by a

[43] This has been well described by J. Kaye and P. Martin: 'In the longer term the company plans to integrate this database of individual genotype profiles with the medical records of almost every Icelandic citizen and publicly available genealogies. These three separate databases will be linked under the administrative structure of the Health Sector Database to allow deCODE to carry out genetic epidemiological research.' J. Kaye & P. Martin. Safeguards for Research using Large Scale DNA Collections. *BMJ* 2000; 321: 1146.

[44] Annas, *op. cit.* note 36, p. 1831.

[45] The new WMA guidelines on health databases declare: 'Patients' consent is needed if the inclusion of their health information on a database implies a disclosure to a third party or would permit access by people other than those involved in the patients' care.' The World Medical Association Declaration on Ethical Considerations regarding Health Databases, Art. 17. http://www.wma.net/e/policy (accessed 15 November, 2002). There is a debate between the Icelandic medical association and deCODE in Iceland as to whether this article applies to the HSD, but they had previously agreed to abide by the WMA statement in the agreement signed 27 August, 2001 (*op. cit.* note 20).

private company for commercial profit, we are in a very different context that goes far beyond the traditional setting of health care research.[46] For whatever reasons, this has not been particularly disturbing to the majority of the Icelandic public who have decided to trust the company.[47] It is preferable, however, to base trust on information rather than ignorance and explicit individual consent would have contributed to more informed decisions in the population.

The third and the weightiest point is that the opting out policy is only suited to competent informed adults. It does not take into account the interests of those – for example the very ill, the demented and mentally handicapped – who are unable to make informed decisions. In fact, presumed consent involves no guarantee that competent people make up their mind at all. To the contrary: health care data about people who have never reflected upon this issue for lack of interest or initiative or general negligence of their own interests are likely to end up in the database. Rather than igniting reflective judgement, the presumed consent policy legitimises carelessness and ignorance among citizens about this important issue. This is contrary to the spirit of contemporary research ethics. Although explicit consent does not secure enlightened decisions, it offers people an opportunity for reflecting. One might add that this policy is rather impolite because it says in effect: 'we will lay hold of your information unless you forbid it', rather than the more civil 'we will lay hold of your information if you allow it.'

This is mildly put. The hard critics of the opting out policy have argued that it violates ethical standards in research on human subjects, namely the requirement of informed consent.[48]

---

[46] Public and private interests have been unhappily mixed throughout this process. The Icelandic government has been unusually favourable to this particular company, probably in the belief that it would bring great benefits to the Icelandic economy.

[47] Two Icelandic lawyers urged people to opt-out of the HSD and offered to act on their behalf to negotiate payments in return for rejoining. Icelanders showed no interest in this and the idea was stillborn. The newspaper: *Dagur* 23 February, 2000. A German philosopher has argued for a contract model between participants and research companies. Such a contract would imply re-compensation in the case of exploitation and sharing of financial profits. H.M. Sass. A 'Contract Model' for Genetic Research and Health Care for Individuals and Families. *Eubios. Journal of Asian and International Bioethics* 2001; 11: 130–132.

[48] See, for example: Greely, *op. cit.* note 1, p. 182.

THE DEMAND FOR INFORMED CONSENT

If we are to preserve a meaningful notion of informed consent for participation in research, it should only be used about specified research where the participants are informed about the aims and methods of a particular research proposal, the foreseeable risks and possible benefits involved, that personal research data will be kept confidential, and that participants have the right to withdraw from the research at any point.[49] These are the ingredients of informed consent.[50] There is no such thing as 'general informed consent.' The more general the consent is, the less informed it becomes. It is misleading to use the notion of informed consent for participation in research that is unforeseen and has not been specified in a research protocol. It is, however, another and an open question whether it is wise to require informed consent for all secondary research purposes.

If we presuppose this standard meaning of informed consent, it seems to me that it is impossible to obtain it from those who intend to participate in HSD. But as critics all too often overlook, this fact is not sufficient to denounce the database project.[51] Let's consider two options for obtaining informed consent. The first option is to obtain informed consent from participants *before* their health care information is placed in the database. But at this point no specific research plans exist, so it is impossible to explain any of the ingredients of informed consent to the prospective participants. There are no specific objectives to be explained, no determinate risks or benefits to be assessed. Informed consent for research before entering the database would, therefore, be empty and senseless. The only specific ingredient that would be possible to explain is the right to withdraw information from the database at any time, that is to say

---

[49] Cf. World Medical Association Declaration of Helsinki: Ethical Principles for Medical Research Involving Human Subjects, Article 22. Adopted by the 18th WMA General Assembly, Helsinki, Finland, June 1964. Amended by the 52nd WMA General Assembly, Edinburgh, Scotland, October 2000. WMA Website: http://www.wma.net (accessed 28 October, 2002).

[50] Moreover, informed consent requires time for dialogue about the research. This is very difficult to facilitate in genetic epidemiological research. The idea of community consultation is more appropriate in that setting.

[51] This has been characteristic of the arguments of the spokespersons of Mannvernd, the Association of Icelanders for Ethics in Science and Medicine, with respect to consent for participation in the database. Cf. the website: http://www.mannvernd.is/english

if the aforementioned agreement between deCODE and the Icelandic Medical Association will be put into practice.

The second option would be to obtain informed consent from individual participants for each particular research *after* entering the database. But because of the heavy emphasis on coding and privacy this would be extremely complicated and cumbersome. Not only would it jeopardise individual privacy but also, according to many scientists, severely limit the research possibilities that the HSD is intended to provide.[52] If these scientists are right, the possible benefits of database research, which requires different methodology and a more free interplay of information than traditional research, would also be lost. In addition, it might be quite difficult to explain this research each time to members of the public in such a way that their consent would count as informed. For these reasons it is not advisable to obtain informed consent from individuals after their health care information have been placed in the database.

If my arguments are sound, it follows that the standard demand for informed consent is not well suited for research on the information in the HSD. The question then is what the implications of this are. The most restrictive one is that if informed consent cannot be obtained from individuals, no research should be allowed on the HSD. In this view, informed consent protects the inalienable rights of research participants and it should never be waived. Another implication would be to say, as Icelandic authorities have done, that since informed consent cannot be obtained, blanket presumed consent will have to suffice. But these are two extremes that certainly do not exhaust the possibilities. There is a viable middle way between informed and presumed consent, as they are generally understood. If we want to be open to these new research possibilities, we need to be ready to find ways other than individual informed consent to secure the participants' interests.

As I argued above, the requirement of informed consent must also be waived in the collection of genetic data for database

---

[52] In a booklet from deCODE genetics it is stated that the demand for informed consent would make it very difficult to realise the idea of HSD. Gagnagrunnur á heilbrigdissvidi. Spurningar og svör. Íslensk erfdagreining: 20. For worries of this kind, although not about the HSD, see for example: L.J. Melton III. The Threat to Medical-Records Research. *NEJM* 1997; 337: 1466–1469; and A. Buchanan. An Ethical Framework for Biological Samples Policy. A Commissioned Paper. Research involving Human Biological Materials: Ethical Issues and Policy Guidance. *National Bioethics Commission* 1999; 2: B19–B20.

research. This is certainly nothing unique but rather in line with a trend that has been forming in the recent years. Legal and moral theorists have increasingly admitted that in this new research environment of multifaceted databases 'too much cannot be expected of individual informed consent, a doctrine that was not designed to deal with scenarios of this type and style.'[53] Stubborn demands for individual informed consent might not only impede the advancements of medical research,[54] but also falsely legitimise complex research because 'consent achieved by overwhelming an agent's cognitive capacities provides no genuine justification.'[55] The principle of informed consent as such is not at stake, but rather the interests that it is intended to protect. The primary harms against which informed consent provides protection (such as non-consensual bodily invasion and disrespectful treatment[56]) need to be analysed in this changed context of consent along with the institutional fabric upon which individuals can place their trust.

This is a formidable task, which I cannot undertake here. I will, in the final section of this paper, describe a way of obtaining consent for participation in the Icelandic database which implies an alternative to the extremes of informed and blanket presumed consent.

AN ALTERNATIVE

In order to avoid confusion of concepts, I will not use the notion of consent in my proposal for an alternative way to obtain consent from individuals for processing their health care information into a coded form to be placed in a central database. Instead, I will use the notion of an explicit written *authorisation* for participation in database research based on general knowledge about the database

---

[53] R. Chadwick. 2001. Informed Consent and Genetic Research. *Informed Consent in Medical Research*. London. BMJ Books: 210.
[54] L.O. Gostin & J.G. Hodge. Genetic Privacy and the Law: An End to Genetic Exceptionalism. *Jurismetrics* 1999; 40: 21–57. H.T. Greely. Breaking the Stalemate: A Prospective Regulatory Framework for Unforeseen Research Uses of Human Tissue Samples and Health Information. *Wake Forest Law Review* 1999; 34: 737–766.
[55] O. O'Neill. Informed Consent and Genetic Information. *Stud. Hist. Phil. Biol. & Biomed. Sci.* 2001; 32: 701. As O'Neill also points out (p. 696), the limits of individual consent are increasing in light of implications of the family in genetic research. See also: Chadwick, *op. cit.* note 53, pp. 203–210.
[56] Buchanan, *op. cit.* note 52, pp. B16–B18.

and the research purposes and practices.[57] The idea is quite simple. No health care data about living individuals should be placed in the HSD without the written authorisation of the individual or his/ her proxy. A proxy authorisation is needed for those who are, for one reason or other, unable to make informed decisions. Parents should authorise the use of health care data about their dead children under the age of 18.[58] Coded health care data about other deceased individuals, who died before the option of entering the database became viable, can be placed in the database without authorisation.[59]

The authorisation implies that an individual permits in writing that health care data will be processed from his/her medical records and moved in a coded form into the HSD. The authorisation also implies that the individual has been informed about, and that he or she claims to have understood, at least the following:

- which information about her/him will be placed into the HSD;
- how privacy will be secured (without going into technical details);
- how the information will be connected to other data;
- who will have access to the information;
- in what context the information will be used and for what purposes;[60]
- how consent for genetic research will be obtained;
- what are the foreseeable risks and benefits of participation;
- how research on the data will be regulated; and

---

[57] Henry Greely uses the term 'permission' in his important proposal of a middle way between informed consent and abandoning consent requirements. Greely argues that the 'requirement of informed consent to the use of non-anonymous information or samples prevents much potentially valuable research.' Greely, op. cit. note 54, p. 761. It is all the more strange, therefore, that in a more recent paper about the Icelandic HSD he states that the 'presumption should be in favor of individual affirmative, informed consent.' Greely op. cit. note 1, p. 182. The idea of authorisation presented here is similar to Greely's proposal but it has been formed in discussions with my colleagues in Iceland in light of the situation there.
[58] There could be exceptional cases where a surviving spouse has that function. It could be argued that there should be a way to opt out of the HSD generally on behalf of the dead, but the question who should have that authority can be become very complex.
[59] A legal challenge to this policy has been in the Icelandic courts. Information about this and other lawsuits testing the database act can be found on http://www.mannvernd.is/English
[60] Legitimate purposes are already stated in the Act on a Health Sector Database no. 139/ 1998, Art. 10: 'Data recorded or acquired by processing on the health-sector database may be used to develop new or improved methods of achieving better health, prediction, diagnosis and treatment of disease, to seek the most economic ways of operating health services, and for making reports in the health sector.'

- that the individual has the right to withdraw the health care data at any time.

This authorisation is in the spirit of informed consent, but it is far more general and open and should, therefore, not be confused with it. This authorisation does not imply a consent to any particular research project. Each research protocol regarding the health care data must be assessed by a Research Ethics Committee. In accordance with the ethics of research concerning human subjects, such a committee would only allow exception from informed consent when the research poses none or minimal risk to the participants. In this way, a Research Ethics Committee would protect the interests of every participant in the HSD, both living and deceased. However, the most important protection for participants in research is the right to withdraw from the HSD at any time.[61] This is technically possible without violating privacy and it is probably the single most significant device against misuse of information and maintaining trust in the HSD.

There is an additional benefit to the proposal about written authorisation for participation in HSD. One of the consequences of the legislation on the HSD is that medical doctors can be required to hand the medical records of patients who have not opted out of the database over to the licensee for processing information into the database. The licensee negotiates with the politically appointed board of each health care institution that has the legal authority to negotiate all transfer of information from medical records.[62] Understandably, the medical profession has reacted strongly to this policy. Not only is their professional autonomy threatened but also their status as guardians of information, which has been created in their confidential interaction with patients. In order to safeguard the trust that is the cornerstone of the

---

[61] This point is especially important because Icelandic political authorities have shown that they want to control the ethical review process. In 1999 the Minister of Health suddenly ousted the National Bioethics Committee whose members had been mainly nominated by academic institutes. Such an action is clearly damaging for the construction of trustworthy institutions, which is crucial for database research. Now the committee is nominated exclusively by the government. See, for example: A. Abbott. 'Strengthened' Icelandic Bioethics Committee comes under Fire. *Nature* 1999; 400: 602.

[62] DeCODE has already completed contracts to this effect with some of the smaller health care institutions in Iceland. Negotiations between deCODE and the National University Hospital have been going on but as I am preparing this paper for publication (November 2002), deCODE has decided to withdraw from these negotiations.

professional-patient relationship and to respect the responsibility of health care professionals, they should not be required to hand over medical records to third parties without their patients' written authorisation.[63] This is especially important when the third party is not involved in the patient's care. Moreover, if this trust is eroded it may affect the data that will be registered in medical records, both because patients could be less willing to unveil information and physicians would be more careful in what the write down, at least in the official records. This would, of course, diminish the quality of the scientific conclusions that will be reached from the HSD.[64]

This idea of a written authorisation could be tailored to fit consent for the use of biological samples in genetic epidemiological research in relation to HSD and the genealogical database. Since participants cannot be informed in advance about the specific aspects of the research normally required for informed consent, they could be asked to sign a written authorisation specifying more general, yet restricted, use of the samples for further research. They would also be informed about purposes of the research, security, access, review procedures, and the right to withdraw at any time and to have the samples destroyed. The main addition for authorisation of coded biosamples for unforeseen research would be about re-contacting sources. In this age of communication and information technology there are several ways to do this, and it could partly be in the hands of ethics committees to decide when there is a reason to re-contact participants (special scrutiny category) who could then opt-out of particular research projects. But the main task is to find effective ways to protect the interests of welfare and autonomy of the participants, which everyone agrees is the main objective of the ethics of research. Forging such a policy is the task of regulatory 'trustworthy institutions' which 'have to offer individuals simple and realistic ways of checking that what they consent to is indeed what happens and what they do not consent to does not happen.'[65]

---

[63] It has been argued (Palsson & Rabinow, *op. cit.* note 37, p. 170) that this position of the Icelandic Medical Association is based on 'a paternalistic and rigid category of knowledge.' True as this description of physicians often is, it fails in this particular case. Icelandic medical doctors should not be expected to 'follow the will of the majority of the Icelandic public' because their primary obligation is towards every single patient.

[64] Cf. Zoëga & Andersen, *op. cit.* note 1, pp. 33–64.

[65] O'Neill, *op. cit.* note 55, p. 702.

CONCLUSION

In this paper, I have considered the issues of privacy and consent in the debate about the Icelandic health sector database. I have examined the prevailing arguments for obtaining consent for the different type of databases that are being set up in Iceland. In particular, I have scrutinised the arguments for presuming consent for the transportation of information from medical records into the HSD. I have not found these arguments convincing. I argued that the traditional requirement for informed consent is not well suited for the collection of information into the HSD. I proposed the idea of a written authorisation, based on clear but general information about the right to withdraw and about the use, protection and purposes of HSD. This I take to be an alternative to both informed and presumed consent worth considering in the new research environment of multifaceted databases.

Giving up the requirement of informed consent for secondary research purposes that cannot be foreseen at the time of collection[66] certainly does not amount to asking individuals for blanket consent for future uses. Such a consent would give researchers optimal freedom for research but it is 'actually a waiver of consent, which is unacceptable for research.'[67] There is a need to search for an alternative to informed consent and uninformed blanket consent, which would strike a balance between respect for the participants and freedom of research. This task is of vital importance in the new research environment of databases that is now being created, not only in Iceland but also throughout the world.

Acknowledgements

This paper was produced as a part of the projects *The Ethical, Legal and Social Aspects of Human Genetic Databases: A European Comparison*, financed between 2002–2004 by the European Commission's Fifth Framework Programme (contract number QLG6-CT-2001-00062) and *The Ethics of Genetic and Medical Information* financed between 2002–2004 by the Nordic Academy for Advanced Study (NorFA). I gratefully acknowledge their support. However, the information provided is the sole responsibility of the author and does not represent the opinion of the European Community or NorFA, and they are not responsible

[66] Of course, informed consent would still be regarded as essential for medical treatment and participation in most primary research and in experimentation, the scenarios for which it was initially constructed.

[67] Annas, *op. cit.* note 36, p. 1832.

for any use that might be made of data appearing in this publication. I also thank the Research Fund of the University of Iceland and the Institute of Philosophy and Science Studies at Roskilde University for their support.

Earlier versions of this paper were read at the IVR conference at Pace University, New York City, USA, June 24–30 1999, and at the Second World Congress of Philosophy of Medicine, Jagiellionian University, Krakow, Polland, August 23–26 2000. I thank Gardar Árnason, Björn Gudbjörnsson, Lena Halldenius, Róbert Haraldsson, Páll Hreinsson, Ingileif Jónsdóttir, Jane Kaye and Sigurdur Kristinsson for useful comments on drafts of this paper. I also thank Ástrídur Stefánsdóttir and Sigurdur Gudmundsson for fruitful discussions about these issues.

PART VII: BEGINNING OF LIFE ISSUES

Chapter 25

IS IT GOOD TO MAKE HAPPY PEOPLE?

STUART RACHELS

It's good for people to be happy. Is it also good for there to be happy people? I will discuss:

Question 1. Would it be good for additional people to exist, assuming they would have lives worth living?

Forms of utilitarianism have been criticized for implying that it would be good. But I will argue that a state of affairs in which more happy people exist is better, other things being equal, than a state of affairs in which fewer happy people exist.[1] This bears not only on population policy but on individual decisions such as whether to abort and whether to treat defective newborns. The question for individual decision is:

Question 2. Does the fact that X would have a life worth living provide a reason for saving/prolonging/not ending X's life? (X could be a zygote or fetus, an embryo or infant, and so on.)

If the answer to Question 1 is Yes, then the answer to Question 2 is Yes because there is always some reason to bring about a better outcome. Thus, we have some reason not to abort most fetuses and to continue treating many genetically unlucky infants. But how much reason? I will discuss:

Question 3. If X would have a life worth living, and this provides a reason for creating or continuing X's life, is this a weak reason, easily overridden, or a strong reason, not easily set aside?

I will argue that the reason is strong but often overridden.

---

[1] I will use 'happy' interchangeably with 'has a life worth living'.

ARGUMENTS AGAINST THE CLAIM THAT IT IS GOOD FOR THERE TO BE ADDITIONAL HAPPY PEOPLE

The no-obligation argument

1. If it would be good for additional happy people to exist, then we would be morally obliged to have children whom we would prefer not to have.
2. We are not morally obliged to have children whom we would prefer not to have.
C. Therefore, it is not the case that it would be good for additional happy people to exist.

The first premise of this familiar argument is questionable. For one thing, creating people who would flourish might be good *in one respect* yet not be obligatory because countervailing considerations ensure that it would not be good *all things considered*. Although the new person might be happy, the consequences of bringing him or her into existence might be bad enough for other people that having the child would not be overall good. Second, creating people might be overall good but not good enough to warrant calling it an 'obligation' just as it is good to buy Girl Scout cookies even though we are not obliged to do so. Third, having children might be good but involve such sacrifices or be so psychologically demanding that it would be supererogatory rather than obligatory. And finally, having children might not be obligatory because there are better ways to use one's time and money. The thousands of dollars required to raise one child can save the lives of many starving children who already exist.[2]

These replies can be circumvented. A variant of the argument goes like this:

1. If it would be good for there to be additional happy people, then, if God exists, God would be obliged to create infinitely many people.
2. If God exists, God would be under no such obligation.
C. Therefore, it is not the case that it would be good for additional happy people to exist.

---

[2] See Peter Unger, *Living High and Letting Die: Our Illusion of Innocence* (Oxford University Press, New York, 1996).

Now I deny the second premise, as would anyone who rejects the conclusion.

Failing to create is bad for no one

It is tempting to argue as follows:

1. If there are reasons against behaving in a certain way, then that behavior is bad for someone.
2. If we do not create additional happy people, our behavior is bad for no one.
C1. Therefore, there are no reasons against not creating additional happy people.
4. But if it would be good for additional happy people to exist, then there would be reasons against not creating them.
C2. Therefore, it is not the case that it would be good for additional happy people to exist.[3]

Derek Parfit's Non-Identity cases show that premise 1 is false.[4] One such case is 'Depletion'. If we adopt a social policy of depleting resources, we both alter the identity of future generations and lower the future quality of life, although life would still be worth living. Depletion is bad for no one because the people who would exist would be happy, and without depletion they wouldn't exist. Nevertheless, there is reason not to deplete.

Following Narveson,[5] Bennett appeals to a principle similar to premise 1:

> The question of whether action A is morally obligatory depends only upon the utilities of people who would exist if A were not performed.[6]

Suppose we must perform either action A or action A_1. A_1 results in depletion and A does not. Is A morally obligatory? If it is, then

---

[3] Similar arguments are developed in Jan Narveson, 'Moral Problems of Population', *Monist*, 57 (1973), pp. 69–78; R.I. Sikora, 'Utilitarianism: the Classical Principle and the Average Principle', *Canadian Journal of Philosophy*, 5 (1975), pp. 413–416; and Thomas Schwartz, 'Obligations to Posterity' in *Obligations to Future Generations*, ed. R. I. Sikora and Brian Berry (Temple, Philadelphia, 1978), pp. 10–12.

[4] See Derek Parfit, *Reasons and Persons* (Oxford University Press, Oxford, 1984), ch. 16.

[5] Jan Narveson, 'Utilitarianism and New Generations', *Mind*, 76 (1967), pp. 62–72.

[6] Jonathan Bennett, 'On Maximizing Happiness' in *Obligations to Future Generations*, ed. R. I. Sikora and Brian Berry (Temple, Philadelphia, 1978), p. 62.

Bennett's principle fails because A would be obligatory because the utilities of those who would exist were it performed would be greater than the utilities of those who would exist if it were not. Alternatively, perhaps there is reason to perform A but A is not 'morally obligatory' – for example, A might be supererogatory, so A_1 would be permissible. This is consistent with Bennett's principle but inconsistent with using it to deduce a negative answer to Question 1. For the position affirms that the utilities of people we could create are relevant to whether we have reason to create them; it merely denies that such reason ever suffices to create obligations. Neither interpretation tends to show that it is not the case that it would be good for additional happy people to exist.[7]

Tooley's appeal to rights and obligations

Michael Tooley advances the general thesis:

> S: An action is prima facie wrong if and only if it involves a failure to fulfill an obligation regarding some individual, when it was possible to do so, or it makes it the case that there is some individual with respect to whom there will be an obligation that cannot be fulfilled.[8]

S revises the idea that, if there are reasons against behaving in a certain way, that behavior is bad for someone. S implies that, if there are reasons against behaving in a certain way, then that behavior is either bad for someone or creates an obligation that cannot be fulfilled. Thus, S implies that 'there is no prima facie obligation to produce additional persons' because 'refraining from producing additional persons does not in itself either violate an obligation with respect to any individual, or make it the case that there is an individual with respect to whom there are obligations that cannot be met'.[9] It is not part of S that it is prima facie wrong to fail to create someone with respect to whom obligations can be satisfied. However, when we create a person whose life must be miserable, our

---

[7] R.I. Sikora shows that Bennett's principle is subject to Non-Identity style counterexamples in 'Is It Wrong to Prevent the Existence of Future Generations?' in *Obligations to Future Generations*, ed. R.I. Sikora and Brian Berry (Temple, Philadelphia, 1978), pp. 162–163, fn. 18.

[8] Michael Tooley, *Abortion and Infanticide* (Oxford University Press, Oxford, 1983), p. 272.

[9] Tooley, *Abortion and Infanticide*, p. 272.

obligation to respect that person's right to life worth living cannot be fulfilled.[10]

Tooley says that S is 'free of unacceptable consequences'.[11] By itself, S has few consequences; it needs to be supplemented with principles specifying obligations. However, S is vulnerable to Non-Identity style counterexamples. Consider the case of Carlo and Jane. A woman trying to get pregnant is in danger of passing along a heart condition to her child – but only to a male child. This condition would be unpleasant at times but not fatal. The woman can take a pill to ensure a female child. Without this pill, she might have a boy named Carlo, and with it, she would have a girl called Jane. To ensure that Carlo and Jane are different people, assume that the pill would alter the timing of her pregnancy. Suppose that, if the woman does hot take the pill and (unluckily) gives birth to Carlo, Carlo would be provided for, but he would not be nearly as happy as Jane would have been.[12] The woman would be prima facie wrong not to take the pill, even though, if she has Carlo, it seems that she would have no unfulfilled obligations with respect to him.

Tooley agrees that the woman should take the pill.[13] However, he believes that there would be an unfulfilled obligation to Carlo. In defending this claim, he appeals to a principle of equal opportunity:

> Every person has a right to an equal chance of enjoying those natural resources, both environmental and genetic, that a person living in his society might enjoy, and that make it possible for one to lead a satisfying life.[14]

Hence, Carlo, with his genetic heart ailment, is denied an equal chance of enjoying at least some important genetic resources.

But there are at least two problems with this view:

---

[10] Tooley, *Abortion and Infanticide*, p. 272.

[11] Tooley, *Abortion and Infanticide*, p. 243.

[12] For a similar example, see Parfit, *Reasons and Persons*, p. 375.

[13] See Tooley, *Abortion and Infanticide*, section 7.33 (especially p. 262) and p. 268.

[14] Tooley, *Abortion and Infanticide*, p. 272. What does Tooley mean by 'those natural resources . . . that make it possible for one to lead a satisfying life?' He does not mean that each natural resource is needed to lead a satisfying life, for then his application of the principle would be invalid. (On p. 273, Tooley uses the principle to show why a woman shouldn't having a handicapped child, even though such a child could lead a satisfying life.) I interpret the principle to mean 'those natural resources . . . that typically make an important contribution to well-being'.

1. Suppose a couple is poor but happy. Would it be prima facie wrong for them to have a child? If we interpret S and the principle of equal opportunity such that they imply that it would be wrong for the woman not to take the pill, then those principles imply that it would be prima facie wrong for poor people to have children. After all, their children would have a less than equal chance of enjoying environmental resources.

One might think this is acceptable, since the poor couple's obligation is only a prima facie obligation that could be overridden. But the prima facie obligation can be easily turned into an absolute obligation. First, bear in mind that, according to S, the fact that a person would be happy is not a reason to create her. And suppose that this child's existence, on the whole, would neither benefit nor harm other people. It then follows that it would be wrong, all things considered, for the poor couple to bring this happy child into the world. This conclusion seems mistaken, especially since the child would be happy, despite enjoying fewer resources than most others.

2. Suppose half the population enjoys all the relevant natural resources. A woman is deciding whether to take a fertility pill with specific side-effects. If she takes the pill, she will have twins. One of those twins (we can't know which) will be healthy and enjoy all the resources, but the other will become sick and won't. Taking this pill is permissible, on Tooley's view, since each twin would have the same chance of enjoying the natural resources as the population at large (one chance in two). (It might count against Tooley's view that taking the same pill would be unacceptable if 52% of the people in the population enjoy the resources, for then each twin would have a less than equal chance of enjoyment.)

Change the example slightly. Call the twins the woman would have 'Lefty' and 'Righty.' Suppose the woman knows that Lefty would be the sick one. Now Tooley's view entails that it is impermissible for the woman to take the pill, since Lefty would not have a fair chance of enjoying health. But suppose that Lefty is the same person who would have become sick in the original example. Then, on Tooley's view, taking the first pill is permissible, while taking the second pill is impermissible, even though (i) they would lead to the same result, and (ii) if the second pill led to a different result, that result would be as bad as what would actually happen (Righty's being sick would be as bad as Lefty's being sick). This implication counts against Tooley's theory.

The no-benefit argument

Some philosophers say that *we do not benefit people by creating them*. This may seem to imply a negative answer to Question 1, in the following way:

1. A person who is created does not benefit from having been created.
2. If a person does not benefit from having been created, then adding that person to the world (even if she would be happy) does not make the world better.
C. Therefore, it is not the case that it would be good for additional happy people to exist.

The first premise is not obviously true; Parfit deftly defends its denial.[15] But that premise is true on some interpretations of 'benefit'. For example, a person does not benefit from being created if benefiting entails that someone's interests are better promoted than they would have been, and if having interests requires existing. However, the second premise would then beg the question, for the opposing camp believes that we have some reason to create happy people even if they don't benefit. Similarly, we have some reason not to create miserable people even if doing so harms no one.

The no-preference argument

Some people might be persuaded by this argument:

1. If it would be good for additional happy people to exist, then creating those people must satisfy some of their preferences.
2. Creating happy people does not satisfy any of their preferences.
C. Therefore, it is not the case that it would be good for additional happy people to exist.

We cannot fully assess this argument unless we know what theory of preference lies behind it. However, we can see that it is unsatisfactory by comparing it with this parallel argument:

1. If it would be bad for unhappy people to exist, then creating unhappy people must frustrate some of their preferences.

---

[15] Parfit, *Reasons and Persons*, pp. 487–490. John Bigelow and Robert Pargetter take a different view in 'Morality, Potential Persons and Abortion', *American Philosophical Quarterly*, 25, (1988).

2. Creating unhappy people does not frustrate any of their preferences.
C. Therefore, it is not the case that it would be bad for additional unhappy people to exist.

The conclusion of this parallel argument is false because it is bad when a person exists whose life contains intense, uncompensated suffering. Where does it go wrong? Since the argument is valid, it must have a false premise. But neither of its premises can be denied without undermining the corresponding premise of the No-Preference Argument. Its second premise may be challenged in two ways: (i) creating unhappy people frustrates desires because those people will prefer not to have been born; (ii) creating an unhappy person frustrates those desires that constitute the person's unhappiness. If either of these claims is true, then we should be able to say, against the second premise of the No-Preference Argument, that (i) creating happy people satisfies desires because those people will prefer to have been born; or (ii) creating a happy person satisfies those desires that constitute the person's happiness. A similar strategy applies to the first premise of the parallel argument. That premise utilizes the principle that *what is bad for people must frustrate their preferences*. It will be hard to defend this while denying that *what is good for people must satisfy their preferences*.

In short, the No-Preference Argument stands or falls with its parallel. Since its parallel falls, it falls.

Contractualism

Some contract theories are egoistic. These hold that morality is based entirely on agreements of mutual benefit. Thus, Gauthier calls contractualism 'the morality of mutual advantage'[16] and says that his theory 'denies any place to rational constraint, and so to morality, outside the context of mutual benefit.'[17] This implies that I have no reason to create additional happy people, unless doing so benefits me.

Contractual egoism is unsatisfactory because moral reasons exist outside the context of such agreements. If I see an animal suffering, and I can help it easily with no cost to myself, I should do so even

[16] David Gauthier, *Moral Dealing: Contract, Ethics and Reason* (Cornell University Press, Ithaca, 1990), p. 5.
[17] David Gauthier, *Morals By Agreement* (Oxford University Press, New York, 1986), p. 16.

though the animal cannot help me. Moreover, humans cannot benefit God, but God has moral reason to help those who suffer.

Turn now to a Rawlsian 'rightness as fairness' framework.[18] The contractors are still self-interested, but they do not know what place (if any?) they will occupy in society. Would they prefer more rather than fewer happy people in society? If fewer, then either:

(a) in the original position, the contractors know they will exist in society. In this case they wouldn't want additional happy people, provided that the base population would be happier than they would be if they had to share their resources with the additional people; or,

(b) the contractors do not know whether they will exist in society, but they are willing to risk not existing in society by allirming principles that do not grant the mere potential for happy existence in society much weight.[19] If (a), then the theory has ludicrous implications. For if the contractors know that they will exist, then they will prefer society X over society Y if each person in X is better off than each person in Y. And this is often unacceptable when all the people in X and Y have lives not worth living. For example, the contractors would prefer a society in which billions of people live in ghastly, repulsive conditions to one in which only a few people live in conditions very slightly worse.[20]

If the contractors do not know whether they will exist in society, it is not clear what population principles they would act on. Maximin alone would be a poor guide. For in a population containing only lives worth living, the least advantaged class would be the nonexistent, if some contractors do not exist in society. The theory would then imply that ten billion and one lives barely worth living are preferable to ten billion lives of very high quality (plus one life not lived) – an unacceptable result. Of course, the contractors could

---

[18] Rawls talks about *rightness as fairness* as a program to apply Rawlsian methods outside the sphere of justice. See *A Theory of Justice* (Harvard University Press, Cambridge, Mass., 1971), pp. 17, 111.

[19] Parfit only considers a version of (b) according to which the contractors do not know whether they will ever exist. This is incoherent because the contractors 'cannot assume that, in the actual history of the world, it might be true that [they] never exist'. (*Reasons and Persons*, p. 392.) But the contractors can assume that they never exist in society. For this reason Parfit's arguments fail to show that the contractualist method cannot be applied to questions of population size.

[20] Parfit makes a similar criticism. (*Reasons and Persons*, p. 393.)

apply principles characteristic of other theories; questions about population do not show the incompleteness of contractualism or Kantian constructivism. However, contractualism does not have a distinctive answer to these questions. And we still have no reason to believe that the contractors would affirm clauses that do not grant potential life in society much weight. We have no reason to believe (b).

The no-sympathy and the less-sympathy arguments

Some philosophers emphasize that we are *unmoved* by thoughts concerning potential people – they do not engage our sympathies in some hard-to-specify but essential way. The problem, it might be said, is not merely that we are insufficiently sympathetic; it is that we are completely unsympathetic, perhaps because, prior to the beginning of life, there is no one with whom to sympathize. Therefore, the interests of potential people don't matter. Alternatively, it may be said, we sympathize with potential people less than living people because we can't see, touch or befriend them; because they have no projects or desires; because they can't help us, harm us or hold us responsible for not creating them.

These arguments benefit from being offered in obscure or 'suggestive' ways. Put baldly, they are less persuasive:

1. We feel no sympathy for potential people.
C. Therefore, it is not the case that it would be good for additional happy people to exist.

1. We have less sympathy for potential people than for living people.
C. Therefore, it would be slightly good for additional happy people to exist.

These arguments are invalid because our sympathies are unreliable. Our capacity for sympathy is notoriously underdeveloped, for example, in connection with animal suffering and human starvation. We find it difficult to sympathize with pigs or people we don't know, but we should oppose factory farming and support human rights. Why shouldn't something similar be true of our lack of sympathy for potential people? Why shouldn't the thought that *if I were to have a child, that child would be happy* move a benevolent adult toward becoming a parent? This thought does not assume that there now exists someone with whom to sympathize.

The Less Sympathy Argument compromises: it concludes that potential people matter but not very much. There is another compromise to consider:

The average utility compromise

Some people believe that insofar as utility matters, what matters is average utility or the average level of well-being. Average utilitarianism implies that it is good for there to be additional happy people, but only when their existence augments average utility. However, this is unacceptable because it yields pairs of judgments such as the following:

- It is good to create someone who is mildly happy in a world in which happiness and unhappiness are balanced.
- It is bad to create someone more than mildly happy in a world in which there is huge average happiness.

Other arguments also show that the principle of average utility is mistaken. If a population lives in writhing agony, it would be better with respect to average utility if someone were added to the population whose agony was just a tiny bit less severe because this would increase the average level of well-being. But one more suffering soul does not improve the universe with respect to utility.[21]

We have now considered the most important arguments and principles entailing that it is not good for additional happy people to exist. These arguments and principles proved unsuccessful.

ARGUMENTS SUPPORTING THE CLAIM THAT IT IS GOOD FOR THERE TO BE ADDITIONAL HAPPY PEOPLE

Appeals to intuition

Some plausible beliefs suggest a positive answer to Question 1:

1. It would have been bad if the happiest million people in human history had never been born.

---

[21] Parfit, *Reasons and Persons*, p. 422. Also see Parfit's other objections to the average principle in this section.

2. It would have been bad if human beings had never evolved.
    (Assuming, here as elsewhere, that the good in human life
    outweighs the bad.)
3. It would be wrong for everyone to take a drug that causes both
    infertility and an indifference to being infertile, thus ensuring
    that the youngest generation alive will be the last.[22]
4. It would be good for God to add ten billion flourishing people
    to a distant part of the cosmos.

If 1–4 are true, the best explanation for their truth is that it would
be good for additional happy people to exist. 1–4 are true; so it
would be good for additional happy people to exist. Against this,
one may offer principles and arguments implying that some of 1–4
are false and the rest are true but not because it is good for happy
people to exist.[23] I won't try to adjudicate this dispute, but I submit
that 1–4 provide some evidence for answering Yes to Question 1.

An implausible consequence of asymmetry

It is bad for people to exist whose lives are not worth living or worse
than nothing. This is not to say that such people should be killed;
but we do believe it would be better, other things being equal, if
such people never came into existence. Consider John Seabrook's
remarks:

> When one thinks of a truly awful genetic disease, like Lesch-
> Nyhan syndrome, a rare mutation in the single X chromosome
> in males which causes mental retardation, extreme physical pain,

---

[22] This comes from Jonathan Glover, *Causing Death and Saving Lives* (Penguin, New York, 1977), p. 69.

[23] To justify something like 3, Bennett says 'someone might accept a principle enjoining the preservation of every species, or every animal species, or every instance of extreme physical complexity, or every form of life which is capable of moral reflection . . .' ('On Maximizing Happiness', p. 65.) Bennett, however, believes 3 because he wants our great biological and spiritual adventure to continue (p. 66). Compare Gregory Kavka on 'the collective enterprises of man' in 'The Futurity Problem' in *Obligations to Future Generations*, ed. R. I. Sikora and Brian Barry, (Temple, Philadelphia, 1978), pp. 196–198. Tooley says that 3 might be believed because one wants humankind's understanding of reality to advance, because one wants improved human interaction, or because one wants greater justice or fairer distribution of goods. (*Abortion and Infanticide*, pp. 257–258) In defense of something like 4, Bennett says, 'I share Leibniz's liking for rich, organic complexity, and so the discovery that our world has more of it than we realized would be good news indeed'. ('On Maximizing Happiness', p. 64.) If so, then it would better for more happy people to exist because then there would be more rich, organic complexity.

and compulsive self-mutilation – children savagely gnaw their fingers and lips unless they are constantly constrained one – wonders whether the child who would have to suffer from this condition has a right *not* to be born.[24]

It is bad for such human beings to exist.

Now suppose you believe that, while it would be bad for additional unhappy people to exist, it would not be good for additional happy people to exist. This combination of beliefs implies that it is wrong, other things being equal, to act with the predictable consequence that (a) 100,000 happy people come to be, if one's behavior also creates a slight chance of (b) one person existing whose life is not worth living.[25] Such behavior would be considered wrong because (b) counts against it while (a) does not count in its favor. Imagine that the one unhappy life would be *barely* not worth living and that everyone else is blissful. Does it not seem that the bliss of the one hundred thousand outweighs the chance of mild misfortune for one? If so, then it is good for those additional happy people to exist.

The symmetry argument

It is bad for people to exist whose lives are not worth living (at least in part) because their conscious states are unpleasant. Analogously, it is good for happy people to exist (at least in part) because their conscious states are pleasant. We can state the Symmetry Argument as follows:

1. The fact that someone's conscious experiences would be unpleasant is a reason against bringing that person into existence.
2. If (1), then the fact that someone's conscious experiences would be pleasant is a reason for bringing that person into existence.
C1. Therefore, the fact that someone's conscious experiences would be pleasant is a reason for bringing that person into existence.
C2. Therefore, it would be good for additional happy people to exist.

[24] John Seabrook, 'All in the Genes', *The New Yorker*, 12 Feb. 1996, p. 81.
[25] R.I. Sikora has a similar example. See 'Utilitarianism: the Classical Principle and the Average Principle', pp. 414–416, and 'Is It Wrong to Prevent the Existence of Future Generations?' p. 114 and elsewhere.

The Symmetry Argument is analogical. Just as pleasant experiences should be avoided, unpleasant experiences should be sought. How strong is the analogy? Pleasant and unpleasant experiences are ontologically similar: they are conscious items (whatever consciousness may be). Also, normally we have the same type of epistemic access to each: we know them by introspection. Furthermore, both have moral significance because of how they feel. If a sensation feels good, then to some extent it is good; and if a sensation feels bad, then to some extent it is bad.

Several objections to this argument rely on positions that I have already criticized. Appealing to Tooley's principle, one might say that we should not create a miserable person because doing so creates obligations that cannot be fulfilled; but there is no analogous reason to create a blissful person. Or one might say that creating a miserable person is bad for someone, but not creating a happy person is bad for no one. I have already addressed these and other challenges.

The analogy between parts of lives and whole lives

Suppose you expect to live many more years of high quality. If tomorrow you were to die tragically in a bizarre gardening accident,[26] this would not merely be worse for you, it would be bad *simpliciter*. Thus, it is worse that one should die rather than live many golden years before dying. Similarly, it is worse that one should not exist rather than live a golden life before dying. This argument is Parfit's:

> Consider someone dying painfully, who has already made his farewells. . . . He might decide that, at some point in the past, if he had known what lay before him, he would or would not have wanted to live the rest of his life. He might thus conclude that these parts of his life were better or worse than nothing. If such claims can apply to parts of lives, they can apply, I believe, to whole lives.[27]

The argument proceeds by analogy: parts of lives can be good (or bad), so whole lives can be good (or bad). Whole lives and parts of lives are the same sort of entity. It is hard to show a relevant

[26] Cf. Rob Reiner's *This Is Spinal Tap*.
[27] Parfit, *Reasons and Persons*, p. 487.

disanalogy between them that does not rely on a principle or argument criticized above.

I have argued in four ways that it would be good for additional happy people to exist. These arguments provide much better evidence than the opposing arguments. Therefore, it is good for additional happy people to exist.

HOW VALUABLE IS POTENTIAL LIFE?

We may approach this issue by asking whether potential people matter as much as adults. Suppose that Cayce, an adult, has a life of neutral value. Further suppose that we must choose between (i) raising Cayce's life to a high level of prosperity and (ii) creating a new person at that high level. Most of us believe that, other things being equal, (i) is better than (ii), and not merely because (i) is better with respect to average utility. Most of us believe that adult potential matters more than the potential of the unconceived. I believe that (ii) is as good as (i). I will argue for the *Strong Thesis*, which holds that potential people matter as much as adults.[28] The Strong Thesis suggests that potential life should weigh heavily in our reasoning. It implies that *this life would be worth living* provides the same sort of reason for creating life as it does for augmenting and prolonging adult life.

The Strong Thesis should be understood to include the claim that *the longer duration of happy life an individual has in prospect, the stronger the reason for creating or saving her*. So, other things being equal, the reason for prolonging life will be stronger if the individual is younger – say, an infant rather than a college student. This does not entail that infant interests normally outweigh adult interests because our resources often stretch further among adults than among the young. This is due to the fact that infants need considerable care before they can provide for themselves.

A. A version of the Symmetry Argument supports the Strong Thesis. Consider:

---

[28] R. M. Hare would support the Strong Thesis. See 'Abortion and the Golden Rule', *Philosophy and Public Affairs*, 4 (1975), reprinted in *Philosophy and Sex*, ed. Robert Baker and Frederick Elliston (Prometheus, New York, 1984), pp. 231–248.

The Strong Thesis As Regards Lives Not Worth Living: Suppose that Cayce has a life of neutral value. Further suppose we must choose between (i) making Cayce terribly miserable and (ii) creating a new person who will be terribly miserable. (i) is not worse than (ii), assuming away any influence the average principle might have on our assessment.[29]

This principle is (plainly) true: potential people becoming actual and suffering is as bad as adults suffering. But if so, then potential people becoming actual and flourishing is as good as adults flourishing. Together these two claims imply the Strong Thesis. It may seem that there are disanalogies that spoil the argument. However, I tried to answer such objections in assessing arguments against the claim that it is good for additional happy people to exist.

B. The analogy between parts of lives and whole lives can be used to support the Strong Thesis:

1. Parts of my life are better or worse than nothing.
2. If a part of my life is better or worse than nothing, then a whole life of similar quality and duration is exactly as good or bad as that part.
C1. Therefore, whole lives matter as much as parts of lives.
C2. Therefore, potential people matter as much as adults.

As before, the argument rests on a comparison between entities of the same sort: whole lives and parts of lives. I have not found satisfactory arguments to block the analogy.

THE POTENTIAL FOR HIGH QUALITY LIFE IS IMPORTANT IN CASES INVOLVING THE VERY YOUNG

The Strong Thesis has unsettling implications. It implies that potential happiness provides a stronger reason for helping infants and potential persons than adults with similar prospects. If there is something bad about a handicapped adult dying (who would have had a rich life), then there is something worse about a fetus with the same abnormality dying. And if there is something bad about your dying, then there is something worse about parents similar to

[29] Sikora agrees: see 'Is It Wrong to Prevent the Existence of Future Generations?' pp. 140–142.

yours not having children. If this last claim seems implausible, it is probably because we value potential life too little and our own lives too much.

How important, practically, is potential? One answer is provided by a thesis I call 'the Preservation of Life Worth Living':

> We should always do whatever is necessary to prolong young life that would be worth living.

This principle is too strong because sometimes it would be better to use our resources on projects other than helping the young and sick. Consider infants with spina bifida or Down syndrome, for example. Gregory Pence notes that 'Spina hifida and Down syndrome are agonizing cases exactly because many of those afflicted can attain lives worth living'.[30] In such a case, when complications arise, great resources should not be expended on the infant, since they can be put to better use. An infant may be allowed to die painlessly, so his mother can have a different child, whose life might be more rewarding both to itself and to others.[31] Alternatively, the mother may be encouraged to use her money to help other children living in poverty. If the objection to letting a sick infant die is lost potential, then more potential can be gained through having another child or helping other people.[32]

This may be thought to imply that it is permissible to allow afflicted adults to die painlessly. However, this reasoning cannot automatically be transferred to adults because, first, adults might have a right to medical treatment that infants do not have. (This is not my approach, but it does not obviously conflict with my arguments.) Second, adults, unlike infants, typically have social networks that would suffer from their deaths. Third, many policies that would let sick adults die would cause regrettable social upheaval. And, fourth, afflicted adults typically need fewer resources before becoming self-sufficient than afflicted infants who need to grow up.

So the Strong Thesis does not entail that lives worth living should always be saved. As R.M. Hare said of abortion, 'if the termination

---

[30] Gregory E. Pence, *Classic Cases in Medical Ethics*, 1st edn (McGraw-Hill, New York, 1990), p. 151.

[31] Hare makes a similar point on p. 240 of 'Abortion and the Golden Rule'.

[32] 'But are human lives, in this way, like money – what matters being not the particular notes, only the total at the bottom of the ledger?' (James P. Griffin, 'Modern Utilitarianism,' *Revue Internationale de Philosophie*, 141 (1982), p. 367.) I answer Yes to the spirit of this question, although I reject the numerical metaphor, 'the total at the bottom of the ledger'.

of this pregnancy facilitates or renders possible or probable the beginning of another more propitious one, it really does not take much to justify it'.[33] Thus, it may seem as though potential lives rarely need to be protected. But I wish to steer away from such a conclusion. Jonathan Glover, who accepts this conclusion, endorses the view that additional happy people augment the world's value. He says, 'This is likely to arouse feelings of horror in many people. . . . We may think of an exhausted mother of eight children feeling obliged to have still more. Or we may think of starvation, shortages and overcrowding caused by overpopulation'.[34] But, says Glover:

> In practice, the disastrous side-effects of people feeling obliged to have children they do not want, and of having too large a population for the world's resources, together with the more problematic happiness of children not really wanted, will nor- mally heavily outweigh the view that, if other things were equal, the more happy people there are the better. Even if we adopted the total view, it seems likely that in many cases the addition to the population of extra people with worth-while lives would often not even increase the total happiness.[35]

This view is probably too pessimistic. Babies may be put up for adoption; aren't they likely to have lives worth living? Consider similar reasoning applied to an adult. Imagine that you must choose between letting an adult die of a disease or saving her. Saving her would be burdensome: it might involve your acting as a nurse for an extended period, after which time her health should return to normal and you can resume your regular life. Also suppose that you are asked to care for this woman because she does not have close friends. Now consider this reasoning:

> In practice, the disastrous side-effects of people feeling obliged to save lives they do not want to save, and of having too large a population for the world's resources, together with the more problematic happiness of adults not really loved by others, will normally heavily outweigh the view that, if other things were equal, the more happy people there are the better. Even if we adopted the total view, it seems likely that in many cases the

---

[33] Hare, 'Abortion and the Golden Rule', p. 247.
[34] Glover, *Causing Death and Saving Lives*, p. 70.
[35] Glover, *Causing Death and Saving Lives*, p. 70. Sikora agrees; see 'Utilitarianism: the Classical Principle and the Average Principle', p. 411.

preservation of people with worth-while lives would not increase the total happiness.

Glover's remarks seem plausible. These remarks do not. But there is no significant difference between them – at least, the fact that one case involves an adult and the other involves a potential person makes no difference. Which view is superior? The Strong Thesis represents a substantial departure from common sense. Normally we think of the prospect of happiness as being *much less* significant for potential persons than for adults. And although we value our own lives too much, we do not normally value the lives of other adults too highly. Hence, we undervalue potential persons more than we overvalue other adults. This suggests that we should put more trust in our assessment of the second case than in Glover's claim that extra happy people would often not increase the total happiness.

We ought to adopt a position between Glover's and the Preservation of Life Worth Living. In practice, the appeal to potential is sometimes decisive and sometimes overridden. Yet it weighs more heavily in the case of infants than in the case of adults. Thus, the value of potential life matters more than most people think in assessing abortion, commercial surrogacy, contraception, eugenics, infanticide, sterilization of the mentally retarded, teenage pregnancy and the question of how vigorously to treat human beings with a variety of handicaps and disorders whose lives would be worth living. We should not always choose to secure more worth-while lives, but securing fewer will always require a strong, overriding reason.

Chapter 26

GENES, EMBRYOS, AND FUTURE PEOPLE

WALTER GLANNON

INTRODUCTION

Recent advances in reproductive biotechnology have given us the ability to intervene in the process of human biological development from embryos to people. One type of intervention is the testing of embryos for genetic defects that cause disease, which enables us to choose between allowing these embryos to result in disabled people or selectively terminating their further development. Alternatively, in the foreseeable future it may become possible to prevent disease by correcting a mutation in embryonic cells or by inserting a normal gene into these cells. It even may become possible to manipulate genes in such a way as to enhance people's normal cognitive and physical functioning. Still another form of intervention in the development of a human organism is the freezing of an embryo in liquid nitrogen to postpone the birth of a person who subsequently will come into existence from that embryo. All of these interventions give us considerable control over how many people will exist, when people will come into existence, and what sort of people there will be.

I shall explore the moral implications of these technologies and argue that we are morally required to intervene in the process of biological development of human organisms by testing and selectively terminating embryos with genetic defects that cause people to exist with severe disease and disability. As a matter of beneficence, we have a duty to prevent avoidable pain and suffering in the people we bring into existence. As a matter of justice, we have a duty not to cause people to exist with cognitive and physical disabilities that will limit their opportunities for achieving a decent minimum level of lifetime well-being. Each of these claims is motivated by the following moral asymmetry thesis: we do not have a moral duty to bring people into existence with good lives; but we do have a moral duty to prevent the existence of people who would experience so much pain and suffering as to make their lives not worth living for them on the whole.[1] Furthermore, in deciding whether to keep embryos frozen for long periods of time, we have to consider the psychological impact on children born from these embryos after the deaths of their biological parents, or when their parents are at an advanced age. In addition, we must consider whether we can justify keeping genetically defective embryos frozen until the time when inserting a missing gene or correcting a mutant gene become feasible practices.

MORAL ASYMMETRY AND HARM

The moral asymmetry thesis that I articulated above rests on three notions. The first is the person-affecting principle, which says that a person is benefited or harmed when her interests in what happens to her are satisfied or defeated.[2] Once a person exists, she has an interest in not experiencing pain and suffering and thus can be harmed if she experiences these over the course of her lifetime. The second notion is the impersonal comparative principle, which says that, other things being equal, it is worse to cause a person to exist if it would be possible to cause a different, better-off, person to exist

---

[1] This thesis derives from Jan Narveson's claim that we do not have a moral duty to make happy people, but only to make people happy. He argues that the benefit of an act is the good it brings to already existing people and does not include the good of people who come into existence as a result of the act. See 'Utilitarianism and New Generations', *Mind* 76 (1967), pp. 62–72, and 'Moral Problems of Population', *Monist* 57 (1973), pp. 62–86. John Broome and Adam Morton discuss different aspects of the moral asymmetry thesis in 'The Value of A Person', *Proceedings of the Aristotelian Society*, Supplementary Volume 68 (1994), pp. 167–98.

[2] Here I follow the definition of harm given by Joel Feinberg in *Harm to Others* (New York, Oxford University Press, 1984), pp. 102–104, and Allen Buchanan and Dan Brock in *Deciding for Others: The Ethics of Surrogate Decision Making* (New York, Cambridge University Press, 1989), pp. 162–169. Broome, *ibid.*, Derek Parfit, *Reasons and Persons* (Oxford, Clarendon Press, 1984), Part IV, and John Harris, *Wonderwoman and Superman: The Ethics of Human Biotechnology* (Oxford, Oxford University Press, 1992), p. 89, define personal harm in comparative terms. That is, a person is harmed when she is made worse off than she would have been otherwise. I avoid using the comparative sense of harm in considering whether being caused to exist with disabilities harms people, because these people would not exist without the disabilities they have, and a coherent comparison can be made only between two states of existence. The comparative sense of harm can be invoked only insofar as people exist and have interests. Otherwise, we should use an impersonal sense of harm, comparing two distinct potential lives of two distinct potential people.

instead.[3] It involves a comparison, not between the existence and non-existence of one person, but rather between two distinct lives of two distinct people. On the impersonal comparative principle, we evaluate two potential lives of two potential people who do not yet exist, while on the person-affecting principle we evaluate the life of one person who already exists. Yet we can appeal to both principles to support the claim that we are morally required to prevent the existence of people with lives that on balance are not worth living. That is, we prevent harm to the individuals we cause to exist by fulfilling their interest in not having to experience pain and suffering, and we avoid adding to the total amount of suffering in the world.[4] The third notion on which the moral asymmetry thesis rests is the metaphysical relation between embryos and persons.

'Person' is a psychological concept, while 'human organism is a biological concept. A human organism, in the form of a single-celled zygote, begins to exist at around the time of conception, when male and female gametes fuse.[5] Thereafter, the zygote develops into a multi-celled embryo, a presentient fetus, a sentient fetus, and then the body and brain of a person. The zygote, embryo, fetus, and person are distinct but biologically related stages in the development of a human organism. Up to about 14 days after fertilization there is the possibility of monozygotic twinning of the fused gametes. When it occurs, twinning causes two genetically identical but numerically distinct individual organisms to exist from the original zygote, and these subsequently develop into two distinct persons with distinct psychological properties. A person begins to exist when the fetal stage of the organism develops the structure and function of the brain necessary to generate and support consciousness and mental life. This is when the fetus becomes

---

[3] Parfit defends this principle in *Reasons and Persons*, Ch. 18, and 'Comments', *Ethics* 96 (1986), pp. 858 ff., as does Jonathan Glover, 'Future People, Disability, and Screening', in Peter Laslett and James Fishkin, eds. *Justice Between Age Groups and Generations* (New Haven, Yale University Press, 1992), pp. 127–143.

[4] This idea is discussed by Parfit, *Reasons and Persons*, and Harris, *Wonderwoman and Superman*, p. 90.

[5] See Michael Lockwood, 'When Does A Life Begin?', in Lockwood, ed., *Moral Dilemmas in Modern Medicine* (Oxford, Oxford University Press, 1985), pp. 9–31, Norman M. Ford, *When Did I Begin?* (Cambridge, Cambridge University Press, 1988), pp. 97 ff., Stephen Buckle, Karen Dawson, and Peter Singer, 'The Syngamy Debate: When Precisely Does A Human Life Begin?', in Singer et al., eds., *Embryo Experimentation* (Cambridge, Cambridge University Press, 1990), Ch. 19, Harris pp. 61–65, and Jeff McMahan, 'The Metaphysics of Brain Death', *Bioethics* 9 (1995), pp. 91–126.

sentient, at around 23–24 weeks of gestation. Because the structure and function of the organism's brain which generate and support the psychological properties essential to personhood develop gradually, persons come into existence gradually. The zygotic, embryonic, and presentient fetal stages of the organism are related to the person who develops from them to the extent that they all have the same DNA in their cells and that the psychological properties of the person causally depend on the biological properties of the organism. But because a person's essential psychological properties are distinct from, and emerge later than, the biological properties that define these other stages in the development of an organism, a person is neither identical with any one of these stages nor with the organism itself.[6] The embryo or presentient fetus is a potential person, not in the sense that it becomes a person, which implies numerical identity, but only in the sense that it has the potential to develop the biological structures and functions necessary to generate the consciousness and mental life constitutive of personhood.[7]

The metaphysical distinction between human organisms and persons has significant implications for the manipulation of genes in embryonic cells. The manipulation of one or more genes in these cells would not disrupt the identity of the *organism*, provided that its basic structure and function remained intact. Yet it would determine the identity of a different *person*. For, as Robert Elliot has pointed out, even slight changes to the biological properties of an organism at the zygotic or embryonic stage would cause different psychological properties to develop and thus select between

---

[6] McMahan draws a similar distinction between persons and human organisms in 'The Metaphysics of Brain Death', as does Robert Elliot in 'Identity and the Ethics of Gene Therapy', *Bioethics* 7 (1993), pp. 27–40, and 'Genetic Therapy, Person-Regarding Reasons and the Determination of Identity', *Bioethics* 11 (1997), pp. 151–60. Compare these accounts with that of Ingmar Persson, who draws a three-fold distinction between a conceptus, a human being, and a person in 'Genetic Therapy, Identity and the Person-Regarding Reasons', *Bioethics* 9 (1995), pp. 16–31. For a defense of the view that we are essentially human animals, see Eric Olson, *The Human Animal: Personal Identify Without Psychology* (Oxford, Clarendon Press, 1996), and 'Was I Ever A Fetus?', *Philosophy and Phenomenological Research* 57 (1997), pp. 43–59.

[7] In *Causing Death and Saving Lives* (Harmondsworth, Penguin, 1977), Glover says that a fetus is a potential person (p. 122), and Harris holds that embryos are potential persons, or 'pre-persons' (p. 58). Buckle subtly discusses the difference between the potential to *become* and the potential to *produce* in 'Arguing from Potential', *Bioethics* 2 (1988), pp. 227 ff. Reprinted in Singer et al., Ch. 9.

which of a number of different people would come into existence.[8] However, once an embryo has developed into a child with consciousness and mental life, genetic manipulation of its body's cells is more likely to be identity-preserving of personhood than identity-determining, since it already has developed a set of psychological properties. If this is correct, then the earlier genetic manipulation occurs in the development of a human organism, the more likely it is to determine that distinct people come into existence from it.

On the plausible assumptions that only beings with interests can be harmed by the defeat of those interests, that having interests presupposes sentience, and that only late-stage fetuses and persons are sentient, it is morally permissible to terminate a human organism at an early stage of development. The termination affects no one who has interests. One might object that having interests does not presuppose sentience. For example, it may be said that future people, who do not yet exist and are not sentient, have an interest not to live in a polluted environment.[9] But the core concept at issue here is harm, and harm consists in the defeat of particular interests of identifiable persons who already exist and can experience the defeat of these interests. Terminating the development of a human organism at the embryonic stage does not kill a person but only prevents a person from coming into existence. There is no one who could be harmed because there is no identifiable individual with particular interests who exists at that time.

Similar reasoning underwrites the claims that we do not have a moral duty to bring people into existence, and that bringing someone into existence by itself does not benefit her, however good her life may be. We cannot say that being caused to exist is better for a person than she otherwise would have been, since otherwise *she* would not have existed. Put differently, there is no one *who* is caused to exist; rather, we make it the case *that* someone exists.

---

[8] Elliot, 'Identity and the Ethics of Gene therapy', and 'Genetic Therapy, Person-Regarding Reasons and the Determination of Identity'. McMahan explores the implications of the differences between genetic techniques that are identity-determining and those that are identity-preserving in 'Cognitive Disability, Misfortune, and Justice', *Philosophy & Public Affairs* 25 (1996), pp. 3–35.

[9] Tom Regan first argued for this position in 'Feinberg on What Sorts of Beings Can Have Rights', *Southern Journal of Philosophy* 14 (1976), pp. 485–498.

Derek Parfit argues that the relation between existence and non-existence does not meet the 'Full Comparative Requirement', which says that we benefit someone only if we do what will be better for him.[10] While causing someone to exist may be good for him, it cannot make him better off since nonexistence is morally neutral and therefore neither good nor bad. We do not have a moral duty to benefit persons by bringing them into existence, because we benefit persons by satisfying their interests, and it is difficult to see how non-existing persons could have an interest in being caused to exist.

However, while it is morally neutral to cause a person to exist with a life that on balance is good, it is morally wrong to bring a person into existence with a life that on balance is bad because of severe pain and suffering. For in this case there *is* someone who actually experiences pain and suffering and who is harmed by being caused to exist in such a condition. And since it is not morally neutral but wrong, we have a moral duty to prevent the existence of a person who would have such a life. Yet there is an air of paradox about the idea that, although we do not benefit people by bringing them into existence with lives that are good on the whole, we harm people by causing them to exist with restricted lives that are bad on the whole.[11] Presumably, we harm someone by causing them to exist with a disability because we make them worse off than they otherwise would have been. But if they did not exist with the disability, then they would not have existed at all. Insofar as a person's life is worth living on the whole, being brought into existence with a cognitive or physical disability cannot be worse for her, because if we terminated the development of the embryo containing the gene that caused the disability, then she would not

---

[10] *Reasons and Persons*, pp. 488–489.

[11] In 'The Paradox of Future Individuals', *Philosophy & Public Affairs* 11(1982), pp. 93–112, Gregory Kavka defines a restricted life as 'one that is significantly deficient in one or more of the major respects that generally make human lives valuable and worth living' (p. 105). Yet Kavka says further that 'restricted lives typically will be worth living, on the whole, for those who live them' (p. 105). When I say that life is or is not worth living for a person, I mean it in the subjective rather than objective sense, or, what it is like for the person who lives it. McMahan offers insightful discussions of this and related issues in 'Cognitive Disability, Misfortune, and Justice', and 'Wrongful Life: Paradoxes in the Morality of Causing People to Exist', in Jules Coleman and Christopher Morris, eds., *Rational Commitment and Social Justice: Essays for Gregory Kavka* (Cambridge, Cambridge University Press, forthcoming).

exist. This is a variant of what Parfit has called the 'Non-Identity Problem'.[12]

Jonathan Glover has devised a strategy to sidestep the NonIdentity Problem. Instead of trying to draw a comparison between the existence and non-existence of one identifiable individual, Glover maintains that the relevant comparison is between two distinct lives of two distinct people. It is 'impersonal' in the sense that 'harm can be done even though identifiable people are no worse off than they otherwise would have been'.[13] Glover uses the following example to illustrate the impersonal comparative principle. Imagine that a factory emits a chemical that causes babies to be born blind. On the Non-Identity Problem, they are not made worse off than they otherwise would have been, since their lives are worth living and otherwise they would not have existed. But 'what we should say here is, not that the pollution made the blind children worse off than they would have been otherwise, but instead that their condition is worse than the condition of the other children who would have been born in the absence of the pollution.'[14] The choice is between bringing different people into existence, while retaining the same number of people who will exist.[15] Both person-affecting and impersonal harm principles give us reasons to bring a normal child into existence rather than a diseased or disabled one. We prevent actual people from experiencing pain and suffering and thereby avoid defeating their interest in having healthy lives, and we avoid adding to the total amount of suffering in the world.

In some genetically caused diseases, severe cognitive and physical disability may make people's lives so restricted that they are not worth living. By definition, these lives fall outside the scope of the

---

[12] *Reasons and Persons*, Ch. 16, and 'Comments', pp. 854–862. Others who address this problem include McMahan, 'Cognitive Disability' and 'Wrongful Life', Kavka, 'The Paradox of Future Individuals', James Woodward, 'The Non-Identity Problem', *Ethics* 96 (1986), pp. 804–31, Matthew Hanser, 'Harming Future People', Philosophy & *Public Affairs* 19 (Winter 1990), pp. 47–70, and David Heyd, *Genethics: Moral Issues in the Creation of People* (Berkeley, University of California Press, 1992), Chs. 4, 6. Robert Adams first articulated the Non-Identity Problem in 'Existence, Self-Interest, and the Problem of Evil', *Nous* 13, (1979), pp. 65–76.

[13] 'Future People, Disability, and Screening', p. 141.

[14] *Ibid.*, p. 142.

[15] I assume that the same number of people will exist in the different outcomes. This avoids complications involving different numbers of people and having to determine which group is better or worse off than others. See Parfit's discussion of 'Same People Choices', 'Same Number Choices', and 'Different Number Choices' in *Reasons and Persons*, pp. 356 ff. See also Hanser, 'Harming Future People', and Heyd, *Genethics*.

Non-Identity Problem. When we can predict that a disease would involve so much disability, pain, and suffering as to make life not worth living on the whole, we are morally required to prevent the existence of people who would have the disease. Or, if we do cause people to exist with such a disease, then we are morally required to either cure them or alleviate the severity of their symptoms, insofar as we are able. The first scenario that I described pertains to the impersonal sense of harm and potential persons, while the second pertains to the personal sense of harm and actual persons. One suggests genetic testing and selective termination of defective embryos as the appropriate strategy to prevent harm. The other suggests that the appropriate strategy to prevent or compensate for harm would be gene therapy or some other form of genetic alteration. A person is a further stage of development of the same human organism of which the embryo is an earlier stage. In this sense, embryos are potential persons, and failing to terminate a genetically defective embryo can cause harm by allowing it to develop into a diseased or disabled person.[16] Because gene therapy is not yet feasible for most diseases, genetic testing and selective termination of genetically defective embryos appears to be the only medically effective and morally defensible way to prevent the sort of harm at issue. Before defending this claim, however, we should examine the different forms of genetic intervention and assess their medical and moral significance.

GENETIC INTERVENTION

There are three basic types of genetic alteration.[17] Gene therapy consists in the correction or addition of genes in the somatic (body)

---

[16] Helga Kuhse and Peter Singer claim that 'we can, of course, damage the embryo in such a way as to cause harm to the sentient being *it* will become, if it lives, but if it never becomes a sentient being, the embryo has not been harmed'. See 'Individuals, Humans, and Persons: The Issue of Moral Status', in *Embryo Experimentation*, p. 82. Furthermore, Harris maintains that 'harm done at the preperson (embryo) stage will be harm done to the actual person *she* becomes. It is a form of delayed-action wrongdoing'. *Wonderwoman and Superman*, p. 153. I believe that persons can be harmed or wronged by what we do or fail to do to embryos even if embryos do not strictly speaking become persons.

[17] Patricia Baird provides an excellent overview of these issues in 'Altering Human Genes: Social, Ethical, and Legal Implications', *Perspectives in Biology and Medicine* 37 (1994), pp. 566–75. See also Leroy Walters and Julie Gage Palmer, *The Ethics of Human Gene Therapy* (New York, Oxford University Press, 1997).

cells of a person to treat a disease the person already has, where the aim of treatment is to cure the disease or alleviate its symptoms. By contrast, genetic alteration of germ cells (gametes; sperm and egg) at the zygotic or embryonic stage of the human organism prevents diseased persons from coming into existence. It is therefore mistaken to call this form of genetic manipulation 'therapy,' because when the gametes are altered, there are no existing persons who might benefit from this act.[18] 'Therapy' implies that there is a disease to be treated or cured, and it is not zygotes or embryos but rather persons or late-term fetuses who are diseased. Defective genes in embryonic cells may be the causes of diseases, but the diseases do not manifest themselves until the organism has developed into a fetus or person. Unlike somatic-cell gene therapy, which preserves the identity of already existing persons who are treated, germ-line genetic alteration determines the identity of the person who would come into existence from the embryo in which a defective gene is corrected or replaced by a normal one. The intervention takes place before the process of cell differentiation and the development of tissues and bodily organs has begun, and thus determines that a biologically and psychologically distinct individual will come into existence from the one who would have come into existence from the same embryo had the defective gene not been corrected or replaced. Genetic enhancement involves non-therapeutic alteration of genes aimed at improving cognitive and physical functioning which already are at or above the normal level for persons.

The three types of genetic alteration which I have mentioned are to be distinguished further from selective termination of embryos after genetic testing has revealed the presence of disease-causing genes, or markers for these genes, in the cells of embryos.[19] Like germ-line genetic alteration, germ-line genetic testing and

---

[18] Elliot and Persson fail to recognize this in their respective uses of 'gene therapy'.

[19] The diseases I discuss involve genetic defects in the nuclei of cells. Genes in the mitochondria of cells can mutate in the same way that the more familiar nuclear genes do. And like nuclear genes, mutations in mitochondrial genes may lead to disease. There are indications that familial Alzheimer disease may be caused by a faulty mitochondrial gene, though the research has not yet yielded any definitive conclusions. Moreover, my concern is with genetic testing rather than genetic screening. '*Genetic testing* denotes the use of specific assays to determine the genetic status of individuals already suspected to be at high risk for a particular inherited condition because of family history of clinical symptoms; *genetic screening* involves the use of various genetic tests to evaluate populations or groups of individuals independent of a family history of a disorder.' Arno Motulsky et al., *Assessing Genetic Risks: Implications for Health and Social Policy* (Washington, D. C., National Academy Press, 1994), p. 4.

termination is not a therapeutic but a preventive strategy designed to avoid the existence of individuals who would be severely disabled and have restricted lives. Let us now further explore the four types of genetic intervention at the embryonic stage of development of a human organism.

Somatic-cell gene therapy is not yet feasible for treating the majority of genetically caused diseases. This is because gene therapy is primarily relevant to single-gene disorders, and chromosomal disorders such as Down syndrome involve large segments of DNA which are not amenable to treatment. Moreover, the single-gene disorders that might be amenable to gene therapy are recessive rather than dominant disorders. Recessive disorders, where a single copy of the normal gene is sufficient for one to function within the normal cognitive and physical range for persons, may be treatable because inserting one copy of a normal gene into someone with a double dose of the defective gene may be enough to raise that individual's functioning or health up to the normal range. Dominant disorders, by contrast, result even when the affected person has only a single copy of the defective gene. These disorders might be prevented or cured by correcting the mutation within the gene. Presently, however, it is not possible to correct a mutation but only to insert an additional normal copy of a gene into cells, and therefore only recessive disorders can be treated through genetic intervention.

In theory, a recessive disorder like cystic fibrosis (CF) could be treated by inserting a normal gene into the relevant cells so that the pancreas produced the necessary enzymes for food absorption, as well as to ensure proper function of the glands in the lining of the bronchial tubes. Similarly, in hemophiliacs, who are unable to produce normal amounts of a factor necessary for blood clotting, the missing gene could be delivered through injections. In practice, though, what has plagued the efforts of gene therapy to cure people of diseases, or at least effectively treat their symptoms, is the lack of suitable vectors to deliver therapeutic genes into human cells and maintain them in working order. Viral vectors have been the method used to date, specifically adenoviruses and retroviruses, which slice copies of their genes permanently into the chromosomes of the cells they enter. Yet this method has been largely unsuccessful because the stripped-down viruses that have been used do not provide a stable platform for the genes to operate efficiently. Some of these viruses are not large enough to carry a full human gene and its switches, while others may provoke an adverse response by the immune system. Work on hemophiliacs, children with severe combined immunodeficiency disease (SCID), and familial hypercholesterolemia has shown some promise. But for the majority of genetically based diseases, gene therapy is not yet an effective cure or treatment.[20]

Germ-line genetic alteration initially may seem more attractive than gene therapy. Manipulation or replacement of genetic abnormalities in germ cells at the zygotic or embryonic stage after *in vitro* fertilization (IVF) would correct a defect before it could manifest itself as a disease in an existing person. This type of alteration would affect the resulting cells in the process of differentiation and in turn the germ line of the person who develops from the embryo. The altered genes would then be passed on to future generations of the person's offspring. But it is questionable whether germ-line genetic manipulation would be desirable from an evolutionary perspective. Some degree of genetic mutation is necessary for species to adapt to changing environmental circumstances, and some genetic disorders confer benefits on certain populations. For example, the gene for sickle-cell anemia provides greater resistance to malaria. Altering a gene or genes at the germ line to correct one disorder may only lead to other disorders. This also raises the question of whether we have a duty to prevent passing on unforeseeable consequences of germ-line alteration to future generations, which is morally significant for two reasons. First, people existing in the future might be adversely affected by a policy to which they did not consent. Second, it would be extremely difficult to determine whether the benefits of such a policy would outweigh its harms, in which case it may be morally preferable to err on the side of caution and prevent such a policy from being implemented. In sum, there may be both medical and moral reasons against germ-line genetic alteration.

---

[20] But see R.M. Blaese et al., 'Treatment of Severe Combined Immunodeficiency (SCJD) Due to Adenosine Deaminase Deficiency with CD34+ Selected Autologous Blood Cells Transduced with a Human ADA Gene', *Human Gene Therapy* 4 (1993), pp. 521–527, M. Grossman et al., 'Successful *Ex Vivo* Gene Therapy Directed to Liver in a Patient with Familial Hypercholesterolemia', *Nature Genetics* 6 (1994), pp. 335–341, R.C. Boucher et al., 'Gene Therapy for Cystic Fibrosis Using El Deleted Adenovirus: A Trial in the Nasal Cavity', *Human Gene Therapy* 5 (1994), pp. 615–639, and Melissa A. Rosenfeld, 'Human Artificial Chromosomes Get Real', *Nature Genetics* 15 (1997), pp. 333–335.

Genetic enhancement is a non-therapeutic form of genetic intervention which aims to raise cognitive and physical capacities above the normal range of functioning for persons. But to the extent that people's actual cognitive and physical functioning enable them to achieve a decent minimum level of well-being, there are no compelling medical or moral reasons for genetic enhancement. Indeed, some would say that there are compelling reasons for prohibiting it. Insofar as genetic enhancement aimed at something over and above disease prevention and health promotion, it would threaten to introduce a program of positive eugenics which would unjustly discriminate against certain groups of people who are moderately disabled and whose lives, though somewhat restricted, are nonetheless worth living. I will return to the eugenics question in the last part of the next section.

My analysis of the different forms of genetic alteration and the problem of their feasibility supports my earlier claim that genetic testing and selective termination of embryos with defective genes that cause people to exist with severe pain and suffering is the only medically effective and morally defensible way to prevent this state of affairs from obtaining. It will be instructive to cite some specific diseases that recommend such a preventive measure.

WHICH LIVES SHOULD BE PREVENTED?

Present biotechnology allows us to test embryonic cells for genetic abnormalities that lead directly to severe early-onset disorders, like Tay-Sachs disease, Hurler syndrome, Lesch-Nyhan syndrome, and Canavan's disease, as well as late-onset disorders like Huntington's disease.[21] We also can test embryos for genes that predispose people to chronic and ultimately fatal conditions like coronary heart disease and cancer. Genetic mutations play a causal role in many diseases by altering a crucial enzyme or other protein. The alteration may occur in differing degrees, depending on the extent of

---

[21] Canavan's is a degenerative disease that strikes infants, leading to the decay of the nervous system and early death. Hurler syndrome involves disruption of cognitive development in early childhood and usually death by age 10. LeschNyhan syndrome causes both mental retardation and compulsive self-mutilation in boys. Philip Kitcher offers an insightful discussion of the genetic causes of these and other diseases in *The Lives to Come: The Genetic Revolution and Human Possibilities* (New York, Simon and Schuster, 1996).

interaction between genes and the environment. In the specific diseases I mentioned above, though, environment plays little or no causal role in their occurrence. Either the defective gene necessarily causes the disease, or else it has a very high probability of causing it (95% with the Huntington's gene).

In Tay-Sachs, for instance, babies appear quite normal at birth. But in the first year of life their nervous systems degenerate, and they usually die by the time they reach 3 or 4. This disease is caused by the presence of two copies of an abnormal gene, or mutant allele, at a particular site on one of the 23 chromosome pairs. Tay-Sachs is an autosomal recessive disorder, which effectively means that the child inherits one mutant allele from each parent. Through the fusion of the gametes in the zygote that develops into the embryo, fetus, and person, the parents transmit the disease to their child.

Ideally, we would use gene therapy by inserting an additional normal copy of the defective gene into the relevant cells and thus cure the disease. But Tay-Sachs, like most recessive (and dominant) disorders, has not proven amenable to therapy. Alternatively, we can test and selectively terminate embryos with genes that cause this or other severely disabling diseases, preventing these diseases by preventing the existence of the people who would have them. This practice can be justified on two grounds. Beneficence requires that we not harm people by causing them to experience pain and suffering over the balance of their lives. In addition, justice requires that we not deny severely disabled people the same opportunities for achieving a good life as are open to others who are healthy or have only moderate cognitive or physical disabilities.[22] Arguably, the justice requirement will apply to only a small number of people, since the idea of equal opportunity for a good life implies a certain number of years to undertake and complete projects for a decent minimum level of well-being, and most people with severe early-onset genetically caused diseases have relatively short lifespans. Perhaps this is not the case with a disease like CF, where people afflicted often live for 30 years or more. But I do not believe that this genetically caused disease is so severely disabling and painful that we can justifiably prevent the lives of the persons who would

---

[22] See Glover, 'Future People, Disability, and Screening', McMahan, 'Cognitive Disability', and Allen Buchanan, 'Equal Opportunity and Genetic Intervention', *Social Philosophy and Policy* 12 (1995), pp. 105–135, and 'Choosing Who Will Be Disabled: Genetic Intervention and the Morality of Inclusion', *Social Philosophy and Policy* 13 (1996), pp. 18–46.

have it. Considerations of justice matter; but what matters more than ensuring equal opportunity for achieving a good life is preventing avoidable severe pain and suffering that people actually experience once they exist. These are what make lives not worth living on the whole. Indeed, it is often the severe pain and suffering associated with disabilities which preclude people from having the opportunities to achieve a decent minimum level of lifetime well-being.

Testing of embryonic cells for genetic abnormalities may be done by extracting cells from preimplantation IVF embryos. To produce extracorporeal IVF embryos for this type of testing, fertility drugs such as Clomid or Pergonal can be given to a woman to induce superovulation and in turn produce a number of eggs that can be recovered for fertilization with sperm. One advantage of producing multiple embryos is that, if genetic abnormalities are detected in any one of the embryos, then it can be selectively terminated and another, normal, embryo can be implanted in the woman's uterus. This would enable parents to have a normal child instead of a disabled one and to avoid any burdens that such a child might have on them or, if they have other children, the rest of the family. Significantly, the capacity to produce multiple JVF embryos is largely what grounds the impersonal harm principle, since at least two embryos must be available for a parent or parents to choose to bring a normal child into existence instead of a disabled one.

Another attractive feature of this method, as Robert Edwards explains, is that 'identifying embryos with genetic abnormalities would offer an alternative to amniocentesis during the second trimester of pregnancy, and the 'abortion' *in vitro* of a defective preimplantation embryo . . . would be infinitely preferable to abortion *in vivo* at twenty weeks of pregnancy or thereabouts as the results of amniocentesis are obtained'.[23] Testing preimplantation IVF embryos for genetic abnormalities would be preferable to testing fetal cells for these abnormalities by amniocentesis or chorionic villus sampling because, unlike these invasive procedures, it would not be painful to the pregnant woman and would avoid certain medical risks. Specifically, putting a needle into the uterus to extract

---

[23] R.G. Edwards & J. Purdy, *Human Conception In Vitro* (London, Academic Press, 1981), p. 373.

cells from either the amniotic fluid or embryonic membrane triggers a miscarriage once in every 50 to 100 pregnancies. Moreover, villus sampling may cause limb deformities in the fetus.

Terminating the development of one embryo and implanting a different embryo would mean that the life of one potential person was not allowed to become actual and that the life of a different potential person became actual instead. The same number of people would exist, but they would be different people. Yet whether one or a different potential person is allowed to exist does not matter morally. Rather, what matters morally is preventing avoidable pain and suffering that actual people will have to experience. And to the extent that an embryo containing a disease-causing gene will result in severe pain and suffering in the person who develops from it, we are morally required to prevent the disease, pain, and suffering by terminating the development of that embryo. What must be emphasized, however, is that the moral requirement to terminate embryos and thereby prevent certain people from coming into existence pertains only to those people who would have *severe*, not just moderately severe, diseases. Only severe diseases make people's lives not worth living on the whole.

One consequence of not preventing genetically defective embryos from resulting in severely diseased or disabled persons is that a child caused to exist in such a condition could file a tort of wrongful life against his parents.[24] Or, if the child is cognitively or physically unable to do so, a different person could file a tort on the child's behalf. Suppose that a boy has Duchenne muscular dystrophy, a recessive disorder traceable to a genetic defect on the X chromosome which adversely affects the dystrophin protein. This defect causes muscles to begin weakening at age 3 and subsequent respiratory failure, which gives children afflicted with the disease an average life expectancy of 16–20 years. If the boy's mother knew that she was a carrier of the defect and that there was a 50% chance of transmitting it to her son, was able to abort the embryo containing the defect, yet allowed the child to be born from that embryo, then the boy could claim that his parents acted in reckless disregard of his welfare, wronged and harmed him, and accordingly owe him

---

[24] See Feinberg, 'Wrongful Life and the Counterfactual Element in Harming', in *Freedom and Fulfillment* (Princeton, Princeton University Press, 1992), pp. 3–36, Heyd, *Genethics*, Ch. 1, Harris, *Wonderwoman and Superman*, Ch. 4, and McMahan, 'Cognitive Disability' and 'Wrongful Life'.

compensation for causing him to exist with a condition that defeats his right and interest in having a life that is not severely restricted. The person-affecting principle would ground the child's claim against his parents.

There would not be grounds for a tort of wrongful life, however, if the child claimed that genetic intervention other than testing and termination at the embryonic stage of development, such as adding a normal copy of the dystrophin gene, would have made a significant difference between the quality of life he actually experiences and what he might have experienced otherwise. For at the time of the intervention, there would not have been any identifiable individual to be benefited or harmed. Genetic alteration at such an early stage of development of the organism would have resulted in a completely different set of biological and psychological properties that would have belonged to a different person. So the child only could claim that the wrong or harm was committed by not terminating the defective embryo from which he developed, not by failing to add a normal copy of the gene. Gene therapy involving somatic cells at an early age after birth also would entail different subsequent biological and psychological properties as the child's life unfolded. Arguably, however, these would not be so radically different from the properties possessed before the therapy that they would be of a different person, since presumably the child who receives the therapy already has a fairly developed biological and psychological life. Although some of his properties would have changed, intuitively there would be enough biological and psychological continuity before and after the therapy to say that the child cured of CF or SCID by gene therapy would remain the same individual. If such a child's parents had access to affordable gene therapy that could cure his disease or treat the symptoms associated with it, but failed to seek such treatment, then perhaps the child could claim that his parents harmed or wronged him by defeating his interest in being cured of or treated for a disease that was amenable to gene therapy. But to the extent that the child already exists with a condition for which his parents are not completely responsible, strictly speaking this case would involve something other than the standard notion of wrongful life.

The cases that I have just discussed involve physical disability. More difficult to assess would be gene therapy to correct severe cognitive disability at a fairly early stage of a person's life. This could have a significant effect on subsequent psychological properties that arguably *would* be those of a different person from the one who underwent cognitive gene therapy for the affected brain cells at an earlier time, given that the brain generates and supports the consciousness and other psychological properties necessary for personhood and personal identity through time. The medical prospects for cognitive gene therapy are even less promising than they are for physical gene therapy, and the moral implications of such therapy are so complex that I cannot address them adequately here. Nevertheless, cognitive and physical disability may very well have different relative weights in determining personal identity through time, as well as in determining whether or to what extent people can be harmed.

I have claimed that the diseases that morally require us to prevent the existence of people who would have them must be so severely disabling that they make their lives not worth living on the whole. This is not the case with moderately severe genetic disorders like Down syndrome, where, although there is some cognitive and physical impairment, the lives of people with this disorder can be fulfilling and thus very much worth living. So there would be no moral grounds for preventing the existence of people with Down syndrome. But there would be no moral requirement to bring them into existence either, given that existence is morally neutral and entails no requirement to cause people to exist with good lives.

A further distinction must be drawn between early-onset genetic disorders of the sort I have been discussing, which affect people from birth or early childhood, and late-onset genetic disorders, like Huntington's disease, which do not affect people until the adult stage of their lives. The onset of symptoms in people afflicted with Huntington's may range anywhere from age 30 to 50, and these include progressive loss of muscle control and dementia. Generally, they die within 15 years after onset. Prior to this time, they usually have normal lives with comparatively high levels of cognitive and physical functioning for a considerable number of years. In trying to determine whether people's lives are worth living on the whole, we should do so by evaluating the quality of their lives in terms of all the stages of their lives. But the radical difference in cognitive and physical functioning before and after the onset of symptoms in diseases like Huntington's makes it difficult to assess overall quality of life for the people who have them.

With severe adult-onset diseases, perhaps the most plausible way to measure lifetime quality is to weigh the level of normal functioning per year lived against the level of disability per year lived and arrive at an average level of well-being for the person's entire lifespan.[25] On this view, the earlier the onset of symptoms in the person's life, the longer the period of time between onset and death, and the more severe the disability, pain, and suffering associated with the disease, the stronger the reason will be for saying that the person's life is not worth living on the whole. Correspondingly, there will be a stronger reason for preventing that life by terminating the embryo with the gene that causes the disease. Thus, for a person afflicted with the degenerative physical and cognitive symptoms of Huntington's disease at age 30, the severity of the pain and suffering he experiences in his last 15 years may be bad enough to outweigh the normal functioning he had in his first 30 years and average out to a level of lifetime well-being which falls below the decent minimum. This in turn may lead us to conclude that his life is not worth living on the whole for him and that, if we could have foreseen this through genetic testing of the embryo from which he developed, then we should have terminated the embryo and thereby prevented him from existing.

Or consider a more controversial variant of the same case. Suppose that genetic testing could predict that symptoms would not manifest themselves until age 50. One might claim that the pain and suffering caused by the disease in the last 10 or 15 years of the person's life would be so severe as to outweigh the good 50 years and thus make the person's average lifetime well-being fall below the decent minimum. Although it would be difficult to sustain, here too there may be a principled reason for terminating an embryo with the Huntington's gene. It may weigh the decision in favor of preventing the existence of a person who would have the disease over causing him to exist with a life that has a wretched last stage. Alternatively, one could take the view that, with adult-onset diseases, it is the victim's responsibility to decide whether to go on living beyond a certain point. This is consistent with the conviction

---

[25] Thomas Hurka presents a model that measures quality of life in terms of averaging achievements in earlier and later stages of life in *Perfectionism* (New York, Oxford University Press, 1993), pp. 70 ff. See also Brock, 'Quality of Life Measures in Health Care and Medical Ethics', in *Life and Death: Philosophical Essays in Biomedical Ethics* (New York, Cambridge University Press, 1993), pp. 268–324.

that the value of a life is determined subjectively by the person whose life it is. But whether this view were to figure in any way in public policy would depend, among other things, on the legal climate in which the afflicted person was living.[26]

Pain and suffering in the last stage or years of a person's life must be weighed against the achievements afforded by normal cognitive and physical functioning in earlier stages. Fifty years of normal functioning should be enough for a person to complete many of the projects in his life plan and make for a life that is worth living. If so, then the fact that a person loses his normal functioning at age 50 by itself is not enough to support the claim that on balance his life is not worth living and that he should not have been allowed to come into existence. Indeed, some people have lives of thirty years that are full of achievements. A shorter life can be very well worth living. But if the pain and suffering in one's last years are severe enough, and if the number of these years is large enough, then this may weigh the decision in favor of preventing the person from coming into existence. The experience of severe pain and suffering, more so than what it implies about limited opportunities for achievement, grounds the claims that a person's life on balance is not worth living for him and that it is morally wrong to cause a person to exist with such a life.

Two objections might be raised against the claim that people with severe disease or disability should not be brought into existence. Disabilities rights advocates might argue that intervention in the form of testing and selectively terminating genetically defective embryos would reduce the number of people with disabilities. Consequently, public support for persons who already have disabilities would erode. It would lead to a devaluation of the lives of the disabled and to discrimination against them. To rebut this objection, we can appeal to Allen Buchanan's point that 'it is not the *people* with disabilities which we devalue, it is the *disabilities*'.[27] Buchanan further says 'we devalue disabilities because we value the opportunities and welfare of the people who have them – and it is because we value people, all people, that we care about limitations on their welfare and opportunities. We also know that disabilities, as such, diminish opportunities and welfare, even when they are *not*

---

[26] I thank a referee for *Bioethics* for raising this issue.
[27] 'Choosing Who Will Be Disabled', p. 32. Emphasis added.

so severe that the lives of those who have them are not worth living'.[28] The underlying rationale for this position is that it is a matter of justice, not only beneficence, that we remove or prevent limitations on an individual's opportunities for a decent life. But the second passage cited from Buchanan leaves open the possibility that it is morally permissible to terminate embryos with genetic defects that would lead to people having lives with limited opportunities that are nonetheless worth living. Against Buchanan, I believe that we should terminate only those embryos with genetic defects that manifest themselves in severe disabilities that make life on balance not worth living.

Still, we have to weigh the relative importance of cognitive and physical functioning for different people in assessing quality of life. Suppose it were discovered that the adult-onset motor neuron disease amyelotrophic lateral sclerosis (ALS) had a genetic cause and that the disease could be prevented only by terminating embryos whose cells contained the defective gene. The case of the brilliant theoretical physicist Stephen Hawking illustrates that a person can suffer from a severe physical disability as a symptom of ALS for well over the balance of his life yet maintain a high level of cognitive functioning which makes life for him very much worth living. It would be difficult to adduce reasons for preventing such a life from coming into existence, despite the fact that ALS is a severely disabling disease. On the other hand, for people who value physical functioning very highly (e.g. athletes, dancers), severe physical disability may lead them to judge that on balance their lives are not worth living, even if their normal cognitive functioning remains intact. Granted, people can adapt their preferences and life plans to adult-onset disabilities and the limited opportunities they entail. But it is not so easy to do this if one has to endure constant pain and suffering over a considerable period of time. Furthermore, in the case of someone like Hawking, if the pain associated with the physical disability were so severe that it adversely affected his cognitive functioning, then we might consider whether he would believe that his well-being was at a level high enough for him to judge that his life was worth living.

A second objection to my view is that any form of genetic intervention is motivated by the desire to improve the human species

---

[28] *Ibid.*, p. 33.

through selection. This amounts to a program of positive eugenics, which would lead to a repeat of the inhumane treatment of people and a violation of their intrinsic worth which have occurred in recent history.[29] To this objection, we can respond by saying that the aim of any medically and morally defensible form of genetic intervention should not be to enhance people's genotype or phenotypic traits, but only to ensure that the people we do cause to exist have normal, or close to normal, cognitive and physical functioning over the balance of their lives. In preventing the existence of people with severe disability, we arc not aiming to enhance or improve lives that already are, or would be, at a decent minimum level of well-being, but only to ensure that the people we do bring into existence will not fall well below this level. This accords with the moral asymmetry thesis. We have no moral duty to bring people into existence with good lives. But if we do bring people into existence, we have a moral duty to ensure that their lives do not contain so much pain and suffering as to be not worth living for them on the whole.

The negative eugenics I am defending has affinities with what Philip Kitcher calls 'utopian eugenics'.[30] This involves a policy guaranteeing that people have reproductive freedom in choosing which embryos they allow to develop and subsequently the people they bring into existence. Their choices must be free of any socially coercive pressure to prevent people from existing for economic reasons or perfectionist ideals. Provided that genetic testing and selective termination of defective embryos are practiced in order to prevent extreme pain and suffering in people, not to enhance their cognitive and physical capacities above the normal range, and that reproductive technologies like IVF and genetic testing are affordable and accessible to all, utopian eugenics is a morally justifiable policy.

---

[29] See, for example, Daniel Kevles, *In the Name of Eugenics: Genetics and the Uses of Human Heredity* (New York, Alfred A. Knopf, 1985), an examination of the history of eugenics in the United States.

[30] *The Lives to Come*, p. 202. See also Glover, *What Sort of People Should There Be?* (Harmondsworth, Penguin, 1984), John A. Wagner, 'Gene Therapy Is not Eugenics', *Nature Genetics* 15 (1997), p. 234, and A. Buchanan, D.W. Brock, N. Daniels and D. Wikler, *From Chance to Choice* (Cambridge, CUP, 2000).

LONG-TERM CRYOPRESERVATION

Another practice made possible by reproductive biotechnology is the storing of frozen embryos in 'embryo banks' of liquid nitrogen. One attractive feature of this type of cryopreservation is that a woman could decide to preserve an embryo produced by IVF from her egg and a man's sperm in such a bank in order to pursue a career and later have the embryo implanted in her uterus for pregnancy and birth. Assuming that long-term storage does not entail a risk of genetic mutation in embryonic cells, she could undertake a later pregnancy without fear of birth defects regardless of her age because the embryo fertilized at the earlier time would be biologically optimal. Moreover, if genetic testing determines that an embryo has a genetic abnormality that likely will result in a severely diseased or disabled person, then storing multiple IVF embryos gives parents the choice to terminate the defective embryo and implant a normal one instead. In addition, cryopreservation of embryos for an extended period of time may make any genetic mutations they contain correctable by the insertion of normal copies of the relevant genes, if such a technique becomes feasible in the near future. This would determine the identity of the person brought into existence free from disease, who would replace the diseased individual who would have existed instead from the same embryo without the altered or additional gene. But it is worth repeating that it is not whether genetic alteration or therapy is identity-determining or identity-preserving which is morally significant, but rather the sort of experience the persons who are brought into existence will have.

There are reasons to be wary of freezing and storing embryos for long periods of time, however. It is unknown whether this process might entail genetic mutations in embryonic cells which might result in disease and premature death in the individuals who come into existence in this way. Also, IVF and cryopreservation of embryos make it possible for a person resulting from such an embryo to have three distinct mothers: (1) the genetic, or biological mother, whose gamete contributes 23 chromosomes to the embryo and determines many of the subsequent biological and psychological properties of the child who develops from the embryo; (2) the gestational mother, in whose uterus the embryo is implanted and who gives birth to the child; and (3) the social mother who raises and cares for the child. The social mother is perhaps the most important of the three with respect to the child's interests, since she is the one who cares for the child when it has the requisite psychological properties for interests, rights, and a biographical self. To the extent that only individuals with interests and rights can be harmed, and these interests and rights can be affected directly by the social mother, she can directly affect the welfare of the child. But the relationship between a child and its biological parents can have a significant psychological impact on the child as well.

If an embryo is frozen and not implanted until many years after fertilization, then it is possible for a child to be born from that embryo and come into existence after the deaths of its biological parents. Even assuming that there are no known genetic abnormalities in the embryo, the prospect of being born after the deaths of its biological parents may have harmful effects on the child's psychological identity, its sense of self. A mature self ordinarily will have a relationship with its biological parents which involves more than mere knowledge of who they are. There may be an even greater sense of harm to a child resulting from an embryo stored for a considerable period of time. Earlier, I said that storing embryos could allow a woman to pursue a professional career before having a child. But suppose that a woman's egg, fertilized when she was 30, is frozen and not implanted in her still normally functioning uterus (or that of a surrogate mother) until she is 60.[31] She becomes pregnant and decides to bring the pregnancy to term. The increasing likelihood of disease with age may mean that the child or adolescent born from this pregnancy would have the burden of caring for her mother or both parents before she was emotionally mature enough to do so. It also would be an obstacle to her own emotional development as a person and thus have a deleterious effect on her overall well-being. With these issues in mind, it will be instructive to consider a well-known legal case in the United States involving frozen embryos.

In December 1988, seven embryos produced *in vitro* from the gametes of Mary Sue Davis and Junior Lewis Davis were placed in

---

[31] Eight years ago, in 'Contemporary and Future Possibilities for Human Embryonic Manipulation', Mark Ferguson wrote 'it is unclear how well the ageing human female reproductive system would cope with such good embryos'. In Anthony Dyson and John Harris, eds., *Experiments on Embryos* (London, Routledge and Kegan Paul, 1990), p. 10. Yet recently a woman of 63 in Los Angeles gave birth to a healthy baby girl. See Gina Kolata, 'A Record and Big Questions as Woman Gives Birth at 63'. *New York Times*, April 24, 1997.

cryogenic storage for possible future implantation.[32] In February 1989, the couple filed for divorce, at which time the question arose as to whether the right of Mrs. Davis (then remarried as Mrs. Stowe) to become a mother outweighed Mr. Davis' right not to become a father. Arguing in Mr. Davis' favor, John Robertson concluded that the right to avoid biological offspring should have priority over the right to reproduce using frozen embryos.[33] While Robertson's argument is persuasive as far as it goes, it pays insufficient attention to the interests of the future children who may be produced from these embryos. More specifically, it does not adequately consider how long-term cryopreservation of embryos may adversely affect the well-being of children born from embryos implanted in surrogate mothers after the deaths of their biological parents, or if children are born when their biological parents are at an advanced age.

These points underscore some of the disturbing implications of what amounts to altering the normal lifespan of a human organism and the normal reproductive cycle. In particular, it forces us to ask whether we have a moral obligation to impose some time limit after which frozen embryos should not be implanted. Indeed, the Human Fertilization and Embryo Act of 1991 in the United Kingdom stipulated a five-year limit on the storage of frozen embryos, after which time they were to be destroyed. Even if time limits on storage resolve the problems involving the length of a biological lifespan and the reproductive cycle, the question remains as to whether disposing of embryos is morally permissible.

Bonnie Steinbock maintains that it matters whether we think that embryos should be preserved because of their symbolic value or because they have a right to life. The import of this question derives from a distinction she draws between moral status and moral value.[34] Moral status is limited to beings with interests of their own, that is, sentient, aware, beings. Moral value concerns the symbolic value of entities, even if they lack moral status. The debate in the United Kingdom may be taken either from the point of view of moral status or from that of moral value. If, as the Church

[32] *Davis v. Davis* 1989 WL 140495 (Tenn Cir 1984) rev'd 842 5. W. 2D 588, 597 (Tenn 1992).

[33] 'Resolving Disputes over Frozen Embryos', *Hastings Center Report* 19 (November-December 1989), p. 11. More recently, Robertson examines this and related issues in *Children of Choice: Freedom and the New Reproductive Technologies* (Princeton, Princeton University Press, 1996).

[34] *Life Before Birth: The Moral and Legal Status of Embryos and Fetuses* (New York, Oxford University Press, 1992), pp. 5–41.

maintains, embryos have moral status and rights, then it is impermissible to deliberately destroy them. But if they lack moral status, then we still can discuss whether respecting them as symbols of human life is consistent with destroying them.[35] By Steinbock's lights, destroying embryos is as respectful of human life as is keeping them frozen for long periods, and this understanding of moral value seems plausible.

Nevertheless, the possibility that deletion of defective genes and insertion of normal genes in embryonic cells will become feasible in the near future may provide a reason for keeping embryos in frozen storage. This would be the case if parents wanted to have a normal child at some point not too late in their lives and were able to produce only one viable but genetically abnormal embryo from their gametes. Yet if they were able to produce multiple embryos and none of them was genetically abnormal, then, given that there is no moral obligation to bring people into existence, there would be no corresponding moral obligation to preserve any of these embryos on the basis of their presumed moral status.

CONCLUSION

I have examined two aspects of reproductive biotechnology – genetic testing and selective termination of defective embryos, and long-term cryopreservation of embryos – and have explored the ethical implications of each. In the first case, I have argued that we are morally required to terminate the development of embryos with genetic defects that cause severe disease or disability in people who develop from them. The moral justification for this view is that it is wrong to cause people to exist when the avoidable pain and suffering they experience make their lives not worth living on the whole. This claim is motivated by both the person-affecting and impersonal harm principles. If we cause these people to exist with severe disease and disability, then we defeat their interest in living without pain and suffering. Or, if we are considering whether to cause people to exist, then it is better, other things being equal, to prevent the existence of a person with severe cognitive and physical disability and instead bring into existence a person with normal cognitive and physical functioning. By doing so, we avoid

---

[35] I thank Bonnie Steinbock for pointing this out.

gratuitously adding to the total amount of suffering in the world. In addition, considerations of justice support this position, because it means that people will not come into existence with a condition that will severely limit their opportunities for achieving a decent minimum level of lifetime well-being. Consistent with the idea of negative eugenics, we should prevent the existence of people who would have severe disease and disability, not in order to raise the average level of people's cognitive and physical functioning, but rather to prevent the pain and suffering that make people's lives not worth living on the whole. The aim of negative eugenics is disease prevention and health promotion, not enhancement of normal capacities.

With respect to long-term cryopreservation of embryos, I have cited reasons for not preserving embryos for too long when it entails harmful psychological effects on a child born after the deaths of its biological parents, or when its parents are at an advanced age. However, if genetic technology develops in the near future to the point of making it feasible to correct genetic defects at the embryonic stage of development, then this may provide medical and moral grounds for preserving them. Such genetic alteration would mean that a biologically and psychologically different person would come into existence from the person who would have come into existence without genetic alteration to the embryo. Yet what matters morally is not *who* comes into existence, but that if we decide to bring a person into existence, we ensure, insofar as we can, that they not experience severe pain and suffering over the balance of their lives.

In time, recessive genetic disorders may become amenable to somatic-cell gene therapy. Perhaps both recessive and dominant disorders will be prevented by germ-line genetic alteration at an early stage of a developing human organism. The latter would have profound medical and moral implications for the evolution of genetic mutation in the human species as well as for our obligations to generations in the distant future. But the genetic technology we presently have already gives us considerable power to determine which people will exist and the sorts of lives they will have in the near future.[36]

[36] I am grateful to Michael Burgess, David Donaldson, Chris McDonald, Bonnie Steinbock, and an anonymous referee for *Bioethics* for very helpful comments on an ancestor of this paper. Work on the paper was supported by a Killam Postdoctoral Fellowship at the Centre for Applied Ethics, University of British Columbia, which also is gratefully acknowledged.

Chapter 27

PROCREATIVE BENEFICENCE: WHY WE SHOULD SELECT THE BEST CHILDREN

JULIAN SAVULESCU

INTRODUCTION

Imagine you are having in vitro fertilisation (IVF) and you produce four embryos. One is to be implanted. You are told that there is a genetic test for predisposition to scoring well on IQ tests (let's call this intelligence). If an embryo has gene subtypes (alleles) A, B there is a greater than 50% chance it will score more than 140 if given an ordinary education and upbringing. If it has subtypes C, D there is a much lower chance it will score over 140. Would you test the four embryos for these gene subtypes and use this information in selecting which embryo to implant?

Many people believe intelligence is a purely social construct and so it is unlikely to have a significant genetic cause. Others believe there are different sorts of intelligence, such as verbal intelligence, mathematical intelligence, musical ability and no such thing as general intelligence. Time will tell. There are several genetic research programs currently in place which seek to elucidate the genetic contribution to intelligence. This paper pertains to any results of this research even if it only describes a weak probabilistic relation between genes and intelligence, or a particular kind of intelligence.

Many people believe that research into the genetic contribution to intelligence should not be performed, and that if genetic tests which predict intelligence, or a range of intelligence, are ever developed, they should not be employed in reproductive decision-making. I will argue that we have a moral obligation to test for genetic contribution to non-disease states such as intelligence and to use this information in reproductive decision-making.

Imagine now you are invited to play the Wheel of Fortune. A giant wheel exists with marks on it from 0–$1,000,000, in $100 increments. The wheel is spun in a secret room. It stops randomly on an amount. That amount is put into Box A. The wheel is spun again. The amount which comes up is put into Box B. You can choose Box A or B. You are also told that, in addition to the sum already put in the boxes, if you choose B, a dice will be thrown and you will lose $100 if it comes up 6.

Which box should you choose?

The rational answer is Box A. Choosing genes for non-disease states is like playing the Wheel of Fortune. You should use all the available information and choose the option most likely to bring about the best outcome.

PROCREATIVE BENEFICENCE: THE MORAL OBLIGATION TO HAVE THE BEST CHILDREN

I will argue for a principle which I call Procreative Beneficence:

> couples (or single reproducers) should select the child, of the possible children they could have, who is expected to have the best life, or at least as good a life as the others, based on the relevant, available information.

I will argue that Procreative Beneficence implies couples should employ genetic tests for non-disease traits in selecting which child to bring into existence and that we should allow selection for non-disease genes in some cases even if this maintains or increases social inequality.

By 'should' in 'should choose', I mean 'have good reason to.' I will understand morality to require us to do what we have most reason to do. In the absence of some other reason for action, a person who has good reason to have the best child is morally required to have the best child.

Consider the following three situations involving normative judgements.

(1) 'You are 31. You will be at a higher risk of infertility and having a child with an abnormality if you delay child-bearing. But that has to be balanced against taking time out of your career now. That's only something you can weigh up.'

(2) 'You should stop smoking.'

(3) 'You must inform your partner that you are HIV positive or practise safe sex.'

The 'should' in 'should choose the best child' is that present in the second example. It implies that persuasion is justified, but not coercion, which would be justified in the third case. Yet the situation is different to the more morally neutral (1).

Definitions

A disease gene is a gene which causes a genetic disorder (e.g. cystic fibrosis) or predisposes to the development of disease (e.g. the genetic contribution to cancer or dementia). A non-disease gene is a gene which causes or predisposes to some physical or psychological state of the person which is not itself a disease state, e.g. height, intelligence, character (not in the sub-normal range).

Selection

It is currently possible to select from a range of possible children we could have. This is most frequently done by employing fetal selection through prenatal testing and termination of pregnancy. Selection of embryos is now possible by employing in vitro fertilization and preimplantation genetic diagnosis (PGD). There are currently no genetic tests available for non-disease states except sex. However, if such tests become available in the future, both PGD and prenatal testing could be used to select offspring on the basis of non-disease genes. Selection of sex by PGD is now undertaken in Sydney, Australia.[1] PGD will also lower the threshold for couples to engage in selection since it has fewer psychological sequelae than prenatal testing and abortion.

In the future, it may be possible to select gametes according to their genetic characteristics. This is currently possible for sex, where methods have been developed to sort X and Y bearing sperm.[2]

[1] J. Savulescu. Sex Selection – the case for. *Medical Journal of Australia* 1999; 171: 373–375.
[2] E.F. Fugger, S.H. Black, K. Keyvanfar & J.D. Schulman. Births of normal daughters after Microsort sperm separation and intrauterine insemination, in-vitro fertilization, or intracytoplasmic sperm injection. *Hum Reprod* 1998; 13: 2367–2370.

Table 1. Behavioural Genetics

Aggression and criminal behaviour
Alcoholism
Anxiety and Anxiety disorders
Attention Deficit Hyperactivity Disorder (ADHD)
Antisocial personality disorder
Bipolar disorder
Homosexuality
Maternal Behaviour
Memory and intelligence
Neuroticism
Novelty Seeking
Schizophrenia
Substance Addiction

Behavioural Genetics

Behavioural Genetics is a branch of genetics which seeks to understand the contribution of genes to complex behaviour. The scope of behavioural genetics is illustrated in Table 1.

AN ARGUMENT FOR PROCREATIVE BENEFICENCE

Consider the *Simple Case of Selection for Disease Genes*. A couple is having IVF in an attempt to have a child. It produces two embryos. A battery of tests for common diseases is performed. Embryo A has no abnormalities on the tests performed. Embryo B has no abnormalities on the tests performed except its genetic profile reveals it has a predisposition to developing asthma. Which embryo should be implanted?

Embryo B has nothing to be said in its favour over A and something against it. Embryo A should (on pain of irrationality) be implanted. This is like choosing Box A in the Wheel of Fortune analogy.

Why shouldn't we select the embryo with a predisposition to asthma? What is relevant about asthma is that it reduces quality of life. Attacks cause severe breathlessness and in extreme cases, death. Steroids may be required to treat it. These are among the most dangerous drugs which exist if taken long term. Asthma can be lifelong and require lifelong drug treatment. Ultimately it can leave the sufferer wheel chair bound with chronic obstructive airways disease. The morally relevant property of 'asthma' is that it is a state which reduces the well-being a person experiences.

Parfitian defence of voluntary procreative beneficence in the Simple Case

The following example, after Parfit,[3] supports Procreative Beneficence. A woman has rubella. If she conceives now, she will have a
blind and deaf child. If she waits three months, she will conceive
another different but healthy child. She should choose to wait until
her rubella is passed.

Or consider the Nuclear Accident. A poor country does not have
enough power to provide power to its citizens during an extremely
cold winter. The government decides to open an old and unsafe
nuclear reactor. Ample light and heating are then available. Citizens
stay up later, and enjoy their lives much more. Several months later,
the nuclear reactor melts down and large amounts of radiation are
released into the environment. The only effect is that a large number
of children are subsequently born with predispositions to early
childhood malignancy.

The supply of heating and light has changed the lifestyle of this
population. As a result of this change in lifestyle, people have
conceived children at different times than they would have if there
had been no heat or light, and their parents went to bed earlier.
Thus, the children born after the nuclear accident would not have
existed if the government had not switched to nuclear power. They
have not been harmed by the switch to nuclear power and the
subsequent accident (unless their lives are so bad they are worse
than death). If we object to the Nuclear Accident (which most of
us would), then we must appeal to some form of harmless wrongdoing. That is, we must claim that a wrong was done, but no one
was harmed. We must appeal to something like the Principle of
Procreative Beneficence.

An objection to Procreative Beneficence in the Simple Case

The following objection to Procreative Beneficence is common.

> 'If you choose Embryo A (without a predisposition to asthma),
> you could be discarding someone like Mozart or an olympic
> swimmer. So there is no good reason to select A.'

---

[3] D. Parfit. 1976. Rights, Interests and Possible People, in *Moral Problems in Medicine*, S.
Gorovitz, et al., eds. Englewood Cliffs. Prentice Hall. D. Parfit. 1984. *Reasons and Persons.*
Oxford. Clarendon Press: Part IV.

It is true that by choosing A, you could be discarding a person like Mozart. But it is equally true that if you choose B, you could be discarding someone like Mozart without asthma. A and B are equally likely (on the information available) to be someone like Mozart (and B is more likely to have asthma).

Other principles of reproductive decision-making applied to the Simple Case

The principle of Procreative Beneficence supports selecting the embryo without the genetic predisposition to asthma. That seems intuitively correct. How do other principles of reproductive decision-making apply to this example?

1. *Procreative Autonomy:* This principle claims that couples should be free to decide when and how to procreate, and what kind of children to have.[4] If this were the only decision-guiding principle, it would imply couples might have reason to choose the embryo with a predisposition to asthma, if for some reason they wanted that.

2. *Principle of Non-Directive Counselling:* According to this principle, doctors and genetic counsellors should only provide information about risk and options available to reduce that risk.[5] They should not give advice or other direction. Thus, if a couple wanted to transfer Embryo B, and they knew that it would have a predisposition to asthma, nothing more is to be said according to Non-Directive Counselling.

3. *The 'Best Interests of the Child' Principle:* Legislation in Australia and the United Kingdom related to reproduction gives great weight to consideration of the best interests of the child. For example, the Victorian Infertility Treatment Act 1995 states *'the welfare and interests of any person born or to be born as a*

[4] R. Dworkin. 1993. *Life's Dominion: An Argument about Abortion and Euthanasia*. London. Harper Collins; J. Harris. Goodbye Dolly? The ethics of human cloning. *Journal of Medical Ethics* 1997; 23: 353–360; J. Harris. 1998. Rights and Reproductive Choice, in *The Future of Reproduction*, J. Harris and S. Holm, eds. Oxford. Clarendon Press; J.A. Robertson. 1994. *Children of Choice: Freedom and the New Reproductive Technologies*. Princeton. Princeton University Press; C. Strong. 1997. *Ethics in reproductive and perinatal medicine*. New Haven. Yale University Press.

[5] J.A.F. Roberts. 1959. *An introduction to human genetics*. Oxford. OUP.

result of a treatment procedure are paramount.[6] This principle
is irrelevant to this choice. The couple could choose the embryo
with the predisposition to asthma and still be doing everything
possible in the interests of *that* child.

None of the alternative principles give appropriate direction in
the Simple Case.

MOVING FROM DISEASE GENES TO NON-DISEASE GENES: WHAT IS THE 'BEST LIFE'?

It is not asthma (or disease) which is important, but its impact on
a life in ways that matter which is important. People often trade
length of life for non-health related well-being. Non-disease genes
may prevent us from leading the best life.

By 'best life', I will understand the life with the most well-being.
There are various theories of well-being: hedonistic, desire-
fulfilment, objective list theories.[7] According to hedonistic theories,
what matters is the quality of our experiences, for example, that we
experience pleasure. According to desire-fulfilment theories, what
matters is the degree to which our desires are satisfied. According
to objective list theories, certain activities are good for people, such
as achieving worthwhile things with your life, having dignity, having
children and raising them, gaining knowledge of the world, developing one's talents, appreciating beautiful things, and so on.

On any of these theories, some non-disease genes will affect the
likelihood that we will lead the best life. Imagine there is a gene
which contributes significantly to a violent, explosive, uncontrolla-
ble temper, and that state causes people significant suffering. Violent outbursts lead a person to come in conflict with the law and
fall out of important social relations. The loss of independence,
dignity and important social relations are bad on any of the three
accounts.

Buchanan et al. argue that what is important in a liberal democracy is providing people with general purpose means, i.e. those

---

[6] The *Human Fertilization and Embryology Act 1990* in England requires that account be
taken of the welfare of any child who will be born by assisted reproduction before issuing a
licence for assistance (S.13(5)).

[7] Parfit, *op. cit.*, Appendix I, pp. 493–502; Griffin. 1986. *Well-Being* Oxford. Clarendon Press.

useful to any plan of life.[8] In this way we can allow people to form and act on their own conception of the good life. Examples of general purpose means are the ability to hear and see. But similarly the ability to concentrate, to engage with and be empathetic towards other human beings may be all purpose means. To the degree that genes contribute to these, we have reason to select those genes.

Consider another example. Memory (M) is the ability to remember important things when you want to. Imagine there is some genetic contribution to M: Six alleles (genes) contribute to M. IVF produces four embryos. Should we test for M profiles?

Does M relate to well-being? Having to go to the supermarket twice because you forgot the baby formula prevents you doing more worthwhile things. Failing to remember can have disastrous consequences. Indeed, forgetting the compass on a long bush walk can be fatal. There is, then, a positive obligation to test for M and select the embryo (other things being equal) with the best M profile.

Does being intelligent mean one is more likely to have a better life? At a folk intuitive level, it seems plausible that intelligence would promote well-being on any plausible account of well-being. On a hedonistic account, the capacity to imagine alternative pleasures and remember the salient features of past experiences is important in choosing the best life. On a desire-fulfilment theory, intelligence is important to choosing means which will best satisfy one's ends. On an objective list account, intelligence would be important to gaining knowledge of the world, and developing rich social relations. Newson has reviewed the empirical literature relating intelligence to quality of life. Her synthesis of the empirical literature is that 'intelligence has a high instrumental value for persons in giving them a large amount of complexity with which to approach their everyday lives, and that it equips them with a tool which can lead to the provision of many other personal and social goods.'[9]

Socrates, in Plato's Philebus, concludes that the best life is a mixture of wisdom and pleasure. Wisdom includes thought,

---

[8] A. Buchanan, D.W. Brock, N. Daniels & D. Wikler. 2000. *From Chance to Choice*. Cambridge. CUP: 167. Buchanan and colleagues argue in a parallel way for the permissibility of genetic manipulation (enhancement) to allow children to live the best life possible (Chapter Five). They do not consider selection in this context.

[9] A. Newson. The value of intelligence and its implications for genetic research. *Fifth World Congress of Bioethics*, Imperial College, London, 21–24 September 2000.

intelligence, knowledge and memory.[10] Intelligence is clearly a part of Plato's conception of the good life:

> without the power of calculation you could not even calculate that you will get enjoyment in the future; your life would be that not of a man, but of a sea-lung or one of those marine creatures whose bodies are confined by a shell.[11]

Choice of means of selecting

This argument extends in principle to selection of fetuses using prenatal testing and termination of affected pregnancy. However, selection by abortion has greater psychological harms than selection by PGD and these need to be considered. Gametic selection, if it is ever possible, will have the lowest psychological cost.

Objections to the principle of Procreative Beneficence applied to non-disease genes

1. *Harm to the child:* One common objection to genetic selection for non-disease traits is that it results in harm to the child. There are various versions of this objection, which include the harm which arises from excessive and overbearing parental expectations, using the child as a means, and not treating it as an end, and closing off possible future options on the basis of the information provided (failing to respect the child's 'right to an open future').

There are a number of responses. Firstly, in some cases, it is possible to deny that the harms will be significant. Parents come to love the child whom they have (even a child with a serious disability). Moreover, some have argued that counselling can reduce excessive expectations.[12]

Secondly, we can accept some risk of a child experiencing some state of reduced well-being in cases of selection. One variant of the harm to child objection is: 'If you select embryo A, it might still get asthma, or worse, cancer, or have a much worse life than B, and you

---

[10] *Philebus* 21 C 1-12. A.E. Taylor's translation. 1972. Folkstone. Dawsons of Pall Mall: 21 D 11-3, E 1-3.

[11] *Philebus* 21 C 1-12.

[12] J. Robertson. Preconception Sex Selection. *American Journal of Bioethics* 1: 1 (Winter 2001).

would be responsible.' Yet selection is immune to this objection (in a way which genetic manipulation is not).

Imagine you select Embryo A and it develops cancer (or severe asthma) in later life. You have not harmed A unless A's life is not worth living (hardly plausible) because A would not have existed if you had acted otherwise. A is not made worse off than A would otherwise have been, since without the selection, A would not have existed. Thus we can accept the possibility of a bad outcome, but not the probability of a very bad outcome. (Clearly, Procreative Beneficence demands that we not choose a child with a low predisposition to asthma but who is likely to have a high predisposition to cancer.)

This is different to genetic manipulation. Imagine you perform gene therapy to correct a predisposition to asthma and you cause a mutation which results in cancer later in life. You have harmed A: A is worse off in virtue of the genetic manipulation than A would have been if the manipulation had not been performed (assuming cancer is worse than asthma).

There is, then, an important distinction between:

- interventions which are genetic manipulations of a single gamete, embryo or fetus
- selection procedures (e.g. sex selection) which select from among a range of different gametes, embryos and fetuses.

2. *Inequality:* One objection to Procreative Beneficence is that it will maintain or increase inequality. For example, it is often argued that selection for sex, intelligence, favourable physical or psychological traits, etc. all contribute to inequality in society, and this is a reason not to attempt to select the best.

In the case of selection against disease genes, similar claims are made. For example, one version of the *Disability Discrimination Claim* maintains that prenatal testing for disabilities such as Down syndrome results in discrimination against those with those disabilities both by:

- the statement it makes about the worth of such lives
- the reduction in the numbers of people with this condition.

Even if the Disability Discrimination Claim were true, it would be a drastic step in favour of equality to inflict a higher risk of having a child with a disability on a couple (who do not want a child with a disability) to promote social equality.

Consider a hypothetical rubella epidemic. A rubella epidemic hits an isolated population. Embryos produced prior to the epidemic are not at an elevated risk of any abnormality but those produced during the epidemic are at an increased risk of deafness and blindness. Doctors should encourage women to use embryos which they have produced prior to the epidemic in preference to ones produced during the epidemic. The reason is that it is bad that blind and deaf children are born when sighted and hearing children could have been born in their place.

This does not necessarily imply that the lives of those who now live with disability are less deserving of respect and are less valuable. To attempt to prevent accidents which cause paraplegia is not to say that paraplegics are less deserving of respect. It is important to distinguish between disability and persons with disability. Selection reduces the former, but is silent on the value of the latter. There are better ways to make statements about the equality of people with disability (e.g., we could direct savings from selection against embryos/fetuses with genetic abnormalities to improving well-being of existing people with disabilities).

These arguments extend to selection for non-disease genes. It is not disease which is important but its impact on well-being. In so far as a non-disease gene such as a gene for intelligence impacts on a person's well-being, parents have a reason to select for it, even if inequality results.

This claim can have counter-intuitive implications. Imagine in a country women are severely discriminated against. They are abandoned as children, refused paid employment and serve as slaves to men. Procreative Beneficence implies that couples should test for sex, and should choose males as they are expected to have better lives in this society, even if this reinforces the discrimination against women.

There are several responses. Firstly, it is unlikely selection on a scale that contributes to inequality would promote well-being. Imagine that 50% of the population choose to select boys. This would result in three boys to every one girl. The life of a male in such a society would be intolerable.

Secondly, it is social institutional reform, not interference in reproduction, which should be promoted. What is wrong in such a society is the treatment of women, which should be addressed separately to reproductive decision-making. Reproduction should not become an instrument of social change, at least not mediated or motivated at a social level.

This also illustrates why Procreative Beneficence is different to eugenics. Eugenics is selective breeding to produce a better *population*. A *public interest* justification for interfering in reproduction is different from Procreative Beneficence which aims at producing the best child, of the possible children, a couple could have. That is an essentially private enterprise. It was the eugenics movement itself which sought to influence reproduction, through involuntary sterilisation, to promote social goods.

Thirdly, consider the case of blackmail. A company says it will only develop an encouraging drug for cystic fibrosis (CF) if there are more than 100 000 people with CF. This would require stopping carrier testing for CF. Should the government stop carrier testing?

If there are other ways to fund this research (e.g., government funding), this should have priority. In virtually all cases of social inequality, there are other avenues to correct inequality than encouraging or forcing people to have children with disabilities or lives of restricted genetic opportunity.

LIMITS ON PROCREATIVE BENEFICENCE: PERSONAL CONCERN FOR EQUALITY OR SELF INTEREST

Consider the following cases. David and Dianne are dwarfs. They wish to use IVF and PGD to select a child with dwarfism because their house is set up for dwarfs. Sam and Susie live a society where discrimination against women is prevalent. They wish to have a girl to reduce this discrimination. These choices would not harm the child produced if selection is employed. Yet they conflict with the Principle of Procreative Beneficence.

We have here an irresolvable conflict of principles:

- personal commitment to equality, personal interests and Procreative Autonomy
- Procreative Beneficence.

Just as there are no simple answers to what should be done (from the perspective of ethics) when respect for personal autonomy conflicts with other principles such as beneficence or distributive justice, so too there are no simple answers to conflict between Procreative Autonomy and Procreative Beneficence.

For the purposes of public policy, there should be a presumption in favour of liberty in liberal democracies. So, ultimately, we should allow couples to make their own decisions about which child to have. Yet this does not imply that there are no normative principles to guide those choices. Procreative Beneficence is a valid principle, albeit one which must be balanced against others.

The implication of this is that those with disabilites should be allowed to select a child with disability, if they have a good reason. But the best option is that we correct discrimination in other ways, by correcting discriminatory social institutions. In this way, we can achieve both equality and a population whose members are living the best lives possible.

CONCLUSIONS

With respect to non-disease genes, we should provide:

- information (through PGD and prenatal testing)
- free choice of which child to have
- non-coercive advice as to which child will be expected to enter life with the best opportunity of having the best life.

Selection for non-disease genes which significantly impact on well-being is *morally required* (Procreative Beneficence). 'Morally required' implies moral persuasion but not coercion is justified.

If, in the end, couples wish to select a child who will have a lower chance of having the best life, they should be free to make such a choice. That should not prevent doctors from attempting to persuade them to have the best child they can. In some cases, persuasion will not be justified. If self-interest or concern to promote equality motivate a choice to select less than the best, then there may be no overall reason to attempt to dissuade a couple. But in cases in which couples do not want to use or obtain available information about genes which will affect well-being, and their desires are based on irrational fears (e.g., about interfering with nature or playing God), then doctors should try to persuade them to access and use such information in their reproductive decision-making.

Chapter 28

THE PROBLEM OF ABORTION: ESSENTIALLY CONTESTED CONCEPTS AND MORAL AUTONOMY

SUSANNE GIBSON

When one thinks about the ethics of abortion, one inevitably thinks about rights, since it is in terms of the concept of rights that much of the debate has been conducted.[1] This is true of overtly feminist as well as non-feminist accounts. Indeed, some early feminist writers – Judith Jarvis Thomson and Mary Ann Warren,[2] for example – employ a model of rights that is indistinguishable, or virtually indistinguishable, from that of their non-feminist counterparts. However, more recent feminist writers have developed a different understanding of 'a woman's right to choose.'

In this paper, I will begin by outlining the non-feminist debate over the moral permissibility of abortion. I will suggest that this debate is irresolvable, since at its heart is an 'essentially contested concept', that of personhood. I will then consider the way in which some feminist writers have attempted to reconceive the terms of the abortion debate and suggest an expanded account of women's right to abortion, drawing on the work of Susan Sherwin.[3] Finally, I will argue that there is a further element to a 'woman's right to choose' that expands on and provides a conceptual link between the feminist[4] and non-feminist understanding of abortion.

From the perspective of mainstream, non-feminist philosophy, the abortion debate can be characterised as follows: the rights of the woman are pitted against those of the foetus. Women have rights

---

[1] An earlier version of this paper was presented at the 'Beijing Symposium on Feminist Approaches to Bioethics', 1–2 November, 2001. I thank my referees from *Bioethics* for their helpful and insightful comments.

[2] Judith Jarvis Thomson. 1984. A Defence of Abortion; Mary Anne Warren. On the Moral and Legal Status of Abortion. Both reprinted in *The Problem of Abortion*. Joel Feinberg, ed. Wandsworth, UK. Wandsworth Publishing.

[3] Susan Sherwin. 1992. *No Longer Patient*. Philadelphia. Temple University Press.

[4] I recognise that there are a wide variety of feminist positions on abortion. In this paper I use the term 'feminist' to refer to the particular feminist position that I am dealing with.

to privacy, self-determination, bodily integrity or rights over property in the person that might or might not outweigh the competing
rights of the foetus. An examination of the literature shows that
there is at least some agreement over what rights a woman possesses, but disagreement over what these rights amount to; this
disagreement arises out of conflicting accounts of the moral status
and consequent moral rights of the foetus. Three basic positions
can be delineated: (i) the foetus has a right to life from the moment
of conception; (ii) the foetus comes into possession of the right to
life at some stage during pregnancy; (iii) the foetus does not at any
stage of gestation have a right to life. These are referred to as the
'conservative', 'moderate' and 'liberal' positions respectively. Where
the foetus has a right to life from the moment of conception, abortion becomes impermissible except in perhaps a small minority of
cases, since whatever rights a woman does have regarding what
happens in and to her own body do not outweigh the right to life.[5]
Similarly, where the foetus comes into possession of the right to life
at some point during pregnancy, abortion becomes impermissible
after that point – in the contemporary debate, the point at which
the foetus becomes viable is often taken to be the significant point.
Finally, where the foetus does not have a right to life, the woman
has a right to abortion at any stage during pregnancy since her
rights are stronger than any lesser rights that the foetus might
possess, if indeed the foetus can be said to possess any rights at all.

The abortion debate, then, becomes a debate not so much over
women's rights but over foetal moral status, and for this reason, I
suggest, it is interminable. Just as foetal rights are grounded in
foetal moral status, this status in turn rests on the concept of 'personhood', and this, I will show, is an example of what W.B. Gallie
terms an 'essentially contested concept.'[6]

An essentially contested concept is a concept over which there is
disagreement regarding its proper use and where 'there is no one
clearly definable general use . . . which can be set up as the correct
or standard use.'[7] However, it is not the case that once the variety
of uses of the term is recognised, the dispute comes to an end – the
participants do not agree to differ, neither are we left with a

---

[5] Thomson's contribution to the debate is a notable exception to this rule.
[6] W.B. Gallie. Essentially Contested Concepts. *Proceedings of the Aristotelian Society* 1956;
LVI: 167–198.
[7] Ibid. p. 168.

relativist account of that term. On the contrary, Gallie states, 'Each party continues to maintain that the special functions which the [concept] fulfils on *its* behalf or on *its* interpretation, is the correct or proper or primary, or only important, function which the term can plainly be said to fulfil. Moreover, each party continues to defend its case with what it claims to be convincing arguments, evidence and other forms of justification.'[8] The dispute over an essentially contested concept, although irresolvable, is a genuine dispute; that is, it is characterised by coherent and sustainable argument.[9] It is not the case, for example, that the same term is being used to refer to two different concepts such that there is no real contest over the true meaning.

Gallie sets out a number of necessary conditions for an essentially contested concept. Conditions (I) to (III) can be summarised as follows: the concept must be appraisive, signifying a valued achievement of an internally complex character, whereby an explanation of its worth refers to 'the respective contribution of its various parts or features.'[10] Condition (IV) states that the achievement in question remains open to modification in the light of changing circumstances; condition (V) that the contest over the use of the concept is recognised by all parties to the dispute. Gallie argues further that in order to distinguish between an essentially contested concept and the confusion of two or more different concepts – in order to establish that the disputants are in some sense referring to the same thing – we need to be able to show that the concept in question has been derived from an 'exemplar', and that this exemplar must be acknowledged by all of the contestants as such.[11] This then is condition (VI). Finally, condition (VII) requires that the competition over the use of the concept sustains or develops the achievement of the exemplar.[12]

I suggest that the concept of personhood is an essentially contested concept. In the context of the abortion debate, the term 'person' is used just because it is appraisive, signifying a valued achievement, that of moral status, which is variously explained in terms of the significance that is attached to its various features.

[8] Ibid. p. 168. Emphasis in original.
[9] Ibid. p. 169.
[10] Ibid. pp. 171–172.
[11] Ibid. p. 176.
[12] Ibid. p. 180.

Thus, those who adopt the conservative position focus on membership of the human species, emphasising its special status. The liberals, on the other hand, relegate species membership to a position of low importance, focusing instead on capacities such as self-consciousness and rational autonomy. The moderate might be said to pick out the capacity for sentience or for independent survival.[13] At the same time, any genuine participant in the debate must recognise that the use of this term is disputed.

Gallie explains condition (IV) in terms of a persistent vagueness in the achievement accredited by the concept in question. In terms of the concept of personhood, this vagueness consists in the fact that we cannot say in advance *exactly* what a person will look like: it is possible that something that we cannot imagine, in a context that we cannot imagine, will meet our criteria. It is also clear that the different conceptions of personhood are derived from an exemplar, that of the human adult, which all parties to the dispute will agree has the requisite moral status. What they disagree over is which features of the human adult confer that moral status. I will argue below that condition (VII) can also be satisfied.[14]

If the concept of personhood is an essentially contested concept, and if it is fundamental to the abortion debate, then that debate is and will remain irresolvable. At the same time, it remains a genuine debate and one with which there is reason to engage. Further, the claim that it is irresolvable does not imply that we cannot reach a conclusion over whether or not women have a right to choose abortion, or over what this right consists in. Indeed, it is my argument that women have the right to choose abortion just because of the essentially contested nature of the concept of personhood.

I will refer again to Gallie's conditions for an essentially contested concept in the final stages of my argument. Next, I want to consider the feminist account of what is at stake in the abortion debate. If the non-feminist account can be characterised in terms of its focus on the moral status of the foetus, then the feminist alternative can

---

[13] For a detailed account of the main perspectives on the status of the foetus, see: Rosalind Hursthouse. 1987. *Beginning Lives*. Oxford. Blackwell Publishing Ltd.

[14] Of course, there are numerous examples of the non-recognition of the moral status of the human adult, for example, the practice of slavery. However, such practices tend to be justified precisely on the grounds of the denial of full membership of the human race for those so treated. Conversely, the practice of slavery becomes unsustainable once it is recognised that the slave is a person 'just like us.' I thank one of my referees for drawing my attention to this point.

be distinguished by the effort to broaden or indeed to shift this focus. As Sherwin puts it:

> The most obvious difference between feminist and nonfeminist approaches to abortion lies in the relative attention each gives in its analysis to the interests and experiences of women. Feminist analysis regards the effects of unwanted pregnancies on the lives of women individually and collectively as the central element in the moral examination of abortion; it is considered self-evident that the pregnant woman is the subject of principal concern in abortion decisions. In many nonfeminist accounts, however, not only is the pregnant woman not perceived as central, she is often rendered virtually invisible. Nonfeminist theorists, whether they support or oppose women's right to choose abortion, generally focus almost all their attention on the moral status of the foetus.[15]

For Sherwin, a feminist perspective on abortion takes the most significant moral feature of pregnancy to be the fact that it is something that takes place in a woman's body, having a profound effect on a woman's life.[16] Putting women at the centre of the abortion debate has a number of implications. At one level, abortion is put in its social and political context. In societies in which women are oppressed, and in which women's options are limited by the structures of patriarchy, abortion becomes a means of responding to the consequences of male domination as well as a means of breaking free from it.[17]

However, what is more important for the purpose of this paper is the implication of a woman-centred account for an understanding of the nature of the abortion decision as it is made by particular women in particular circumstances. Here the difference between the feminist and non-feminist approaches lies in a shift away from an abstract account of abortion that can be applied to any woman and any foetus, to a more contextual understanding that recognises the uniqueness of each pregnancy. The abortion decision is still a moral decision, but it is one that resists formulation in abstract, generalised terms. To quote Sherwin again:

---

[15] Sherwin, *op. cit.* note 3, p. 101.
[16] Ibid. p. 104.
[17] See, for example: Rosemarie Tong. 1997. *Feminist Approaches to Bioethics: Theoretical Reflections and Practical Applications*. Boulder, CO. Westview Press: 132–146.

Women's personal deliberations about abortion involve contextually defined considerations that reflect their commitments to the needs and interests of everyone concerned, including themselves, the fetus they carry, other members of their household, and so forth. Because no single formula is available for balancing these complex factors through all possible cases, it is vital that feminists insist on protecting each woman's right to come to her own conclusions and resist the attempts of other philosophers and moralists to set the agenda for these considerations. Feminists stress that women must be acknowledged as full moral agents, responsible for making moral decisions about their own pregnancies.[18]

A woman's right to choose, then, is a right to make a decision about the morality of continuing or terminating a pregnancy in just this particular case. It is a moral decision, but not one that can be generalised to apply to any other woman making the same decision in her own particular case.

Thus conceived, the feminist approach to abortion brings the woman, as a particular moral agent, back into the picture. However, it is not the case that the foetus disappears. Although feminists like Sherwin want to expand the terms of the debate, there is still a conception of the moral status of the foetus, and of personhood, embedded in this account. This can be termed a 'relational' conception of moral status. Rather than viewing the foetus and the woman as two independent beings whose moral claims have to be balanced against one another, the focus is on the relationship between the foetus and the woman. The ontological and moral status of the foetus is unique in that a foetus exists only in relationship with a particular other on whom it is entirely dependent for support. It is because of this relationship that the foetus is morally significant, since it is out of relationships that our moral obligations arise. However, since the only direct relationship it can have is with the woman inside of whom it is developing, and since no one else can do anything directly to the foetus without also doing something to the woman, the decision to continue or to discontinue nurturing the foetus lies solely with the woman.[19] Hence the specific status of a foetus will vary according to the value ascribed to it by the woman

---

[18] Sherwin, *op. cit.* note 3, p. 102.
[19] Ibid. p. 110.

in whose womb it is developing. Foetuses do not have absolute value because they have no existence independent of this one relationship. Their value is the kind of value that attaches not to an individual human being, but to a human relationship. Because there can be no abstract account of the absolute value of human relationships, but only of particular relationships, there can be no abstract account of the absolute value of foetuses.

I argued above that the non-feminist debate is irresolvable because it centres on the essentially contested concept of personhood. Sherwin claims that foetuses are not persons because they lack morally significant development with regard to their capacity for social relationships.[20] Nevertheless, it is clear that this still presupposes a conception of personhood, just as the parties to the non-feminist debate each presuppose a conception of personhood. Personhood is here understood in terms of social relations. According to Sherwin, 'humans are fundamentally relational beings.'[21] The self is relational in that each of us develops as a person through our relationships with others. It is the variety of relationships and roles that a human being participates in – their membership of a community – that gives them their value as persons. The foetus is not a person because it cannot have this variety of roles; following birth, however, a human being immediately begins to develop into a person by virtue of its ability to participate in an increasing range of relationships with other persons.

The feminist conception of foetal moral status might be seen as having something in common with each of the conservative, moderate and liberal positions. Like the conservatives, the humanness of the foetus is valued; like the moderates, foetal value develops through pregnancy, as the relationship develops; however, like the liberals, the foetus is denied personhood prior to birth. At the same time, it is clear that this relational conception of personhood picks out a different feature of the exemplar – the human adult – as the relevant feature of what it is to be a person and thus to have moral value. In this case it is our capacity to participate in a variety of relationships that is constitutive of our personhood.

Is it the case, then, that the feminist conception of what it is to be a person is the one true conception, such that personhood is not in fact an essentially contested concept after all? I do not think that

---

[20] Ibid. p. 111.
[21] Ibid. p. 110.

454   **Susanne Gibson**

this is the case. Without entering into the details of what such an argument would look like, it seems evident that someone who values genetic humanness, or self-consciousness, or the capacity for independent survival might still dispute the feminist account. However, I stated above that any dispute over an essentially contested concept is a genuine dispute, and it is because the dispute over the concept of personhood is a genuine dispute that there is a further aspect to women's moral agency with regard to abortion and therefore to a woman's right to choose abortion, understood as a right to make a moral decision.

By referring again to Gallie, it can be seen that where there is a genuine dispute over an essentially contested concept, then there are good reasons to continue to engage in that dispute. Indeed, it might be said that simply by adopting a particular conception, one is necessarily engaged in the dispute. That this is the case arises out of conditions (V) and (VII). Condition (V) states that where a concept is essentially contested then it is:

> not only that different persons or parties adhere to different views of the correct use of [the concept] but . . . that each party recognizes the fact that its own use of it is contested by those other parties, and that each party must have at least some appreciation of the different criteria in the light of which the other parties claim to be applying the concept in question. More simply, to use an essentially contested concept means to use it against other uses and to recognize that one's own use of it has to be maintained against these other uses.[22]

Condition (VII) is that:

> continuous competition for the acknowledgement as between the contestant users of the concept [should enable] the original exemplar's achievement to be sustained and/or developed in optimum fashion.[23]

I take this to mean that in using the concept of personhood to defend a position on the ethics of abortion, we are also necessarily defending that conception of personhood against those other conceptions that we reject but nevertheless take seriously enough to engage with. Further, in doing so, we somehow advance not only

---

[22] Gallie, *op. cit.* note 6, p. 172.
[23] Ibid. p. 180.

our understanding of personhood, but also our own personhood – we become more human, in the evaluative sense of that term.

What I want to suggest, then, is that when a particular woman makes a decision about abortion, insofar as she exercises her moral agency, she necessarily exercises that agency in the realm of the abstract as well as in the realm of the particular. This is not to make an empirical claim about the way in which women in fact make the decision to have or not have an abortion, nor about the way in which they might conceive of that decision. Rather, it is an aspect of the logic of moral agency. In making a judgement about the moral value of this particular foetus or this particular pregnancy, a woman must in some sense formulate or adopt (or be prepared to formulate or adopt) a more general conception of personhood, which she must then be prepared to defend against alternative conceptions, at least in principle. Indeed, Sherwin implicitly acknowledges this point when she says that '[w]omen may sometimes make mistakes in their moral judgments' with regard to abortion.[24] The concept of a moral mistake implies a set of standards against which the judgement can be assessed external to the woman herself, even if it is the same woman who later comes to think that it is she who has made a mistake. In this respect, it might be said that there is no such thing as a private morality.

However, Sherwin then goes on to claim that even though women might make such mistakes, 'no one else can be assumed to have the authority to evaluate and overrule their judgments.'[25] My argument in this respect is that a distinction needs to be drawn between evaluating a judgement on the one hand and overruling that judgement on the other. Whereas, in the case of abortion, it can be argued that no one has the authority to overrule a woman's judgement, it does not follow that it cannot be evaluated. Indeed, insofar as a judgement regarding an abortion decision is a moral judgement, then it is necessarily evaluative. This can be understood by returning to the concept of moral agency, or moral autonomy. In the traditional Kantian conception of moral autonomy, the moral agent is self-legislating, but in such a way that when she legislates for herself she legislates for all others in relevantly similar circumstances. There is no sense in which one can make a moral judgement regarding one's own actions without making a judgement regarding the

---

[24] Sherwin, *op. cit.* note 3, p. 102.
[25] Ibid.

actions of others, real or hypothetical. I have already suggested one way in which a woman making a decision regarding abortion might engage in this kind of abstract reasoning: that is, in adopting a particular conception of personhood. It should be noted, however, that feminist philosophers have been critical of Kantian moral theory, precisely because of its tendency towards abstraction and away from the context and contingency of real lives. The Kantian focus on the rational individual as the source of morality also obscures the significance of personal and social relationships and the effects that they give rise to.[26] Thus it is more in keeping with a feminist approach to put this point in terms of the concept of 'relational autonomy.'

The concept of relational autonomy is a reworking rather than a rejection of the Kantian, or more broadly the liberal-individualist ideals of personal and moral autonomy, building upon the relational conception of personhood outlined above. Autonomy is still viewed as something that resides in the individual self, but as the self is constituted and re-constituted within a network of relationships, so too is the capacity for autonomy. Further, as Anne Donchin has pointed out, since the self is fundamentally relational, the relational component of autonomy is inherent in the meaning of the term.[27] In her own account of relational autonomy, Sherwin points to the social and political context in which autonomy is developed and exercised, signalling the ways in which the capacity for autonomy is both constrained and facilitated by more or less oppressive social circumstances. Under conditions of oppression, an individual's autonomy can be undermined both by denying that individual the opportunity to exercise her autonomy and by undermining her confidence in herself as an autonomous agent.[28]

---

[26] Marilyn Friedman. 2000. Feminism in Ethics: Conceptions of Autonomy. In *The Cambridge Companion to Feminism in Philosophy*. Miranda Fricker & Jennifer Hornsby, eds. Cambridge. Cambridge University Press: 212. Friedman also points out that contemporary mainstream conceptions of autonomy acknowledge the ways in which necessarily socialised, dependent human beings nevertheless remain autonomous (p. 218).

[27] Anne Donchin. 2000. Autonomy and Interdependence: Quandaries in Genetic Decision Making. In *Relational Autonomy: Feminist Perspectives on Autonomy, Agency and the Social Self*. Catriona Mackenzie & Natalie Stoljar, eds. Oxford. Oxford University Press: 239.

[28] Susan Sherwin. 1998. A Relational Approach to Autonomy in Health Care. In *The Politics of Women's Health: Exploring Agency and Autonomy*. S. Sherwin, F. Baylis, M. Bell, M. De Koninck, J. Downie, A. Lippman, M. Lock, W. Mitchinson, K. Pauly Morgan, J. Mosher, B. Parish, eds. Philadelphia. Temple University Press: 35–36.

Thus understood, moral autonomy as much as personal autonomy is developed and exercised in a social and political context. Under what kind of conditions, then, might one develop, or fail to develop as a moral agent? Paul Benson has argued for a relational account of moral responsibility, drawing a connection between moral responsibility and self worth.[29] Moral responsibility means being prepared to answer for one's actions and as such it depends upon a sense of one's worthiness to do so. Thus it is founded in certain kinds of social relationship. Fundamentally, answerability requires that there be others to whom one is answerable, others who can criticise and who can expect reasons and explanations offered in terms of publicly shareable norms. It is not enough simply to decide for oneself when one has or has not made a mistake, in terms of one's own account of what constitutes a good or a bad reason for abortion. The sense of self-worth is developed precisely by being held responsible, as well as by holding oneself responsible. According to Benson, 'being responsible is itself a matter of occupying a certain social position, having *the status of an eligible participant in a community of moral dialogue.*'[30] This in turn means that the morally autonomous agent is appropriately subject to attitudes of blame and so on when she fails to behave in the way in which she might reasonably have been expected to behave.

Indeed, Sherwin acknowledges the importance of self-respect in the development of autonomy, and the way in which diminished expectations can easily result in a diminished capacity for autonomy.[31] From this perspective it might be said that moral agency cannot be developed or exercised in isolation. To be refused entry into a community of moral dialogue is to be denied the conditions for a sense of one's own worthiness to answer for one's actions. Similarly, to refuse to explain and defend one's own decisions or to refuse to engage evaluatively with the decisions of others is to sever the moral relationships that are constitutive of moral identity.

I hold, therefore, that we are committed in respect of our (relational) moral autonomy to answering for our own abortion decisions and being prepared to evaluate the decisions of others.

---

[29] Paul Benson. 2000. Feeling Crazy: Self-worth and the Social Character of Responsibility. In *Relational Autonomy: Feminist Perspectives on Autonomy, Agency and the Social Self*, *op. cit.* note 27, pp. 72–93.

[30] Benson, *op. cit.* note 29, p. 83. Emphasis in the original.

[31] Sherwin, *op. cit.* note 28, p. 37.

However, I claimed above that while there is this necessity to evaluate, Sherwin is correct in arguing that no one has the authority to
overrule the abortion decision of another. It is not my contention
that overruling another's decision is always impermissible: that is, I
am not arguing for moral subjectivism. However, as I argued above,
the dispute over abortion is based on a dispute over an essentially
contested concept, that of personhood. Just because there is no
resolution to the dispute over what it is to be a person, there is no
foundation for the authority to overrule the decision to have an
abortion, and therefore it remains the case that it is the woman's
right to choose abortion. Indeed, it is a particularly robust right,
since it is grounded in the nature of the dispute rather than in the
conclusions of any of its participants.

The right to abortion is understood by the liberals as a right to
bodily self-determination, and by feminist writers as a right to make
a moral decision regarding the continuation of a particular relationship. The additional aspect to this right that I am positing is the
right to act as a moral agent, whether understood in terms of a
Kantian self-legislator, engaging in and acting on the application of
abstract moral reasoning, or perhaps more plausibly, as a relation-
ally autonomous moral agent, participating in membership of a
network of moral relationships. Further, in this way, the feminist
account of abortion is reintegrated with the non-feminist account:
the defence of abortion remains an important part of the defence
of a particular conception of personhood, and therefore the feminist and non-feminist theorists are necessarily engaged in the same
dispute, broadly speaking.

Chapter 29

THE INJUSTICE OF UNSAFE MOTHERHOOD

REBECCA J. COOK AND BERNARD M. DICKENS

DIMENSIONS AND CAUSES OF UNSAFE MOTHERHOOD

The differential incidence of unsafe motherhood has been described as marking the greatest discrepancy in any health statistic between developed and developing countries of the world.[1] The most recent World Health Organization and associated agencies' estimate is that every year worldwide, about 515 000 women die of complications of pregnancy and childbirth,[2] a rate of over 1400 maternal deaths each day. Further, at least 7 million women suffer serious health problems when they survive childbirth, and an additional estimated 50 million women suffer adverse health effects after childbirth.[3] Statistics are incomplete because many countries lack vital statistics registries and systematic examinations of causes of maternal deaths, and many women are unattended by health care professionals or other adequately skilled personnel during pregnancy, labour, childbirth and their resulting death or morbidity. Nevertheless, it is estimated that almost 99% of these tragic and often preventable consequences of unsafe motherhood occur in developing countries. It has been observed that 'Almost 90% of these deaths occur in sub-Saharan Africa and Asia' alone.[4]

The ends of the spectrum of maternal mortality and morbidity are not easily determined, but representative figures are that the estimated probability of pregnancy-related death faced by an average woman over her reproductive life-span is 1 in 8,700 in Canada, and

---

[1] A. Starrs. 1998. *The Safe Motherhood Action Agenda: Priorities for the Next Decade.* New York. Family Care International: 1.
[2] World Health Organization, United Nations Children's Fund and United Nations Population Fund. 2001. *Maternal Mortality in 1995. Estimates Developed by WHO, UNICEF, and UNFPA.* Geneva. World Health Organization (WHO/RHR/01.9).
[3] United Nations Population Fund. 1999. *The State of the World Population 1999, 6 Billion: A Time for Choices.* New York. UNFPA: 30.
[4] A. Starrs, *op. cit.* note 1, p. 1.

1 in 7 in Ethiopia, 1 in 6 in Rwanda and Sierra Leone.[5] Canadian statistics may conceal different rates between aboriginal and non-aboriginal women, in the same way that the United States of America's rate of 1 in 3500 conceals differences between black, white and hispanic women and members of rural and urban populations.[6] By way of general contrast and comparison, however, the average rate in sub-Saharan Africa is 1 in 14 but 1 in 70 in South Africa, the average rate in South-East Asia is 1 in 47 but 1 in 1100 in Thailand, 1 in 60 in the Eastern Mediterranean but 1 in 430 in Tunisia and 1 in 1,300 in Europe, ranging from 1 in 4600 in the United Kingdom to 1 in 1000 in Romania and 1 in 450 in Kazakhstan.[7]

Causes of unsafe motherhood may in theory be separated into medical, health system, social and other causes, but in practice they often overlap. For instance, many pregnant women in developing countries suffer from anemia, which compromises their survival and health status associated with pregnancy and childbearing in general, and particularly when heavy blood loss occurs. Where food resources are inadequate due, for instance, to regional drought and famine or family poverty, the nutritional disadvantages of girl children may be aggravated by their devaluation in their homes and cultures. Food allocation practices within families that give priority to feeding husbands and sons before wives, then other family dependents such as elderly parents and lastly daughters,[8] may condemn girl children to malnutrition in the form of undernourishment, with associated anemia.

Similarly, early marriage, perhaps when adolescents are below the minimum age for marriage prescribed by law,[9] followed by

---

[5] See World Health Organization *op. cit.* note 2, and R.J. Cook et al. 2001. *Advancing Safe Motherhood Through Human Rights.* Geneva. World Health Organization: Appendix I, pp. 93–95.

[6] In the US the black population has a relative risk of maternal death 4.3 times higher than the nonblack population: H.K. Atrash et al. Maternal Mortality in Developed Countries: Not Just a Concern of the Past. *Obstetrics and Gynecology* 1995; 86: 700–705.

[7] See World Health Organization and R.J. Cook et al., *op. cit.* note 5.

[8] See e.g. J. Kabeberi-Macharia. 1998. Reconstructing the Image of the Girl-Child. In *Law, Culture, Tradition and Children's Rights in Eastern and Southern Africa.* W. Ncube, ed. Aldershot. Ashgate/Dartmouth: 47–56 at 47.

[9] For instance the Child Marriage Restraint Act in India sets the minimum age of marriage for girls at 18, but it has been recorded that about 50% of women enter their first union before their eighteenth birthday and almost 30% have their first child by age 18. See Alan Guttmacher Institute. 1998. *Into a New World: Young Women's Sexual and Reproductive Lives.* New York. AGI: 18.

premature and repeated pregnancy, create medical circumstances inimical to survival and health. These are conditioned, however, by social forces that favour or even require girls' early marriage, and fecundity. Conditioning factors include families' concerns regarding dowry payments, fears of family dishonour due to daughters' premarital loss of virginity, whether by their sexual adventure or victimization by rape, and husbands' requirement of births of sons and of evidence of their virility.

Infections such as malaria, that may be more associated with geographical rather than social considerations, pose a medical risk in pregnancy, endangering health and life itself. Equally, women with the genetic sickle-cell trait may face health hazards due to pregnancy. However, some other medical risks aggravated by pregnancy are socially conditioned. Prominent among these is HIV/AIDS, to which women are often exposed because of their powerlessness to resist sexual intercourse with infected men or to require men to wear condoms, or their lack of access to such protection because of financial, legal, health system or other barriers. Pregnancy naturally reduces women's immunity to infection, and their vulnerability is considerably increased when HIV/AIDS has already compromised their immune systems. In some religions and cultures, female genital cutting, often described judgmentally as mutilation, also contributes to unsafe motherhood in causing medical complications antenatally, and in early labour and childbirth, including prolonged labour and, for instance, post partum hemorrhage, and death.[10]

Health system failures often add significantly to the burden of unsafe motherhood. It has been explained that in the course of pregnancy, labour and delivery, women '. . . in every country and every population develop complications, but women in developing countries are much less likely to get prompt adequate treatment, and are therefore more likely to die.'[11]

The scarcity of physicians, trained nurses or midwives and often of skilled birth attendants, in urban as well as rural settings,

---

[10] Department of Women's Health, Family and Community Health, World Health Organization. 2000. *A Systematic Review of the Health Complications of Female Genital Mutilation, including Sequelae in Childbirth.* Geneva. World Health Organization (WHO/FCH/WMH/00.2): 48.

[11] D. Maine et al. 1997. *The Design and Evaluation of Maternal Mortality Programs.* New York. Center for Population and Family Health, School of Public Health, Columbia University: 4.

accounts for much of the incidence of maternal mortality and morbidity.[12] Social factors and customs may also be involved, however. Where prenatal and maternity care are available, for instance, women may not be allowed to travel to them alone. Further, husbands' consent or consent of unmarried adolescents' parents may be required before women can receive care, for instance because male health care providers are present, or pregnant women lack independent means to ensure that service fees will be paid. Cost itself is often a barrier to access to available care among impoverished families that seek it.

PUBLIC HEALTH BIOETHICS AND UNSAFE MOTHERHOOD

The United Nations' International Conference on Population and Development, held in Cairo in 1994, and World Conference on Women, held in Beijing in 1995, both recognized that reproductive health failures embodied in unsafe motherhood raise concerns that transcend clinical medicine, and must be addressed in addition as public health concerns. The public health implications of developing country urbanization have come to be recognized in recent years,[13] but the public health dimensions of unsafe motherhood, and public health potential for its reduction, have escaped general attention, except for recognition that the consequences of unskilled abortion, both where abortion is legally permissible and where it is not, should be addressed less as a moral than as a public health concern.[14]

It has been conventional to observe that unsafe motherhood is strongly associated with pregnancies that come too early, too late, too often and too closely spaced in women's reproductive lives. This observation has no prognostic value in the clinical care of any

[12] W.J. Graham, J.S. Bell & C.H.W. Bullogh. 2001. Can Skilled Attendance at Delivery Reduce Maternal Mortality in Developing Countries? In *Safe Motherhood Strategies: A Review of the Evidence.* V. DeBrouwere and W. VanLerberghe, eds. Antwerp. ITG Press: 97–130.

[13] See World Health Organization, Centre for Health Development, Kobe, Japan. 1996. *Urbanization: A Global Health Challenge.* Geneva. WHO (WHO/WCK/SYM/96.1).

[14] See the Programme of Action of the International Conference on Population and Development, Cairo, Egypt 5–13 September 1994, para 8.25, in Report of the International Conference on Population and Development, U.N. Doc. A/CONF.171/13/Rev.1, U.N. Sales No. 95. XIII. 18 (1995).

individual adolescent or woman, but remains an epidemiological or public health truism. Safe motherhood depends on women's avoidance of untimely and otherwise inappropriate pregnancy, for instance by means of women's education and power to decide whether, when, with whom and in what ways to be sexually active. It also requires access to natural and assisted means of fertility control, and, for example, women's unimpaired access to medical and related care during pregnancy, labour and childbirth and the immediate and longer post-partum period. These goals are most effectively advanced through public health strategies, which may be implemented through public health law. Public health law has recently been defined as:

> [T]he study of the legal powers and duties of the state to assure the conditions for people to be healthy (e.g. to identify, prevent, and ameliorate risks to health in the population) and the limitations on the power of the state to constrain the autonomy, privacy, liberty, proprietary, or other legally protected interests of individuals for the protection or promotion of community health.[15]

In formulating this definition, Gostin, justly celebrated for his pioneering work to advance civil liberties in the UK, Europe and the US, is conscious that his acknowledgment of 'the power of the state to constrain the autonomy . . . of individuals,' though limited, itself runs counter to a key ethical value in the US and beyond.[16] A prominent bioethicist, however, noting that '[a]utonomy has become a dominant bioethical value in the Western world,'[17] has pointed to instances in which individual autonomy has traditionally been subordinated to community values. An instance is social action to prevent a competent person's suicide, on the justifications that 'a person's death diminishes others as well and that therefore society is permitted to intervene'[18] This reflects the historical observation of the English poet and cleric John Donne (1572–1631) that '[a]ny man's death diminishes me, because I am involved in

---

[15] L.O. Gostin. 2000. *Public Health Law: Power, Duty, Restraint.* Berkeley, CA. University of California Press; New York. The Milbank Memorial Fund: 4.

[16] Ibid. Preface: xxi.

[17] S.M. Glick. Unlimited Human Autonomy A Cultural Bias? *NEJM* 1997; 336: 954–956 at 954.

[18] Ibid. at 955.

mankind; and therefore never send to know for whom the [grave-
yard] bell tolls; it tolls for thee.'[19]

The social sense of diminution has not been raised in many
countries, however, by the incidence of maternal mortality. It is
observable that:

[T]hese hundreds of thousands of avoidable deaths each year are
continuing evidence and condemnation of the unstated presumption on which many societies are organized, namely that lives of
mothers are expendable and that women do not matter.[20]

Making mothers and all women's lives, and health, matter, goes
beyond individualistic ethics and bioethics of autonomy, to impli-
cate macroethical and community values. These are expressed in
some bioethical literature, especially by feminist writers,[21] but particularly in human rights principles, many of which are embodied
in national and international laws.

The late Jonathan Mann identified contrasts and synergies, or
complementarities, between medicine and public health,[22] the
former focussing on individual, clinical care and cure, the latter on
population health and prevention of health hazards, but both pursuing health as defined by the World Health Organization, namely
as a state of physical, mental and social well-being.[23] Similarly he
proposed, in a memorable keynote address opening the International Association of Bioethics' Third World Congress of Bioethics
in San Francisco in 1996, that the equivalent of the role of bioethics
in medicine is the role of human rights in public health. The Summer 2001 edition of the *Cambridge Quarterly of Healthcare Ethics*,
dedicated to his memory, is appropriately entitled *Keeping Human
Rights on the Bioethics Agenda*.

The initial paper of this edition, an appreciation of Jonathan
Mann,[24] addresses the significance of human rights in opening the

[19] J. Donne. 1624. Devotions upon Emergent Occasions-Meditation no. 17.
[20] R.J. Cook. 2001. Advancing Safe Motherhood Through Human Rights. In *Giving Meaning to Economic, Social and Cultural Rights*. I. Merali and V. Oosterveld, eds. Philadelphia.
University of Pennsylvania Press: 109–123 at 109.
[21] R. Tong. 1996. Feminist Approaches to Bioethics. In *Feminism and Bioethics: Beyond
Reproduction*. S.M. Wolf, ed. New York. Oxford University Press: 67–94.
[22] J.M. Mann. Medicine and Public Health, Ethics and Human Rights. *Hastings Center
Report* 1997; 27(3): 6–13.
[23] Constitution of the World Health Organization, Preamble, para. 2.
[24] J.C. d'Oronzio. The Integration of Health and Human Rights: An Appreciation of
Jonathan M. Mann. *Cambridge Q. Health Care Ethics* 2001; 10: 231–240.

public health agenda to ethical perceptions, observing that '[t]he conceptualization of the health and human rights movement reso- nates with ideas that the bioethics movement b[r]ought to medicine. Indeed, a conceptual parallel between this movement and bioethics is to be found in how each views the field and goals of medicine.'[25] This insight shows links between human rights and bioethics, par- ticularly as bioethics progress beyond their contemporary US and more general Western preoccupation with individual autonomy. It constitutes a creative response to Mann's critique of the narrowness of bioethics emerging from medical or clinical experience. Writing in the US in 1997, Mann noted that:

> [T]he contribution of medicine to health, while undeniably important (and vital in certain situations) is actually quite lim- ited. For example, it is estimated that only about one-sixth of the years of life expectancy gained in this country during this century can be attributed to the beneficial impact of medicine, medical care, and medical research. And it has been estimated that only about 10% of preventable premature deaths are associated with a lack of medical care.[26]

Accepting that 'none of these data . . . suggest that medical care is irrelevant; rather they suggest its limits,'[27] Mann looked beyond those limits for explanations of health differences among popula- tions, and found explanatory materials at the public and community health levels. He concluded that the conventional understanding linking socioeconomic status to health status is inadequate, and noted that:

> Other measures, such as the extent of socioeconomic inequality within a community, the nature, level and temporal pattern of unemployment, societal connectedness and the extent of involve- ment in social networks, marital status, early childhood experi- ences, and exposure to dignity-denying situations have all been suggested as powerful potential components of a 'black box' of societal factors whose dominant role in determining levels of preventable disease, disability, and premature death is beyond dispute.[28]

[25] Ibid. at 231.
[26] J.M. Mann, *op. cit.* note 22, at p. 7.
[27] Ibid.
[28] Ibid. at p. 8.

It is a tragic irony that Jonathan Mann's own premature death in September 1998, while flying from New York to Geneva to attend a meeting at the World Health Organization, robbed him and us of his further exploration of how public health strategies inspired by human rights values can promote population health. A legacy, however, is his focus on how social inequality, economic powerlessness, societal exclusion and denials of human dignity condition preventable disease, disability and premature death. These factors relate directly and indirectly to women's high rates of maternal mortality and morbidity.

RELIGIOUS MORALITY AND UNSAFE MOTHERHOOD

The laws and social customs that have often conditioned unsafe motherhood and condemned generations of women to suffer pregnancy-related death and disability may have their roots in religiously-guided perceptions of morality. The demographically-driven Biblical imperative to the people of the Bible to 'be fruitful and multiply,' for instance, has cast a long moral shadow over artificial contraception. Contraceptive means frequently remain critical to women's self-defence against life- and health-endangering pregnancies, but until 1969, for example, the Canadian Criminal Code punished distribution of means and knowledge of contraception as a 'crime against morality.' The Roman Catholic Church maintains its prohibition of contraceptive means such as condoms, opposing distribution even in the face of the international HIV/AIDS pandemic.

This inflexible historical prohibition in fact was transformitive three decades ago in the emergence of modern, secular bioethics from traditional ethics rooted in often intransigent moral philosophy. Catholic theologians and ethicists, whose advice on contraception the Catholic Church requested in the 1960s and then discarded, became the pioneers, when their hopes and expectations to modernize religious doctrine were frustrated. An historian of that time has recorded that:

> Fertility control was the major issue that spawned bioethics, more than any other single issue – certainly more than any high-technology-related issue in medicine. It was an issue that directly affected hundreds of millions of people; it dealt with

quintessentially human suffering and fulfillment . . . The theologians, who were the first ethicists working in bioethics, cut their teeth on contraception/sterilization and abortion debates; and in a very real sense, much of the great energy that was turned toward bioethics around 1970/71 was energy that was diverted from the then-increasingly futile church debates on fertility control.[29]

The futility of proposing change in the moral doctrine of the Catholic Church remains, particularly since, in 1870, the Church adopted the concept of papal infallibility in pronouncements made *ex cathedra*, so that no new revelation can be accepted unless shown consistent with earlier teaching. There can be no reversal on the basis that earlier policies were erroneous.

Proponents of religiously-based morality are unpersuaded by evidence of the harmful consequences of their policies. The spread of HIV/AIDS attributable to the prohibition of condom distribution, and for instance of maternal mortality and morbidity due to Church pressure to maintain prohibitions against contraceptive methods, sterilization and abortion, are of no account to them. The deontological orientation of much religiously-based thinking rejects utilitarianism and consequentialism. Adherents to Church teaching feel no institutional or personal responsibility for preventable disease, disability or death that is a consequence of application of the doctrines of their faith, since such doctrines are considered to be founded on truths revealed to their divinely-appointed, infallible leader within schemes of supernatural mystery and mercy.

Many European powers of the colonial period based their laws on restrictive, ecclesiastically-derived religious morality, after as well as before the Protestant Reformation of the 16th century. It has been observed that:

> The canon law of the later Middle Ages was the first modern legal system of the West, and it prevailed in every country of Europe. The canon law governed . . . a great many aspects of the lives of the laity. The new hierarchy of church courts had exclusive jurisdiction over laymen in matters of family law, inheritance, and various types of spiritual crimes.[30]

---

[29] W.T. Reich. The 'Wider View': André Helleger's Passionate, Integrating Intellect and the Creation of Bioethics. *Kennedy Institute of Ethics J* 1999; 9: 25–51 at 37.
[30] H.J. Berman. 1974. *The Interaction of Law and Religion.* New York. Abingdon Press: 58.

In part protective and paternalistic, but also moralistic and puni-
tive, these laws in time became predominant in certain affairs as 'the
church . . . took legal jurisdiction over sins, and it influenced the
secular law to conform to [its] moral principles.'[31] They applied to
exclude women not only from religious ordination and authority in
church life but also from political, professional, economic and
scholarly life and, *inter alia*, from access to voluntary sterilization
and abortion procedures.

In recent years, such European countries have largely liberalized
their sterilization and abortion laws[32] in favour of accommodation
of reproductive self-determination. However, the laws that they
historically applied in the overseas territories they settled or conquered, by power of imperial legislative domination, have proven
curiously tenacious in the post-colonial, independent countries that
have re-emerged or arisen in these territories, including by successful rebellion against European rule. Retention of these laws restrictive of women's rights in general and of their reproductive choice
in particular is due in part to the remaining colonial legacy of
influential European-derived religious institutions that support
them. This is reflected to some extent in sometimes grossly differential rates of maternal mortality and morbidity that are not due
to economic differences alone between the post-imperial European
countries and those in the territories they once dominated. A recent
global comparison between countries in regions with restrictive and
accommodating abortion legislation has noted that 'The risk of
death from unsafe abortion is about 1 in 150 procedures in Africa,
and 1 in 150,000 in the USA and Europe.'[33]

A recent echo of religiously moralistic hostility to women's reproductive self-determination was heard at the two UN Conferences
on Population and Development, and on Women, held respectively
in Cairo in 1994 and Beijing in 1995. The Vatican employed the

---

[31] Ibid. at p. 61.

[32] See for instance the UK Abortion Act 1967, in France the 1975 Law 75–17 and 1979 Law
79–1204, in Portugal the 1984 Law 6 of 11 May, and in Spain the 1985 Organic Law 9 of 5
July; see generally R.J. Cook and B.M. Dickens. A Decade of International Change in
Abortion Law: 1967–77. *Amer. J. Public Health* 1978; 68: 637–644; R.J. Cook & B.M.
Dickens. International Developments in Abortion Laws: 1977–88. *Amer. J. Public Health*
1988; 78: 1305–1311; R.J. Cook, B.M. Dickens & L.E. Bliss. International Developments in
Abortion Law from 1988 to 1998. *Amer. J. Public Health* 1999; 89: 579–586.

[33] P.F. Thonneau. 2001. Maternal Mortality and Unsafe Abortion: A Heavy Burden for
Developing Countries. In *Safe Motherhood Strategies: A Review of the Evidence.* V. DeBrouwere, W. VanLerberghe, eds. Antwerp. ITG Press: 151–173, at 151.

specious and increasingly contested statehood of the Holy See,[34] which privileges the Roman Catholic Church over other Christian denominations and different religions, to maximize its representatives' attendance, and to limit the development of legal recognition of women's human rights to fertility control. At the latter conference, the Church adopted the view that its enemies' enemies could be its friends, and sought to achieve solidarity with its historical religious adversaries, particularly the more reactionary Islamic countries, to resist 'feminist' initiatives in support of what both conferences defined as reproductive health.

REPRODUCTIVE HEALTH, ABORTION AND SAFE MOTHERHOOD

Building on the World Health Organization definition that 'health' is a state of physical, mental and social well-being, the Programme of Action developed at the Cairo conference proposed a definition of reproductive health that was endorsed at the International Conference on Women held the following year in Beijing. The definition reads:

> Reproductive health is a state of complete physical, mental and social well-being and not merely the absence of disease or infirmity, in all matters relating to the reproductive system and to its functions and processes. Reproductive health therefore implies that people are able to have a satisfying and safe sex life and that they have the capability to reproduce and the freedom to decide if, when and how often to do so. Implicit in this last condition are the right of men and women to be informed and to have access to safe, effective, affordable and acceptable methods of family planning of their choice, as well as other methods of their choice for regulation of fertility which are not against the law, and the right of access to appropriate health-care services that will enable women to go safely through pregnancy and childbirth and provide couples with the best chance of having a healthy infant.[35]

The establishment of a claim of access to methods for regulation of fertility had to be limited to methods 'which are not against the law,'

---

[34] See internet http://www.seechange.org.
[35] *Op. cit.* note 14, para 7.2.

since conferences that are UN initiatives cannot usually recommend illegal conduct. However, many countries maintain laws and practices that obstruct achievement of reproductive health as described in the earlier part of the definition, and the ethical status of such laws and practices is open to question on grounds of justice. Many women lack access to 'a satisfying and safe sex life,' reproductive freedom and methods of family planning, because of oppressive laws that make them dependent on the economic support of men, expose them to sexual and other violence, in their homes and outside and, for instance, leave them at risk of life- and health-endangering pregnancies.

Implicit in the above definition, because, for political reasons, it could not be stated explicitly, is the right to lawful abortion which, when available under skilled and timely medical management, is likely to be safely conducted. Religious authorities that oppose abortion in principle, such as in the Roman Catholic, Islamic and Hindu faiths, tend to allow termination of pregnancy in a clinical case when continuation of pregnancy poses an immediate threat to the survival of a particular woman. In the Catholic tradition, for instance, the doctrine of 'double effect'[36] allows the ending of an ectopic and other life-endangering pregnancy not to be characterized as abortion, in the same way that removing a man's cancerous testicles is not characterized as sterilization, notwithstanding that sterility is a secondary effect of the life-saving surgery. Laws often remain, however, that prohibit abortion where pregnancy poses an epidemiological, statistical or population-based risk to women in general but not to any one in particular. That is, even where women face a 1 in 7 or a 1 in 6 risk of maternal death in their reproductive life-span,[37] they have at least a 6 in 7 or a 5 in 6 likelihood to survive a particular pregnancy.

Unsafe or otherwise unwanted pregnancy that results in unsafe abortion, because abortion is not legally and therefore safely available, or is legally available but qualified practitioners decline to provide it,[38] raises macroethical, community-wide concerns.

---

[36] D.P. Sulmasy & E.D. Pellegrino. The Rule of Double Effect: Clearing-up the Double Talk. *Annals of Internal Medicine* 1999; 159: 545.

[37] *Op. cit.* note 5.

[38] In India, abortion has been legally available through medical practitioners on liberal grounds since 1972, but subject to cumbersome conditions; of the estimated 6.7 million abortions in India each year, about 4 million are performed by non-physicians, primarily using drugs, indigenous methods and insertion of objects into the uterus. An estimated 15–20,000 abortion-related deaths occur each year. See A. Starrs, *op. cit.* note 1, p. 57.

Governments endorsing the 1994 Cairo Programme of Action resolved: 'to strengthen their commitment to women's health to deal with the health impact of unsafe abortion as a major public health concern and to reduce the recourse to abortion through expanded and improved family planning services.'[39]

Similarly, the 1995 Beijing Conference developed a Platform for Action which recognized that: 'Unsafe abortions threaten the lives of a large number of women, representing a grave public health problem as it is primarily the poorest and the youngest who take the highest risk.'[40]

This is the case not only within countries but also among countries. That is, the highest rates of maternal mortality and morbidity due to unsafe abortion tend to be experienced in the world's poorest and younger independent countries,[41] many of which retain oppressive abortion laws inherited from colonization.

The injustice of these restrictive laws is not simply that they disrespect women as decision-makers in their own lives, but that their aim is to compel women to continue pregnancies, perhaps initiated by rape, incest or otherwise coerced sexual intercourse, to serve fetal interests or state interests in fetal life, while no other persons are required to give the resources and services of their bodies to preserve the lives of others, including their own voluntarily conceived children. When children's lives are at risk due, for instance, to liver disease, leukemia or anemia, their parents and others are not compelled by law to provide liver segments for transplantation or even far less invasive bone-marrow or blood donations. The common legal requirement that parents provide their dependent children with the 'necessaries of life' is limited to financially affordable food, shelter, clothing and medical care, and has never been considered to cover even blood transfusion, which is usually a paradigm minimum-risk procedure considerably less risk-laden than continuation of routine pregnancy.

It has long been recognized that restrictive abortion laws are frequently legally avoided by women of means or influence, who receive safe, legal procedures by travelling abroad or obtaining medical explanations for local care that ends inconvenient or otherwise

---

[39] *Op. cit.* note 14, para 8.25.
[40] United Nations. 1995. Report of the Fourth World Conference on Women. New York. UN: para 97.
[41] *Op. cit.* notes 2 and 5.

unwanted pregnancies,[42] but that such laws deny safe services to poor and powerless women, of all ages. Beyond resourceful avoidance, women of means may also simply evade restrictive laws. It has been observed that 'for example in Latin America, private physicians often perform safe abortions for relatively high medical fees, and the law is rarely enforced.'[43] The main effect of restrictive laws is not to reduce the numbers of abortions, but primarily to channel them into the least skilled, least safe hands, including those of desperate women who self-induce their abortion by primitive means. A leading obstetrician/gynecologist with wide-ranging international experience has observed that:

> Analysis of available data reveals that there is no direct correlation between the prevalence of induced abortion and how restrictive or liberal a country's abortion law may be . . . Abortion rates seem to be more directly related to the number of unwanted pregnancies. The number of unwanted pregnancies will be greater where the desired fertility is low, and where effective methods of contraception (including emergency contraception)[44] and family-planning information and education services are not available or easily accessible. In this situation, restricting access to abortion will only increase the number of illegal and unsafe abortions. The choice will not be between allowing or preventing abortion. The choice will be between decriminalizing abortion, or allowing it only to be performed as an illegal procedure.[45]

The burden of restrictive laws, which falls primarily on the poor and the powerless, can also have racial dimensions. The introductory language of South Africa's 1996 Choice on Termination of Pregnancy Act acknowledges that the country's former, restrictive law applied inequitably between women of European and African races, in stating that the new law is enacted: 'Recognizing the values of human dignity, the achievement of equality, security of the person, non-racialism and non-sexism and the advancement of

---

[42] A. Jenkins. 1961. *Law for the Rich: A Plea for the Reform of the Abortion Law.* London. Victor Gollancz.

[43] M.F. Fathalla. 1997. *From Obstetrics and Gynecology to Women's Health: The Road Ahead.* New York. Parthenon: 238.

[44] Post-coital contraception, within 72 hours of unprotected intercourse or of malfunction of pre-coital means.

[45] M.F. Fathalla, *op. cit.* note 43, p. 239.

human rights and freedoms which underlie a democratic South Africa.'

The denial of human dignity implicit in legally compelled involuntary continuation of pregnancy, particularly but not only when it is life- and health-endangering, was recognized in 1995, when the Beijing Platform for Action analogized it to rape in its comprehensive condemnation of 'forced pregnancy.'[46] Indeed, the International Criminal Court at The Hague, considering the denial of abortion for pregnancy following rape as included within 'forced maternity,'[47] approaches it as a war crime committed not only by rapists but also by governments and states themselves.[48] The Rome Treaty of 1998, constituting the Court and its jurisdiction, defines rape, sexual slavery, enforced prostitution, forced pregnancy and other forms of sexual violence as both war crimes and crimes against humanity,[49] equal, for instance, to torture and the most egregious international crimes against humanitarian law.

THE MULTIPLE INJUSTICES OF UNSAFE MOTHERHOOD

Restrictive abortion laws are perhaps the most obvious, but only one of many instances of how women, particularly in developing countries, are denied safe options in their reproductive lives. They are often compelled by such abortion laws to choose between continuing a life- or health-endangering pregnancy or resorting to illegal termination, conducted by an unskilled person, frequently in unsanitary conditions. Risks to life and health are not only medical. In several countries and regions of the world, women caught in adultery[50] or found pregnant before or outside marriage face injury

---

[46] United Nations, *op. cit.* note 40, at paras 114, 132 and 135.

[47] See Finalized Draft Text of the Elements of Crimes, Preparatory Commission for the International Criminal Court, UN Doc. PCNICC/2000/JNF/3/Add.2(2000).

[48] K.D. Askin. 1997. *War Crimes Against Women: Prosecution in International War Crimes Tribunals.* The Hague, Netherlands. Kluwer Law International.

[49] Rome Statute of the International Criminal Court. 1998. U.N. Doc. A/CONF. 183/9, Articles 7 and 8.

[50] The 1960 Penal Code of Jordan, article 340, No. 16 has been translated to provide 'He who discovers his wife or one of his female unlawfuls committing adultery with another, and he kills, wounds or injures one or both of them is exempt from any penalty'; see The Center for Reproductive Law and Policy. 2000. *Reproductive Rights 2000: Moving Forward.* New York. CRLP: 47.

or death at the hands of their family members.[51] Laws against so-called 'honour killings' are not uncommonly unenforced, or applied with sentences of such leniency as to constitute them of no deterrent effect.

Injustices are aggravated when women have little or no control over their sexual availability to men. Beyond instances of pregnancy following rape, for instance in military conflicts and civil turmoil, or when women are in police or comparable custody,[52] women denied education and economic opportunities, including rights of legal inheritance, may lack any feasible options in life to early marriage and repeated childbearing. When women cannot resist their husbands' demands and have no access to contraception, for instance because it is too costly, or because their husbands refuse them access to available means or refuse themselves to use condoms, their risks of unsafe motherhood mount. Availability of contraceptive drugs in their communities is often of little avail to young girls of whose vulnerability and perhaps dependency older men take sexual advantage, even while the men are affected by sexually transmitted diseases such as HIV/AIDS. In developed as well as developing countries, high percentages of adolescent girls have been shown to become pregnant due to intercourse imposed by older men they have no social or other practical means to resist.[53]

More contentious than contraception has been sterilization. Restrictive laws and religions have generally come to allow this to women on strictly established medical grounds, but it often remains denied as a reproductive choice. Husbands and family members may also deny women that choice, even when medically indicated, particularly when the son(s) required in their culture have not yet

---

[51] The Penal Code of Syria, article 548, has been translated to provide 'He who catches his wife or one of his ascendants, descendants or sister committing adultery or illegitimate sexual acts with another and he killed or injured one or both of them benefits from an exemption of penalty'; ibid.

[52] See e.g. Asia Watch, Women's Rights Project. 1992. *Double Jeopardy: Police Abuse of Women in Pakistan.* New York. Human Rights Watch.

[53] It has been estimated for instance from Peru that only 72 cases of sexual abuse are reported of the 360 that occur each day and that 60% of pregnancies among 12 to 14 year old girls result from rape by family members or persons close to the victims; S. Tuesta. 2000. *The Search for Justice.* Lima. Movimiento Manuela Ramos: 5. The US Department of Justice reported that there were 330,088 rapes and sexual assaults in 1998 on victims aged 12 and above, the 12–19 age group suffering twice as many as victims aged over 25; F. McLellan. US Paediatricians Advised to Ask About Sexual Assault. *The Lancet* 2001; 357: 1951.

been born. Young women's health and survival can be compromised when, instantly on marriage, they are pressured to have successive pregnancies until sons are born. The attitude of husbands and of the families into which women marry, that women's primary role is as bearers of children, especially sons, presents one of the 'dignity-denying situations' that Jonathan Mann identified as a societal factor that conditions women s 'preventable disease, disability and death.'[54] His vision of finding solutions through human rights is enlightened, but some human rights initiatives illustrate the problem as much as they may offer a solution. For instance, the International Covenant on Economic, Social and Cultural Rights provides in Article 10(2) that: 'Special protection should be accorded to mothers during a reasonable period before and after childbirth.'[55]

This provides for legal effect to be given to Article 25(2) of the 1948 Universal Declaration of Human Rights, which states that 'Motherhood and childhood are entitled to special care and assistance.'[56]

Necessary though these provisions are, they link protection of women to their pregnant status and childbearing role. This reinforces the perception that protection of women's health is an instrumental means of serving children, rather than an inherent right for women to enjoy for themselves. Valuing women as mothers risks their devaluation or invisibility in other aspects of their lives as girl children, adolescents, unmarried and non-pregnant women and widows. Unsafe motherhood is gaining attention, for instance in the Safe Motherhood initiative pioneered by the World Health Organization,[57] but it remains only an epitome of the socially-constructed multiple injustices that many women suffer throughout their lives.

---

[54] *Op. cit.* note 22, p. 8.
[55] See I. Brownlie, ed. 1992. *Basic Documents on Human Rights* (3rd edition). Oxford. Clarendon Press: 117. See also J. Stanchieri, I. Merali and R.J. Cook. 2000. *The Application of Human Rights to Reproductive and Sexual Health,* http://www.acpd.ca/compilation.
[56] I. Brownlie, ibid., p. 26.
[57] See World Health Organization. 1995. *Mother-Baby Package: Implementing Safe Motherhood in Countries.* Geneva. WHO (WHO/FHE/MSM/94.11).

CONCLUSION

The over half a million maternal deaths that occur each year, in all but about five thousand cases in developing countries,[58] are more a consequence than an isolated cause or expression of gender inequity and injustice to women. These deaths have become rare in countries and communities in which women's power of self-determination approaches equality with that of men, but remain pandemic where women's equal rights are not respected in their societies. Vulnerability to social, economic, religious and related repression denies women an effective voice in the decisions that affect their initiation and continuation of pregnancy, and their access to medical and other appropriate services before and during pregnancy, and at and following childbirth. An approach to relief through improved prenatal care, birth assistance and post-partum care is necessary but not sufficient to resolve the injustice of unsafe motherhood. Attention should be directed to such conditioning factors as women's inability to regulate their conception in particular and their reproductive and sexual lives in general. Unsafe motherhood condemns political, economic, religious, judicial and comparably influential social institutions not just for their disregard for motherhood, but for their disregard for and systemic discrimination against women.

[58] *Op. cit.* note 1.

Chapter 30

THE LIMITS OF CONSCIENTIOUS OBJECTION TO ABORTION IN THE DEVELOPING WORLD

LOUIS-JACQUES VAN BOGAERT

INTRODUCTION

The legalisation of voluntary abortion raises the ethical problem of the right to conscientious refusal. In turn, conscientious refusal raises the problem of the moral obligation of health care providers to assist women to obtain a right sanctioned by the law. At first glance, this might appear as a non-issue in most developing countries with liberal abortion laws and readily available and accessible abortion services. In these conditions, the duty of the conscientious objector to abortion is to refer the woman to a non-objecting colleague or institution. In developing countries with liberal abortion laws, however, the right to abortion is often limited by various local constraints: education, information, accessibility of health care facilities, social stigma, and last but not least, conscientious refusal.[1] In such cases, whereas the law ensures the right to abortion, access to abortion is limited by the mentioned reality factors.

In order to meet the two conflicting rights, two alternatives may be considered: 1) limiting the right to conscientious objection; or 2) recruiting and employing non-objecting personnel to staff the facilities designated by the state. The first option involves a strong restriction on individual rights; the second does not. However, what the first option does in developing countries is to put women's health and lives in peril. The second option is fraught with practical problems.[2]

---

[1] C. Bateman. Abortion: damned if you do or you don't. *South African Medical Journal* 2000; 90: 750–751.

[2] M. Berer. Reproductive Rights, Advocacy and Changing the Law. *Reproductive Health Matters* 2000; 8: 6–9; P. Varkey, S. Fonn and M. Kethlapile. The Role of Advocacy in Implementing the South African Abortion Law. *Reproductive Health Matters* 2000; 8: 103–111; S.J. Varkey and S. Fonn. Termination of Pregnancy. *South African Health Review* 1999. Health Systems Trust Pretoria: Chapter 26 at: http://www.hst.org.za/sahr/99/chap26.htm

Therefore, we have to consider the two following questions. To what extent is the exercise of different 'free' choices dependent on the local reality factor of infrastructure? Which choice is morally more binding: to avoid 'innocent' deaths by refusing to participate in abortion, or to prevent the potential death of a pregnant woman?

CONSCIENTIOUS OBJECTION

In its broadest sense, conscientious objection is to object in principle to a legally required or permitted practice. The issue of moral obligations of laws has been a matter of controversy from times immemorial. In the *Crito,* Plato explored the question. Closer to us, Martin Luther King invited civil disobedience in his 'Letter from Birmingham City Jail.' This was followed by widespread conscientious objection during the Vietnam War and later the Gulf War.[3]

Conscientious objection finds its roots in Biblical principles and in classical natural law theory. The Bible teaches that God institutes human authority. In case of conflict, his commands take precedence and ought to be obeyed. The religious version of the natural law theory, associated with Aquinas and the subsequent scholastic tradition, is an offshoot of the Biblical teaching: the natural law is the expression of God's will for the creation. The secular version, as first promoted by Hugo Grotius, sees the natural law as an objective set of principles that can be discovered by reason.[4]

There is a wide range of situations where conscientious objection to the law or to the state is involved. One of the most popular has always been the problem of the 'just war' and the objection to the bearing of arms where a compulsory draft law does exist. As an alternative to bearing arms, conscientious objectors in some countries have been given the choice of a 'national service' which entails a lengthier civilian service.[5] More recently, since the legalisation of abortion in a large number of countries, conscientious objection to abortion has come to the fore. The question is whether conscientious objection is an inalienable and unlimited right, or whether it

---

[3] C.E. Bertha. Is Selective Conscientious Objection Tenable? Available online: http://www.usafa.af.mil/dfpfa/CVs/Bertha/Sco.html.

[4] S. Blackburn. 1996. *Oxford Dictionary of Philosophy.* Oxford & New York. Oxford University Press: 256.

[5] Bertha, *op. cit.* note 3.

should be limited in certain circumstances. Can the question be answered affirmatively without compromising personal rights and integrity?

In the context of military obligations, Bertha[6] argues that, from a Hobbesian perspective, the fact that the state has spent enormous amounts of money in the training (of soldiers) puts duties to fulfil a contract. Therefore, conscientious objection is not tenable, and, he argues, a government should be very conservative in granting conscientious objection statuses. Following Bertha's line of thinking one could equally (arguably) say that, in a Hobbesian perspective, the state has spent enormous amounts of money to train doctors. Hence, in this view, their right to conscientious objection should be limited.

One should make a distinction between conscientious objection against war and bearing weapons, and conscientious objection in medicine. In the former, having a person refuse to carry a weapon and/or to take part in combat does not directly affect the life of a fellow human being. The latter, however, does. In medicine, abortion is an exception to the general obligation to treat *all* categories within the limits of one's competence.[7] (Another exception to the duty of assistance is the request for physician-assisted suicide.)

Guidelines for a doctor's conscience

According to the *Declaration of Lisbon on the Rights of the Patient*, adopted by the 34th World Medical Assembly (1981), a physician should always act according to his or her conscience and always in the best interest of the patient.[8] The *Declaration of Lisbon's* intent was to place emphasis on the medical profession's independence from legislations and governments. As a rule, the legalisation of abortion aims at providing abortion seekers the lawful opportunity for voluntary abortion in proper and safe medical conditions. Also as a rule, the abortion laws equally protect the professional's independence to provide or to deny the service. The refusal, however, puts a legal obligation on the professional to refer the woman to

[6] Ibid.

[7] K.M. Boyd, R. Higgs & A.J. Pinching. 1997. *The New Dictionary of Medical Ethics.* London. BMJ Publishing Group: 54–55.

[8] W.T. Reich, ed. 1995. Declaration of Lisbon on the Rights of the Patients. *Encyclopedia of Bioethics.* London. Simon & Schuster and Prentice Hall International: 2261.

an abortion service provider. Hence, abortion laws are in keeping with the spirit of the *Declaration of Lisbon.*

Limits to conscientious objection in medicine

According to Christie & Hoffmaster, 'a physician's role is to subordinate moral beliefs to moral obligations, for the ultimate commitment is to the patient even if that necessitates the violation of one's moral views'.[9] In Wicclair's view:

> Appeals to conscience can have a significant moral weight even when physicians have conscience-based objections to practices which are endorsed by established norms of medical ethics. However, since other values and interests, such as patient autonomy, dignity, and well-being, are also at stake, it is unwarranted to give physicians more or less blanket permission to withdraw from patient care in such cases.[10]

It does not follow, however, from the legalisation of abortion that it is endorsed by established norms of medical ethics. The old adage that what is legal is not always moral (and vice versa) also applies to the abortion debate. Christie & Hoffmaster remind us:

> A physician cannot ignore the problem [of a request deemed immoral]. He or she must choose between some degree of complicity and rejection . . . and should back off when there is genuine value conflict.[11]

It seems impossible to be at the same time an accomplice and to retreat when a conflict of values arises. Complicity is to be a partner in a 'wrongdoing'; to back off is to refuse such partnership. To back off is to keep one's hands clean; to compromise is to make one's hands dirty. To back off is to keep one's integrity, regardless of the consequences affecting others. To back off is to hide behind conscientious objection, whatever may happen to the victim of a back street abortion. To compromise is to accept the *aporia* of responsibility, to use Jacques Derrida's vocabulary.[12] Aporia (from the Greek *poria*, path; and the *alpha privativum*, absence, lack) means

[9] R.J. Christie & B.C. Hoffmaster. 1986. *Ethical Issues in Family Medicine.* New York & Oxford. Oxford University Press: 143.
[10] M.R. Wicclair. Conscientious Objection in Medicine. *Bioethics* 2000; 14: 205–207.
[11] Christie & Hoffmaster, *op. cit.* note 9.
[12] J. Derrida. 1995. *The Gift of Death.* Chicago. Chicago University Press: 60–68.

the lack of a path to follow; it also means a question. Is there an answer? Is there a path to follow? Is moral purity and self-integrity the answer? As Murphy writes: 'If moral purity means never choosing anything which one will have to regard as in some sense wrong and regret for all one's days, the moral purity may be impossible in a complex world.'[13]

One of the mainstream moral theories of medical ethics is the so-called 'principlism', based on the principles of autonomy, beneficence, non-maleficence, and justice. But, as pointed out by Pellegrino:

> The most radical reorientation in the Hippocratic tradition is that, in the last 25 years, autonomy has superseded beneficence ... Autonomy as a moral guide has its limitations. Moral minimalism (contractualism) minimises the obligation of beneficence ... To be beneficent, respect for the patient's values and choices is essential.[14]

If the practice of medical ethics leans too much on the contract between patient and physician, a conscientious objector has every right to refuse to be part of that contract, to be an 'accomplice' in a request deemed immoral. In that case, however, the duty to respect a patient's request/choice is negated. In *Abortion and Moral Theory*, Sumner writes: 'It is in general preferable not to require doctors and nurses to perform tasks that deeply offend their moral principles, at least as long as others are willing to meet patients' needs'.[15] In other words, the right to conscientious objection is limited by the circumstances within which it arises. The reasons for this are:

> Any institution that is publicly funded is obliged to provide a suitable wide range of public services. Individual persons may opt out of performing abortions without thereby rendering abortions unavailable, but if the entire hospitals do so, substantial numbers of women may have no meaningful access to the service.[16]

---

[13] J.G. Murphy. 1994. Is Killing the Innocent Absolutely Immoral? In *Killing and Letting Die*, 2nd ed. B. Steinbock and A. Norcross, eds. New York. Fordham University Press: 199.
[14] E.D. Pellegrino. 1990. The Relationship of Autonomy and Integrity in Medical Ethics. In *Ethics in Medicine. Individual Demands versus Demands of Society*. P. Allebeck and J. Bengt, eds. New York. Raven Press: 3–15.
[15] L.W. Sumner. 1981. *Abortion and Moral Theory*. Princeton. Princeton University Press: 21.
[16] Quoted in R.J. Cook and B.M. Dickens. Human Rights and Abortion Laws. *International Journal of Gynecology & Obstetrics* 1999; 65: 81–88.

Individual limits to conscientious objection to abortion

The *British Abortion Act* (1967: section 4[2]) states that conscientious objection is inapplicable when the continuation of pregnancy poses a serious danger to life, or health, physical or mental.[17] The *European Code of Medical Ethics* (1987: art.18) states: 'It is ethical for a doctor, by reason of his own beliefs, to refuse to intervene in the process of termination of pregnancy, and to suggest consultation of other doctors.'[18] The *Medical Termination of Pregnancy Act* N7 (1995) of Guyana precludes conscientious objection where women's lives are at risk.[19] The *Committee on the Elimination of Discrimination against Women* (CEDAW) of the United Nations (1999: art. 12 §11) states that it is the government's duty to ensure access to care that some physicians conscientiously object to providing.[20] This implies that governments must ensure the availability of non-objecting physicians who are prepared to render the service. Swedish law provides no right of conscientious objection and imposes a contractual obligation to assist in the termination of a pregnancy.[21] The South African *Choice on Termination of Pregnancy Act* 92 (1996: section 10) makes provision for penalties for obstructing the law:

> Any person who prevents the lawful termination of pregnancy or obstructs access to a facility for the termination of pregnancy, shall be guilty of an offence and liable on conviction to a fine or to imprisonment for a period not exceeding 10 years.[22]

The shortcomings of this section of the act is, first, that it seems to address only the physical obstruction to the access to an abortion service facility and not the health hazards (i.e. the morbidity) and life threats (i.e. the mortality) caused by conscientious objectors who willingly neglect women undergoing a termination of pregnancy. Second, it does not mention the right to conscientious objection or the lack thereof (or limits to conscientious objection).

---

[17] Ibid.
[18] W.T. Reich, ed. European Code of Medical Ethics (1987). *Encyclopedia of Bioethics.* London. Simon & Schuster and Prentice Hall International: 2681.
[19] Quoted in Cook and Dickens, *op. cit.* note 16.
[20] Ibid.
[21] P. Saunders. 1996. Abortion and conscientious objection. *Nucleus.* January. Available at: http://www.cmf.org.uk/pubs/nucleus/nucjan96/consc.htm.
[22] Government Gazette. 1996. *Choice on Termination of Pregnancy Act 92.* Pretoria. Government Printers.

Still, in the South African context, the health portfolio committee indicated in parliament its concern about the preventable death of women from botched illegal abortions. The minister of health's response was: 'Health care workers should place their duty before their beliefs.' At the same session, the chief director for maternal & child health services stated: 'Health care workers should not use their beliefs to deny people access to services.'[23]

Institutional limits to conscientious objection

Abortion is a personal choice, as it is emphasised in the title of the South African Act: *choice* on termination of pregnancy. Whose choice is it? The woman's, the lawmaker's, the physician's, the nurse's? Is the choice guaranteed? What hampers the making of the choice? Is it a choice limited by the local circumstances? On one view (call it the personal choice to be anti-choice, to refuse the right to choose to others), the right to conscientious objection is inalienable and unrestricted.[24] To be morally flawless, this view will have to 'justify' the 600 000 annual deaths from 'unsafe' abortion globally.[25] On the other view (call it pro-choice), one has the moral obligation to prevent these avoidable deaths. To be morally flawless, this view should have to 'justify' the 50 million abortions that are induced annually worldwide.[26] The irony is that, whatever the choice, both stances lead to a dead end and end in death. In the end, it is a matter of choice between the woman's or the unborn's life. Therefore, the lawmaker's perspective on abortion boils down to a public health matter rather than an ethical one.

The points made by Sumner are important for three reasons. First, he emphasises that conscientious objection, where applicable, is an individual right but not an institutional right. Second, he insists on the fact that even private health facilities, by virtue of the fact that they provide services to the public under the auspices of governmental agencies 'cannot refuse ethically or legally a service unless they provide a reasonable access to such services through

---

[23] Bateman, *op. cit.* note 1.

[24] H. Barratt. 2001. Conscientious objection to abortion. *Nucleus* January. Available at: http://www.cmf.org.uk/pubs/nucleus/nucjan01/abortion.htm

[25] Varkey et al., 2000, *op. cit.* note 2.

[26] J.G. Schenker and J.M. Cain. FIGO Committee for the Ethical Aspects of Human Reproduction and Women's Health. *International Journal of Gynecology & Obstetrics* 1999; 64: 319.

other facilities.'[27] And finally, he notes that 'public hospitals must guarantee that at least some of their medical staff will perform abortions, or will refer to others who do.'[28]

GLOBAL VIEW ON ABORTION

In an ideal world, one should wish that all pregnancies would be planned and welcome, and that contraception would eliminate the need for voluntary abortion. Currently, however, half of all pregnancies in developed countries are still unplanned, and half of the unintended ones are terminated.[29] On the other hand, the increase in involuntary infertility is addressed by reproductive technologies that result in supernumerary embryos and multiple pregnancies. The former poses the ethical problem of the 'disposal' of tens of thousands of unclaimed or unwanted embryos, not to mention the ethics of cloning. The latter poses the problem of fetal 'reduction.' For all these reasons, contraception on its own is unlikely, in the foreseeable future, to eliminate the need for abortion. Thus, the reality of abortion (in its broadest sense) is likely to stay with us for a while, whether we like it or not.

In the developing world, the need for 'safe' abortion results from different socio-economic factors and circumstances. For a host of reasons – culture, education, poverty, tradition, sexism, gender bias, etc.[30] – contraception has not yet made a significant impact on the need for abortion. Therefore, in an attempt to curb the morbidity and mortality from 'unsafe' abortions, the procedure has been legalised in more than 100 countries worldwide.[31]

Arguments pro and con abortion

A common, but arguably simplistic, view on abortion is limited to the two antipodean but straightforward stances: pro-choice/pro-life

[27] Sumner, *op. cit.* note 15.
[28] Ibid.
[29] Schenker and Cain, *op. cit.* note 26.
[30] Gender Bias: Perspectives from the Developing World. Available at: http://advocatesforyouth.org/publications/factsheets/fsgender.htm
[31] G. Benagiano and A. Pera. Decreasing the Need for Abortion. Challenges and Constraints. *International Journal of Gynecology & Obstetrics* 2000; 70: 35–48; R.J. Cook & B.M. Dickens. Human Rights and Abortion Laws. *International Journal of Gynecology & Obstetrics* 1999; 65: 81–88.

(anti-choice). The former rests its case on the premise that women have the right to dispose of their own bodies; neither rights nor moral standing are granted to the unborn. The latter rests its case on the inalienable right to life of the unborn; no right is granted to the woman.

As Benjamin writes, 'the main strength of the absolute pro-choice is the philosophical limitation of the absolute pro-life stance – that is, its inability to provide a plausible secular justification of the absolute sanctity of life.'[32] While Benjamin has a point, it does, however, not follow from the weakness of the pro-life argument that the pro-choice counter-argument is valid. The real philosophical conundrum arising from the dispute is, according to Oddie, 'the extraordinary difficulty of achieving some kind of rational consensus on the moral status of the unborn.'[33] The same difficulty applies to the pro-choice argument. As pointed out by Chervenak & McCullough, 'there is no clearly convincing moral argument that the woman's life is more important than that of the fetus.'[34]

There is a third argument on the morality of abortion that focuses on public health and demographic concerns. In Western Europe, abortion is regulated as a public health need with the medical profession as its gatekeepers. Access to abortion is legal when the physician decides that it is indicated on health and/or socio-economic grounds. In North America, abortion is part of an individual's right to bodily integrity, privacy, or autonomy, which cannot be infringed by the state except to protect conflicting rights.[35] South Africa's *Choice on Termination of Pregnancy Act* addresses abortion as a matter of social equity and justice, rather than on health grounds (but includes medical indications).[36] It declares that the law was enacted 'recognising the values of human dignity, the achievement of equality, security of the person, non-racialism and non-sexism and the advancement of human rights and freedom.'[37] Making

---

[32] M. Benjamin. 1990. *Splitting the Difference. Compromise and Integrity in Ethics and Politics.* Lawrence. University Press of Kansas: 104.

[33] G. Oddie. 1994. Moral Uncertainty and Human Embryo Experimentation. In *Medicine and Moral Reasoning.* K.W.M. Fulford, G.R. Gillett and J.M. Soskice, eds. Cambridge. Cambridge University Press: 153.

[34] F.A. Chervenak and L.B. McCullough. Perinatal Ethics: a Practical Method of Analysis of Obligations to Mother and Fetus. *Obstetrics & Gynecology* 1985; 66: 442–446.

[35] Berer, *op. cit.* note 2.

[36] Government Gazette, *op. cit.* note 22.

[37] Berer, *op. cit.* note 2.

abortion strictly a matter of women's rights leaves little, if any, room for conscientious objection. Moreover, as mentioned earlier, the act makes provision for indictment in case the access to this human right is obstructed. What, then, are the 'justifications' of the public health stances on abortion?

The 'reality factor'

A global survey of the situation of abortion in the year 2000 shows that 60% of humanity lives in countries where voluntary abortion – that is, abortion on demand – is legal. This represents more than 100 countries; 28 of them are in Europe, and only two in Africa (Tunisia and South Africa). In the remaining 39%, 14% permit abortion only to protect a woman's physical health, and 21% only to save a woman's life. In 4% of countries, abortion is still absolutely prohibited (e.g. Ireland).[38]

There are globally 50 million induced abortions each year.[39] According to the World Health Organization, it is estimated that there are 20 million 'unsafe' abortions globally each year, and that 600 000 women die each year from the complications of 'unsafe' abortions. Most 'unsafe' abortions happen in the developing world.[40] Indeed, abortion is not only an ethical issue; it is a very serious health matter. Why is that?

Many factors affect the rates of abortion. What is clear is that the legal prohibition of abortion is no deterrent. On the contrary, there is ample evidence showing that the legalisation of abortion does result in a significant decrease in abortion rates. It is equally clear that the decriminalisation of abortion leads to a significant drop in morbidity and mortality from 'unsafe' abortion procedures. Education, availability of and easy access to contraception, and the availability of proper health care have all contributed to the decrease in abortion rates in the developed world.[41] Hence, from a strict public health point of view, there is a need to legalise abortion. But that does not solve the issue of conscientious objection/refusal.

In the developing world, however, things are different. I wish to limit the discussion to the South African reality. At the time of the

---

[38] Benagiano & Pera, *op. cit.* note 31.
[39] Schenker & Cain, *op. cit.* note 26.
[40] Varkey et al., 2000, *op. cit.* note 2.
[41] Benagiano & Pera, *op. cit.* note 31.

enactment of the act, in February 1997, the national department of health designated 246 public and 138 private facilities to provide legal abortion services. Since then, around 50 000 legal abortions are performed annually. An equal number (and most likely even more) of 'unsafe' – that is, 'technically illegal' (as they are performed outside of the designated facilities) – abortions are performed. The South African particular also indicates that 30% of avoidable maternal deaths result from 'unsafe' abortions. The 1997 confidential enquiries into maternal deaths revealed that 575 deaths resulted from pregnancy-related sepsis or incomplete (that is, 'unsafe') abortions.[42] In 1998, the same enquiries showed that 60.5% of early pregnancy deaths and 38.8% of deaths from pregnancy-related sepsis were due to 'unsafe' abortions.[43]

Why is it that, in spite of the legalisation of abortion, more women still do resort to unsafe practices instead of safe ones? Ignorance of the law, unavailability of the services (for whatever reason), taboos and stigmatisation undoubtedly play a role.[44] A recent survey has shown that only 53% of all South African women were aware of the Act, and that 61 % of rural women were totally unaware of the availability of legal abortion. It also showed that, in rural communities, 58% of women are unable to negotiate for protected sex.[45] In addition, I would argue that, in South Africa, appeal to conscientious objection by health care providers in state-run facilities is a major contributor to the high number of 'unsafe' abortions. It is known that only 28% of the designated facilities are effectively on-line, and that 95% of them are in cities and towns.[46] This leaves almost half of the female population (that is, those living in rural areas) with little or no access to a constitutional right. The designated facilities that do not provide the service invoke the right to conscientious objection.[47] The state does not prosecute those who provide 'technically illegal' abortion because 'unsafe' abortions have become 'safe' or 'safer' (that is, the medically induced

---

[42] Department of Health. 1997. Report on Confidential Enquiries into Maternal Deaths in South Africa. Pretoria.
[43] Department of Health. 1998. Report on Confidential Enquiries into Maternal Deaths in South Africa. Pretoria: 51–62.
[44] Berer, *op. cit.* note 2.
[45] Varkey et al., 2000, *op. cit.* note 2.
[46] Varkey et al., 1999, *op. cit.* note 2.
[47] Bateman, *op. cit.* note 1.

abortions have much less morbidity and mortality than the 'surgically-induced' ones).

Much has been said about the limits of conscientious abortion as it relates to where a health care provider starts involving or withdrawing him or herself. In Britain, for instance, the *Janaway vs Salford Health Authority* was about a doctor's secretary who refused to type the referral letter for an abortion on grounds of conscientious objection.[48] The British Medical Association regards the situation as similar to that in France, Italy and Norway: doctors are not legally required to authorise or to perform abortions, but are obliged to be involved in pre-operative care and referral.[49] In Denmark and the Netherlands, one can conscientiously object to being involved in pre-operative care, but there is nonetheless a legal obligation to refer the woman seeking an abortion to another colleague.[50] It could, however, be argued that the current situation with 'medical' abortion differs from the traditional 'surgical' abortion. In other words, in most cases abortion is induced by the oral intake and/or the vaginal application of a drug that induces uterine contractions. The drug is self-administered by the woman. The role of the health care provider is to prescribe the drug and to hand it over to the woman seeking an abortion. The real active role player in the induction of the process is the woman herself. A staunch conscientious objector could also argue that the janitor who sweeps the operating theatre floor after the evacuation of retained products of conception has the right to conscientious objection and to refuse to sweep the floor. Where does participation start and end?

In developing countries with liberal abortion laws, an unlimited right to conscientious objection not only denies women a constitutional right, but also puts their health and life at risk. The local circumstances do not ensure access to a legitimate and legal request. Therefore, the right to conscientious objection to abortion is not absolute. The only way to protect the conscientious objectors' right would be to staff the designated facilities with non-objecting health care providers.

---

[48] Saunders, *op. cit.* note 21.
[49] British Medical Association. 1993. *Medical Ethics Today. Its Practice and Philosophy.* BMA's Ethics, Science and Information Division: 107–109.
[50] Saunders, *op. cit.* note 21.

CONCLUSION

Where abortion is decriminalised, women's right to abortion often conflicts with health care providers' right to conscientious objection. One has to keep in mind that the right to conscientious objection is an individual right and not an institutional right. Health facilities, private and public, have the moral duty to ensure that women seeking abortion are provided the service they are entitled to by the law. Although it is not clear where the right to conscientious objection starts and ends, the duty to refer is both a moral and legal obligation that can easily be fulfilled in developed countries. In developing countries, however, often the local circumstances do not ensure access to safe abortion. Therefore, the right to conscientious objection should be balanced against the health hazards resulting from 'unsafe' practices. It could also be said that the state that passed abortion laws simultaneously has the duty to ensure access to safe abortion to all women seeking an abortion. In South Africa, 72% of the designated state-run facilities claim conscientious refusal. Therefore, more than half of abortions are still 'unsafe.' Since conscientious objection is not an institutional right, the state has the moral and legal duty to enforce the law in the institution it has designated. This places a limit to conscientious objection. Moral purity is difficult in a complex world.

Chapter 31

SURROGATE MOTHERING: EXPLOITATION OR EMPOWERMENT?

LAURA M. PURDY

INTRODUCTION

'Pregnancy is barbaric'[1] proclaimed Shulamith Firestone in the first heady days of the new women's movement; she looked forward to the time when technology would free women from the oppression of biological reproduction. Yet as reproductive options multiply, some feminists are making common cause with conservatives for a ban on innovations. What is going on?

Firestone argued that nature oppresses women by leaving them holding the reproductive bag, while men are free of such burden; so long as this biological inequality holds, women will never be free. (Firestone, 198–200) It is now commonplace to point out the naivety of her claim: it is not the biological difference, per se, that oppresses women, but its social significance. So we need not change biology, only attitudes and institutions.

This insight has helped us to see how to achieve a better life for women, but I wonder if it is the whole story. Has Firestone's brave claim no lesson at all for us?

Her point was that being with child is uncomfortable and dangerous, and it can limit women's lives. We have become more sensitive to the ways in which social arrangements can determine how much these difficulties affect us. However, even in feminist utopias, where sex or gender are considered morally irrelevant except where they may entail special needs, a few difficulties would remain. Infertility, for instance, would exist, as would the desire for a child in circumstances where pregnancy is impossible or undesirable.

[1] Shulamith Firestone, *The Dialectic of Sex*, (New York: Bantam Books, 1970), p. 198. A version of this paper was given at the Eastern SWIP meeting, 26 March 1988. I would like especially to thank Helen B. Holmes and Sara Ann Ketchum for their useful comments on this paper; they are, of course, in no way responsible for its perverse position! Thanks also to the editors and referees of *Bioethics* for their helpful criticisms.

At present, the problem of infertility is generating a whole series of responses and solutions. Among them are high-tech procedures like IVF, and social arrangements like surrogate motherhood. Both these techniques are also provoking a storm of concern and protest. As each raises a distinctive set of issues, they need to be dealt with separately, and I shall here consider only surrogate motherhood.

One might argue that no feminist paradise would need any practice such as this. As Susan Sherwin argues, it could not countenance 'the capitalism, racism, sexism, and elitism of our culture [that] have combined to create a set of attitudes which views children as commodities whose value is derived from their possession of parental chromosomes.'[2] Nor will society define women's fulfilment as only in terms of their relationship to genetically-related children. No longer will children be needed as men's heirs or women's livelihood.

We will, on the contrary, desire relationships with children for the right reasons: the urge to nurture, teach and be close to them. No longer will we be driven by narcissistic wishes for clones or immortality to seek genetic offspring no matter what the cost. Indeed, we will have recognized that children are the promise and responsibility of the whole human community. And childrearing practices will reflect these facts, including at least a more diffuse family life that allows children to have significant relationships with others. Perhaps childbearing will be communal.

This radically different world is hard to picture realistically, even by those like myself who – I think – most ardently wish for it. The doubts I feel are fanned by the visions of so-called 'cultural feminists' who glorify traditionally feminine values. Family life can be suffocating, distorting, even deadly.[3] Yet there is a special closeness that arises from being a child's primary caretaker, just as there can be a special thrill in witnessing the unfolding of biologically-driven traits in that child. These pleasures justify risking neither the health of the child[4] nor that of the mother; nobody's general well-being should be sacrificed to them, nor do they warrant hugh social investments. However, they are things that, other things being

---

[2] Susan Sherwin, 'Feminist Ethics and In Vitro Fertilization,' *Science, Morality and Feminist Theory*, ed. Marsha Hanen and Kai Nielsen, *The Canadian Journal of Philosophy* supplementary volume 13, 1987, p. 277.

[3] Consider the many accounts of the devastating things parents have done to children, in particular.

[4] See L. M. Purdy 'Genetic Diseases: Can Having Children be Immoral?' *Moral Problems in Medicine*, ed. Samuel Gorovitz, (N.J.: Prentice-Hall, 1983), 377–84.

equal, it would be desirable to preserve so long as people continue to have anything like their current values. If this is so, then evaluating the morality of practices that open up new ways of creating children is worthwhile.[5]

MORAL OR IMMORAL?

What is surrogate mothering exactly? Physically, its essential features are as follows: a woman is inseminated with the sperm of a man to whom she is not married. When the baby is born she relinquishes her claim to it in favour of another, usually the man from whom the sperm was obtained. As currently practiced, she provides the egg, so her biological input is at least equal to that of the man. 'Surrogate' mothering may not therefore be the best term for what she is doing.[6]

By doing these things she also acts socially – to take on the burden and risk of pregnancy for another, and to separate sex and reproduction, reproduction and childrearing, and reproduction and marriage. If she takes money for the transaction (apart from payment of medical bills), she may even be considered to be selling a baby.

The bare physical facts would not warrant the welter of accusation and counter-accusation that surrounds the practice.[7] It is the social aspects that have engendered the acrimony about exploitation, destruction of the family, and baby-selling. So far we have reached no consensus about the practice's effect on women or its overall morality.

I believe that the appropriate moral framework for addressing questions about the social aspects of contracted pregnancy is

---

[5] Another critical issue is that no feminist utopia will have a supply of 'problem' children whom no one wants. Thus the proposal often heard nowadays that people should just adopt all those handicapped, non-white kids will not do. (Nor does it 'do' now.)

[6] I share with Sara Ann Ketchum the sense that this term is not adequate, although I am not altogether happy with her suggestion that we call it 'contracted motherhood' (New Reproductive Technologies and the Definition of Parenthood: A Feminist Perspective', paper given at the 1987 *Feminism and Legal Theory Conference*, at the University of Wisconsin at Madison, summer 1987, p. 44ff.) It would be better, I think, to reserve terms like 'mother' for the social act of nurturing. I shall therefore substitute the terms 'contracted pregnancy' and 'surrogacy' (in scare quotes).

[7] This is not to say that no one would take the same view as I: the Catholic Church, for instance, objects to the masturbatory act required for surrogacy to proceed.

consequentialist.[8] This framework requires us to attempt to separate those consequences that invariably accompany a given act from those that accompany it only in particular circumstances. Doing this compels us to consider whether a practice's necessary features lead to unavoidable overridingly bad consequences. It also demands that we look at how different circumstances are likely to affect the outcome. Thus a practice which is moral in a feminist society may well be immoral in a sexist one. This distinction allows us to tailor morality to different conditions for optimum results without thereby incurring the charge of malignant relativism.

Before examining arguments against the practice of contracted pregnancy, let us take note of why people might favour it. First, as noted before, alleviating infertility can create much happiness. Secondly, there are often good reasons to consider transferring burden and risk from one individual to another. Pregnancy may be a serious burden or risk for one woman, whereas it is much less so for another. Some women love being pregnant, others hate it; pregnancy interferes with work for some, not for others; pregnancy also poses much higher levels of risk to health (or even life) for some than for others. Reducing burden and risk is a benefit not only for the woman involved, but also for the resulting child. High-risk pregnancies create, among other things, serious risk of prematurity, one of the major sources of handicap in babies. Furthermore, we could prevent serious genetic diseases by allowing carriers to avoid pregnancy. A third benefit of 'surrogate mothering' is that it makes possible the creation of non-traditional families. This can be a significant source of happiness to single women and gay couples.

All of the above presuppose that there is some advantage in making possible at least partially genetically-based relationships between parents and offspring. Although, as I have argued above, we might be better off without this desire, I doubt that we will soon

---

[8] The difficulty in choosing the 'right' moral theory to back up judgments in applied ethics, given that none are fully satisfactory continues to be vexing. I would like to reassure those who lose interest at the mere sight of consequentialist – let alone utilitarian – judgment, that there are good reasons for considering justice an integral part of moral reasoning, as it quite obviously has utility.

A different issue is raised by the burgeoning literature on feminist ethics. I strongly suspect that utilitarianism could serve feminists well, if properly applied. (For a defence of this position, see my paper 'Do Feminists Need a New Moral Theory', to be given at the University of Minnesota, Duluth, at the conference *Explorations in Feminist Ethics: Theory, and Practice*, 8–9 October 1988.)

be free of it. Therefore, if we can satisfy it at little cost, we should try to do so.

IS SURROGATE MOTHERING ALWAYS WRONG?

Despite the foregoing advantages, some feminists argue that the practice is *necessarily* wrong: it is wrong because it must betray women's and society's basic interest.[9]

What, if anything is wrong with the practice? Let us consider the first three acts I described earlier: transferring burden and risk, separating sex and reproduction, and separating reproduction and childrearing. Separation of reproduction and marriage will not be dealt with here.

Is it wrong to take on the burden of pregnancy for another? Doing this is certainly supererogatory, for pregnancy can threaten comfort, health, even life. One might argue that women should not be allowed to take these risks, but that would be paternalistic. We do not forbid mountain-climbing or riding a motorcycle on these grounds. How could we then forbid a woman to undertake this particular risk?

Perhaps the central issue is the transfer of burden from one woman to another. However, we frequently do just that – much more often than we recognize. Anyone who has her house cleaned, her hair done, or her clothes dry-cleaned is engaging in this procedure;[10] so is anyone who depends on agriculture or public works such as bridges.[11] To the objection that in this case the bargain includes the risk to life and limb, as well as use of time and skills, the answer is that the other activities just cited entail surprisingly elevated risk rates from exposure to toxic chemicals or dangerous machinery.[12]

Furthermore, it is not even true that contracted pregnancy merely shifts the health burden and risks associated with pregnancy from one woman to another. In some cases (infertility, for example,) it

---

[9] See for example Gena Corea, *The Mother Machine*, and Christine Overall, *Ethics and Human Reproduction*, (Winchester, Mass.: Allen and Unwin, 1987).

[10] These are just a couple of examples in the sort of risky service that we tend to take for granted.

[11] Modern agricultural products are brought to us at some risk by farm workers. Any large construction project will also result in some morbidity and mortality.

[12] Even something so mundane as postal service involves serious risk on the part of workers.

makes the impossible possible; in others (for women with potentially high-risk pregnancies) the net risk is lowered.[13] As we saw, babies benefit, too, from better health and fewer handicaps. Better health and fewer handicaps in both babies and women also means that scarce resources can be made available for other needs, thus benefiting society in general.

I do think that there is, in addition, something suspect about all this new emphasis on risk. Awareness of risks inherent in even normal pregnancy constitutes progress: women have always been expected to forge ahead with child bearing oblivious to risk. Furthermore, childbearing has been thought to be something women owed to men or to society at large, regardless of their own feelings about a given – or any – pregnancy. When women had little say about these matters, we never heard about risk.[14] Why are we hearing about risk only now, now that women finally have some choices, some prospect of remuneration?[15] For that matter, why is our attention not drawn to the fact that surrogacy is one of the least risky approaches to non-traditional reproduction?[16]

Perhaps what is wrong about this kind of transfer is that it necessarily involves exploitation. Such exploitation may take the form of exploitation of women by men and exploitation of the rich by the poor. This possibility deserves serious consideration, and will be dealt with shortly.

Is there anything wrong with the proposed separation of sex and reproduction? Historically, this separation – in the form of contraception – has been beneficial to women and to society as a whole. Although there are those who judge the practice immoral. I do not think we need belabour the issue here.

It may be argued that not all types of separation are morally on a par. Contraception is permissible, because it spares women's health, promotes autonomy, strengthens family life, and helps make

---

[13] The benefit to both high-risk women, and to society is clear. Women need not risk serious deterioration of health or abnormally high death rates.

[14] See Laura Purdy, 'The Morality of New Reproductive Technologies', *The Journal of Social Philosophy*, (Winter 1987), pp. 38–48.

[15] For elaboration of this view, consider Jane Ollenburger and John Harnlin, ' "All Birthing Should be Paid Labor" – A Marxist Analysis of the Commodification of Motherhood', *On the Problem of Surrogate Parenthood: Analyzing the Baby M Case*, ed. Herbert Richardson, (Lewiston, N.Y.: The Edwin Mellen Press, 1987).

[16] Compare the physical risk with that of certain contraceptive technologies, and high-tech fertility treatments like IVF.

population growth manageable. But separation of sex and reproduction apart from contraception is quite another kettle of fish: it
exploits women, weakens family life, and may increase population.
Are these claims true and relevant?

Starting with the last first, if we face a population problem, it
would make sense to rethink overall population policy, not exploit
the problems of the infertile.[17] If family strengthing is a major
justification for contraception, we might point out that contracted
pregnancy will in some cases do the same. Whether or not having
children can save a failing marriage, it will certainly prevent a man
who wants children from leaving a woman incapable of providing
them. We may bewail his priorities, but if his wife is sufficiently
eager for the relationship to continue it would again be paternalistic
for us to forbid 'surrogacy' in such circumstances. That 'surrogacy'
reduces rather than promotes women's autonomy may be true
under some circumstances, but there are good grounds for thinking
that it can also enhance autonomy. It also remains to be shown that
the practice systematically burdens women, or one class of women.
In principle, the availability of new choices can be expected to
nourish rather than stunt women's lives, so long as they retain
control over their bodies and lives. The claim that contracted pregnancy destroys women's individuality and constitutes alienated
labour, as Christine Overall argues, depends not only on a problematic Marxist analysis, but on the assumption that other jobs available to women are seriously less alienating.[18]

Perhaps what is wrong here is that contracted pregnancy seems
to be the other side of the coin of prostitution. Prostitution is sex
without reproduction; 'surrogacy' is reproduction without sex. But
it is difficult to form a persuasive argument that goes beyond mere
guilt by association. Strictly speaking, contracted pregnancy is not
prostitution; a broad-based Marxist definition would include it, but
also traditional marriage. I think that in the absence of further
argument, the force of this accusation is primarily emotional.

Perhaps the dread feature contracted pregnancy shares with prostitution is that it is a lazy person's way of exploiting their own

---

[17] Infertility is often a result of social arrangements. This process would therefore be especially unfair to those who already have been exposed to more than their share of toxic
chemicals or other harmful conditions.

[18] Christine Overall, *Ethics and Human Reproduction*. (Winchester, Mass.: Allen & Unwin,
1987), ch. 6. Particularly problematic are her comments about women's loss of individuality,
as I will be arguing shortly.

'natural resources'. But I suspect that this idea reveals a touchingly naive view of what it takes to be a successful prostitute, not to mention the effort involved in running an optimum pregnancy. Overall takes up this point by asserting that it

> is not and cannot be merely one career choice among others. It is not a real alternative. It is implausible to suppose that fond parents would want it for their daughters. We are unlikely to set up training courses for surrogate mothers. Schools holding 'career days' for their future graduates will surely not invite surrogate mothers to address the class on advantages of 'vocation'. And surrogate motherhood does not seem to be the kind of thing one would put on one's curriculum vitae. (p. 126)

But this seems to me to be a blatant *ad populum* argument.

Such an objection ought, in any case, to entail general condemnation of apparently effortless ways of life that involved any utilization of our distinctive characteristics.

We surely exploit our personal 'natural resources' whenever we work. Ditchdiggers use their bodies, professors use their minds. Overall seems particularly to object to some types of 'work': contracted pregnancy 'is no more a real job option than selling one's blood or one's gametes or one's bodily organs can be real job options.' (p. 126) But her discussion makes clear that her denial that such enterprises are 'real' jobs is not based on any social arrangements that preclude earning a living wage doing these things, but rather on the moral judgement that they are wrong. They are wrong because they constitute serious 'personal and bodily alienation'. Yet her arguments for such alienation are weak. She contends that women who work as 'surrogates' are deprived of any expression of individuality, (p. 126) are interchangeable, (p. 127) and that they have no choice about whose sperm to harbor. (p. 128) It is true that, given a reasonable environment (partly provided by the woman herself), bodies create babies without conscious effort. This fact, it seems to me, has no particular moral significance: many tasks can be accomplished in similar ways yet are not thought valueless.[19]

It is also usually true that women involved in contracted pregnancy are, in some sense, interchangeable. But the same is true,

---

[19] Men have been getting handsome pay for sperm donation for years; by comparison with childbearing, such donation is a lark. Yet there has been no outcry about its immorality. Another double standard?

quite possibly necessarily so, of most jobs. No one who has graded mounds of logic exams or introductory ethics essays could reasonably withhold their assent to this claim, even though college teaching is one of the most autonomous careers available. Even those of us lucky enough to teach upper level courses that involve more expression of individual expertise and choice can be slotted into standardized job descriptions. Finally, it is just false that a woman can have no say about whose sperm she accepts: this could be guaranteed by proper regulation.

I wonder whether there is not some subtle devaluing of the physical by Overall. If so, then we are falling into the trap set by years of elitist equations of women, nature and inferiority.

What I think is really at issue here is the disposition of the fruit of contracted pregnancy: babies. However, it seems to be generally permissible to dispose of or barter what we produce with both our minds and our bodies – except for that which is created by our reproductive organs. So the position we are considering may just be a version of the claim that it is wrong to separate reproduction and childrearing.

Why? It is true that women normally expect to become especially attached to the product of this particular kind of labour, and we generally regard such attachment as desirable. It seems to be essential for successfully rearing babies the usual way. But if they are to be reared by others who are able to form the appropriate attachment, then what is wrong if a surrogate mother fails to form it? It seems to me that the central question here is whether this 'maternal instinct' really exists, and, if it does, whether suppressing it is always harmful.

Underlying these questions is the assumption that bonding with babies is 'natural' and therefore 'good'. Perhaps so: the evolutionary advantage of such a tendency would be clear. It would be simpleminded, however, to assume that our habits are biologically determined: our culture is permeated with pronatalist bias.[20] 'Natural' or not, whether a tendency to such attachment is desirable could reasonably be judged to depend on circumstance. When infant mortality is high[21] or responsibility for childrearing is shared

---

[20] See Ellen Peck and Judith Senderowitz, *Pronatalism: The Myth of Mom and Apple Pie*, (New York: Thomas Y. Crowell Co., 1974).

[21] As it has been at some periods in the past: see for example information about family relationships in Philippe Ariès, *Centuries of Childhood: A Social History of Family Life*, trans. Robert Baldick, (New York, 1982), and Lloyd DeMause's work.

by the community, it could do more harm than good. Beware the naturalistic fallacy![22]

But surely there is something special about gestating a baby. That is, after all, the assumption behind the judgement that Mary Beth Whitehead, not William Stern, had a stronger claim to Baby M. The moral scoreboard seems clear: they both had the same genetic input, but she gestated the baby, and therefore has a better case for social parenthood.[23]

We need to be very careful here. Special rights have a way of being accompanied by special responsibilities: women's unique gestational relationship with babies may be taken as reason to confine them once more to the nursery. Furthermore, positing special rights entailed directly by biology flirts again with the naturalistic fallacy and undermines our capacity to adapt to changing situations and forge our destiny.[24]

Furthermore, we already except many varieties of such separation. We routinely engage in sending children to boarding school, foster parenting, daycare, and so forth; in the appropriate circumstances, these practices are clearly beneficial. Hence, any blanket condemnation of separating reproduction and childrearing will not wash; additional argument is needed for particular classes of cases.

John Robertson points out that for the arguments against separating reproduction and childrearing used against contracted pregnancy are equally valid – but unused – with respect to adoption.[25] Others, such as Herbert Krimmel, reject this view by arguing that

---

[22] Consider the arguments in chapter 8 of *Women's Work*, by Ann Oakley, (New York: Vintage Books, 1974).

[23] One of the interesting things about the practice of contracted pregnancy is that it can be argued to both strengthen and weaken the social recognition of biological relationships. On the one hand, the pregnant woman's biological relationship is judged irrelevant beyond a certain point; on the other, the reason for not valuing it is to enhance that of the sperm donor. This might be interpreted as yet another case where men's interests are allowed to overrule women's. But it might also be interpreted as a salutary step toward awareness that biological ties can and sometimes should be subordinated to social ones. Deciding which interpretation is correct will depend on the facts of particular cases, and the arguments taken to justify the practice in the first place.

[24] Science fiction, most notably John Wyndham's *The Midwich Cuckoos*, provides us with thought-provoking material.

[25] John Robertson, 'Surrogate Mothers: Not so Novel After All', *Hastings Center Report*, vol. 13, no. 5 (October 1983). This article is reprinted in *Bioethics*, ed. Rem B. Edwards and Glen C. Graber, (San Diego, California: Harcourt, Brace Jovanovich, 1988). Krimmel's article ('The Case Against Surrogate Parenting') was also orginally published in the *Hastings Center Report* and is reprinted in *Bioethics*. References here are to the latter.

there is a big moral difference between giving away an already existing baby and deliberately creating one to give away. This remains to be shown, I think. It is also argued that as adoption outcomes are rather negative, we should be wary of extending any practice that shares its essential features. In fact, there seems to be amazingly little hard information about adoption outcomes. I wonder if the idea that they are bad results from media reports of offspring seeking their biological forbears. There is, in any case, reason to think that there are differences between the two practices such that the latter is likely to be more successful than the former.[26]

None of the social descriptions of surrogacy thus seem to clearly justify the outcry against the practice. I suspect that the remaining central issue is the crucial one: surrogacy is baby-selling and participating in this practice exploits and taints women.

IS SURROGACY BABY-SELLING?

In the foregoing, I deliberately left vague the question of payment in contracted pregnancy. It is clear that there is a recognizable form of the practice that does not include payment; however, it also seems clear that controversy is focusing on the commercial form. The charge is that it is baby-selling and that this is wrong.

Is paid 'surrogacy' baby-selling? Proponents deny that it is, arguing that women are merely making available their biological services. Opponents retort that as women are paid little or nothing if they fail to hand over a live, healthy child, they are indeed selling a baby. If they are merely selling their services they would get full pay, even if the child were born dead.

It is true women who agree to contracts relieving clients of responsibility in this case are being exploited. They, after all, have

---

[26] One major difference between adoption and contracted pregnancy is that the baby is handed over virtually at birth, thus ensuring that the trauma sometimes experienced by older adoptees is not experienced. Although children of contracted pregnancy might well be curious to know about their biological mother, I do not see this as a serious obstacle to the practice, since we could change our policy about this. There is also reason to believe that carefully-screened women undertaking a properly-regulated contracted pregnancy are less likely to experience lingering pain of separation. First, they have deliberately chosen to go through pregnancy, knowing that they will give the baby up. The resulting sense of control is probably critical to both their short- and long-term well-being. Second, their pregnancy is not the result of trauma. See also Monica B. Morris, 'Reproductive Technology and Restraints', *Transaction/SOCIETY*, March/April 1988, pp. 16–22, especially p. 18.

done their part, risked their risks, and should be paid – just like the physicians involved. Normal childbearing provides no guarantee of a live, healthy child – why should contracted pregnancy?

There are further reasons for believing that women are selling their services, not babies. Firstly, we do not consider children property. Therefore, as we cannot sell what we do not own, we cannot be selling babies. What creates confusion here is that we do think we own sperm and ova. (Otherwise, how could man sell their sperm?) Yet we do not own what they become, persons. At what point, then, does the relationship cease to be describable as 'ownership'?

Resolution of this question is not necessary to the current discussion. If we can own babies, there seems to be nothing problematic about selling them. If ownership ceases at some time before birth (and could thus be argued to be unconnected with personhood), then it is not selling of babies that is going on.

Although this response deals with the letter of the objection about babyselling, it fails to heed its spirit, which is that we are trafficking in persons, and that such trafficking is wrong. Even if we are not 'selling', something nasty is happening.

The most common analogy, with slavery, is weak. Slavery is wrong according to any decent moral theory: the institution allows people to be treated badly. Their desires and interests, whose satisfaction is held to be essential for a good life, are held in contempt. Particularly egregious is the callous disregard of emotional ties to family and self-determination generally. But the institution of surrogate mothering deprives babies of neither.[27] In short, as Robertson contends, 'the purchasers do not buy the right to treat the child . . . as a commodity or property. Child abuse and neglect laws still apply.' (p. 655)

If 'selling babies' is not the right description of what is occurring. then how are we to explain what happens when the birth mother hands the child over to others? One plausible suggestion is that she is giving up her parental right to have a relationship with the child.[28]

---

[27] There may be a problem for the woman who gives birth, as the Baby M case has demonstrated. There is probably a case for a waiting period after the birth during which the woman can change her mind.

[28] Heidi Malm suggested this position in her comment on Sara Ann Ketchum's paper 'Selling Babies and Selling Bodies: Surrogate Motherhood and the Problem of Commodification', at the Eastern Division *APA* meetings, 30 December 1987.

That it is wrong to do this for pay remains to be shown. Although it would be egoistic and immoral to 'sell' an ongoing, friendly relationship, (doing so would raise questions about whether it was friendship at all), the immorality of selling a relationship with an organism your body has created but with which you do not yet have a unique social bond, is a great deal less clear.[29]

People seem to feel much less strongly about the wrongness of such acts when motivated by altruism; refusing compensation is the only acceptable proof of such altruism. The act is, in any case, socially valuable. Why then must it be motivated by altruistic considerations? We do not frown upon those who provide other socially valuable services even when they do not have the 'right' motive. Nor do we require them to be unpaid. For instance, no one expects physicians, no matter what their motivation, to work for beans. They provide an important service; their motivation is important only to the extent that it affects quality.

In general, workers are required to have appropriate skills, not particular motivation.[30] Once again, it seems that there is a different standard for women and for men.

One worry is that women cannot be involved in contracted pregnancy without harming themselves, as it is difficult to let go of a child without lingering concern. So far, despite the heavily-publicized Baby M case, this appears not to be necessarily true.[31]

Another worry is that the practice will harm children. Children's welfare is, of course, important. Children deserve the same consideration as other persons, and no society that fails to meet their basic needs is morally satisfactory. Yet I am suspicious of the objections raised on their behalf in these discussions: recourse to children's alleged well-being is once again being used as a trump card against women's autonomy.

---

[29] Mary Anne Warren suggests, alternatively, that this objection could be obviated by women and children retaining some rights and responsibilities toward each other in contracted pregnancy. Maintaining a relationship of sorts might also, she suggests, help forestall and alleviate whatever negative feelings children might have about such transfers. I agree that such openness is probably a good idea in any case. (Referee's comment.)

[30] Perhaps lurking behind the objections of surrogacy is some feeling that it is wrong to earn money by letting your body work, without active effort on your part. But this would rule out sperm selling, as well as using women's beauty to sell products and services.

[31] See, for example, James Rachels, 'A Report from America: The Baby M Case', *Bioethics*, vol. 1, n. 4 (October 1987), p. 365. He reports that there have been over six hundred successful cases; see also the above note on adoption.

First, we hear only about possible risks, never possible benefits, which, as I have been arguing, could be substantial.[32] Second, the main objection raised is the worry about how children will take the knowledge that their genetic mother conceived on behalf of another. We do not know how children will feel about having had such 'surrogate' mothers. But as it is not a completely new phenomenon we might start our inquiry about this topic with historical evidence, not pessimistic speculation. In any case, if the practice is dealt with in an honest and commonsense way, particularly if it becomes quite common (and therefore 'normal'), there is likely to be no problem. We are also hearing about the worries of existing children of women who are involved in the practice: there are reports that they fear their mother will give them away, too. But surely we can make clear to children the kinds of distinctions that distinguish the practice from slavery or baby-selling in the first place.

Although we must try to foresee what might harm children, I cannot help but wonder about the double standards implied by this speculation. The first double standard occurs when those who oppose surrogacy (and reproductive technologies generally) also oppose attempts to reduce the number of handicapped babies born.[33] In the latter context, it is argued that despite their problems handicapped persons are often glad to be alive. Hence it would be paternalistic to attempt to prevent their birth.

Why then do we not hear the same argument here? Instead, the possible disturbance of children born of surrogacy is taken as a reason to prevent their birth. Yet this potential problem is both more remote and most likely involves less suffering than such ailments as spina bifida, Huntington's Disease or cystic fibrosis, which some do not take to be reasons to refrain from childbearing.[34]

Considering the sorts of reasons why parents have children, it is hard to see why the idea that one was conceived in order to provide a desperately-wanted child to another is thought to be problematic. One might well prefer that to the idea that one was an 'accident',

[32] Among them the above mentioned one of being born healthier.

[33] To avoid the difficulties about abortion added by the assumption that we are talking about existing foetuses, let us consider here only the issue of whether certain couples should risk pregnancy.

[34] There is an interesting link here between these two aspects of reproduction, as the promise of healthier children is, I think, one of the strongest arguments for contracted pregnancy.

adopted, born because contraception or abortion were not available, conceived to cement a failing marriage, to continue a family line, to qualify for welfare aid, to sex-balance a family, or as an experiment in childrearing. Surely what matters for a child's well-being in the end is whether it is being raised in a loving, intelligent environment.

The second double standard involves a disparity between the interests of women and children. Arguing that surrogacy is wrong because it may upset children suggests a disturbing conception of the moral order. Women should receive consideration at least equal to that accorded children. Conflicts of interest between the two should be resolved according to the same rules we use for any other moral subjects. Those rules should never prescribe sacrificing one individual's basic interest at the mere hint of harm to another.

In sum, there seems to be no reason to think that there is anything necessarily wrong with 'surrogate mothering', even the paid variety. Furthermore, some objections to it depend on values and assumptions that have been the chief building blocks of women's inequality. Why are some feminists asserting them? Is it because 'surrogacy' as currently practiced often exploits women?

IS 'SURROGATE MOTHERING' WRONG IN CERTAIN SITUATIONS?

Even if 'surrogate mothering' is not necessarily immoral, circumstances can render it so. For instance, it is obviously wrong to coerce women to engage in the practice. Also, certain conditions are unacceptable. Among them are clauses in a contract that subordinate a woman's reasonable desires and judgements to the will of another contracting party,[35] clauses legitimating inadequate pay for the risks and discomforts involved, and clauses that penalize her for the birth of a handicapped or dead baby through no fault of her own. Such contracts are now common.[36]

One popular solution to the problem of such immoral contracts is a law forbidding all surrogacy agreements; their terms would then be unenforceable. But I believe that women will continue to engage

---

[35] What this may consist of naturally requires much additional elucidation.
[36] See Susan Ince, 'Inside the Surrogate Industry', *Test-Tube Women*, ed. Rita Arditti, Renate Duelli Klein, and Shelley Minden, (London: Pandora Press, 1984).

in surrogate mothering, even if it is unregulated, and this approach leaves them vulnerable to those who change their mind, or will not pay. Fair and reasonable regulations are essential to prevent exploitation of women. Although surrogate mothering may seem risky and uncomfortable to middle-class persons safely ensconced in healthy, interesting, relatively well-paid jobs, with adequate regulation it becomes an attractive option for some women. That these women are more likely than not to be poor is no reason to prohibit the activity.

As I suggested earlier, poor women now face substantial risks in the workplace. Even a superficial survey of hazards in occupations available to poor women would give pause to those who would prohibit surrogacy on the grounds of risk.[37]

Particularly shocking is the list of harmful substances and conditions to which working women are routinely exposed. For instance, cosmeticians and hairdressers, dry cleaners and dental technicians are all exposed to carcinogens in their daily work. (Stellman, Appendixes 1 and 2) Most low-level jobs also have high rates of exposure to toxic chemicals and dangerous machinery, and women take such jobs in disproportionate numbers. It is therefore unsurprising that poor women sicken and die more often than other members of society.[38]

This is not an argument in favour of adding yet another dangerous option to those already facing such women. Nor does it follow that the burdens they already bear justify the new ones. On the contrary, it is imperative to clean up dangerous workplaces. However, it would be utopian to think that this will occur in the near future. We must therefore attempt to improve women's lot under existing conditions. Under these circumstances it would be irrational to prohibit surrogacy on the grounds of risk when women would instead have to engage in still riskier pursuits.

Overall's emphatic assertion that contracted pregnancy is not a 'real choice' for women is unconvincing. Her major argument, as I suggested earlier, is that it is an immoral, alienating option. But she

---

[37] See, for example, Jeanne Mager Stellman, *Women's Work, Women's Health*, (New York: Pantheon 1977).

[38] See George L. Waldbott, *Health Effects of Environmental Pollutants*, (St. Louis: The C.V. Mosby Co., 1973); Nicholas Ashford, *Crisis in the Workplace: Occupational Disease and Injury*, (Cambridge: MIT Press, 1976); *Cancer and the Worker*, The New York Academy of Science, 1977); *Environmental Problems in Medicine*, ed. William D. McKee, (Springfield, Ill.: Charles C. Thomas, 1977).

also believes that such apparently expanded choices simply mask an underlying contraction of choice. (p. 124) She also fears that by 'endorsing an uncritical freedom of reproductive choice, we may also be implicitly endorsing all conceivable alternatives that an individual might adopt; we thereby abandon the responsibility for evaluating substantive actions in favour of advocating merely formal freedom of choice.' (p. 125) Both worries are, as they stand, unpersuasive.

As I argued before, there is something troubling here about the new and one-sided emphasis on risk. If nothing else, we need to remember that contracted pregnancy constitutes a low-tech approach to a social problem, one which would slow the impetus toward expensive and dangerous high-tech solutions.[39]

A desire for children on the part of those who normally could not have them is not likely to disappear anytime soon. We could discount it, as many participants in debate about new reproductive technologies do. After all, nobody promised a rose garden to infertile couples, much less to homosexuals or to single women. Nor is it desirable to propagate the idea that having children is essential for human fulfilment.

But appealing to the sacrosancity of traditional marriage or of blood ties to prohibit otherwise acceptable practices that would satisfy people's desires hardly makes sense, especially when those practices may provide other benefits. Not only might contracted pregnancy be less risky and more enjoyable than other jobs women are forced to take, but there are other advantages as well. Since being pregnant is not usually a full-time occupation, 'surrogate mothering' could buy time for women to significantly improve their lot: students, aspiring writers, and social activists could make real progress toward their goals.

Women have until now done this reproductive labour for free.[40] Paying women to bear children should force us all to recognize this process as the socially useful enterprise that it is, and children as socially valuable creatures whose upbringing and welfare are critically important.

---

[39] These are the ones most likely to put women in the clutches of the paternalistic medical establishment. Exploitation by commercial operations such as that of Noel Keane could be avoided by tight regulation or prohibition altogether of for-profit enterprises.

[40] The implications of this fact remain to be fully understood; I suspect that they are detrimental to women and children, but that this is a topic for another paper.

In short, 'surrogate mothering' has the potential to empower women and increase their status in society. The darker side of the story is that it also has frightening potential for deepening their exploitation. The outcome of the current warfare over control of new reproductive possibilities will determine which of these alternatives comes to pass.

PART VIII: END OF LIFE

Chapter 32

THE METAPHYSICS OF BRAIN DEATH

JEFF McMAHAN

Advancing knowledge of the functions of different areas of the brain, together with recent innovations in brain imaging techniques, has now made it possible to know with reasonable certainty that certain comas are irreversible. Even as recently as a few decades ago, however, this knowledge was not available and doctors were obliged to assume that recovery from coma was possible until the cessation of cardiac and pulmonary functions assured that it was not. It had to be assumed, in other words, that the irreversible cessation of brain functions, and in particular the loss of the brain's capacity to support consciousness and mental activity, coincided with the irreversible cessation of cardiac and pulmonary functions. But along with advances in our understanding of the brain came new technologies for sustaining cardiopulmonary functions and together these made it possible in many cases for heart and lung functions to continue after the point at which one could be confident that the capacity for consciousness had been lost and indeed after clinical criteria indicated that the whole brain had irreversibly ceased to function.

This alone might not have been sufficient to motivate the shift from the traditional criterion of death as the irreversible cessation of cardiac and respiratory functions to the now dominant view that death consists in the death of the whole brain. But social and moral factors also contributed to the pressure to reassess our understanding of death. Patients in whom all possibility of consciousness had been lost were increasingly being sustained for lengthy periods at considerable cost in terms of the consumption of scarce medical resources, though without apparent benefit to the patients themselves. And the indefinite support of patients in this condition also meant that other patients who might have been saved by organ transplantation instead died for want of donors. The concept of brain death provided a ground for distinguishing among the former patients in such a way that at least some of them could be declared dead and thus be disconnected from expensive life-support systems without doctors having to fear legal liability, thereby also freeing the patients' organs for use in transplant operations. These concerns were explicitly acknowledged as important factors leading to the adoption of brain death as the criterion of death in the influential report of the group that became known as the Harvard Brain Death Committee.[1]

But, even though these social and moral concerns created incentives for revising our understanding of death, one may still wonder why we settled so readily on what I will call 'the dominant conception of brain death' – that is, the death of the whole brain (or, in Britain, the death of the brain stem, which at present is an immediate and infallible precursor of the death of the whole brain) – as the criterion of death. In what follows I will offer an explanation of why the dominant conception of brain death has seemed so attractive but will argue that this appeal is specious. I will suggest that no single conception of death can satisfy the requirements that the dominant conception of brain death has been supposed to satisfy. To meet these requirements, we need to distinguish two concepts of death: the death of the person, or self, and the death of the physical organism. I will propose and defend a particular conception of the former and will conclude by drawing out some of its implications for various practical moral problems.

I. THE DOMINANT CONCEPTION OF BRAIN DEATH

Much of the intuitive force of the idea that a person dies when her entire brain, or even just her brain stem, dies derives from the fact that both these conditions involve the irreversible loss of the capacity of consciousness and mental activity. For it is intuitively plausible to suppose that the capacity for subjectivity, for consciousness and mental activity, is essential to our existence – in other words, that one cannot exist without at least the capacity for consciousness or mental activity of some sort. Thus, writing about the historical development of the notion of brain death, one

---

[1] The Ad Hoc Committee of the Harvard Medical School, 'A Definition of Irreversible Coma', *Journal of the American Medical Association* 205 (1968): 337–340; reprinted in Samuel Gorovitz, et al., eds., *Moral Problems in Medicine*, second edition. Englewood Cliffs: Prentice-Hall, 1983: 419–424. for discussion, see Peter Singer, *Rethinking Life and Death: The Collapse of Our Traditional Ethics*, Melbourne: Text, 1994; chapter II.

scholar has commented that he has 'little doubt that the impact of loss of consciousness on acceptance of brain death has been considerable'.[2]

If, however, one were to identify the death of a person with the person's loss of the capacity for consciousness, then it would be a mistake to insist that the death of the whole brain, or even of the brain stem, is necessary for a diagnosis of brain death. For there are other conditions involving considerably less destruction of the brain that nevertheless cause the irreversible loss of the capacity for consciousness. One of these is *cerebral death*, which has been defined as the 'irreversible destruction of both cerebral hemispheres exclusive of the brain stem and cerebellum'.[3] Another is *neocortical death*, which involves 'the destruction of cortical neurons bilaterally while deep structures of the cerebral hemispheres such as the thalamus and basal ganglia may be intact along with the brain stem and cerebellum'.[4] Individuals who have suffered cerebral or neocortical death are commonly said to be in a *persistent vegetative state*. In many cases, a persistent vegetative state may persist only as a result of mechanical life support; in other cases, however, the survival and continued functioning of the brain stem is sufficient to ensure the continuation of spontaneous respiratory and thus cardiac function even in the absence of the capacity for consciousness. But, if the capacity for consciousness were essential for our existence, then cerebral death or even, apparently, neocortical death would be sufficient for the patient's ceasing to exist.

There are various explanations of why the death of the whole brain was adopted as the definition of death for clinical and legal purposes in preference to either cerebral or neocortical death. One appeals to the practical difficulty – more serious in the past than now, though still formidable in may cases – of determining when the damage to the cerebral hemispheres or cortical neurons is sufficiently extensive to preclude any possibility of consciousness. In short, a case might be made for the dominant conception on purely practical grounds: namely, that it is only when the entire brain is

---

[2] Peter McCullagh, *Brain Dead, Brain Absent, Brain Donors: Human Subjects or Human Objects?* Chichester: John Wiley & Sons, 1993, p. 15.

[3] Julius Korein, ed., *Brain Death: Interrelated Medical and Social Issues.* New York: New York Academy of Sciences, 1978, p. 7; quoted in Karen Grandstand Gervais, *Redefining Death*, New Haven: Yale University Press, 1986, p. 11.

[4] Korein, *Brain Death*, p. 8; quoted in Gervais, *Redefining Death*, p. 11.

dead that we can be fully confident that all capacity for consciousness has been lost.

But any complete explanation of the appeal of the dominant conception will also have to take account of the perceived requirement that a criterion of death should serve as a plausible marker of the biological death of the human organism as a whole. Thus advocates of the dominant conception of brain death have contended that brain death is equivalent to the death of the organism by arguing, for example, that the brain is the irreplaceable 'master control' that regulates and integrates the functions of the various parts of the organism.[5] Since the human organism can spontaneously maintain respiratory, cardiac, and other functions indefinitely after cerebral or neocortical death, these latter conditions have seemed less plausible as criteria for the death of the organism.

It has become increasingly evident, however, that even the death of the entire brain is not equivalent to the biological death of the human organism. We have, it seems, a unitary conception of death as the loss of those properties necessary and sufficient for a being to be *alive*, a *living* being. In the case of organisms (as opposed, say, to organs), death, or the loss of life, is generally held to consist in the irreversible cessation of integrated functioning by the organism as a whole. (This definition is probably insufficiently specific to be quite right; but the precise details are unnecessary for our purposes.) This general characterization of biological death says nothing about the brain, which is unsurprising given that most living organisms do not have brains. And even in the case of those that do, the brain is only one of the organism's many organs and thus cannot be identical with the organism itself. Hence it would be surprising if the death of the brain were one and the same thing as the death of the organism.

In the case of the human organism, it is clear that the death of the whole brain is neither necessary nor sufficient for the death of the organism – that is, for the cessation of integrated functioning of the system as a whole. Suppose that a living, functioning human brain were surgically extracted from the body and then kept alive for a certain period, either by being suspended in a tank of fluid or by being transplanted into the skull of a different human organism. The brains of nonhuman animals have been removed and kept

---

[5] See David Lamb, *Death, Brain Death and Ethics*, Albany: State University of New York Press, 1985, chapter 4, esp. p. 37. For discussion, see McCullagh, *Brain Dead*, pp. 13–20.

briefly alive in both of these ways and it seems in principle possible that a human brain could be kept alive and indeed conscious even when severed from its source of sensory inputs. But, if this is in principle possible, then brain death is not necessary for the death of the organism, since in this case the organism could clearly die even though its brain would continue to live. (The organism would of course be 'brain dead' according to clinical indicators, but in this case that would not show that the brain itself was dead.) This shows that brain death is not necessary for the death of the human organism.

Nor is the death of the whole brain sufficient for the death of the human organism. While it is true that a human organism, left to its own devices, will very quickly cease to function when the whole of its brain dies, it has long been known that mechanical ventilation can enable a human organism to maintain functional integrity for a certain time beyond the death of the whole brain. While until recently it was widely believed that this interval during which functions could be artificially sustained was measured only in hours or days, it is now well established that mechanical ventilation can sustain cardiac and other functions in a human organism for well over three months following a reliable diagnosis of brain death. In some cases, the bodies of pregnant women diagnosed as brain dead have been sustained in this way for several months in order to allow the fetus to mature.[6] In those cases in which the fetus was nourished and sustained for several months in its mother's mechanically ventilated body and then delivered alive by caesarian section, it seems implausible to say that it was incubated in a corpse. If an organism can circulate blood, metabolize food, and perform its other characteristic functions with sufficient efficiency to support the growth of a fetus, that seems evidence enough that it is functioning in an integrated manner.

The defender of the dominant conception of brain death may reply that, as was noted earlier, it is part of the point of the criterion of brain death to distinguish between patients who remain alive and those who are dead and whose bodily functions can therefore be maintained only artificially and temporarily. Yet it is important to notice that, in functional terms, the difference between the body of a pregnant woman in a persistent vegetative state and the mechanically ventilated body of a pregnant woman who has been diagnosed

[6] See McCullagh, *Brain Dead*, pp. 35–39, and Singer, *Rethinking Life and Death*, Chapter I.

as brain dead is that, in the former case, respiration is artificially induced while it may occur spontaneously in the latter. But is the fact that an array of seemingly vital functions are triggered artificially rather than spontaneously of decisive biological significance in determining whether an organism is dead? Certainly there are cases in which it is not – for example, cases in which a lesion on the respiratory center in the brain stem prevents spontaneous respiration in persons in whom other brain functions, including cognition, remain unimpaired. Even though these persons have to be sustained by mechanical ventilation, no one is tempted to declare them dead.[7] We might, indeed, imagine a case in which an individual in a persistent vegetative state (i.e., an individual who has suffered cerebral or neocortical death) whose respiration has until now been spontaneous develops a lesion on the respiratory center of the brain stem and thus comes to require mechanical ventilation. This individual would not be brain dead according to the dominant conception, since much of the brain stem would remain alive and functional. But now compare this individual with another whose entire brain has died but whose various bodily functions are maintained by mechanical ventilation. Neither organism is capable of supporting consciousness or mental activity and neither is capable of spontaneous respiratory function (nor, therefore, any other spontaneous vital functions), though both continue to carry out a vast range of functions characteristic of living human organisms. The difference is that there is some residual brain stem activity in one but not in the other. This is an insufficient basis for the claim that the one organism is alive while the other is dead.[8]

There is, in fact, an easier way to think about this. The claim that a human organism cannot be alive unless at least some of its functions are regulated by the action of its brain implies that human embryos are not alive. For the vital processes of an early human embryo are not only not governed by its brain but are also crucially dependent on life-support from the body of the pregnant woman in whose womb it is located. Yet human embryos are clearly living human organisms. This shows that a human organism can be alive even when it altogether lacks brain functions and when its vital functions cannot be sustained independently of external support.

---

[7] See Gervais, *Redefining Death*, p. 33.
[8] One of the referees for the journal, Daniel Wikler, has called my attention to the fact that a similar example appears in his 'Brain Death: A Durable Consensus?' *Bioethics* 7 (1993), p. 243.

I therefore conclude, as many others have done, that the death of the whole brain is not equivalent to the death of the human organism. The dominant conception of brain death is an unstable compromise between those views that make the irreversible loss of the capacity for consciousness the criterion for human death and those that insist that the death of a human being, like the death of any other organism, consists in the irreversible loss of functional integrity by the organism. Some critics had concluded that we must either accept that it is the loss of the capacity for consciousness that is decisive and thus embrace cerebral or neocortical death as the criterion of death or else focus on the biological characteristics of the organism and accept a broader criterion of death that is applicable even to organisms that lack brains.[9] I believe that this is a mistake. I will argue that, while the irreversible cessation of integrated functioning by the human organism is indeed death, cerebral death is also death. They are both valid criteria of death, though each is a criterion of the death of a different thing.

II. PERSONS AND ORGANISMS

Much of the confusion in the debate about brain death arises from the failure to understand, or even to consider, the nature of the relation that we bear to our physical organisms. I should confess at the outset that I do not myself understand the nature of this relation. Where I differ from many participants in the debate is that I explicitly base my account of brain death on the claim that the relation is *not identity*. I have an organism, I exist in association with it, am intimately related to it in ways that are hard to explain; but I am not identical with it. The same is true of all other members of my kind; indeed it is true of all beings that possess the capacity for consciousness and mental activity. None of these is identical with its physical organism.

There are various arguments for the claim that we are not identical with our organisms (or, as I will say, that we are not organisms). I will mention two. First, the idea that we are identical with our organisms has implausible implications about when we begin to exist and when we cease to exist. For it implies that we begin to exist and cease to exist when our organisms do. Thus, if we assume

---

[9] See, for example, Gervais, *Redefining Death*, p. 160 and elsewhere.

that my organism began to exist at the time of its conception, then we must accept that I began to exist at conception. (Two qualifications are necessary. First, conception is not a momentary event but is instead a process lasting about 24 hours. It is arguable that the human organism does not begin to exist at least until syngamy, the point at which the genetic materials from the sperm and egg have fused.[10] Second, some human organisms do not begin to exist until well after syngamy. In the case of monozygotic twinning, a single zygote divides within fourteen days of conception to form two qualitatively identical embryos. Since it cannot be the case that both subsequent embryos are identical with the original zygote, and since it seems arbitrary to say that one of the subsequent embryos is identical with the original zygote while the other is not, it seems reasonable to conclude that the original zygote ceases to exist when it splits and that two new embryos, and thus two new organisms, begin to exist at that point. If this is right, then identical twins have organisms that began to exist slightly later in the process of gestation than those of the rest of use. This also suggests an objection to the idea that we are organisms. For, if we are organisms, then one of us ceases to exist whenever monozygotic twinning occurs. If it is bad when one of us ceases to exist, thereby losing the whole of a life that would have been worth living, then twinning is bad. But no one believes this.[11])

Many of us, however, find it hard to believe that we began to exist at conception. Surely, we think, *I* could never exist as a thing so humble as a single cell! To appreciate the force of this doubt, imagine that the process of human biological development were reversed in some of us. We would begin to grow younger, in physical terms. Eventually some of us would revert to being babies. These people would soon have to be placed in artificial uteruses in order to survive. As their brains reverted to the infantile and fetal stages of their development, their mental lives would become increasingly rudimentary and would eventually disappear altogether when their brains ceased to be capable of supporting consciousness. Suppose now that one were to face this prospect. When during the process

---

[10] See Stephen Buckle, Karen Dawson, and Peter Singer, 'The Syngamy Debate: When *Precisely* Does a Human Life Begin?' in Peter Singer, et al., eds., *Embryo Experimentation: Ethical, Legal and Social Issues.* Cambridge: Cambridge University Press, 1990: 213–25.

[11] There is a lot that could be said in response to this argument but it is not worth pursuing here.

of biological regression would one cease to exist? Would one survive to the very end of the process, when one's organism would have reverted to a single-celled entity?

If we are identical with our organisms, then not only do we begin to exist when they do but we do not cease to exist until they do. This means that in most cases we do indeed survive death, since in most cases our organisms do not cease to exist when they die but instead continue to exist as corpses. According to this view, therefore, most of us survive death as corpses. Again, however, this is not what most of us believe. Unless we believe that we are immortal souls, we accept that the death of a person's organism is a sufficient condition of the person's ceasing to exist, even if the organism continues to exist as a corpse.

There are two ways in which those who believe that we are organisms can attempt to salvage their view without being committed to accepting that we can exist as corpses. One is to hold that, when a human organism dies, it ceases to exist. That is, one might hold that the living organism and the corpse are not one and the same thing. The corpse is not a phase in the history of a body that was once alive; rather, it is a different substance altogether, one that pops into existence upon the death of the organism. I assume, however, that this is even less plausible than the idea that we may continue to exist after death as corpses.[12]

The other way of attempting to reconcile the view that we are organisms with the view that we do not survive death as corpses is to claim that we are essentially functional organisms. In that case one would cease to exist when one's organism ceased to function – that is, to be alive. It is not clear, however, whether this view is really coherent. If there really is some thing that ceases to exist when the organism ceases to function, then that thing is not identical with the organism, since the organism continues to exist. The alternative is to suppose that we really are not things, or substances, at all, but are just phases in the histories of our organisms. But in that case there is no thing that ceases to exist when the organism ceases to function.

Even if the metaphysics of this last view could be made coherent, the view would still succumb to the second main argument against

---

[12] For discussion, see W.R. Carter, "Death and Bodily Transfiguration", *Mind* XCIII (1984): 412–418.

the view that we are organisms. This argument appeals to a thought-experiment involving a brain transplant.[13] Suppose that the entire brain of a person, P, is transplanted into the body of his identical twin brother, whose brain was irreparably damaged and has been removed. Suppose that surgical techniques have advanced well beyond what is now considered possible and that all the connections between P's brain and the nerve pathways in his twin's body can be established. Following the operation, a person is brought to consciousness. He has P's memories, beliefs, and dispositions of character. He believes himself to be P. But he has the body of P's brother. Most of us believe that this person is P. On another operating table in the room lies the organism from which P's brain was removed. Perhaps it has been left decerebrate and thus has died; or it may have received a brain stem transplant, in which case it might be alive, though lacking the capacity for consciousness; or it might have received a whole brain transplant so that it is now 'inhabited' by a new person. The point is that, although it may have been mutilated or altered in various ways, it clearly remains P's organism (or, more precisely, it remains the same thing as that which was his organism, since he now has a new organism). But if P is lying on one table babbling amazedly about finding himself with a different body while his organism lies on a different table, he is not now identical with his organism. And if he is not now identical with his organism, then he never was identical with it. For a thing cannot cease to be itself and yet continue to exist.[14]

---

[13] Other authors have appealed to this thought-experiment to show that, as Mark Johnston puts it, we are not 'essentially human organisms'. See Johnston, 'Human Beings', *Journal of Philosophy* 84 (February 1987), pp. 75–76. More recently I have found a briefer version of the same argument in Michael Lockwood, 'Warnock Versus Powell (and Harradine): When Does Potentiality Count?' *Bioethics* 2 (July 1988), p. 200. While working on this paper I have read certain papers, or in some cases reread papers about which I had forgotten, which I have discovered together contain many of the elements of my overall argument, which itself is drawn from work done years ago on a manuscript entitled *Killing at the Margins of Life*, New York: Oxford University Press, forthcoming. If this paper has a virtue, therefore, it is not novelty but the fact that it synthesizes scattered elements from different areas of metaphysics and moral theory into a single coherent conception of brain death and personal identity.

[14] This claim has been challenged by George Myro, who argues that identity statements are implicitly temporally indexed, so that one might be identical with one's organism at one time but not another. He attempts to work out the logic of a temporally indexed concept of identity in 'Time and Identity', in Richard E. Grandy and Richard Warner, eds. *Philosophical Grounds of Rationality: Intentions, Categories, Ends.* Oxford: Clarendon Press, 1986: 383–409.

As I noted, this second argument also disposes of the suggestion that we are functional organisms. For in this case P survives while his organism ceases to function. Hence P is not a functional organism.

If I am not identical with my organism, then there are two things here: I am here and this organism is also here. I seem to share a great many properties with it. But, if I am not identical with it, then I can have properties that it does not have and *vice versa*. Most importantly for our purposes, while my organism and I may cease to exist simultaneously (for example, if a nuclear bomb lands on me), it is possible that I may cease to exist at one time while it will cease to exist at another. This, as I have indicated, is in fact what many of us believe: that I will very likely cease to exist when my organism dies while it may continue to exist until it disintegrates as a result of the process of decay.

Normally, the ceasing to exist of a person coincides with the biological death of his or her organism. But, not only is it possible for the person to cease to exist before the organism ceases to exist, it is also possible for the person Lo cease to exist before the organism dies. And it is in principle possible for the organism to die and perhaps even to cease to exist before the person ceases to exist. This happens, for example, in the variant of the brain-transplant case cited above in which P continues to exist in association with a new body while his decerebrate organism is left to die.

Since it is not necessarily the case that we cease to exist either when our organisms die or when they cease to exist, the fact that a person's organism can be kept alive after his whole brain has died or ceased to function does not show that the dominant conception of brain death is not death. It shows only that brain death is not equivalent to the death of the organism. Thus the fact that the death of my whole brain and the death of my organism are not one and the same thing is compatible with the claim that *my* death *is* equivalent to the death of my whole brain.

III. PERSONAL IDENTITY

It is *possible* that my death is equivalent to the death of my whole brain; but is it *really?* How can one tell? One must begin by clarifying what one means by 'my death'. Some commentators have claimed that 'death is a biological concept. Thus in a literal sense, death can be applied directly only to biological organisms and not to persons. We do not object to the phrase "death of a person", but the phrase in common usage actually means the death of the organism which was the person'.[15] The authors of this passage claim that their understanding of the notion of death is faithful to 'our ordinary use of the term'.[16] But the idea that we are not identical with our organisms is not a wild new idea that requires a departure from ordinary ways of speaking. Anyone who is skeptical of the idea that we begin to exist at conception, or of the idea that most people continue to exist after death as corpses, believes that it is a coherent possibility that we are not identical with our organisms. Therefore ordinary language should have the resources to enable us to articulate the distinction between *my* ceasing to exist and the death of my organism. And it is, in fact, entirely natural to say that when I cease to exist I die, even if I am not an organism. The only alternative, if we deny that I am identical with my organism, is to say that I cease to exist without dying. But since, when I will cease to exist, I clearly will not be alive, this alternative seems to commit us to the view that I am not now alive – for, if I will *cease* to be alive when I cease to exist, then that seems a sufficient ground for saying that I will have died. It is, I concede, possible to argue that, if I am not an organism, then I am not a biological entity and thus essentially biological predicates such as 'alive' and 'dead' cannot apply to me. But that is clearly inconsistent with ordinary language.

It seems, therefore, that we must distinguish two concepts of death, both of which, I believe, are found in ordinary language. One is the concept of the biological death of a living being – an organism or perhaps an organ, a piece of tissue, or a cell. It is in this sense that an organism dies when it irreversibly loses the capacity for integrated functioning. The other is the concept of the death of the conscious or potentially conscious being whose existence is supported by the functioning of the organism. *My* death will be a death of this second sort and will consist in my ceasing to exist, which may or may not coincide with the biological death of my organism.

What are the essential conditions of my death, or ceasing to exist? Would the death of my whole brain be equivalent to, or a necessary

---

[15] Charles M. Culver and Bernard Gert, *Philosophy in Medicine*, New York: Oxford University Press, 1982, p. 183. Their view is echoed by David Lamb, who writes that 'the concept of "death" can only be applied to organisms, not persons'. See Lamb, *Brain Death*, p. 93.
[16] Culver and Gert, *Philosophy in Medicine*, p. 181.

and sufficient condition of, my death? To answer these questions with confidence, one requires an account of personal identity – that is, an account of what is necessarily involved in our continuing to exist. What is required is not a *de dicto* account of what is necessarily involved in being or continuing to exist as a *person*. For we might (as I in fact believe) be persons only contingently – that is, we may be able to exist while not being persons. Instead, what is required is an account of the conditions for the existence of things of our kind, whatever kind of thing we essentially are.

In this section I will sketch what I think is the best account of personal identity. While it is not possible here to present the arguments for the account, or to indicate its advantages over rival accounts, I have attempted to provide a defense elsewhere.[17]

This account of personal identity captures the intuition that I have suggested was among the considerations that motivated the shift to the current understanding of death as brain death – namely, the intuition that the capacity for consciousness and mental activity is essential to our existence. This intuition is, I believe, best articulated by the claim that each of us is essentially a mind. This, of course, requires elucidation. What is a mind? And how is it related to the brain?

Unfortunately, it is easier to say what the mind is not than to be confident about what exactly it is. It is, for example, generally recognized that the mind is not a Cartesian nonmaterial substance with identity conditions independent to those of the brain.[18] Nor is it simply a collection of causally related mental states. For, if each of us is a substance and each is essentially a mind, then minds are substances, at least in whatever sense in which it is true that you and I are substances. So the mind should not be identified simply with its particular contents. Nor can we say simply that the mind is the brain. For, when the entire brain dies, that is certainly sufficient for the ceasing to exist of the mind but not, in the normal case, of the ceasing to exist of the brain. A dead, nonfunctional brain is still a brain. Finally, it also does not seem quite right to say that the mind is just the brain (or even certain parts of the brain) in

---

[17] In Chapter III of *Killing at the Margins Life*. Other arguments for accounts that are extremely close to that which I defend may be found in Thomas Nagel, *The View From Nowhere*, New York: Oxford University Press, pp. 37–43, and Johnston, 'Human Beings'.
[18] This view is effectively criticized in Derek Parfit, *Reasons and Persons*. Oxford: Oxford University Press, corrected edition, 1986, sections 81 and 82.

certain functional states. For, again, when the brain altogether stops working, the mind no longer exists. But is there anything in the brain that ceases to exist rather than merely ceasing to function? Perhaps this temptation to reify the mind is just a feature of the way we talk that is without deep significance. Yet many of the other things that we regard as substances in their own right bear a similar sort of relation to the physical matter in which they are realized. We believe, for example, that a statue is a substance that is distinct from – i.e., not identical to – the lump of bronze of which it is composed, so that the statue may cease to exist when the lump of bronze merely undergoes a certain change (for example, when it is melted).

Although my sympathies lie with 'dual aspect' theories of the mind and mental states, I am reluctant (because incompetent) to issue pronouncements about the precise nature of the relation between the mind and the brain.[19] But I suspect that it is not necessary, for present purposes, to commit oneself to a particular position on the mind-brain problem. For the essential point is one that the adherents of most rival schools of thought – property dualists, dual aspect theorists, functionalists, and even materialists who would prefer to drop the word 'mind' from their vocabularies – can agree on. This is that what in ordinary language is called the mind is *either* generated by *or* identical with the states and operations of the brain and hence cannot be tracked or traced independently of the brain. Assuming, then, that we are minds, my continuing to exist must consist in the continued existence of my (i.e., this) mind. And, since the continued existence of my mind is a matter of the continued existence and functioning of my brain, it follows that my continued existence necessarily consists in the continued existence and functioning of my brain.[20]

This, however, is insufficiently specific. We need to know how much of the brain and, more particularly, which areas of the brain must survive and remain functional in order for one and the same mind to continue to exist. As a first approximation, we can say that enough of the brain must survive in order to retain the capacity for supporting consciousness and mental activity. The emphasis here is

---

[19] A dual aspect theory is defended in Nagel, *The View From Nowhere*, chapter III.

[20] Most theories of personal identity, such as that advanced by Derek Parfit, that deny that one's continuing to exist *necessarily* consists in the continued existence and functioning of one's brain accept that one's continued existence *in fact* consists in or depends on the continued functioning of one's brain. See Parfit, *Reasons and Persons*, Part III.

on capacity. Consider a mind that has been sustained by the operations of a particular brain. If the brain were injured in such a way that it became dormant or inactive, in the sense that it ceased to generate conscious or even unconscious mental activity, the same mind would nevertheless continue to exist provided that the brain retained the capacity to generate consciousness and mental activity. This would be true for two reasons. First, the possibility of restoring consciousness to the brain just is the possibility of reviving or reactivating the same mind. The regeneration of consciousness would, in other words, count as the emergence or recovery of the person from the coma. Thus, unless we think of the existence of the mind as in this case discontinuous, the mind must continue to exist in a dormant state during the interval between periods of past and future, or potential future, activity. Second, elements of the mind would in fact persist throughout the period of coma in the form of unconscious mental states. Assuming that the micro-organization of certain parts of the brain were preserved, the neurological bases for particular memories, desires, and so on would remain intact. So, for example, during the period of coma it would remain true that the individual continued to believe certain things, to have certain desires, and so on, albeit unconsciously.[21]

The claim that the retention by the brain of the capacity to generate consciousness and mental activity is necessary and sufficient for the continued existence of the mind is, as I noted, only a first approximation. It requires clarification and refinement. For there are cases in which there is a clear sense in which the brain loses the capacity to support consciousness and mental activity while the individual mind nevertheless survives. There is an area of the brain, located primarily in the brain stem, called the *ascending reticular activating system* or, less cumbersomely, the 'reticular formation'. If this system is damaged, for example by a lesion, coma ensues; consciousness and mental activity cease to occur. Since, given the current state of medical technology, it is not possible to restore the functions of the system by healing such a lesion or by replacing the damaged system, either with transplanted tissue or a mechanical replacement, there is a clear sense in which an individual whose reticular formation is damaged thereby loses the capacity for consciousness and mental activity. And the loss is, in practice,

---

[21] For a plausible analysis of the nature of unconscious mental states, see John R. Searle, *The Rediscovery of the Mind*. Cambridge: MIT Press, 1992, chapter 7.

irreversible. Does this mean that the mind associated with the individual's brain has ceased to exist?

I believe that it does not. The reticular formation seems to function like an on-off switch. Without it, consciousness is not possible. But, when it functions, it does not appear to affect or contribute to the contents of the mind. The locus of consciousness and mental activity, the area in which consciousness and mental activity occur or are generated, is the upper brain – specifically, certain areas of the cerebral hemispheres. It is here that the neurological correlates of the actual or potential contents of consciousness are located. This, in short, is the area of the brain in which mental states, and thus the mind itself, are realized. The reticular formation, by contrast, is an essential support system for the parts of the brain where mentation occurs but its tissues are not tissues in which the mind or any of its elements are realized. Because of this, it is possible for those areas of the brain in which the mind is realized to remain intact and potentially functional even when the reticular formation is nonfunctional. In this case, while there is a sense in which the cerebral hemispheres retain the capacity for consciousness, there is another sense in which the brain as a whole lacks this capacity. I think the best way to understand what happens in this case is to say that the mind survives even though it cannot be activated.

A familiar distinction between two types of capacity is relevant here. In the case just cited, the parts of the brain that once directly produced consciousness and mental activity remain intact and potentially functional. Because of this, the brain *in principle* retains the capacity to generate consciousness and mental activity. There *is* something that would count as reviving this same mind although at present we lack the knowledge or technical means necessary to bring it about. Because the lack of capacity is contingent rather than necessary, we say that *in practice* the brain lacks the capacity for supporting consciousness and mental activity. If, by contrast, the tissues of the cerebral hemispheres were destroyed, the brain would necessarily or in principle lack the capacity to support consciousness. Replacement of the tissues through the transplantation of new hemispheres might make consciousness possible, but this would not count as reviving the same mind, even if the new hemispheres were perfect duplicates of those that had been destroyed. There would instead be a new and different mind.

Would there also be a new and different brain? Probably so; but this would not be necessary for there to be a new mind. It is tempting to say that for there to be a different mind there must be a different brain, since the continued functioning of one and the same brain is sufficient for the continued existence of one and the same mind. But we must recall that the mind appears to be realized only in certain parts of the brain. Thus what we need to say is that the continued functioning of *those parts* of the brain is sufficient for the continued existence of the same mind. But it is conceivable that one and the same brain could in principle survive the replacement of those parts. This would be suggested if, for example, a brain could *lose* those parts and yet continue to exist as the same brain. But, if a brain could survive the replacement of those parts by functional substitutes, then after the replacement that brain would support the existence of a different mind from that which it supported before.

There are, in summary, two different types of irreversible coma, each corresponding to one of the two forms of incapacity. A coma that leaves the cerebral hemispheres largely intact – e.g., one induced by a lesion on the reticular formation – is in practice irreversible though in principle reversible. By contrast, a coma caused by the destruction of the cerebral hemispheres or the neocortex is in principle irreversible. Since the areas of the brain in which the mind was previously realized have been destroyed, the revival of that same mind is necessarily impossible.

These observations about the notions of capacity and irreversibility have implications for the debate about brain death. It is not uncommon for those advocating a revisionist conception of brain death (such as cerebral death or neocortical death) to assert that 'death is the irreversible loss of the capacity for consciousness'.[22] Let us assume that this is proposed as a definition of the death of the person or self – that is, according to the view proposed here, as a definition of the ceasing to exist of the mind – and not as a definition of the biological death of the human organism. It is still inadequate if 'irreversible loss of the capacity for consciousness' is intended to cover cases in which the absence of capacity is traceable to the malfunctioning of some support system such as the reticular formation rather than to the destruction of the locus of consciousness – that is, cases in which the irreversibility of the loss of capacity is contingent rather than necessary.

---

[22] Dr. Robert Troug, quoted in Singer, *Rethinking Life and Death*, chapter III.

We must therefore refine our understanding of what is necessarily involved in the continuing to exist of the mind. Retention of the brain's capacity in practice to sustain consciousness and mental activity is not necessary for the survival of the mind. What is necessary is instead the survival, in a potentially functional state, of those areas or tissues of the brain that directly generate consciousness and mental activity – i.e., those areas in which the mind is realized. In short, the continued existence of the mind, and thus of the self, consists in the survival of enough of the cerebral hemispheres to be capable in principle, or in conjunction with relevant support mechanisms, of generating consciousness and mental activity.

This account of self- or personal identity is still imprecise. Various qualifications may be necessary in order to deal with challenges posed, for example, by science-fiction cases involving the grafting of neural tissues from one brain to another. But these refinements are unnecessary for present purposes.

I have been assuming – and this seems, on all the available evidence, to be correct – that most or all of the particular elements of an individual's mental life are realized in the upper brain. Our knowledge of the brain is, however, still rudimentary and it is possible that we will discover that the brain stem contributes to the character and content of an individual's mental life in various ways. In that case, we might have to think of the mind as being realized in part in the brain stem. We can distinguish several possibilities. First, it might be that the brain stem can actually support consciousness or mental activity on its own, even in the absence of a functional upper brain. This is of course most improbable. But if it turned out to be the case, then the mind could survive even if the organism were in a persistent vegetative state. It is very unlikely, however, that such a life could be worth living. If indeed an individual in a persistent vegetative state were actually conscious at some level, it is more likely that his or her life would be worse than no life at all. There might, in short, be positive reason not to prolong such an individual's life, provided of course that the coma were clearly irreversible.

Second, a somewhat more realistic possibility is that, although the brain stem is in principle incapable of generating consciousness on its own, certain particular mental states are nevertheless directly realized in its tissues – that is, the neurological bases for certain conscious states might be located there. In that case, it might be true that certain unconscious mental states could survive in the brain stem even after the hemispheres had died. We should, however, consider whether, if unconscious mental states were to survive in the brain stem following the death of the hemispheres, they would be in principle as well as in practice inaccessible to consciousness? Would they together constitute a mind, albeit an unconscious one. These are difficult issues that would need to be resolved in order, for example, to determine the plausibility of the revisionist conceptions of brain death; but they cannot be addressed here. One point is, however, worth noting. If elements of our mental lives are realized in the brain stem, then the brain stem might not, as I have been assuming, be in principle replaceable. A brain stem transplant would not, for example, involve merely the replacement of a support system for the mind. Rather, elements of one mind would be fused with those of another and it might be unclear, and perhaps indeterminate, whether either of the original minds would survive at all.[23] This would depend on how many or what proportion of the constitutive elements of the mind were realized in the brain stem.

A third and final possibility is that the brain stem contributes in subtle ways to the character of the contents of the mind. It might, for example, modulate the emotional hue of certain experiences or memories. This, in fact, appears to be the likeliest of the three possibilities. But, if the brain stem contributes only marginally to the contents of character of the mind, then it does not seem that the continued existence and functioning of the brain stem is in principle (though of course it is in practice) necessary for the continued existence of the same mind.

Next, it is important to distinguish the account of personal identity I am developing from a related and influential view. I have argued that those areas of the brain whose survival and functional integrity are essential to the continued existence of the mind are the areas in which the elements of mental life are realized. This insistence on the preservation of the neurological bases of mental life may suggest that my account holds that it is necessary for an individual's survival that some proportion of the neurological bases of *the particular contents and continuities* of his or her mental life be preserved. This is in fact the view of a number of those who have written about personal identity. For example, in their seminal and

---

[23] For related discussion of the possibility of 'fusing' different persons, see Parfit, *Reasons and Persons*, sections 100 and 101.

important paper on personal identity and brain death, Michael B. Green and Daniel Wikler claim that 'the ordinary causal processes which link events in a personal history involve more than spatio-temporal continuity of brain tissue. They also require continuity of certain brain *processes*, carried out through microstructural and microfunctional registrations in the brain tissue. Two body-stages which fail to be linked by continuity of these processes will fail to be stages of the same person, even if identity of the brain is preserved'. They then elucidate this claim by noting that the relevant processes are those that 'normally underlie that person's psychological continuity and connectedness'.[24]

One might interpret this as meaning that some degree of psychological continuity is required for individual survival. This interpretation is, however, repudiated by Green and Wikler.[25] Their claim is not that psychological continuity itself is necessary for an individual's survival, but rather that what is necessary is the integrity of those neurological processes that in the normal case underlie psychological continuity. It is not clear, however, whether there is a significant distinction here. For how could there be continuity of the relevant processes without psychological continuity? Green and Wikler cite a case in which 'Jones is hypnotized and made to think, feel, and otherwise resemble Smith in all mental respects'.[26] This, one assumes, is intended to be a case in which the relevant brain processes are preserved while psychological continuity is not. But, if Jones's original memories, dispositions, and so on remain configured in the tissues of his brain, then this is not in fact a case in which psychological continuity is lost. For the contents of Jones's original mental life are preserved. They are, admittedly, present only in an unconscious form, but that is true of most of the elements of our

---

[24] Michael B. Green and Daniel Wikler, 'Brain Death and Personal Identity', *Philosophy and Public Affairs* 9 (1980), pp. 125–26 and 127. Emphasis in the original. Green and Wikler (p. 119, n. 27) credit the writings of John Perry as the source of their view. What appears to be the same view is advanced by Michael Lockwood in 'When Does a Life Begin?' in Michael Lockwood, ed., *Moral Dilemmas in Modern Medicine*. Oxford: Oxford University Press, 1984, esp. p. 23 and in 'Warnock Versus Powell', esp. p. 206, where he claims that an individual cannot survive 'too radical a *dis*continuity of organisation in the parts of [his or her brain] that subserved mental functioning', even if the brain were to continue to support consciousness and mental activity. A further statement of essentially the same view appears in Parfit's *Reasons and Persons*, p. 207, labeled as the *Narrow Psychological Criterion*. A possible difference is that Parfit is explicit in requiring a strong form of psychological continuity for the preservation of identity.

[25] In Wikler's comments on the original draft of this paper.

[26] Green and Wikler, 'Brain Death', p. 126, n. 36.

mental lives at any given time. It seems, in short, that the preservation of the relevant processes is sufficient for psychological continuity; if so, and if the preservation of the processes is necessary for survival, then the preservation of psychological continuity is necessary as well.

Let us, however, focus on the brain processes themselves. While it is compatible with a person's survival that a certain proportion of these brain processes, or patterns of neural organization, should be disrupted or destroyed, there is also, on this view, some degree of loss that the person could not survive. Thus Green and Wikler claim that, if a person's brain were 'unwired' in such a way that the neural bases of the various elements of her particular mental life were reconfigured, thereby rendering the mental life generated by the brain radically discontinuous, the person would cease to exist. This could be true, on their view, even if her brain continued to support consciousness and mental activity.[27]

The implausibility of this view can be seen by considering actual cases in which the causal processes or patterns of organization that underlie psychological continuity are severely disrupted. In the case of a patient with Alzheimer's Disease, for example, the 'processes . . . which normally underlie that person's psychological continuity and connectedness' are gradually destroyed. Yet the capacity of the patient's brain to sustain consciousness and rudimentary mental activity may persist well beyond the point at which the loss of neural organization has become so great that, on Green and Wikler's view, the patient will have ceased to exist. The idea that the patient ceases to exist at this point is implausible, for two reasons.

First, the view that the patient survives at least until he irreversibly loses consciousness is intuitively quite compelling.[28] If, for example, a person in the early stages of Alzheimer's Disease knew that in the later stages, after virtually all of his memories, beliefs, and so on had been eliminated, his body would be subjected to

---

[27] Green and Wikler, 'Brain Death', p. 125. Compare Lockwood, 'Warnock Versus Powell', p. 206.

[28] An alternative and perhaps equally plausible view is that the patient ceases to exist gradually, by degrees, as her brain and mind disintegrate. This view, however, requires the revision of various traditional assumptions and concepts – for example, the assumption that existence is all-or-nothing and cannot be partial, that there is no intermediate state between existence and nonexistence. For the beginnings of a defense of the view that existence is not all-or-nothing, see Warren Quinn, 'Abortion: Identity and Loss', *Philosophy and Public Affairs* 13 (1984), section II.

terrible physical trauma without the possibility of anesthesia, we believe that it would be rational for him now to feel at least some fear of that future pain. On Green and Wikler's view, by contrast, it would be irrational for him to fear the future pain, at least for egoistic reasons, since he will have ceased to exist by the time the pain occurs.

The second reason why Green and Wikler's view is implausible in this case is that it implies that, at the point at which the destruction of the neural states and processes that underlie psychological continuity advances so far that the patient ceases to exist, a *new* subject of consciousness must begin to exist in association with the patient's body. For, in this case, even after the neural basis of psychological continuity has been destroyed, the brain continues to generate consciousness and mental activity. If this is not the mind of the original patient, then it must be a new mind that has popped into existence simultaneously with the death or ceasing to exist of the original patient.[29] The only other alternative, it seems, is to say that, although the original *person or self* ceases to exist when the relevant processes are disrupted, his *mind* nevertheless continues to exist and becomes the mind of a new individual who has supplanted him in his body. There would, in short, be two distinct individuals not overlapping in time but sharing the same mind. Since this latter possibility is doubtfully coherent, I assume that the former offers the best account that Green and Wikler's view can give of what happens in cases of advanced dementia.

For these reasons, I reject the commonly accepted requirement that the preservation of the neurological bases of some degree of psychological continuity is necessary for personal identity or for the survival of the same mind. The continued existence of one and the same mind requires the preservation of various mental powers or capacities in the areas of the brain in which consciousness and mental activity occur, but not the preservation of the particular contents of the mind – that is, the various particular mental states configured in the tissues of the cerebral hemispheres.

There is one final detail of this account of personal identity that should be noted. It arises from consideration of certain science fiction examples that are frequently discussed in the literature on personal identity. Imagine, first, that one's cerebral hemispheres

---

[29] Parfit's view, which makes psychological continuity itself the criterion of personal identity, also has this implication.

could be surgically detached from one's brain stem and then attached to the waiting brain stem in another organism from which the hemispheres had been removed. Assuming that the brain stem is just a support system for the parts of the brain in which the mind is realized, most of us intuitively accept that this is a case in which one would continue to exist in a new organism. Next imagine a case in which one of one's cerebral hemispheres is destroyed while the other is transplanted into a new body from which the hemispheres have been removed. On reflection, most of us believe that this too is a case in which one would survive in a new body. For we know that it is possible to survive the loss of a single hemisphere: this happens both when a hemispherectomy is performed and in some instances in which a stroke kills an entire hemisphere. Thus, if one could survive in a new body if both of one's hemispheres were transplanted into it, then one could also survive in that body if only one of one's hemispheres were transplanted into it. But now imagine a third case in which one's hemispheres are detached from one's brain stem, separated from each other, and separately transplanted into different bodies from which the hemispheres have been removed but in each of which the waiting brain stem is alive and functional. This third case is relevantly like the second except that there are two single-hemisphere transplants rather than one. If the original individual survives in the second case, what happens in the third?

Call the person whose brain is divided A and the two persons who wake up following the operation, each of whom has one of A's hemispheres, B and C. It cannot be the case that both B and C are identical with A, for that would imply that B and C are identical with each other. And it is arbitrary to say that either B or C is A while the other is an entirely new individual. We should therefore conclude that neither B nor C is A. A has ceased to exist.

This is Derek Parfit's response to this case.[30] Parfit's insight is that what this case shows is that identity is not the basis for egoistic concern about the future. Rather, the ground for concern about oneself in the future is whatever relation is constitutive of identity in the normal case. But it is possible that this relation may obtain when identity does not. When this is the case, it can be rational to have a concern that is relevantly like egoistic concern though it is for the future of, someone who will not be oneself. (I will refer to

---

[30] Parfit, *Reasons and Persons*, chapter 12.

this as 'egoistic concern', with the stipulation that this concern need not be for *oneself*.) Thus, while A should recognize that he will not *be* either B or C, he has as much reason to care about what will happen to each of them as he would have to be concerned about his own future if the operation were not going to occur and he were going to survive in the normal way. For the basis for egoistic concern is surely preserved in his relations to both B and C. This is shown by the fact that the relation he bears to both B and C would have been sufficient to make him identical with either one *had the other not existed*. And in either case – that is, if either B or C had existed but not the other – it would clearly have been rational for A to be egoistically concerned about the single-hemisphered person he would have become. In the actual case, the presence of C makes it implausible to say that A *is* B, but surely the mere presence of C does not affect whether it is rational for A to be egoistically concerned about B.

The claim that it is not identity but the relation that is constitutive of identity that provides the basis for egoistic concern is of profound significance for understanding individual self-interest. Again I follow Parfit in thinking that, if it is the relation that is constitutive of identity that is the basis for egoistic concern about the future, and if this relation may be present to a greater or lesser degree, then the strength of one's present interests in future events or states of affairs may vary with the degree to which this relation holds between oneself now and oneself in the future. This, however, is a different topic.[31] Where my account of personal identity diverges from Parfit's is in its understanding of what the relevant relation is. I have contended that what is constitutive of one's identity over time is the continued existence of enough of the cerebral hemispheres to be capable, in conjunction with relevant support mechanisms, such as those in the brain stem, of generating consciousness and mental activity. What the case involving the separate transplantation of both hemispheres shows, however, is that the presence of this relation is not always sufficient for *identity*. For, as this case shows, the relation may, at least in principle, take a 'branching' form. When it does, the resulting minds cannot be identical with the original, since they are not identical with one another. The criterion of personal *identity* must therefore be the survival, *in nonbranching form*, of

---

[31] For a fuller discussion of these issues, see Parfit, *Reasons and Persons*, chapters 12–15.

enough of the cerebral hemispheres to be capable, in conjunction with relevant support mechanisms, of generating consciousness and mental activity. Call this the *Continuity of Mind* account of personal identity.

The case involving branching, which reveals the need for this final qualification in the account, is drawn from science fiction. But there may be certain 'real life' instances of branching – cases in which alterations in the structure of the brain may possibly result in more than one center of consciousness and thus, perhaps, more than one mind. Possible examples here include 'split brain' patients in whom the connecting tissues between the cerebral hemispheres have been surgically severed and psychiatric patients with multiple personality disorder. These cases raise important questions about how many distinct minds, and therefore how many individual persons, a single brain is capable of supporting.[32] While it is important for the Continuity of Mind account to have a criterion for individuating minds at a single time as well as a criterion for tracking a single mind over time, I will not pursue the former problem here since it is not relevant to the practical concerns that have prompted the debate about brain death. If, for example, a split brain patient suffers a stroke that kills an entire hemisphere, there is a genuine issue about whether a mind, and therefore a person, has died or ceased to exist. And a similar problem is raised by 'cures' of multiple personality disorder that succeed by eliminating all but one of the personalities. But, as long as at least one mind is left behind in these cases, there is no question of declaring anyone dead for legal or medical purposes.

IV. SOME OBJECTIONS AND PROBLEMS

Like all views in this area, the Continuity of Mind account of personal identity is vulnerable to a variety of objections. Many people will object, for example, that it reintroduces a variant of a thoroughly discredited dualistic metaphysic. For, although it rejects Cartesian dualism, which conceives of the mind as a substance with identity conditions that are entirely distinct from those of the brain or body, it nevertheless holds that, wherever one of us is, there are

---

[32] See, for example, Kathleen V. Wilkes, *Real People: Personal Identity Without Thought Experiments*. Oxford: Clarendon Press, 1988, chapters 4 and 5.

in fact two substances there: the mind, or self, and the organism. It therefore embraces a form of mind-body dualism.

It is worth stressing that mind-*body* dualism need not entail mind-brain dualism. The mind might not be distinct from the brain and yet be distinct from the body as a whole, since brain and body are obviously not identical. Yet I do not wish to rule out the idea that the mind is a substance that, while dependent for its existence on the operations of the brain, is not reducible to the brain. There are, therefore, two puzzling relations here: the relation of the mind to the brain and the relation of the mind to the body (i.e., the relation of the self to the organism). My focus will be on the latter, which is puzzling enough. For it seems contrary to educated scientific common sense to suppose that I am a substance distinct from my body. This view may seem, in the old phrase, to multiply entities without necessity.

It is not, however, unusual to find two distinct substances existing in the same location. Recall the earlier example of the bronze statue. There are, it seems, two things there: the statue and the lump of bronze of which it is made. These two things are intimately related but are not identical. The relation that one bears to one's body might be analogous to the relation that the statue bears to the bronze.

One response to this suggestion is to say that the statue is not really a substance at all. It has no independent existence but is just a phase in the history of the lump of bronze. If this is the case, then nothing goes out of existence when the lump is melted; it merely changes from a statue to an amorphous shape. This response, however, implicitly denies the independent existence of many things that we take to be substances: tables, cars, and so on. Even the lump of bronze is threatened. If I cut the lump in half, there will no longer be a lump but the collection of molecules of which it was composed will continue to exist. One might conclude that the lump was never really a substance but was just a phase in the history of the collection of molecules, one form that the collection took for a certain time.

Let us assume, then, that the statue and the lump of bronze are distinct substances. It may seem that, despite their distinctness, they share a range of properties: each has the same shape, same weight, and so on. Is this true in the case of a person and his organism? If it is, then this is the basis of a slightly different objection to the Continuity of Mind account (or, rather, to all views that deny that we are identical with our organisms) that has been pressed by W.R. Carter. Suppose that, just as the statue and the lump of bronze are both the same color, I and my organism are both now conscious. That means there are now two conscious entities sitting in my chair, both of which are experiencing a toothache. But 'how many toothaches are in question in such a case? Those of us who believe that there is only one toothache in the works, and who also believe that different beings do not (ordinarily at least) feel the same toothache, will say that we *are* our organisms'.[33]

It seems to me that the appropriate response to this objection is to deny that my organism is conscious – indeed, that it has any psychological properties at all. For, if the various psychological predicates that apply to me also apply to my organism, so that it is now self-conscious, experiencing the pain of a toothache, thinking about philosophy, and so on, then it would seem that it must itself *be* a person. And if it is a person, then either that person is me, in which case I am identical with my organism, or it is not me, in which case there are two persons here, which is absurd. Since the Continuity of Mind account denies that I am identical with my organism, it must, it seems, accept that our application of psychological predicates to organisms is only a *façon de parler*. We say, for example, that my body is hungry or feels pain, but this must be interpreted as a figurative way of expressing the observation that *I* am in these states.

There are two objections to this response. One has been advanced by Carter. 'There is reason to think', he writes, 'that "higher forms" of animal life can and do feel pain (hunger, fear, etc.) and so reason to think that a variety of physical organisms are in some sense *conscious* beings. Surely there is no plausibility to the thesis that non-human organisms are conscious beings and human organisms are not.'[34] What this shows, I think, is not that psychological predicates must apply to human organisms but that they do not apply to any organisms. Wherever there is a conscious being, a being with a mind, that being is distinct from its organism. While it makes no sense to distinguish between a plant and its organism, or an amoeba and its organism, it always makes sense to distinguish between a

[33] W.R. Carter, 'DO Zygotes Become People?' *Mind* XCI (1982), p. 94. Emphasis in the original. Also see W.R. Carter, 'Once and Future Persons', *American Philosophical Quarterly* 17 (1980), p. 63.
[34] Carter, 'Do Zygotes Become People?', p. 94.

conscious subject and its organism. Suppose, for example, that I
have a Golden Retriever called Rufus whose brain is transplanted
from his own body into that of another Golden Retriever. I believe
that the Golden Retriever that now has Rufus's brain – the one that
jumps up and licks me when he sees me, responds when I call the
name "Rufus", and so on – is Rufus. Thus Rufus is not now and
never was identical with his original organism. Although there is a
temptation to assume that nonhuman animals are identical with
their organisms and that we therefore employ a bodily continuity
criterion for tracking them through time, this example suggests that
this is a mistaken assumption and that the Continuity of Mind
account applies to most animals as well as to persons – that is, to
all conscious or potentially conscious beings. This, I believe, is a
virtue of the account (one that is not shared by a number of other
accounts).

The second objection to the idea that psychological predicates do
not apply to organisms but only to the minds that animate organisms is that this suggests that the situation is symmetrical with
respect to the attribution of an organism's physical properties to the
conscious being whose organism it is. If, for example, my mind does
not occupy all of the space that my organism occupies and I am my
mind and not my organism, then it seems that I do not occupy all
of the space my organism occupies. Similarly, although my organism weighs 150 pounds, I may weigh considerably less than that, if
I weigh anything at all. In short, the objection is that the Continuity
of Mind account, and indeed any other account of personal identity
that denies that we are identical with our organisms, seems to
commit us to a conception of the organism as what Warren Quinn
has called a 'subentity'. Quinn writes that, 'so conceived, it is our
body that digests, that converts nourishment to protoplasm, that
sweats, that jerks when struck in certain ways, and *we* (human
beings) are seen to metabolize, jerk, sweat, or even simply to occupy
physical space only because our bodies do. According to this conception, we supervene upon, contain, or bear some other exotic
relation to a distinguishable source of activities which then become
attributable to us by a kind of logical courtesy'.[35]

It seems to me that, if we reject the idea that we are identical with
our organisms, then we may have to accept both that mere organisms do not have psychological properties and that at least some of

---

[35] Quinn, 'Abortion: Identity and Loss', pp. 28–29.

the properties of our physical organisms are not, strictly speaking, attributable to us. We can go on speaking in the normal ways but only with the understanding that the predication of psychological properties to organisms and the predication of certain of the properties of organisms to the minds that animate them constitute natural but nevertheless figurative uses of language. Acknowledging this may, in fact, help us to achieve greater clarity in our understanding of death. Earlier I distinguished two concepts of death: the death of the self and the death of the human organism. Distinguishing the properties of organisms from those of the minds that animate them helps us to see that the two concepts of death correspond to two concepts of life. There is life in the biological sense, which is what our organisms have when they are functioning in an integrated way. And we too are alive, though in an extended or perhaps derivative sense. To say that a person is alive is just to say that she exists – for which, as things stand at present, it is a necessary but not sufficient condition that her organism be biologically alive. An organism dies when it ceases to be alive in the biological sense. A person dies when he or she ceases to exist.

Other writers have, of course, distinguished between different senses or understandings of 'life'. James Rachels, for example, distinguishes between *being alive*, which involves only life in the biological sense, and *having a life*, which involves life 'in the biographical sense' and requires a conscious subject.[36] Rachels, however, believes that in the normal case both types of life, biological and biographical, can be predicated of one and the same thing: the individual self. Thus he also believes that there are cases – for example, cases of persistent vegetative state – in which a person ceases to have a life in the biographical sense but does not die because he remains alive in the biological sense. His distinction is therefore quite different from the one I have drawn. In my view, only the organism has biological life and only the self has a biography. Thus most of the cases that Rachels says involve an individual's remaining alive only in the biological sense are in my view cases in which the self or conscious subject dies (and thus has no life of any sort) while his or her organism continues to live. (This is not to deny that there are cases in which an individual ceases to have a biographical life in Rachels's sense and yet remains alive.

[36] James Rachels, *The End of Life*. Oxford: Oxford University Press, 1986, pp. 5–6 and 24–27.

Cases in which a persistent vegetative state results from damage to the reticular formation are cases of this sort.)

All this is, of course, quite odd, and is difficult to accept with equanimity. One is reluctant to become committed to these results. Hence virtually all of those who have claimed that some form of brain death is the death of the person though not necessarily of the organism have nevertheless failed explicitly to embrace any form of mind-body dualism. Yet attempts to articulate the idea that the death of the person is compatible with the continued life of the organism that fail openly to acknowledge that there are two non-identical substances – the person (or mind or self) and the organism – tend to result in incoherence. Green and Wikler, for example, begin by stipulating that they will use the term 'patient' 'neutrally to designate the entity in the hospital bed.' They then sketch a case in which the patient 'entered the hospital as Jones' but in which 'the patient ceases to be Jones when brain death strips the body of its psychological traits'.

After this happens, however, the 'living patient' is still there, for 'brain-dead patients can nevertheless be alive'.[37] This, I think, is their way of saying that the person, Jones, ceases to exist when brain death occurs even though his organism continues to live.

What they actually say, however, is different – and doubtfully coherent. The references to the patient's ceasing to be Jones suggest that there is only one entity or substance here: the patient, who is Jones for a while but then ceases to be Jones. The dualistic metaphysic is thus happily avoided. But, if the patient is a substance and can cease to be Jones, then Jones cannot be a substance. To say that the patient can cease to be Jones must be like saying that the patient can cease to be an adolescent or a squash player. The adolescent and the squash player are not substances in their own rights; they are just phases in the life of a single substance – the patient. Hence there is nothing that dies or ceases to exist (except perhaps metaphorically) when the patient ceases to be an adolescent or a squash player. Similarly, if the patient can cease to be Jones, Jones must be simply a phase in the career of the patient. Since Jones is not a substance, nothing dies or ceases to exist when the patient ceases to be Jones. Hence, if brain death simply causes the patient to cease to be Jones, then brain death is not the death of anything.

---

[37] Green and Wikler, 'Brain Death', p. 118.

Green and Wikler, however, clearly need for brain death to be the death or ceasing to exist of some thing. If that thing is Jones, then Jones is a substance. But the patient must also be a substance; for it cannot be just a phase in the history of Jones if it can continue to exist as 'the entity in the hospital bed' after Jones has ceased to be. If, however, there is only one substance, then Jones and the patient must be identical. But then the patient cannot cease to be Jones and continue to exist. Either the idea that the patient ceases to be Jones is literally nonsense or it means that Jones, and hence the patient, ceases to exist (since Jones and the patient are identical).

The only interpretation that is compatible with the idea that Jones dies or ceases to exist while the patient continues to live is that Jones and the patient are both substances but are not identical. In short, there are two substances: Jones and the patient or, in other words, the person (or self or mind) and the organism. The dualistic metaphysic, with its attendant problems in accommodating the assumption the physical properties of our organisms are attributable to us, seems unavoidable.

I will note just one further challenge to the Continuity of Mind account.[38] This account of personal identity, along with most others, is premised on the rejection of the idea that we are identical with our physical organisms. These theories therefore face the challenge of specifying the precise nature of the relation that we do bear to our organisms. One suggestion is that our organisms stand to us in the relation that logicians call 'constitution'. This view has been elaborated by Sydney Shoemaker as follows:

> One can allow that there is a sense of 'is' in which a person is an animal. But this will not be the 'is' of predication or of identity; it will be, perhaps, the sort of 'is' we have in 'The statue is a hunk of bronze' – it will mean something like 'is composed of the very same stuff as'. Arguably, the statue and the hunk of bronze are not one and the same thing, since if the hunk of bronze were hammered into another statue, the statue we had originally would no longer exist, but the hunk of bronze would still be there. So two things, the statue and the hunk of bronze, can occupy the same place and share the same matter and the same non-historical properties. . . . The suggestion is that a person 'is' an

[38] I address other objections – for example, those advanced in the appendix to Parfit's *Reasons and Persons* entitled 'Nagel's Brain' – in *Killing at the Margins of Life*, chapter III.

animal, not in the sense of being identical to one, but in the sense of sharing its matter with one.[39]

This is an appealing proposal, but it is not without problems. One problem arises from the assumption that, if a person is his organism, where 'is' here is the 'is of constitution' explained by Shoemaker, then the person and his organism will share the same non-historical properties. This, at any rate, is what is suggested by the analogy with the statue and the lump of bronze. But, if my organism shares my psychological properties – e.g., if it is conscious, hungry, experiencing the pain of a toothache – then we are back to our earlier problem that this implies that there are two distinct conscious beings now sitting in my chair, which is absurd.

There is, in fact, a problem with this solution even as it applies to the case of the statue and the lump of bronze. If the lump of bronze has all the non-historical properties of the statue – e.g., the same shape, size, weight, and so on – then why is it not *itself* a statue? How can it have all the properties that make a thing a statue without *being* a statue? But, if it is a statue, then how many statues are there?

While the analogy with the statue and the lump of bronze is suggestive, the relation that the one bears to the other may not be quite like that between a person, or mind, and his or her organism. The latter relation may, indeed, be *sui generis*, unlike any other relation. In any case, the appeal to the relation of constitution does not seem to solve to our problem. To my knowledge, no one who denies that we are identical with our organisms has been able adequately to explain what exactly the relation is if not identity. Although this is not a decisive objection to the Continuity of Mind account, since it does not show that a solution cannot be found, it is nevertheless a serious challenge.

V. SOME IMPLICATIONS

Rejection of the dominant conception of brain death

When those parts of the brain in which consciousness and mental activity are realized are destroyed or rendered irreversibly nonfunctional, the mind ceases to exist – that is, the person dies. To the best

---

[39] Sydney Shoemaker, 'A Materialist's Account', in Sydney Shoemaker and Richard Swinburne, *Personal Identify*. Oxford Basil Blackwell, 1984, p. 113.

of our knowledge, the relevant parts of the brain are all in the cerebral hemispheres. Hence cerebral death – the death or destruction of the cerebral hemispheres – is sufficient for the death of the person. Neocortical death is presumably also sufficient, though there is perhaps some room for doubt about whether all capacity for consciousness is lost while some areas of the hemispheres remain intact and functional. Lacking sufficient knowledge about these matters, I will remain agnostic on the question whether neocortical death is always sufficient for the death of the person.

What is clear, however, is that the dominant conception of brain death as the death of the whole brain is inadequate as a criterion of death. While it is certainly sufficient for the death of the person, it is not necessary. It is, as I remarked earlier, an unstable compromise that seems intended, whether consciously or unconsciously, to satisfy intuitions both about the deaths of persons and about the deaths of organisms without requiring a dualistic metaphysic. That, I think, is its key attraction: it seems, on superficial examination, to offer a conception of death that captures the decisive significance we intuitively attribute to the irreversible loss of the capacity for consciousness while also doing justice to our beliefs about what counts as the biological death of an organism. If there is a single account that satisfies both requirements, then the pressure to embrace a dualistic metaphysic does not arise. In reality, of course, the dominant conception has neither of these virtues. For a person may irreversibly lose the capacity for consciousness, thereby ceasing to exist, without having suffered the death of the whole brain; and the death of the whole brain is, as I argued earlier, neither necessary nor sufficient for the biological death of the human organism. Separate criteria are required for the deaths of persons and the deaths of organisms. (The foregoing comments apply equally to the official British conception of death as the death of the brain stem.)

It should be reemphasized that cerebral death is here advanced as the criterion of the death or ceasing to exist of the person and not for the death of the human organism. It is, however, the death of the person and not that of the organism that is of moral significance. Mere organisms do not have interests and cannot be harmed or benefited in the relevant sense, though (as I will suggest shortly) a person who has ceased to exist may have a surviving or posthumous interest in what happens to his or her organism.

In many cases in which a patient enters a persistent vegetative state, what has happened is that the person has died or ceased to exist while the organism, sustained by the operations of the brain stem, remains alive. In these cases, provided that one's action is compatible with the wishes of the person when he or she was alive, there is no direct moral objection to disconnecting the organism from life-support systems or even to killing it in order to obtain its organs for transplantation.

It should be borne in mind, however, that not every case in which a person lapses into a persistent vegetative state is a case in which the person dies or ceases to exist. In cases in which the lack of capacity for consciousness is contingent – for example, when it is a result of a problem with the support mechanisms in the brain stem – the person may continue to exist even though the coma is in practice irreversible. While this case is thus very different in metaphysical terms from that in which a persistent vegetative state is the result of the death of the cerebral hemispheres, it is not significantly different in moral terms. While in this case the person does continue to exist, he will in fact never regain consciousness and his life has thus ceased to be worth living. While there may or may not be a reason to kill or allow the organism to die for the sake of the person himself, it is hard to imagine a reason for keeping it, and therefore him, alive for his sake.

If the existence of each human mind is dependent on the functioning of the cerebral hemispheres, then anencephalic infants, who are born without cerebral hemispheres, are without minds. Since you and I and all others of our kind are essentially minds, anencephalic infants are a fundamentally different sort of thing from us. They are simply organisms – permanently unoccupied human organisms. Whereas in a normal infant's cot there are two substances – a human organism and the infant mind or self that will eventually become a person – there is only one substance in the cot of an anencephalic infant. This organism may well be alive but it will never support the existence of a mind, self, or person. There are, therefore, even fewer moral constraints on the use of the anencephalic infant – for example, as a source of organs or tissue for transplantation – than there are in the case of the living organism of someone who has suffered cerebral death. For, in the latter case, the organism once belonged to a person who may have a surviving interest in what is done to it or may have expressed preferences about what should be done with it. But in the case of an anencephalic infant, there is never anyone whose organism it is. The only people whose interests can be affected by what is done with the infant organism are its parents and those who might benefit from the use of its organs or tissues.

Brain death and brain life

It has frequently been suggested that our understanding of when life begins should be symmetrical with our understanding of when it ends. I believe that, with certain qualifications, this is correct. But, just as the dualistic metaphysic requires that we have two distinct accounts of death, or the end of life, one for the person and another for the organism, so it requires that we have two accounts of the beginning of life.

Because the death of an organism and its ceasing to exist are not one and the same thing, it is in principle possible that its beginning to exist and the onset of its life are also different. But, since the human organism is in an important sense functional from the start (though of course its characteristic functions increase in complexity as it matures), it seems that its life begins at the same time that it begins to exist. As we have seen, with the exception of cases involving monozygotic twinning, this probably occurs around the time of conception, perhaps at syngamy. There are in fact interesting issues here but they are not important for our present purposes.[40] The most interesting and morally important issues have to do with when *we* begin to exist and cease to exist.

Numerous writers have proposed criteria of 'brain life' corresponding to various criteria of brain death. These proposals all seem extremely implausible if there is any suggestion that they pick out the beginning of the existence or the life of the human organism. If brain life is to be symmetrical with brain death, then brain life must be understood as marking the beginning of the existence of the mind or self, not the organism.

The idea that brain life marks the beginning of our existence will also seem implausible if the conception of brain death to which the notion of brain life corresponds is itself implausible as the criterion for the ceasing to exist of the mind or self. We have seen, for example, that the death of the whole brain cannot be the criterion for the ceasing to exist of the self. Because of this, proposals for brain life that are based on the dominant conception of brain death

---

[40] For example, Quinn argues that human organisms may come into existence gradually. See Quinn, 'Abortion: Identity and Loss', section II.

are themselves implausible. If one says that a person ceases to exist when his entire brain dies, or the last signs of life in the brain disappear, then one will be led to assume that brain life occurs when the first signs of life appear in the brain. This, however, seems entirely arbitrary. Interestingly, it is a useful test of the plausibility of a conception of brain death to see whether the corresponding conception of brain life is plausible.

According to the Continuity of Mind account, the mind or self ceases to exist when the cerebral hemispheres irreversibly lose the capacity to support consciousness and mental activity. The corresponding account of brain life is that the mind or self begins to exist when the cerebral hemispheres develop the capacity to support consciousness and mental activity. I defend the plausibility of this view in detail elsewhere.[41]

Potential

This account of when we begin to exist has implications that are important for understanding the morality of abortion. I will briefly summarize them here, though they are spelled out in greater detail elsewhere.[42] If I began to exist only when my brain developed the capacity to support consciousness and mental activity, then all that existed in my mother's womb prior to that point was an unoccupied, developing human organism. If, prior to that point, my mother had had an abortion, that would not have involved killing me, for the obvious reason that I would have had to exist in order for it to have been possible for the abortion to kill me. The abortion would instead have prevented me from coming into existence. Thus an early abortion – one that is performed prior to the coming into existence of a mind or self – is relevantly like an act of contraception. Unlike certain forms of contraception, it does kill a human organism but, again, mere organisms do not have interests and cannot be harmed in the morally relevant sense.

Many have argued that, even if the embryo is not yet a person, it nevertheless has the potential to become a person. This, it might be thought, is a reason for rejecting the idea that the embryo cannot have interests or be harmed. For it may be harmed by being prevented from realizing its potential.

---

[41] See *Killing at the Margins of Life*.
[42] *Ibid.*

Given the dualistic metaphysic, however, these claims are false. To see this, we must distinguish two types of potential.[43] In one sense, X has the potential to become Y only if X and Y are identical. Call this *identity-preserving potential*. It is in this sense that Prince Charles has the potential to become the King of England. In another sense, X has the potential to become Y even though X and Y are not identical. Call this *nonidentity potential*. It is in this sense that my desk has the potential to become a pile of sawdust and a sperm and egg have the potential to become a zygote.

Most previous discussions have assumed that potential of the human embryo to become a person is identity-preserving. But, given the assumption that we are not identical without physical organisms, the human embryo has the potential to become a person only in the sense in which becoming does *not* imply identity. This is, of course, a very odd sort of 'becoming'. It is natural to say that the desk becomes sawdust or that the sperm and egg become a zygote because in these cases the same matter is transmuted from one substance (or pair of substances) into another. By contrast, when the fetal organism 'becomes' a person, this is not a process in which matter is restructured in such a way that one substance ceases to exist while another is realized in the same matter. Instead, in this process of 'becoming', the original entity continues to exist (though it soon ceases to be an embryo, a fetal organism, and so on) while generating and sustaining a *new* entity – the mind or self. We call this a process of becoming only because, as noted, we have hitherto wrongly assumed that only one substance is involved. If I am right, however, the fetal organism has the potential to 'become' *two* things. It has the nonidentity potential to 'become' (i.e., causally generate) a new substance – the self – and the identity-preserving potential to become a mature or adult human organism.

The embryo or fetal organism cannot, however, have an interest in realizing its nonidentity potential to become a person. This is true for two reasons. First, it is only if X's potential to become Y is identity-preserving that it can be good for X, or in X's interest, to become Y. Second, mere organisms devoid of psychological properties are not the sort of thing that can have interests or be

---

[43] Similar distinctions are drawn in Jim Stone, 'Why Potentiality Matters', *Canadian Journal of Philosophy* 17 (1987), p. 818, and in Stephen Buckle, 'Arguing From Potential', *Bioethics* 2 (1988), pp. 230–231.

benefited or harmed. Thus, even though the fetal organism has the identity-preserving potential to become a mature organism, it cannot have an interest in realizing this biological potential.

The various potentials involved in the early stages of human development may be summarized as follows. The sperm and egg have the nonidentity potential to become a zygote. The zygote has the identity-preserving potential to become an embryo, a fetal organism, a juvenile organism, and an adult organism. It also has the nonidentity potential to 'become' a fetal mind or self, which itself has the identity-preserving potential to become a person. Of these various potentials, only the last gives rise to an interest in the realization of the potential. Because the fetal mind or self, which is a substance distinct from the fetal organism, has the identity-preserving potential to become a person, it can have an interest in becoming a person and can be harmed by having this potential thwarted. This is, in fact, only a cumbersome way of saying that the fetal self may have an interest in its own future life. (I argue elsewhere that this interest cannot be a strong one. This fact, together with certain other assumptions, shows that, while a late abortion may be against the interests of the fetus, this does not constitute a strong moral objection to late abortion.[44])

Brain death and euthanasia

The question whether it is acceptable to terminate life-support for an individual in a persistent vegetative state is often considered to be a question of euthanasia. To determine whether this is correct, we first need a definition of euthanasia. Let us say that euthanasia is an act of killing or of letting die that is intended to benefit and actually succeeds in benefiting the individual who is killed or allowed to die. An act that fortuitously benefits the individual killed or allowed to die but was not intended to do so is clearly not an instance of euthanasia. And an act that actually harms the individual who is killed or allowed to die, even though it was intended to benefit her, is only an instance of intended or attempted euthanasia. When killing an individual or letting her die is actually harmful to her, it is not euthanasia.

---

[44] *Killing at the Margins of Life.*

Recall that, according to the Continuity of Mind account, there are two distinct types of persistent vegetative state, one in which the person survives in a permanently unconscious condition and another in which the person or mind has altogether ceased to exist. Let us consider these in turn.

When a person continues to exist in a state of permanent unconsciousness, his life has, as I noted, ceased to be worth living. It is also, however, not a burden to the person, for he is aware of nothing. He cannot feel pain, suffer, or regret his present state. The main reasons for terminating his life-support systems therefore have to do with the interests of others: for example, that continuing to support his life drains resources away from valuable purposes and uses them in a way that benefits no one. If life-support is withdrawn for this reason, this is not euthanasia, though it may nevertheless be justifiable.

It can be argued, however, that life in this state is objectively degrading even if it is subjectively unobjectionable. If so, then the termination of life-support with the intention of releasing the unconscious person from an objectively degrading state may count as euthanasia.

Finally, consider the case in which a persistent vegetative state is the result of the death of the cerebral hemispheres. In that case the person has already ceased to exist; consequently he can be neither killed nor allowed to die. In a literal sense, euthanasia is no longer possible. His organism may, of course, be killed or allowed to die, but since a mere organism cannot be the subject of benefits or harms, it is not a possible candidate for euthanasia. This is a matter of conceptual necessity, in the same way that it is of necessity not possible to practice euthanasia on a plant.

There remains, however, one possibility. Most of us care what happens to our bodies after we die. One feels that it would be degrading, for example, if one were to donate one's body for use in medical research only for it to be mutilated and made an object of derision by medical students. Similarly, one may have a deep aversion to having one's living body sustained indefinitely by artificial means after one has oneself ceased to exist. It is therefore arguable that terminating life-support for, or even actively killing, the living organism of a person who has ceased to exist benefits that person posthumously. This would, of course, be a case in which the beneficiary and the thing killed or allowed to die would be different. And normally if this is the case then the act of killing or letting die cannot be euthanasia. But, given the extremely close (though here unspecified) relation between a person and his or her organism, it is surely acceptable to extend the boundaries of the concept so as to include this as an instance of euthanasia.[45]

---

[45] I am very grateful to Dr. George Khoury of the Medical College of the University of South Carolina for comments and discussion and to Daniel Wikler for comments and references to the literature.

Chapter 33

ADVANCE DIRECTIVES, AUTONOMY AND UNINTENDED DEATH[1]

JIM STONE

Living wills typically have two defects. First, most living wills fail to enable people to effectively avoid unwanted medical intervention. Second, most living wills have the potential of ending your life in ways you never intended, years before you had to die. Policy issues surrounding advance directives often seem pretty obvious and simple, when in fact they are demonically complicated and difficult. Partly as a consequence, living wills and other advance directives tend to be ill-crafted, vague, and confusing to lay people, lawyers, and the medical professionals who implement them – though usually nobody is aware of the confusion until a crisis, if then. People generally do not understand the implications of the advance directives they sign, or, for that matter, create.

Philosophers and others with the critical skills to recognize the inadequacies of most living wills seldom give them careful attention. Perhaps this is because advance directives are thought to represent a welcome protection of individual autonomy – something to be supported, even promulgated, not criticized. Certainly living wills are being sold aggressively to the public: I have attended church meetings where well-intentioned doctors peddled truly frightening instruments, urging the audience to sign 'before you go home'. President Bill Clinton and First Lady Hillary Clinton are asking Americans to sign living wills. The national organization *Choice in Dying* is campaigning to persuade 1,000,000 Americans to sign advance directives in 1994. For better or worse, advance directives are the wave of the future. But if that future is to be better rather than worse, philosophers had better give such instruments a critical examination, before millions of innocents sign on the dotted line.

---

[1] This is a revised and much expanded version of 'Living Wills, Autonomy, and Unintended Death', which appeared in *The American Philosophical Association Newsletter on Philosophy and Medicine*, Fall, 1991; Volume 90:3, 41–45.

Consider, as a case in point, the living will published in the *American Philosophical Association Newsletter on Philosophy and Medicine* (Fall 1990), an effort of the Midwest Bioethics Center and the Kansas City Metropolitan Bar Association, submitted by Joan D. Killion of Midwest Bioethics Center, who writes: 'You may make as many copies of the document found on the next two pages as you would like to share with others'.[2] The *APA Newsletter* has published a full-page copy of the will, to facilitate its widespread distribution. Editor Rosamond Rhodes writes: 'This document, reproduced at the end of the article, satisfies the stringent require-ments of both Missouri and Kansas and also allows each will writer to customize the document to meet personal needs'.[3] In the first part of this paper, I propose that we subject the Midwest Bioethics Center Living Will (as I will call it) to the scrutiny we would give a contract concerning a used car, not to mention a matter of life and death. I believe you will find the exercise illuminating, far more than any abstract discussion could be.

Of course, advance directives do not operate in a Platonic realm: they need to be evaluated against the background of the institutions in which they will actually be implemented. Yet this is almost never done. For example, few philosophers can imagine the incompetence and confusion concerning advance directives in many nursing homes, though it is in nursing homes that many advance directives will be implemented. In the second part of this paper, I want to relate some of my experiences in trying to protect the life of a severely disabled woman, my sister, who has lived in hospitals and nursing homes for the last twenty years. Here I will consider both living wills and resuscitation orders. Again, I believe you will find the story more illuminating than any abstract discussion could be.

In the third part, I will consider a recent alternative to traditional living wills, namely, advance directives establishing durable power of attorney for health care.

I

The MBC Living Will consists of a standard living will declaration followed, on the second page, by Optional Additional Instructions

---

[2] *APA Newsletter on Philosophy and Medicine* Fall, 1990; Volume 90:1, 10.
[3] *APA Newsletter*, 5.

so that we can 'customize' the document to meet our personal needs. The substance of the living will declaration is this:

> If at any time I should have an incurable injury, disease, or illness certified to be a terminal condition by two physicians who have personally examined me, one of whom shall be my attending physician, and the physicians have determined that my death will occur whether or not life-sustaining procedures are utilized, and where the application of life-sustaining procedures would serve only to artificially prolong the dying process, and I am unable to participate in decisions regarding my medical treatment, I direct that such procedures be withheld or withdrawn, and that I be permitted to die naturally with only the administration of medication or the performance of any medical procedure deemed necessary to provide me with comfort.[4]

This statement invites some obvious questions. First, if two physicians must 'certify' that I am in a 'terminal condition', how are they to do it? Doctors have never been asked to 'certify' such things; naturally they may be concerned about legal liability. The will provides no hint of a suitable procedure or instrument, which is an impediment to its being implemented. Also, the statement is sufficiently convoluted grammatically to make it unclear what it is both physicians must certify. It appears that both must certify that my death will occur whether or not life-sustaining procedures are utilized (unfortunately, this is formulated so that it is satisfied vacuously for all people at all times). But must both physicians (or, for that matter, anyone) 'certify' that I am 'unable to participate in decisions regarding my medical treatment'? This constitutes a determination of mental incompetence, a judgement that has been reserved to the courts. How are they to 'certify' that? Would it involve a formal statement? Must both doctors 'certify' that the application of life-sustaining treatment would serve 'only to artificially prolong the dying process'? What does that mean, anyway? The attending physician, who must explain to a colleague what to certify and how to certify it *before* the will can be implemented, is left wholly at sea. Indeed, the MBC Living Will may result in your continued futile treatment while the attending physician, who otherwise would have let you die on the traditional ground that doctors have no duty to impose futile therapies on patients who cannot

---

[4] *APA Newsletter*, 11.

consent, hunts about for a willing colleague and legal advice so that he can without liability satisfy the conditions of the will.

Second and more serious, what is the meaning of the operative term 'terminal condition'? Remarkably, the MBC Living Will is wholly silent on this point. *Tabor's Cyclopedic Medical Dictionary* defines 'terminal illness' as 'illness that because of its nature can be expected to cause the patient to die; usually a chronic disease for which there is no known cure'.[5] This certainly captures what many people have in mind when they sign a living will – for instance, most would agree that acquired immune deficiency syndrome is a terminal condition, for it is bound sooner or later to terminate your life. On this reading, the MBC Living Will could end your life years before the 'terminal condition' would have killed you. A different account: The Long Term Care Facility Ombudsman of a western state recently sent me the third draft of a new brochure explaining living wills, prepared by an attorney, the ombudsman, and several medical professionals, which defined 'terminal condition' as 'any injury, disease, or illness from which you will not recover'. On this account, it is not required that a terminal condition be life-threatening or even serious. Rheumatism is included, along with chronic allergies. This is an instance of the confusion that surrounds the operative terms in living wills: lawyers and medical professionals are sure they know what the terms mean, though they often give substantially different (not to mention hair raising) accounts.

Joan Killion kindly informed me in a telephone conversation that in Kansas and Missouri 'terminal condition' is legally defined as 'a condition where death will occur in a short period of time whether or not life-sustaining procedures are given'. The law does not specify how short the period of time must be. (Consequently a physician nervous about implementing the will need only judge that the time remaining may not be sufficiently short.) However she cautioned me that the term (and consequently the MBC Living Will) might well have a different meaning elsewhere in the country. Then why distribute the MBC Living Will nationwide without defining the operative term? Signing this living will may have different consequences in different states, and the meaning of the document may shift over time. If legislation defining 'terminal condition' is passed

---

[5] *Tabor's Cyclopedic Medical Dictionary*, Editor, Clayton L. Thomas, M.D. Philadelphia: F.A. Davis, 1989, 1836.

in your state and then modified later the will may have one meaning when you sign it and a very different meaning when it is implemented. Equally important: Without a definition of 'terminal condition' in the living will itself, most signers will only vaguely understand the circumstances in which the will applies (or they will have a significantly mistaken idea), though they probably will be unaware of this. And it is my experience that physicians, family members, and clergy with whom they may discuss the document will be no better off. It is improbable that anyone involved will be acquainted with the local legal definition of 'terminal condition', if there is one. Indeed, it will never occur to most signers that there is a question or problem here at all. And the two physicians who must 'certify' that the patient is in a 'terminal condition' before the will can be implemented, will probably themselves not be clear on what the term means, not to mention what the signer had in mind when she signed the document years before, perhaps in another state. Sherrill Whately, R.N., who works in an ICU in Tucson, wrote in correspondence:

> It is very difficult to make the term 'terminal' stick: it is frequently not applied due to vagueness. I have seen many people with living wills die on ventilators against their will due to the vagueness of the term 'terminal'. They feel misled . . .

It is a serious and obvious defect of the MBC Living Will that there is no account at all of the operative term.

Indeed, I believe the term 'terminal condition' cannot be defined to meet the purposes of living wills. And the problem iterates for the second operative term in the MBC Living Will, 'life-sustaining treatment', which is also unexplained. Consider California's newest amended Living Will statute, the Keene Natural Death Act (1991), which gives these definitions:

> 'Terminal condition' means an incurable and irreversible condition that, without the administration of life-sustaining treatment will, within reasonable medical judgement, result in death within a relatively short time.[6]

> 'Life-sustaining treatment' means any medical procedure or intervention that, when administered to a qualified patient, will

---

[6] *California Natural Death Act*, Senate Bill No. 980, 1991, chapter 3.9, sec 7186, (j).

serve only to prolong the process of dying or an irreversible coma or persistent vegetative state.[7]

'Qualified patient' means a patient 18 or more years of age who has executed a declaration and who has been diagnosed and certified in writing by the attending physician and a second physician who has examined the patient to be in a terminal condition or a permanent unconscious condition.[8]

Note that 'terminal condition' is defined in terms of 'life-sustaining treatment', which is defined in terms of 'qualified patient', which is defined in terms of 'terminal condition'. The definitions move in a circle. Further, the critical phrase 'relatively short time' is virtually meaningless. Relative to what? (The Hastings Center suggests that a 'relatively short time' might be defined as one year.[9]) The California statute leaves the matter wholly to the doctor's discretion.[10] Old age would qualify.[11] Worse, the definition of 'terminal condition' is incoherent, given a plain reading of the law, for it implies that there may be treatments available that will preserve the life of a terminally ill person for more than a 'relatively short time', that is, in plain English, for a long time, perhaps for years. But a treatment that preserves someone's life for a long time does not serve 'only to prolong the process of dying', if that phrase has any clear sense, so it is *not* 'life-sustaining treatment', which is what the statute calls it. Indeed, the existence of such treatment implies that the terminal condition is 'reversible', or at least that its progress can be slowed markedly, which for the purposes of a living will should amount to the same thing.

The deep problem is that if we take the phrases 'without the administration of life-sustaining treatment' and 'relatively short time' out of the definition, so that a terminal condition must kill you quickly no matter what the doctors do, then you will not be in a terminal condition if you can be kept alive a long time on a respirator, say. So the will cannot be implemented under the circumstances for which it was designed. To do its work, the will must allow that you can be in a terminal condition *even though* your life

---

[7] *California Natural Death Act*, sec 7186, (d).
[8] *California Natural Death Act*, section 7186, (h).
[9] *Hastings Center Guidelines On The Termination of Life-Sustaining Treatment and The Dying*, Hastings Center, 1987, 141.
[10] *California Natural Death Act*, section 7190.5, (a) and (b).
[11] Nothing in the *California Natural Death Act* precludes this.

can be preserved for a long time by measures you choose in advance to forego. But measures that preserve your life for a long time do not 'serve only to prolong the dying process', if that phrase has any clear sense. So they are not 'life-sustaining treatments'. It follows that someone who can be kept alive for a long time on a respirator is not terminally ill, according to the California statute, for his life can be preserved a long time without resorting to 'life-sustaining treatments'. Again the will cannot be implemented.

The only escape from this dilemma is to broaden the range of 'life-sustaining treatments'. For example, the Hastings Center defines 'life-sustaining treatment' as 'any medical intervention that is administered to a patient in order to prolong life and delay death', which captures what most people think the term means.[12] Chemotherapy, insulin, dialysis, blood transfusions, intravenous food and water are life-sustaining treatments. The President's Commission for the Study of Ethical Problems in Medicine writes:

> 'Life-sustaining treatment', as used here, encompasses all health care intervention that has the effect of increasing the lifespan of the patient, including physical therapy, nursing support for activities of daily living, and special feeding procedures, provided that one effect of the treatment is to prolong the patient's life.[13]

But California cannot count *all* of these as 'life-sustaining treatments', obviously. Too many conditions will qualify as terminal (e.g., kidney disease where death can be forestalled for a decade by dialysis, metastatic cancers where life can be prolonged for many years by intermittent chemotherapy); and it is unlikely that a person who signs a living will intends to forego all of the above if two doctors declare her 'terminal' and the attending physician thinks that she 'can no longer make decisions regarding her medical treatment' – another matter the statute leaves wholly to the physician's discretion.[14]

---

[12] *Hastings Center Guidelines*, 140.

[13] *President's Commission for the Study of Ethical Problems in Medicine and Biomedical and Behavioural Research – Deciding to Forego Life-Sustaining Treatment*, US Government Printing Office, March 1983, 3.

[14] The Declaration included in the statute includes the condition that 'I am no longer able to make decisions regarding my medical treatment'. *California Natural Death Act*, sec 7186.5, (b). As far as the statute is concerned, this condition is satisfied if the attending physician thinks it is; and nothing need be recorded anywhere saying that this is what he thinks. The physician is absolved of all liability if he 'believes in good faith' that his action 'is consistent with this chapter and the desires of the declarant expressed in the declaration'. *California Natural Death Act*, sec 7190.5, (b).

The upshot is this: if the California statute is to be implemented under the circumstances for which it was designed, without being overly broad, there must be a proper subset of medical treatments and interventions that can preserve life for a long time but, which, nonetheless, 'serve only to prolong the dying process'. These are the class of 'life-sustaining treatments'. But now the notion of a treatment that 'serves only to prolong the dying process' is unconstrained, indeed, it has no clear sense. In fact, what the statute amounts to is this: if you are in a condition that will probably cause your death sooner or later (unless something else kills you first) and the attending physician believes your life is not worth preserving, then you are in a 'terminal condition', and any medical intervention that prolongs your life, even for years, is 'life-sustaining treatment', including antibiotics, dialysis, and artificial hydration. If, under the same conditions, the attending physician thinks your life is worth preserving, then medical intervention that prolongs your life is not 'life-sustaining treatment' and you are not in a 'terminal condition'. In general, signing a living will does not preserve your autonomy; rather, it places you entirely at the mercy of doctors, who decide whether you are competent to participate in treatment decisions, how long a 'relatively short time' is, whether you are 'terminally ill', and what counts as the 'life-sustaining treatment' to be foregone. As Thomas J. Marzen observes: 'Execution of a declaration is more of an act of faith than an act of will – an essentially symbolic gesture that effectively delegates decisions on all crucial matters to the discretion of an attending physician'.[15]

Matters get worse on the second page of the MBC Living Will where Optional Additional Instructions are provided to enable us to customize the will to meet our personal needs. Of course, many signers will stop at the declaration on the first page, satisfied that it expresses their wishes. The Optional Additional Instructions begin:

> The following (or photocopy thereof) is a statement of my treatment wishes if I lack the capacity to make or communicate decisions regarding my medical treatment and there is no reasonable expectation that I will regain a meaningful quality of life.

---

[15] Thomas J. Marzen, J.D. 'The "Uniform Rights of the Terminally Ill Act": A Critical Analysis', in *Issues in Law and Medicine*, Vol. 1, No. 6, May 1986, 470. This is an excellent critique (which has certainly influenced this paper) of the attempt in 1985 by the National Conference of Commissioners on Uniform State Laws to promote uniformity in state living will statutes.

I direct all life-sustaining procedures be withheld or withdrawn if I have:

a terminal condition, or

a condition, disease or injury without hope of significant recovery, or

extreme mental deterioration, or

other _____ [16]

The MBC Living Will states that all 'life-sustaining procedures' are to be withheld or withdrawn under any of these circumstances unless the signer draws a line through and adds her initials. (As 'life-sustaining procedures' can now be withheld or withdrawn even when I am not in the process of dying, the phrase cannot mean 'procedure that serves only to prolong the dying process', but 'any procedure that sustains or prolongs life'.) The direction to withdraw or withhold all life-sustaining procedures becomes operative when two conditions are satisfied: I lack the capacity to make or communicate decisions regarding my medical treatment, and there is no reasonable expectation that I will regain a 'meaningful quality of life'. But this statement is extraordinarily and dangerously unclear, for two reasons. First, if I lack temporarily the capacity to make or communicate decisions regarding my treatment, is the first condition satisfied? Or is it required that the incapacity be judged something permanent (or at least indefinite)? Suppose I become quadriplegic, and later catch pneumonia so that I am too sick to communicate my decisions. My doctors judge that I will get well enough in a few days to communicate *if* they give me antibiotics. Otherwise I will die. Should they judge the first condition satisfied and go on to ponder whether quadriplegics have a 'meaningful quality of life', or should they judge the first condition unsatisfied and save me? Or suppose a quadriplegic suffers a stroke and cannot communicate, though the doctors judge that she will probably regain that capacity in a week or so if they keep her on a respirator. Reading the will literally, the first condition is satisfied in both cases. I submit that it is irresponsible in evaluating a document dealing with a matter of life and death, to suppose the implementers will not take it to mean what it literally says. Here the will endangers

[16] *APA Newsletter*, 12.

the autonomy it is designed to protect. But those who sign the statement will not understand this implication; few would sign who did.

Second, the phrase 'quality of life' is virtually meaningless, and the expression 'meaningful quality of life' is worse. In *Clinical Ethics*, Jonsen, Siegler, and Winslade observe:

> The phrase 'quality of life' is frequently heard in clinical discussions about ethical problems. Frequent use has given the phrase neither any precise meaning nor any definite application.
>
> It seems an attempt to put a value upon some feature, or collection of features, of human experience. As such it is highly subjective; yet the phrase is often used by someone other than the person who is living the life being evaluated.[17]

A good way to destroy public trust in the medical profession is to encourage doctors to make highly subjective decisions, based on an empty phrase, concerning who lives and who dies – an outcome the MBC Living Will invites on a large scale. By what standard can a doctor judge that my life will not regain a 'quality' that is 'meaningful'? And note that the requirement that at least two physicians agree about any of this has fallen away, though this statement is far stronger than the previous one, potentially directing the withdrawal of all 'life-sustaining procedures' in cases where I am not even 'terminally ill'. Many physicians will not touch this statement with a ten-foot pole, rendering it ineffective; those undeterred are liable to make judgements the signer might well consider idiosyncratic. (Remember that for many signers the directive will finally be implemented, perhaps scores of years hence, by a physician they may never even have met.) I recall a neurosurgeon apologizing sincerely to a young woman's family for saving her life; now she would be a cripple, he said. More than a few doctors believe mild retardation in an infant deprives his life of sufficient 'meaning' to warrant surgery to correct intestinal blockage. Many doctors automatically consider any nursing home resident terminally ill, mentally incompetent, and lacking a 'meaningful quality of life'. (Note that the standard living will declaration is triggered under these circumstances.) I once saw a respected internist no-code a 41-year-old,

---

[17] Albert R. Jonsen, Mark Siegler, William Winslade, *Clinical Ethics, Second Edition*, Macmillan, 1986, 102.

healthy, manifestly happy disabled woman residing in a nursing home, simply because she was *there* – without informing anyone he had done so.[18] Any seriously injured young person, temporarily unable to communicate, who will be significantly disabled after the doctors save him, can lose his life as a consequence of signing this will. Any elderly or disabled person in a nursing home will be at risk. Few who sign will understand the implications.

The framers of the will provide an additional statement in the middle of page 2:

> A meaningful quality of life means to me that: (*This does not need to be filled in for the instructions to be valid.*)[19]

Sadly, the emphasis is in the original. Those undiscouraged who go on to the unnecessary bother of completing this entry, must wrestle without guidelines with 'meaningful quality of life', a phrase with 'neither precise meaning nor definite application'. Naturally much of what is written will share the defect; a good deal will be dangerously broad, vague, and confused. Many will not understand the lethal implications of what they have written.

Matters get worse still. Remember the Optional Additional Instructions continued:

> I direct all life-sustaining procedures be withheld or withdrawn if I have:
>
> a terminal condition

This term is undefined in the MBC Living Will, and I hardly need repeat that it may have different meanings in different times and places, as well as for different doctors and patients.

> a condition, disease, or injury without hope of significant recovery

Note that the condition, disease, or injury without hope of significant recovery need not be life threatening or even serious. Blindness qualifies, along with arthritis and chronic eczema. Few who sign will realize this. And remember, *all* life-sustaining procedures (e.g., antibiotics, insulin, blood transfusions) are directed to be withheld or withdrawn under this circumstance *unless* Uncle Henry takes the

---

[18] My sister, in fact; more about this later.
[19] *APA Newsletter*, 12.

trouble to draw a line through it *and* sign his initials. The MBC Living Will errs grossly on the side of death. Let this one get by you and you may be denied life-saving surgery if you are too sick to communicate, you are permanently blind or disabled, and a doctor makes an idiosyncratic judgement about the 'quality' of your life.

extreme mental deterioration

Note that the mental deterioration need not be permanent or irreversible for this condition to be satisfied. Your mental condition 'deteriorates' just in case it 'becomes worse.' What gets bad can get better, so there can be temporary extreme mental deterioration. The term 'extreme' is vague and subjective (is loss of short-term memory plus all comprehension of dates, times, and numbers 'extreme'?), and 'mental deterioration' is sufficiently general to include psychosis and the immediate aftermath of a stroke.

The MBC Living Will is dangerously defective in ways that few who sign it will recognize. But I believe it is better than most of the living wills now being distributed zealously. I propose that we resist the popular contention that dangerous advance directives are the price of enabling people to avoid unwanted medical intervention. Directives are dangerous because they are nebulous and confused, and a muddled directive will not effectively enable you to avoid unwanted intervention; indeed, it can have the opposite effect. I observed earlier, however, that advance directives must be evaluated against the background of the institutions in which they will actually be implemented. Living wills may be alarming, but they represent only the surface of a far more dangerous situation, invisible to most signers. What will happen to the advance directive you sign?

II

In 1974 my sister Michele, the mother of a two-year-old, suffered a stroke due to an aneurism, which left her permanently brain damaged, quadriplegic, and barely able to speak. She was twenty-eight. Michele was twice resuscitated after the stroke and she was in a persistent vegetative state for six months, the doctors insisting that she would never talk again – until she began talking again. Relatives described my sister's condition as 'a fate worse than death', but this was not so, for over the next two years Michele reemerged as a feisty, funny, indomitable woman, *sans* numbers and dates, her short-term memory impaired, unable to read or write, yet more than ever before herself. When her husband divorced her and remarried, Michele grieved for months – until one day I found her cheerful and smiling. 'Plenty of fish!' Michele said. When he refused to allow her visitation with her daughter, maintaining that Michele was a vegetable, she went to court, singing in her wheelchair on the witness stand when she could not speak, defeating him. 'You've changed a lot since the stroke' I once observed. 'Better!' Michele responded. 'How better?' 'Grew up!'

Michele gave me durable power of attorney to deal with her affairs, with the understanding that I would do what she wanted. In that capacity, I stayed in close touch with her nursing home and with her physician. In 1986 I received a Fulbright to teach in India, and I visited Michele to say goodbye. She had formed a close friendship with another resident, a retired attorney, but she drew the line at marriage. 'Too tall!' Michele complained. 'Not Jewish!' 'Of course, you will save her if anything goes wrong', I told the charge nurse on Michele's floor on my way out of the facility, 'We can't do that', the brave nurse said, and she showed me the DNR order Michele's doctor had put in her chart six months before, without informing us. I had ordered him explicitly the previous year to resuscitate Michele if ever it became necessary. It transpired that the medical director of the facility had phoned the residents' attending physicians, asking them to record a decision about resuscitation in each resident's chart. The doctors had come in and no-coded everybody, without consulting or informing the residents or their families. (As I observed earlier, for many physicians it is a foregone conclusion that the life of a nursing home resident is not worth preserving.) The charge nurse understood perfectly the force of the no-code: if something went seriously wrong, she would stand aside and let Michele die.

I tore the code out of the chart. The social service worker happened to be standing near the nurse's station. Social service workers typically have the job of discussing resuscitation with incoming residents, and helping them to sign an advance directive. 'We don't have to worry about resuscitation here', she explained to me. 'We don't have the facilities to do that sort of thing.' 'You mean the nurses don't know CPR, and you don't have oxygen?' I asked. The social service worker became visibly confused and perplexed. She looked at the nurse questioningly. It became plain that she did not know what the word 'resuscitation' means. This level of incompetence may be difficult to believe, but it is hardly uncommon. The average tenure of a social service worker in a nursing home is six months.[20] The job is demanding and poorly paid; and it often tends to attract young college graduates (many of whom have no background in social work) who are not career oriented.[21] In rural areas the college-degree requirement can be waived to allow the position to be filled. Some social service workers in nursing homes – especially more mature women – are very good. Others have trouble writing sentences; functional illiteracy is not uncommon even among American college graduates. Social service workers in nursing homes especially do not understand advance directives, and they often have little conception of the gravity of the decisions involved. Some are zealous, inventing their own advance directives for all incoming residents to sign, the principal words misspelled. Others repeatedly question healthy residents who have opted for resuscitation, 'to see if they have changed their minds'. If you enter a nursing home, the social service worker will collect your living will.

I wheeled Michele to the nursing home director's office, who defended the placing of the DNR order in Michele's chart. 'We can put any order we want in anyone's chart', she insisted. 'There is no obligation to ask or inform anyone. The onus is on the family to make their wishes known. Till then I can do as I choose.' Later I saw the director accost a resident, asking bluntly: 'DO you want to be resuscitated?' The resident had no idea what the question meant. The average tenure of a nursing home director is one year; having shepherded my sister through five facilities in twenty years, I have known quite a few. Few understand advance directives well, or resuscitation policy, which they often set for their facility, assisted by the social service worker. Generally, in the last decade in nursing homes, the job of raising the resuscitation question and setting

---

[20] This is my own conclusion based on two decades of experience, confirmed by conversations with Ron Tryon, the present director of my sister's facility, who himself worked for several years as a social service worker in nursing homes. Jobs in nursing homes are hard; the social service worker position is especially so. She must deal with abusive residents, grieving families, resident's financial problems, getting people new false teeth, lots of paper work, and the nursing staff may view her as intruding on their affairs. Mr Tryon also confirms my observation (stated in the next sentence in the text) that many people in the social service position are there without adequate preparation, primarily because they need a job.

[21] Because of the low pay, social workers with MSW degrees are rare in American long term care facilities.

policy has tended to pass from nurses and doctors to non-medical personnel.

In 1989, Michele's facility was acquired by a national chain.[22] The central office in Florida adopted an advance directive for all of its fifty-three facilities, to be signed by every resident on admission. I found the same directive in use in other chains with hundreds of facilities. The social service worker in Michele's nursing home posted me a copy, requesting that I sign it, so she could 'send it along to the doctor'.

RESUSCITATION ORDERS

In the event that my physical condition declines to the point that I have a cardiac and/or pulmonary arrest, I hereby request that the staff of _____
will attempt or not attempt cardiopulmonary resuscitation (CPR).

Circle one

I understand that if I choose for the staff to attempt CPR, CPR will be initiated by the staff, the emergency medical team will be called and I will be transported to the hospital.

This decision shall bind myself, all other members of my family and all legal and personal representatives until revoked by me in writing.

The order is to be signed on admission by the patient and a witness, or by the 'Responsible Party' for the patient; then it is sent along to the attending physician, who signs it to 'acknowledge concurrence'.

If ever there was a clear and effective advance directive, this certainly would seem to be it. What could be more simple? The Vice President for Operations informed me in correspondence that the order was the result of 'long deliberation by attorneys, nursing home administrators, and insurance executives'. Yet this directive is dangerously confused and misleading. The language about 'declining physical condition' suggests that the order concerns cardiac or pulmonary arrest in the final stages of a terminal condition.

---

[22] I prefer not to identify the chain because my sister is still in one of its facilities.

The directive appears to raise a straightforward question: if you are someday in the last stages of a terminal disease like cancer, or perhaps just terminal old age, and you finally expire, do you want people banging on your chest, giving you electric shocks, and so on, trying to revive you? Naturally most people opt against resuscitation. What they do not realize is that the order goes into the chart *immediately*, they will be no-coded as soon as the attending physician posts it back to the social service worker, many years before they are in a terminal condition. In fact, most people who enter a nursing home are not terminally ill; many are not terribly old, some are in their twenties – you go to a nursing home when you need full-time nursing care. (There are intelligent, charming old people in nursing homes, there can be quite a bit of sex, people fall in love: for many nursing home residents life goes on.) Once the no-code is in the resident's chart, it is unlikely that she will ever discover it. Hence the no-code may end her life years before she became terminally ill; for if she suffers arrest as a result of being given the wrong medication, an electric shock, drowning in the bath, choking, or any of the reasons any of us might stop breathing at anytime, the nurses are under orders to stand aside and let her die. Further, as a matter of policy, nursing staff will try aggressively to transfer the no-code to any hospital the resident ever enters for any reason (e.g., surgery to remove an impacted wisdom tooth), so that – if they succeed – the hospital staff will let her die if there is an accident with anaesthetic, say, or cardiac arrest due to an embolism.

In general, when you ask people who are not terminally ill to sign a resuscitation order, no matter how it is worded they assume that it will go into effect only when they are dying. The alternative never occurs to them. I mentioned this to the wife of a philosophy professor in Colorado, who went to her mother's facility and found that her mother had been no-coded for two years: she never dreamed when she signed the form on admission that her mother would be no coded *before* she was dying. As I write, I believe that thousands of nursing home residents have DNR orders in their charts without knowing or wanting it, because they did not understand the implications of the advance directive they were requested to sign – along with numerous other forms – on admission.

Note that the form gives no indication that the resident or responsible party know what the resuscitation order is about, have considered the risks and benefits of CPR, or are aware of the resident's prognosis and the consequences of CPR for someone in his particular condition. The social service worker has no medical training. The form is completed by the resident on admission, without medical counsel, then forwarded to the attending physician, who functions as a rubber stamp. Consequently the signing of the order cannot constitute informed consent (note that most living wills are also signed without medical counsel). Also, the policy is coercive. Signing the form is likely to be perceived as a condition of admission. The family member who insists on thinking things over is apt to get a letter saying: 'We need you to fill out this form'. In my own case, visits to my sister became difficult because the nurses would request me to sign the order 'before you leave'. Note too that the order is all or nothing, allowing the resident only two options: to accept or to decline all CPR, regardless of the circumstances. And there is no provision for periodic review. This can lead to the futile resuscitation of the dying against their wishes. Mr Smith must make a decision upon admission; as he is in good health, he requests that the staff attempt CPR. Later he becomes incompetent, and later still terminally ill. When he finally suffers arrest due to the primary illness, the staff, confronted with Mr Smith's order (which binds him, his family, and all legal and personal representatives until he revokes it in writing) resuscitates him repeatedly, something he never would have wanted – this because there was no way he could express the conditional request that he be resuscitated *except* in the last stages of a terminal illness.

This policy is not part of an evil scheme to allow the elderly and the disabled to asphyxiate at the earliest opportunity; rather, it flows from confusion on the part of the people who created it. For example, the resuscitation policy statement for the chain (which the social service worker is supposed to review with the resident on admission) defines 'resuscitation' as 'an extraordinary, "heroic" means employed to maintain the life of a patient'. Note that vague and subjective terms like 'extraordinary' and 'heroic' are likely to prejudice the resident against choosing resuscitation. Worse, the crucial requirement is omitted that resuscitation must aim at reviving someone who has suffered cardiac or pulmonary arrest. Placing an alert resident who has suffered renal failure on dialysis is 'resuscitation' by this definition, if the measure is considered 'extraordinary' or 'heroic'. The definition, which appears prominently in the policy statement, potentially invites the removal of anything that preserves a resident's life, *before* she suffers cardiac or pulmonary arrest, if she has signed a DNR order.

In fact, nursing homes and hospitals are quite confused about what such an order entails. In a 1993 article in *American Journal of Critical Care*, Celine Marsden, R.N. writes: 'In addition to differing interpretations of the meaning of CPR/DNR, nurses and physicians are often confused about what care is to be provided for patients with a written DNR order'.[23] Mildred Simmons, the Long-Term Care Facility Director for the Colorado Department of Health, at a meeting in 1989 called to discuss these issues, told me that a wide range of 'life-preserving means' were being withheld in Colorado facilities from residents who had opted against CPR. Some had been allowed to choke to death; in some facilities, she said, residents had been denied food and water. Such stories can make the papers when the victim is newsworthy. I quote from a 1993 newspaper account of the death of an Indian woman, Mary Jo Estep, a survivor of one of the West's last Indian massacres.

> The story begins with a medication mix-up the morning of Dec. 19 at Good Samaritan Health Care Center in Yakima. Estep, 82, was accidentally given three doses of prescription medicine intended for another resident.
>
> Although the error was discovered less than a half hour later, she would never be told the severity of the accident, nor be given the option of seeking emergency treatment. Nursing home officials say Estep's attending physician . . . ordered no corrective measures because of the woman's advance directive barring heroic measures to keep her alive. In medical jargon, she was a 'no-code' patient.
>
> Estep had remained coherent and alert during the first eight hours following the medication error, . . . But by late afternoon her heart rate and pulse began falling. Sixteen hours after swallowing the wrong pills, Estep was pronounced dead.
>
> 'It really disturbs me that they took her like that,' said one of Estep's closest friends, . . . 'She was very well, very alert, and you can't tell me that being "no-code" means being left to die like that.'[24]

---

[23] Celine Marsden, R.N., ' "Do Not Resuscitate" Orders and End-Of-Life Care Planning', *American Journal of Critical Care*, Vol. 2, No. 2, 1993, 177–179.

[24] David Wasson, ' "No Code" Nightmare', *Yakima Herald-Republic*, March 14, 1993, 1.

Now we can address the question: What will happen to your living will after you sign it? The Patient Self-Determination Act of 1990 requires every hospital and nursing home to ask every patient at admission if they want to fill out a living will. (Note that the sick patient can hardly consider the advance directive intelligently at check-in, another reason why signing it is not informed consent.) The hospital or nursing home must also ask if you already have a living will, and record it in your medical record. There the advance directive is liable to function as, or be translated directly into, a DNR order, even though you are neither incompetent nor terminally ill. Doctors and nurses cannot be relied upon to distinguish living wills from DNR orders, whether you are in a hospital or a nursing home. (In nursing homes, as I mentioned earlier, there is the risk that the directive will be triggered simply by your being there, so that you will be denied all 'life-sustaining treatment'.) In an article in the magazine *Nursing Spectrum*, Diane Majka-Grandstrom, R.N. writes:

> A retired nurse was admitted to the hospital for steroid therapy for multiple sclerosis. Aware of the Patient Self-Determination Act (PSDA), she brought along her living will. Her physician, upon reading it, wrote a do not resuscitate order on her chart.
>
> If you find nothing unusual in this scenario, you may be one of many who confuse living wills with DNR orders. The nurse did, in fact, state in her living will that she did not want CPR or a long list of other treatments. However, she knew that the will would only go into effect if she became terminally ill and unable to communicate, or permanently unconscious. Multiple sclerosis is not a terminal condition. And the nurse was communicating quite well.[25]

'Why do people confuse living wills with DNR orders?' Majka-Grandstrom asks. 'As a result of the PSDA, health care professionals are informing consumers about their right to make advance directives, but the general public and health care professionals are both unclear or uninformed about the timing and process of advance directives.'[26]

[25] Diane Majka-Grandstom, R.N., 'Living Wills Are Not DNR Orders', *Nursing Spectrum*, April 19, 1993, 6.
[26] Diane Majka-Grandstrorn, 6.

This confusion can have lethal consequences. I quote from a recent letter by Phyllis J. Robb, of Fort Wayne, Indiana, to *The American Medical Association News*:

> My mother, at 73 and in excellent health, entered the hospital for her second hip replacement. After six days, she left the hospital and entered a transitional care unit. On entry she was given a standard living will for her consideration. She signed it, not adding any special instructions; she did not take it seriously enough to even mention to us.
>
> In our state, the living will takes effect only if the person is terminally ill and unable to communicate. It is a short simple form, and the language is clear. Regardless, a staff person wrote on mother's record 'no-code, patient's request'. The family was not informed.
>
> On the 11th day after surgery, mother suffered cardiac arrest due to an embolism. The staff did not call a doctor or attempt to treat her in any way; they did not wish to 'go against her wishes'. They stayed by her side for 20 minutes while she died. My reaction was shock and disbelief.[27]

Robb, formerly a strong supporter of living wills, concludes that she would not sign a living will or allow information about her wishes to be entered into a facility's records. She writes: 'Now I know that, to many professionals, a patient who has a living will "wants to die". All the fine points elude them'.[28]

The bottom line, then, is that advance directives are often dangerously confused, even when they least appear to be, and those who implement them are often more so, though they usually do not know it. Consequently signing a living will or a resuscitation order is imprudent, because – at the very least – you risk putting yourself at the mercy of people who do not know what it means. Given the procedural chaos, incompetence, and high turnover endemic to many of the institutions in which advance directives are implemented, the situation is unlikely to improve enough to make signing one more than a fool's gamble. You risk losing your life, and the directive does not effectively or reliably enable you to determine

---

[27] Phyllis, J. Robb, 'Bitter Lesson On Living Wills', *The American Medical Association News*, July 12, 1993, 21.
[28] Phyllis J. Robb, 21.

your future treatment. Philosophical questions aside, why die stupidly? There has to be a better way.

III

In recent years many states have passed laws enabling people to designate a proxy to supervise their treatment in case they become incompetent. This is largely the result of a three-pronged effort by *Choice In Dying* to pass in each state a living will statute, a durable power of attorney for health care statute, and an automatic surrogacy statute. The last establishes a pecking order of relatives and friends whom a health care facility must ask to represent an incompetent patient who has never signed an advance directive. In some states, Oregon for instance, this representative can remove all life sustaining procedures (including artificial nutrition and hydration) from an incompetent patient who is in a terminal condition, though she has never expressed a wish that this be done; and the surrogate may be a complete stranger.[29] Obviously, automatic surrogacy provides a powerful incentive to sign an advance directive; at the very least, most people can think of family members whom they would not want directing their medical care.

I have talked to lawyers who predict that directives designating a health care proxy will replace living wills, which are on their way out. This is unrealistic, for several reasons. First, living wills are easy to sign and, as I observed earlier, they are being very widely distributed. *Choice In Dying* has already given out between 15 and 20 million advance directives, most of them living wills. The organization is now distributing both kinds of directives in every state.[30]

---

[29] Oregon Revised Statutes, 127.635. At the bottom of the list of individuals the health care facility must ask to represent an incompetent patient, is 'any adult relative or adult friend'. It is not required that the adult relative know the patient. The list also includes 'any adult designated by the others listed in this subsection who can be so located, if no person listed in this subsection objects to the designation'. Further, 'life-sustaining procedures may be withheld or withdrawn upon the direction and under the supervision of the attending physician' if the patient is in a terminal condition and no representative can be found. This also applies to a patient who has been diagnosed as 'permanently unconscious'. In Oregon, therefore, there are circumstances in which a doctor can, without the consent of a representative or evidence that it is his patient's wish, starve her to death.

[30] Jeffrey Harrison, a telephone counsellor for *Choice in Dying*, also was kind enough to inform me that his organization estimates that 10% of Americans have signed advance directives. Because durable power of attorney directives are more recent, most of these are probably living wills.

Second, many people will sign a living will because they cannot find a suitable health care representative. Third, many who sign a power of attorney will also sign a living will in order to instruct and constrain their proxy (who is legally bound to honor such declarations), as well as the attending physician in case the proxy quits or is himself incapacitated.

Increasingly popular are 'hybrid' advance directives, which combine a durable power of attorney with a living will; you can sign either or both documents. The Oregon document (which constitutes the 'state of the art' for hybrids) defines 'life support' as 'any medical procedure, pharmaceutical, medical device or medical intervention that maintains life by sustaining, restoring, or supplanting a vital function'.[31] This includes virtually every important medical intervention short of comfort care. The durable power of attorney continues:

INITIAL IF THIS APPLIES:

___ My representative MAY decide about life support for me. (If you don't initial this space, then your representative MAY NOT decide about life support.)[32]

As the definition of 'life support' is so very broad, your representative will have little to do unless you initial the statement. But then he has apparently unlimited discretion to end your life whenever you (even temporarily) cannot direct your health care – the sole condition for his taking over. By statute, the proxy has priority over anyone other than the signer in making health care decisions, including the attending physician. He can hire and fire doctors, for instance. Your physician's only recourse, if he thinks the proxy is not acting in your best interest, is to seek judicial review – something many doctors are loathe to do. The document provides three lines for 'Special Conditions or Instructions' to the proxy, followed by the prominent statement:

INITIAL IF THIS APPLIES:

___ I have executed a Health Care Instruction or Directive to Physicians. My representative is to honor it.[33]

[31] Oregon Revised Statutes, 127.505, 16.
[32] Oregon Revised Statutes, 127.531.
[33] Oregon Revised Statutes, 127.531.

Naturally, many will go on to sign the living will, which follows immediately the durable power of attorney.

The result of a hybrid directive, consequently, will often be a living will (or 'Directive to Physicians') that also binds a proxy, whose duty will be to implement it. This preserves some of the chief dangers of living wills. Most notably, someone in the future must implement a nebulous and dangerously confused advance directive.[34] Some instructions may be virtually meaningless; others may have unintended lethal consequences upon which the proxy will act. Family members usually have far less grasp of medical issues and terminology than do doctors, and little practical experience in medical crises. Also, the proxy is more likely to become distraught. Consequently, representatives will often be even less capable than doctors of rationally interpreting an advance directive. Ideally, proxy and physician will together interpret the will; but the test of a directive can hardly be what will happen ideally. Doctors often tell stories in which, say, a 70-year-old woman has a stroke and is put on a respirator, an irate family member arrives flapping a living will and demanding that it be implemented, the doctor refuses, the woman recovers completely and says she never dreamed the will might have this sort of result. When the family member is the proxy, it will be far more difficult for the doctor to refuse. Also, as any medical facility you enter will record the hybrid, there is the danger that the living will sooner or later will function in the minds of staff as a DNR order. As Ms. Robb observes 'all the fine points elude them'.

Of course, finding a sensible, caring, and assertive individual to look out for you if you become incompetent is a very good idea. (Better still, find two or more, and designate an order of succession.)

---

[34] For example, the Oregon living will (ORS, 127.531) gives the signer the option of filling out specific instructions, or 'you may use the general instruction provided by Item 5'. This reads:

> ___ I do not want my life to be prolonged by life support. I also do not want tube feeding as life support. I want my doctors to allow me to die naturally if my doctor and another knowledgeable doctor confirm I am in any of the medical conditions listed in Items 1 to 4 above.

(Items 1 to 4 are labeled 'Close to Death', 'Permanently Unconscious', 'Advanced Progressive Illness', and 'Extraordinary Suffering'.) This statement is dangerously ambiguous and unclear. 'Life support', remember, is defined in Oregon so that you do not need to be in any of the conditions listed in Items 1 to 4 for medical intervention to count as life support. Note that the first two sentences in the statement are not clearly constrained by the third. Indeed, the statement can be read as three separate directions, in which the first two sentences inform the last one. For example, the second sentence can be easily construed by a proxy as a blanket prohibition against tube feeding.

Arrange a conference with this person and your doctor at which you can discuss your preferences; but saddling her with a living will is a mistake. There is little need to worry that, without a living will, she will lack sufficient authority to refuse futile treatment when you are dying. It is unlikely that any physician will refuse a legal representative's request to withdraw or withhold futile or painful treatment from a plainly incompetent patient; and the proxy can fire any doctor. (I could no-code my sister today, despite the fact that she is still young, healthy, and competent; her attending physician would not bat an eye.[35]) To the contrary, your representative may spend her time demanding second opinions, firing incompetent or uncaring doctors, checking your chart for negligent DNR orders, and generally fighting to preserve your life and health.

If you are in a PVS or an 'irreversible coma', several states may not allow your proxy to withdraw life support until he produces 'clear and convincing evidence' that you would want this done.[36] People often sign living wills partly because they fear these conditions, hence it is worth noting that the prospect of ending up in either is statistically remote: you probably have more to fear from signing a living will. Patients so diagnosed sometimes regain consciousness; if you choose not to wager that you will be one of them, give a signed, witnessed, and notarized statement to your proxy saying so.[37] Include the written instruction that the affidavit must

---

[35] My power of attorney was an arrangement that I concocted with a lawyer in 1976, to protect my sister. It did not involve an advance directive or any mention of mental incompetence.

[36] Missouri, Illinois, Connecticut, New York, Maine, New Jersey, and Ohio are some of them.

[37] A version of Pascal's wager applies to the PVS and the 'irreversible coma'. People in such conditions are not suffering. There remains a small possibility that they will wake up, as some do, or that medical advances will enable doctors to help them. (The term 'irreversible' is, at best, relative to the state of the medical art.) Consequently you have everything to win and nothing to lose if you gamble on staying alive: you may wake up and, if you do not, unconscious life is no worse than being dead. The argument concludes that it is in your interest to stay alive if you are comatose, the more *so* the younger you are. One difficulty is that you may be severely disabled if you wake up. Severe disability, however, while not as good as normalcy, is usually better than being dead. That is what the severely disabled typically say, anyhow. We generally do not think they are better off dead; but that judgement should guide decisions about ourselves. Another difficulty is that unconscious life may be worse than being dead if, for example, your financial resources, needed to support your family, will be exhausted. Note that in the famous cases of comatose patients (e.g., Karen Quinlan) insurance or social security paid the bills. I submit that anyone who opts for death if he becomes comatose, without first considering this argument, has not made a reasoned and informed decision. Further, if you are the guardian of a comatose young person, where your first concern must be to do what is in her interest, your duty is clear.

remain in his possession and not be given to any facility. Also, as your proxy may come under pressure from doctors and administrators to withdraw treatment, providing him a signed and notarized list of prohibitions will help him to resist. For example, if you do not want artificial nutrition and hydration withdrawn, or you do not want to be no-coded before you are dying, a statement prohibiting him from doing so would be helpful. As active euthanasia may be legal before you die, you may choose to prohibit your proxy from exercising that right in your behalf. Finally, if you cannot find a suitable representative and feel that you must have an advance directive, draft a document that begins 'I want all treatment, except . . .'. Then enumerate as clearly as you can, with the help of your doctor, the treatments you do not want and the circumstances under which you do not want them. The positive statement at the beginning may help prevent you from being perceived as someone who 'wants to die'.

To conclude: instruments concerning matters of life and death should all be subjected to the sort of critical review we have given the MBC Living Will, resuscitation orders, and directives creating durable power of attorney for health care. Unfortunately this is seldom done. Philosophers have the critical skills to recognize the defects of these directives, if only we will use them. When next you see an advance directive, I appeal to you to read it with care. If it is defective, bring this to the attention of the framers and to those who might sign it uncritically. If you do not, you can be certain that no one else will, for almost no one else can. If we lack the wisdom to make us kings, surely philosophers have sufficient technical insight to function as guardians of the elderly and the disabled as our society ages, The life you save may be your own.[38]

[38] I am indebted to Kathi Hamlon, Ed Johnson, Phil Fuselier, Thomas Marzen, Jane Brockmann, and Dorothy Crane for helpful conversations, and to Judith Crane and Sherrill Whately for their comments.

Chapter 34

END OF LIFE CARE IN HIV-INFECTED CHILDREN WHO DIED IN HOSPITAL

LESLEY D. HENLEY

Knowledge of current end of life practices is necessary to improve terminal care for children dying in hospital. Evidence from well-resourced countries highlights gaps in the care of dying children, some of whom suffer pain and distress,[1] and receive poorly coordinated palliation[2] or aggressive care in intensive care units until the last few days of life.[3] Apart from limited research and commentary[4] from the United States on pain management and palliation, little is known about end of life practices in children with HIV/AIDS. In South Africa (SA) where HIV/AIDS accounts for an escalating proportion of paediatric admissions and deaths,[5] no published data exist on the care of children dying in public hospitals. This study examined end of life care among hospitalized HIV-infected children.

---

[1] J. Wolfe, H.E. Grier, N. Klar, et al. Symptoms and suffering at the end of life in children with cancer. *N Engl J Med* 2000; 342: 326–333.

[2] D. Parker, I. Maddocks & L.M. Stern. The role of palliative care in advanced muscular dystrophy and spinal muscular atrophy. *J Paediatr Child Health* 1999; 35: 245–250.

[3] Wolfe, *op. cit.* note 1; Parker et al. *op. cit.* note 2; W.M. Robinson, S. Ravilly, C. Berde & M.E. Wohl. End-of-life care in cystic fibrosis. *Pediatrics* 1997; 100: 205–209.

[4] L.M. Czarniecki, M. Boland & J.M. Oleske. Pain in children with HIV disease. *PAAC Notes* 1993; 5: 492–495; A. Anand, L. Carmosino & A.E. Glatt. Management of recalcitrant pain in a pediatric acquired immunodeficiency syndrome patient. *Pediatr Infect Dis J 1993*; 12: 159–160; S. Hirschfeld, H. Moss, K. Dragisic, W. Smith & P.A. Pizzo. Pain in pediatric human immunodeficiency virus infection: incidence and characteristics in a single-institution pilot study. *Pediatrics* 1996; 98: 449–452; E. Wishnie & S.J. Weisman. Children with AIDS – pain syndromes and unique issues of assessment and management. *Child Adolesc Psychiatr Clin N Am* 1997; 6: 863–878; J.M. Oleske & L. Czarniecki. Continuum of palliative care: lessons from caring for children infected with HIV-1. *Lancet* 1999; 354: 1287–1291.

[5] R. Bobat, H. Coovadia, D. Moodley & A. Coutsoudis. Mortality in a cohort of children born to HIV-1 infected women from Durban, South Africa. *S Afr Med J* 1999; 89: 646–648; R.J. Zwi, J.M. Pettifor & N. Soderlund. Paediatric hospital admissions at a South African urban regional hospital: the impact of HIV, 1992–1997. *Ann Trop Paediatr* 1999; 19: 135–142; S. Yeung, D. Wilkinson, S. Escott & C.F. Gilks. Paediatric HIV infection in a rural South African district hospital. *J Trop Pediatr* 2000; 46: 107–110; C. Bateman. Can Kwazulu-Natal hospitals cope with the HIV/AIDS human tide? *S Afr Med J* 2001; 91: 364–368.

PATIENTS AND METHODS

Patients and setting

The study population included all patients who died from HIV/AIDS-related causes between February 1998 and June 2000 in Red Cross War Memorial Children's Hospital in Cape Town, SA. The hospital is a secondary and tertiary teaching facility providing comprehensive medical care to an ethnically diverse, predominantly low-income population. Rotating registrars and senior house officers under consultant supervision provide most medical and surgical care. Limited multidisciplinary services including physiotherapy and social work are provided. The sample was drawn from a computerized register of deaths of children who died at the hospital or whose death at home was certified by a hospital doctor. Only patients who died in the in patient medical, surgical and intensive care wards were included. Patients were excluded if they died at home or in the hospital's emergency services. Of the 211 HIV-related deaths during the study period, 167 patients were eligible for inclusion.

Methods

A structured questionnaire was used to collect data from patients' medical and nursing records and medicine charts. Data included age at death, disease severity, length of stay, documented do not resuscitate (DNR) orders and comfort care plans, diagnostic and therapeutic interventions in patients' last 24 hours, documented pain and distress in patients' last 48 hours, and social work intervention. Data extraction was limited to the terminal hospitalization.

DNR orders were defined as explicit orders to limit the use of cardiopulmonary resuscitation (not for CPR) in the event of cardiac arrest and or mechanical ventilation in the event of respiratory arrest (Not for IPPV – not for intermittent positive pressure ventilation). Orders restricting admission to the paediatric intensive care unit (PICU) were also interpreted as decisions to withhold ventilation since this intervention only takes place in the intensive care setting in this hospital. Presence of a comfort care plan was determined by instructions such as 'comfort care only', 'supportive measures only' and 'tender loving care (TLC)'.[6] Pain and distress were inferred from descriptive reports such as 'crying+++', 'mouth very sore', 'buttocks excoriated', 'penile ulceration', 'distressed+++', and self-reported pain. Social work visits were noted if there was a direct entry by these services in the medical record or mention of their intervention by another discipline.

A paediatric consultant determined disease severity (A-mild, B-moderate, C-severe)[7] for 102 (62%) of patients. The remaining patients were classified as falling into Category C based on written use of this category in the notes or reference to patients as having terminal or end-stage AIDS. Twelve completed questionnaires were reviewed by a paediatric consultant to evaluate content validity and reliability of data collection. Consensus regarding the presence of comfort care plans was reached through discussion. Agreement on other areas was high although inter-rater reliability was not statistically assessed.

Analysis

Quantitative data were analyzed using Epi Info Version 6. Frequency and percentage distributions, single and multiple cross tabulations, and Kruskall-Wallis one-way analysis of variance were the most common statistical analyses. Mantel Haenszel chisquare, Fisher's Exact Test (when expected values were less than five) and Kruskall-Wallis chi square equivalent were used respectively to test the statistical significance of associations between categorical variables and differences between medians of ordinal data. A probability level of less than 0.05 was used to establish statistical significance. Qualitative data were categorized according to themes and counted.

Ethical considerations

Since data were extracted anonymously, parental consent was not obtained for the study. Permission to undertake the study was

---

[6] J.J. Fins, F.G. Miller, C.A. Acres, M.D. Bacchetta, L.L. Huzzard & B.D. Rapkin. End-of life decision-making in the hospital: current practice and future prospects. *J Pain Symptom Manage* 1999; 17: 6–15.
[7] Centers for Disease Control and Prevention. 1994 revised classification system for human immunodeficiency virus infection in children less than 13 years of age. *MMWR* 1994; 43: 1–19.

obtained from the Chief Medical Superintendent of Red Cross War Memorial Children's Hospital, the Head of the School of Child and Adolescent Health, and the Research Ethics Committee of the Health Sciences Faculty of the University of Cape Town.

RESULTS

Sample characteristics

One hundred and sixty five (99%) out of 167 eligible patients were included in the final sample. Two patients were excluded because one folder could not be traced and one set of medical notes was missing. Respectively, 79% and 21% of patients died in general wards and the PICU. The mean and median age of patients was ten months and four months respectively. Of the patients, 80% were under one year of age. Less than 10% of patients were older than two years. Respectively, 69% and 30% of patients had severe (Category C) and moderate (Category B) disease. Only one patient fell in Category A. The mean and median length of hospitalization was 11 days and six days respectively. Whereas 26% of patients survived on average only three days, 23% had an average length of stay of 28 days. Three-quarters of patients were hospitalized for less than two weeks.

Do not resuscitate orders

Of the patients, 84% (N = 138) had a DNR order. Less than two-thirds (N = 85) of DNR orders had a documented rationale. Advanced AIDS with progressive symptomatology, and no improvement despite the best available treatment, were the most common reasons for writing a DNR order (53/85, 62%). Terminal illness, poor prognosis, and end stage or Category C disease were offered as rationales in a further 34% (29/85) of orders. Futility was given as justification in only two patients who died in the PICU. One patient was awaiting confirmation of brain death.

In almost two thirds (N = 87) of folders there was no record of whether the DNR order had been discussed with parents or a caretaker. The DNR order appeared in both medical and nursing notes in 41% of folders. DNR orders were recorded in medical or nursing notes only in 56% and 3% respectively of folders. About half (31/57) of the DNR orders appearing synchronously in medical and nursing notes were identical. Discrepant orders occurred in the remaining folders (26/57): for instance, directives such as 'Not for IPPV' and 'Not for CPR' were documented in the medical and nursing notes of the same patient.

Comfort care plans

Of the patients, 44% (N = 73) had a comfort care plan. Instructions to provide TLC (41%), to keep patients comfortable (20%), and to provide supportive care (20%) characterized most plans. About one in ten plans specified palliation and analgesia only, and a general directive to manage conservatively underpinned the remaining 8% of plans. In addition, two thirds of plans included orders to withhold specific interventions such as invasive diagnostic procedures, blood products or intravenous (IV) therapies, or to add therapies such as morphine. Documented comfort care plans were discussed with 56% (41/73) of parents or caretakers.

Severity, age and length of hospitalization were significantly associated with having a comfort care plan. One in two patients with a comfort care plan fell in Category C compared to less than one in three patients in Category B (51% versus 30%, P = 0,0135). Patients with a comfort care plan were older (median age of six months versus four months, P = 0,0052) and had longer hospital stays (median stay of nine days versus five days, P = 0,0006).

The median time from admission to documentation of a DNR order and or a comfort care plan was four days and seven days respectively.

Interventions in the last 24 hours of life

The frequency of interventions received by at least 10% of patients in their last 24 hours of life is shown in Table 1. IV fluids and IV antibiotics were the most common interventions having been administered to at least three-quarters of patients. Other interventions received by at least 40% of patients included nasogastric feeds, Nystatin (an antifungal treatment for thrush), and head box oxygen for respiratory distress. Analgesia was the next most frequent intervention. Approximately one in four patients received oral antibiotics and nasal prong oxygen or had blood drawn in their final 24 hours. A sizeable minority of patients was ventilated, resuscitated

Table 1. Frequency and Percentage Distribution of Interventions[a] in the Last 24 Hours of Life (N = 165)

	N	%
Intravenous fluids	133	81
Intravenous antibiotics	122	75
Nasogastric feeds	99	60
Nystatin	88	53
Headbox oxygen	68	41
Morphine	63	38
Paracetamol	51	31
Oral antibiotics	44	27
Nasal prong oxygen	44	27
Venipuncture	40	24
Steroids	35	21
Nebulization	31	19
Ventilation	29	18
Sedation	28	17
X-rays	27	16
Cardiopulmonaiy resuscitation	24	14
Ringers lactate	24	14
Inotropes	21	13
Oral feeds	20	12
Anticonvulsants	16	10

[a] Received by at least 10% of patients.

and received resuscitation fluid (Ringers lactate) and cardiac support (inotropes).

The frequency of interventions received by patients in their last 24 hours was also examined according to the presence of a comfort care plan (Table 2).

Pain and distress in the last 48 hours of life

Excluding deaths in the PICU, pain and distress were documented in medical and nursing entries of 55% (N = 72) of patients, of whom about half (N = 38) had a documented comfort care plan. Pain and distress were documented in both medical and nursing entries in 29% (N = 21) of folders, in 53% (N = 38) of nursing notes only, and in 18% (N = 13) of medical notes only. Respiratory distress and painful skin conditions accounted for most discomfort among patients with and without a comfort care plan (Table 3). Phrases such as 'battling to breathe', 'laboured breathing', 'extremely exhausted', 'distressed+++', and 'working very hard' indicate that shortness of breath caused considerable distress in over one in four children (35/131) in the general wards. Vivid descriptions such as

Table 2. Frequency and Percentage Distribution of Interventions[a] in the Last 24 Hours of Life According to Presence of a Comfort Care Plan (N = 73)

	N	%
Intravenous fluids	53	73
Nasogastric feeds	48	66
Intravenous antibiotics	45	62
Nystatin	41	56
Morphine	34	46
Head box oxygen	29	40
Oral antibiotics	24	33
Paracetamol	20	27
Nasal prong oxygen	19	26
Nebulization	14	19
Oral feeds	12	16
Venipuncture	11	15
Sedation	10	14
Anticonvulsants	10	14
X-rays	9	12
Steroids	9	12
Ringers Lactate	8	11

[a] Received by at least 10% of patients.

Table 3. Pain and Distress in the Last 48 Hours of Life According to Presence or Absence of a Comfort Care Plan (N = 72)[a]

Symptomatology[b]	Comfort Care Plan N = 38 N	No Comfort Care Plan N = 34 N	All Patients N = 72 N(%)
Respiratory distress	15	20	35 (49)
Oral and oesophageal candidiasis	11	16	27 (37)
Perianal ulceration and dermatitis	11	2	13 (18)
Herpes, skin lesions and abscesses	9	1	10 (14)
Abdominal distension	2	9	11 (15)
Other[c]	4	3	7 (10)

[a] Excludes patients who died in paediatric intensive care unit.
[b] Multiple symptomatology in some patients.
[c] Includes, for example, otitis media, anxiety, self-reported pain.

'riddled with candida (thrush)', 'skin excoriated', 'nappy rash with deep sores', 'very miserable baby – cries when handled', 'abscess and distinct lesions – painful to touch', 'weak cry though in great pain', 'mouth and buttocks very sore', 'dry bloody crusts on both lips', 'buttocks and vaginal area too sore for urine bag to stick' further illustrate the extent of morbidity. Though less common, abdominal distension (for example, 'abdomen distended+++, seems in pain') caused discomfort in 15% (11/72) of patients with pain and distress.

Respectively 19% (14/72) and 37% (27/72) of patients with documented pain and distress received paracetamol and/or morphine in their last 24 hours. Conversely, half (36/72) the patients with documented pain and distress, including 16 with a comfort care plan, received no analgesia. Almost half (13/27) the patients received their first, and often only, dose of morphine shortly before death. Despite verbatim reports of pain and distress spanning at least two days, only three patients received morphine for three days or more. Although patients with a comfort care plan were significantly more likely to receive morphine (P = 0.0053), in eight patients morphine was recommended in the comfort care plan but never written in the medicine charts.

Social work intervention

Social work intervention took place in 38% (N = 63) of families. The purpose of almost half the social work interviews was pre- and post-test counseling. Supportive counseling and grief counseling accounted for 29% and 22% of interventions, respectively. On parental request, clergy were present at the death of three (2%) patients in the PICU.

DISCUSSION

Improving terminal care requires a shift in goals from prolonging life to a primary concern for palliation. This cannot be easy in the case of very young children. Nevertheless, doctors made tough end of life decisions that included writing DNR orders in the majority of patients and comfort care plans in a significant minority.

Do not resuscitate orders

Even though many patients had a DNR order, documentation and communication of these decisions was inadequate. DNR orders appeared simultaneously in only 41% of medical and nursing entries. This meant the resuscitation status of about two-thirds of patients was not written in the nursing notes. In the event of a cardiac or respiratory arrest, and in the absence of a DNR order, nurses have a legal duty to offer patients full medical treatment including CPR.[8] Due to failed communication between doctors and nurses, terminally ill children risked receiving highly invasive, burdensome interventions. Inconsistent use of terminology in the DNR orders compounded the potential for miscommunication between doctors and nurses. An identical instruction (for example, 'Not for IPPV' or 'Not for CPR') appeared in only 54% of medical and nursing notes. Conversely, 46% of patients had discrepant DNR directives. On busy hospital wards with rotating staff-in-training, it is ill-advised to assume a shared understanding of instructions implying limitation of different interventions.[9] Furthermore, discussion of the DNR order with parents or a guardian was documented in less than 40% of folders. Not only does unilateral decision making ignore parental values and preferences, it disregards professional[10] and local[11] guidelines that stipulate parents as principal decision makers regarding treatment for their children. Language barriers exacerbated by too few interpreters may have impeded communication between parents and clinicians. Alternatively parents, many of whom are poverty stricken, may have visited infrequently and a medical decision not to resuscitate had to be taken urgently.

If DNR orders mean no resuscitation or ventilation in the event of arrest, clinicians should also consider patients' other needs.[12] Since most DNR orders in this study were justified on grounds of imminent death, writing a DNR order should prompt doctors to rethink all the goals of therapy. To this end, several adult studies[13]

---

[8] L. Doyal & D. Wilsher. Withholding cardiopulmonary resuscitation: proposals for formal guidelines. *RMJ* 1993; 306: 1593–1596.

[9] R.F. Uhlmann, C.K. Cassel & W.J. McDonald. Some treatment-withholding implications of no-code orders in an academic hospital. *Crit Care Med* 1984; 12: 879–881.

[10] American Academy of Pediatrics. Guidelines for forgoing life-sustaining medical treatment. *Pediatrics* 1994; 93: 532–536; Royal College of Paediatrics and Child Health. 1997. *Withholding or withdrawing life saving treatment in children. A framework for practice.* London. RCPCH.

[11] S.R. Benatar, C. Abels, R. Abratt, et al. Statement on withholding and withdrawing life-sustaining therapy. *S Aft Med J* 1994; 84: 254–256.

[12] D.P. Sulmasy, G. Geller, R. Faden & D.M. Levin. The quality of mercy: caring for patients with 'do not resuscitate' orders. *JAMA* 1992; 267: 682–686.

[13] J.A. Mittelberger, B. Lo, D. Martin & R.F. Uhlmann. Impact of a procedure-specific do not resuscitate order form on documentation of do not resuscitate orders. *Arch Intern Med* 1993; 153: 228–232; E.E. O'Toole, S.J. Youngner, B.W. Juknialis, B. Daly, E.T. Bartlett & C.S. Landefeld. Evaluation of a treatment limitation policy with a specific treatment-limiting order page. *Arch Intern Med* 1994; 154: 425–432; J.E. Heffner, C. Barbieri & K. Casey. Procedure-specific do-not-resuscitate orders. *Arch Intern Med* 1996; 156: 793–797.

and one anecdotal report in children[14] confirm the usefulness of structured and procedure-specific DNR orders to minimize problems of communication in the health care team, and to improve the quality of terminal care.[15]

Interventions in the last 24 hours of life

Examination of interventions in patients' last 24 hours shows many children received invasive diagnostic and therapeutic interventions even though they were dying. Since the median length of stay was less than one week, the intensity of interventions was most likely determined by diagnostic and prognostic uncertainty. Furthermore, rapid deterioration in at least one-quarter of patients, coupled with clinical uncertainty, would have made a decision to withdraw life-saving care in favour of palliative care difficult. In the face of clinical uncertainty, much aggressive care focused on reversible illnesses such as diarrhoea and pneumonia[16] will appear non-beneficial only after death when the perspective is quite different. Unsurprisingly then, patients with comfort care plans were older, more likely to have clinically proven AIDS and to have spent longer in hospital. Decisions regarding appropriate treatment goals require factual information about a patient's diagnosis and prognosis, the stability of the condition over time, and the likelihood and extent of improvement. Generally, this information takes time to collect.

Comfort care plans

To serve the terminally ill child's best interests, the American Academy of Pediatrics recommends an individualized plan of care that focuses on comfort and symptom relief rather than provision of life-saving medical therapy.[17] The low rate of comfort care plans suggests doctors had difficulty making the transition from life-prolonging to palliative care. Trained to cure, doctors persisted with

[14] J.P. Burns & R.D. Truog. Ethical controversies in pediatric critical care. *New Horiz* 1997; 5: 72–84.
[15] Sulmasy et al., *op. cit.* note 12.
[16] H.J. Zar, D. Hanslo, E. Tannenbaum et al. Aetiology outcome of pneumonia in human immunodeficiency virus-infected children hospitalized in South Africa. *Acta Paediatr* 2001; 90: 119–125.
[17] American Academy of Pediatrics. Palliative care for children. *Pediatrics* 2000; 106: 351–357.

procedures and treatments neither meant for, nor likely to promote patients' comfort. Indeed, despite having a comfort care plan, 73% of patients continued to receive IV fluids, almost twice as many received IV rather than oral antibiotics, and 15% and 12% respectively underwent veni-punctures and X-rays for diagnostic purposes. Patients with a comfort care plan were as likely as those without to receive oral feeds and only slightly more likely to receive morphine. In short, designating patients to receive TLC or comfort care only did not always correspond with care subsequently given.

The high rate of DNR orders compared to comfort care plans underscores previous findings[18] that health care professionals are more comfortable withholding than withdrawing life-saving interventions. Understandably, for psychological reasons, doctors may feel more responsible if a patient dies following withdrawal of a life-sustaining intervention.[19] Yet, critical information may become known only once treatment has started, particularly if decisions to initiate life-saving treatment are made when a patient's prognosis is uncertain. If clinicians could not stop a treatment once it has begun, they might be reluctant to attempt treatment that might be beneficial. Rather than rely on an invalid moral distinction between withholding and withdrawing treatment, clinicians should examine the potential benefits and harms of a particular intervention for a particular patient. Arguably, withdrawal of life-sustaining treatment that proves futile or contrary to a patient's best interests is morally preferable to not having tried at all.[20]

Even so, decisions to limit care can be difficult where treatment may prolong life but it is unclear if doing so benefits the patient. Antibiotic drugs, for instance, may promote comfort by reducing adverse symptoms such as shortness of breath and cough caused by infection.[21] However, if a patient has no distress from the infection, use of antibiotics may prolong dying and add to a child's discomfort by requiring IV access and further laboratory tests. In

[18] M.Z. Solomon, L.O. O'Donnell, B. Jennings, et al. Decisions near the end of life: professional views on life-sustaining treatments. *Amer J Pub Health* 1993; 83: 14–23; P.V. Caralis & J.S. Hammond. Attitudes of medical students, housestaff, and faculty physicians toward euthanasia and termination of life-sustaining treatment. *Crit Care Med* 1992; 20: 683–690; D.L. Dickenson. Are medical ethicists out of touch? Practitioner attitudes in the US and UK towards decisions at the end of life. *J Med Ethics* 2000; 26: 254–260.

[19] Burns, Truog, *op. cit.* note 14.

[20] Ibid.

[21] E. Bruera & C.M. Neumann. Management of specific symptom complexes in patients receiving palliative care. *CMAJ* 1998; 158: 1717–1726.

contrast, decreased use of non-beneficial IV lines would reduce procedural pain as well as the risk of needle stick injuries among junior medical staff who struggle to find veins in extremely wasted infants. If continued use among terminally ill children is medically justified, antibiotics should be administered orally rather than intravenously.

Findings that 73% and 66% of patients with a comfort care plan received IV fluids and nasogastric feeds, compared to only 16% on oral feeds, indicate decisions to withdraw artificial nutrition and hydration are especially problematic given strong emotional and cultural ties attached to eating and drinking. Although it is argued that artificial nutrition and hydration must be given because they represent humane and basic care, these interventions lack the pleasurable oral sensations and interpersonal contact associated with food and fluid intake,[22] particularly in infants. In addition, they are medical interventions that carry complications and require skilled nursing. Paradoxically, availability of skilled nursing along with time pressures in busy hospitals may lead to overuse of artificial nutrition and hydration. If replacing an empty drip is less time consuming than hand feeding, artificial feeding may do more to lessen the nursing load than provide fitting care to a dying child. Moreover, if present, a mother would surely benefit from hand feeding her dying child. Hand feeding is an act of nurturing during which the caregiver can talk to and play with the child. If artificial nutrition and hydration only prolong life in an imminently dying child, treatment produces more harm than good. Still, decisions to limit artificial nutrition and hydration are controversial[23] and doctors should consider clinical review by an impartial senior colleague who is not part of the treatment team.

Head box oxygen administered to 41% of infants with comfort. care plans in their last 24 hours would have prevented parents holding their dying babies. Similarly, head box oxygen would discourage use of oral feeding since access to the mouth would require removal of a child from high concentration oxygen, which might increase respiratory distress. Whilst increased use of nasal prong oxygen would give a parent more access to their child, the oxygen

---

[22] B. Lo & L. Dornbrand. Guiding the hand that feeds. *N Eng JMed* 1984; 311: 402–404.
[23] L. Doyal & V.F. Larcher. Drafting guidelines for the withholding or withdrawing of life sustaining treatment in critically ill children and neonates. *Arch Dis Child Neonatal Ed* 2000; 83: F60–F63.

requirements of these terminal infants are often higher than nasal prong oxygen can deliver. However, if morphine were optimally used, these infants may have been less distressed allowing the use of nasal prong oxygen, thereby giving parents more physical contact with their dying child, as well as facilitating oral feeding.

In 44% of patients with a comfort care plan there was no record of whether doctors had discussed the decision to change from life-prolonging to palliative care with the family. A decision that the burdens of life-sustaining treatment outweigh the benefits includes the non-medical determination of how valuable it is to continue living and the degree of a patient's suffering. Doctors should not make these judgments independently, since they may be influenced by their own professional, religious and sociological backgrounds. In line with ethical and professional norms,[24] doctors are expected to make these decisions in partnership with parents, according to the best interests standard. However, without adequate staff resources including trained interpreters, doctors and nurses will struggle to deliver optimal terminal care. Furthermore, without adequate multidisciplinary support, the broader goals of palliative care concerned with families' psychological, psychosocial and spiritual needs cannot be addressed.

Pain and distress in the last 48 hours

In their last 48 hours, 55% of patients dying in general wards experienced pain and distress that was not treated, was under treated or was treated too late. In the face of clinical uncertainty a mixed management approach[25] combining the goals of cure and palliation is medically and morally indicated in patients not designated for comfort care only. Indeed, international guidelines[26] on palliation specifically reject rigid distinctions between curative, life-prolonging treatment and comfort care precisely because they hinder timely and appropriate provision of palliation and symptom relief. Strikingly, despite documented suffering, many patients with a comfort care plan either failed to receive analgesia or received their first dose of morphine shortly before dying. If achieving the best quality of life and symptom relief are fundamental goals of

[24] AAP, RCPCH, *op. cit.* note et al., *op. cit.* note 11.
[25] Oleske and Czarniecki, *op. cit.* note 4.
[26] AAP, *op. cit.* note 17.

palliative care, palliation failed in many patients with a comfort care plan.

It can only be speculated why pain and distress were sub-optimally managed. Importantly, many clinicians lack experience in providing palliation and symptom relief to dying children. Indeed, prior to the HIV/AIDS pandemic, deaths in general pediatric wards were relatively uncommon in this hospital. Further, compared to nurses, doctors spend less time with patients and may not observe first-hand the degree of suffering. Painful penile and perianal ulceration, for example, is most apparent during nappy changes. Nor do doctors routinely refer to nurses' notes which explicitly detail patients' discomfort. Thus, ignorance that very young children experience pain, together with doctors' failure to identify symptoms of discomfort, may account for poor symptom control,[27] the more so since most patients were too young to verbalize their suffering.

Another significant barrier to administering adequate pain medication, especially morphine, is fear of hastening death.[28] Yet, according to expert opinion,[29] morphine, the most studied, widely used and cheapest opiate available, is perfectly safe even for use in neonates. Provided there is adequate monitoring and adherence to published guidelines, respiratory depression in children receiving opiates is highly unlikely. If prolonging life is no longer in a child's best interests and promoting comfort is the primary goal, clinicians should not hesitate to use full and effective doses of analgesia. Pain and symptom relief is almost always in a child's best interests and should be the standard of care in the absence of strong and explicit indications to the contrary.[30]

Finally, enactment of legislation proposed by the SA Law Commission[31] relating to end of life decisions would clarify doctors'

[27] P.J. McGrath. Attitudes and beliefs about medication and pain management in children. *J Palliat Care* 1996; 12: 46–49; S. Liben. Pediatric palliative medicine: obstacles to overcome. *J Palliat Care* 1996; 12: 24–28.

[28] Liben, *op. cit.* note 27; R.M. Vazirani, S.J. Slavin & J.D. Feldman. Longitudinal study of pediatric house officers' attitudes toward death and dying. *Crit Care Med* 2000; 28: 3740–3745.

[29] I. James & S. Scuplak. 1999. Analgesia and sedation. In: *Care of the critically ill child.* A. Macnab, D. Macrae, R. Henning, eds. London. Churchill Livingstone: 432–446.

[30] J. Wolfe. Suffering in children at the end of life: recognizing an ethical duty to palliate. *J Clin Ethics* 2000; 11: 157–163.

[31] South African Law Commission. 1999. Project 86: Report on Euthanasia and the Artificial Preservation of Life. Pretoria, South Africa.

and nurses' legal, if not ethical, duties regarding relief of dying patients' pain and distress.

CONCLUSION AND RECOMMENDATIONS

Clinical uncertainty, compounded by a relatively short terminal hospital stay, made it difficult for doctors to know when and in what circumstances to limit life-sustaining treatment in HIV-infected children. Even when designated for comfort care only, children continued to receive life-prolonging interventions. Yet, no ethical principle supports continued use of invasive diagnostic and therapeutic interventions that merely increase suffering and prolong dying. On the contrary, once it becomes clear a child will die soon and a DNR order should be issued, there can be few instances where it is in the child's best interests to continue life-sustaining medical care. Concurrently with a DNR order, a decision should be made to discontinue or limit life-saving interventions and substitute comfort care. Goals of care should shift from prolonging life to providing palliation.

Accordingly, it is recommended clinicians strive to: (i) increase the proportion of patients with comfort care plans to more closely reflect the proportion of DNR orders; (ii) make comfort care plans more coherent so dying patients receive only treatment promoting comfort;[32] (iii) make pain and discomfort a fifth vital sign requiring routine monitoring along with pulse, blood pressure, respiration and heart rate.[33] However, given generally low patient : staffing ratios in public hospitals, attempts to raise the quality of terminal care that rely exclusively on improving individual doctor-patient decision making may be ineffective. Improving end of life practices also requires system level change,[34] particularly reforms that integrate palliative care within mainstream hospital practice. Where feasible, hospitals should develop structured plans[35] for HIV-infected children covering a spectrum of care (Table 4). Whilst some elements will not be immediately appropriate for every patient, such plans would prompt the health care team to think about pain and

[32] Fins et al., *op. cit.* note 6.
[33] J. Lynn, J.L. Schuster & A. Kabcenell. 2000. *Improving care for the end of life: a source book for health managers and clinicians.* New York. Oxford University Press: 37–58.
[34] J. Lynn et al., *op. cit.* note 33.
[35] Fins et al., *op. cit.* note 6.

Table 4. Elements of a Care Plan

- Patient's clinical condition
- Prognosis
- Goals of care (cure, prolong life, comfort palliation, mixed)
- Intended level of medical intervention, including DNR status
- Therapies to be instituted or continued
- Existing therapies to be withdrawn and order in which this will be done
- Review of symptoms (for example, pain, shortness of breath, excessive crying or irritability)
- Prescribed palliative treatments and degree of symptomatic relief
- Family's awareness of the plan and their preferences regarding end of life care
- Availability of family support, including telephone numbers
- Cultural, psychosocial and spiritual issues
- Planned social work or pastoral care interventions

symptom relief for patients still receiving life-prolonging interventions.[36]

Lastly, findings in this study are limited by problems inherent in retrospective chart review, such as the quality of medical record keeping and the extent of missing data.[37] During times of stress and crisis, documentation of end of life decisions may be incomplete. For instance, in some cases, clinicians may have discussed DNR orders and comfort care plans with parents but failed to record their doing so. It is also possible the researcher's subjective interpretation of pain and distress, particularly respiratory symptomatology, was inaccurate. Additionally, the study was limited to children who died in a single, specialized teaching institution and findings may not be generalizable to other hospitals or settings. Still, despite its shortcomings, this study is one of the first to examine terminal care for hospitalized, HIV-infected children. However, because many, if not most, HIV-infected children in developing countries will die at home, future research needs to investigate parental preferences for, as well as benefits and burdens of, home-based terminal care.

Acknowledgements

I thank Terry Fleischer and Dr Tony Westwood for scholarly support.

[36] Oleske and Czarniecki, *op. cit.* note 4.
[37] D.P. Sulmasy, M. Dwyer & E. Marx. Do the ward notes reflect the quality of end-of-life care? *J Med Ethics* 1996; 22: 344–348.

INDEX

Printed and bound by CPI Group (UK) Ltd, Croydon, CR0 4YY

08/12/2025

14787497-0001

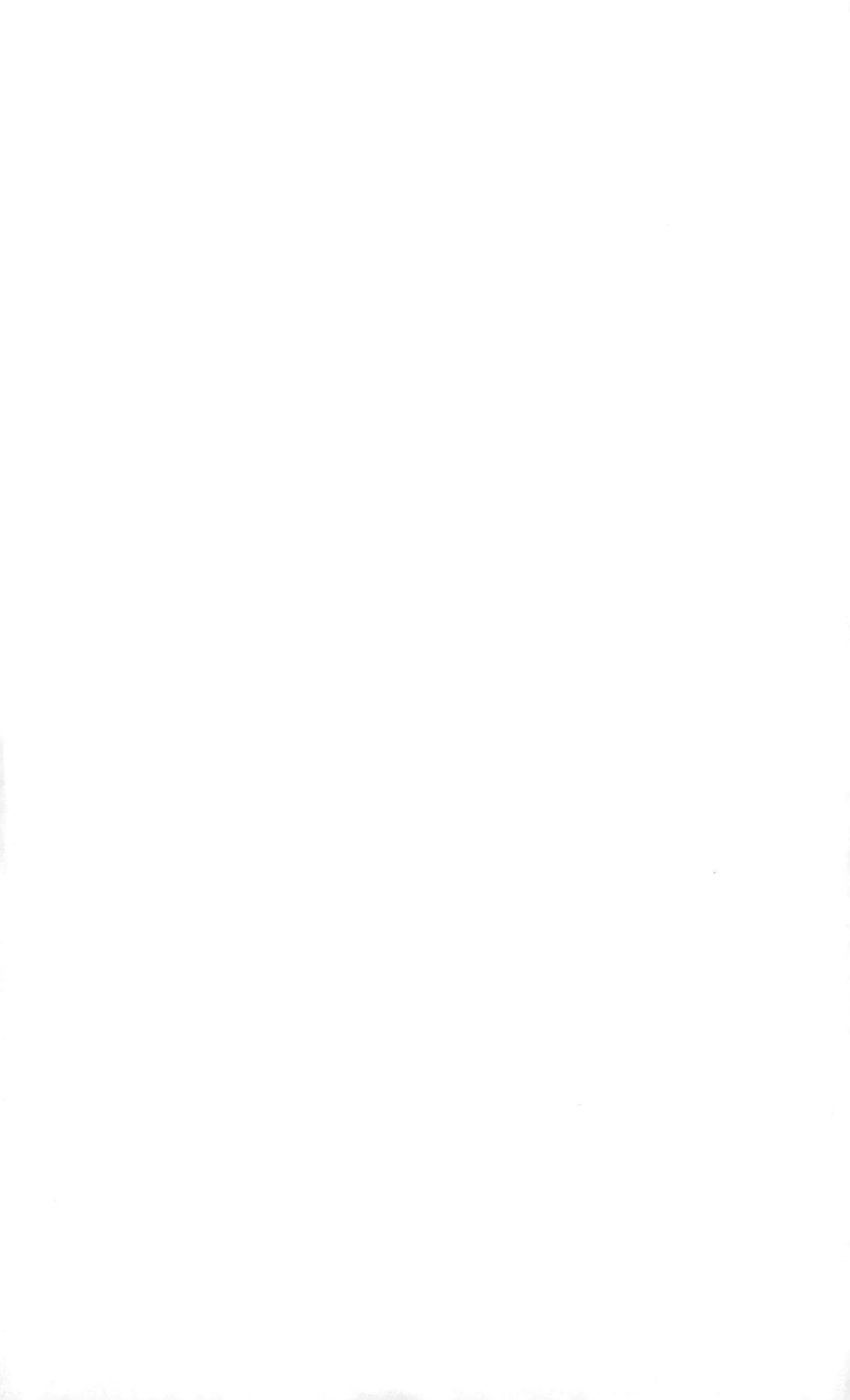